Auriculotherapy Manual

For Elsevier
Content Strategist: Claire Wilson, Kellie White
Content Development Specialist: Carole McMurray
Project Manager: Caroline Jones
Designer/Design Direction: Miles Hitchen
Illustration Manager: Jennifer Rose

FOURTH EDITION

Auriculotherapy Manual

Chinese and Western Systems of Ear Acupuncture

Terry Oleson PhD

Professor of Psychology, Ryokan College;
Director of Doctoral Studies, Emperor's College of Traditional Oriental Medicine,
Los Angeles, California, USA

Foreword by
Richard C. Niemtzow

Illustrations by
Justin Schaid and Andrew Dickinson

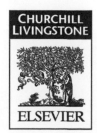

Edinburgh London New York Oxford Philadelphia St Louis Sydney Toronto 2014

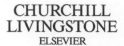

CHURCHILL LIVINGSTONE
ELSEVIER

First edition 1990
Second edition 1998
Third edition 2003
Fourth edition 2014

ISBN 978-0-7020-3572-2

British Library Cataloguing in Publication Data
A catalogue record for this book is available from the British Library

Library of Congress Cataloging in Publication Data
A catalog record for this book is available from the Library of Congress

Notices

Knowledge and best practice in this field are constantly changing. As new research and experience broaden our understanding, changes in research methods, professional practices, or medical treatment may become necessary.

Practitioners and researchers must always rely on their own experience and knowledge in evaluating and using any information, methods, compounds, or experiments described herein. In using such information or methods they should be mindful of their own safety and the safety of others, including parties for whom they have a professional responsibility.

With respect to any drug or pharmaceutical products identified, readers are advised to check the most current information provided (i) on procedures featured or (ii) by the manufacturer of each product to be administered, to verify the recommended dose or formula, the method and duration of administration, and contraindications. It is the responsibility of practitioners, relying on their own experience and knowledge of their patients, to make diagnoses, to determine dosages and the best treatment for each individual patient, and to take all appropriate safety precautions.

To the fullest extent of the law, neither the Publisher nor the authors, contributors, or editors, assume any liability for any injury and/or damage to persons or property as a matter of products liability, negligence or otherwise, or from any use or operation of any methods, products, instructions, or ideas contained in the material herein.

ELSEVIER your source for books,
journals and multimedia
in the health sciences

www.elsevierhealth.com

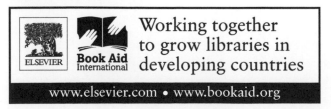

Working together
to grow libraries in
developing countries

www.elsevier.com • www.bookaid.org

The
Publisher's
policy is to use
**paper manufactured
from sustainable forests**

Printed in Great Britain
Last digit is the print number: 14

Contents

Foreword

I am humbled and honored to have the privilege to write the Foreword for Terry Oleson's 4th Edition of *Auriculotherapy Manual: Chinese and Western Systems of Ear Acupuncture*. Since 1994, over a span of 19 years, I have referred to and marveled over his various editions gaining in-sight and knowledge to the vast field of auriculotherapy. If suddenly I was transported to a remote place in the world to practice auriculotherapy and only allowed one book, this is it! The development and design of my own well-known "Battlefield Acupuncture" and "Xerostomia" techniques which has favorably impacted thousands of patients around the world were significantly influenced by his well organized, in-depth and rational information found in previous manuals. I am one of the many thousands of clinicians that will keep re-turning to his manuals for its vast repository of wisdom.

How does the 4th edition of the *Auriculotherapy Manual* compare to the 3rd edition? In other words, how does one make a superb manual even better? The overall organization of this book into specific chapters on the history of this field, microsystem theories, auricular anatomy, auricular zone systems, auricular diagnosis, auriculotherapy treatments, the location and function of individual ear points, clinical case reports, and treatment protocols, all remain essentially the same. At the same time, each chapter has been reorganized to include specific objectives, updated information based upon international conferences held in 2010 and 2012, a succinct definition of terms used in that chapter, and review questions to assess one's understanding of the material.

What is new in this edition of the *Auriculotherapy Manual?* Chapter 1 has included additional information regarding the history of auricular acupuncture in both China and in Europe. Chapter 2 has been revised to highlight the intriguing relationship between the holographic model and the energetic theories of classical acupuncture, and there is more recent scientific research demonstrating the neurobiological basis of acupuncture. As a practicing clinician, the clinical case reports presented in chapter 8 are particularly inspiring to see specific applications of auriculotherapy for difficult health conditions for which alternative treatment options are not available. The most note-worthy change in chapter 3 was to add sophisticated 3-D images of the ear and to add 5 more auricular landmarks that indicate the relationship between the different depths and contours of the external ear. As a result of the utilization of this 3-D ear imagery, there is greater detail to assist the clinician in identifying the specific localization of auricular acupuncture points. This feature of incorporating 3-D images of the auricle has allowed greatly improved identification of the ear images presented in chapter 7 and chapter 9 to the actual ears of human patients. These updates reflect the fact that modern auriculotherapy is not a stagnating discipline, but one in constant evolution.

There are many journeys to take in the field of acupuncture. In particular, auriculotherapy will astonish you. There are many intriguing concepts to learn and clinical skills to acquire. Think of Terry Oleson as your master personal guide. He will lead and expedite you through every facet of auriculotherapy that will be enjoyable and intriguing. It will be an invigorating and enlightened journey as you read through chapter after chapter. You will enjoy the coherent and succinct reading with many pictures and illustrations. It will be a lengthy, but smooth trip. One that will make many stops, but you will ultimately finish with a modern integrative perspective of auriculotherapy. Most intriguing will be where Terry Oleson's impetus will lead us next in future editions of auriculotherapy.

Richard C. Niemtzow, MD, Ph.D, MPH
Director
United States Air Force Acupuncture Center
Joint Base Andrews, Maryland

Preface

When I was first asked to develop a fourth edition of the *Auriculotherapy Manual: Chinese and Western Systems of Ear Acupuncture*, neither I nor the publisher realized what an extensive endeavor that would lead to. While the field of auricular acupuncture has remained essentially the same as when I developed the first edition of this text in 1990, the clinical and basic research on auriculotherapy has continued to grow since the first scientific study that I conducted on auricular diagnosis was published in the medical journal *Pain* in 1980. Besides reorganizing the structure of each chapter in this book to allow for an initial outline of topics, chapter objectives, updated information on auriculotherapy, and a section on the definition of key terms used in that chapter, I have added educational sample questions at the end of the chapters. A major revision has been to develop images of the external ear based upon 3-D technology that is able to reveal hidden surfaces of the auricle from different perspectives. With the addition of close-up photographs of the external ears of a number of individuals and the inclusion of these 3-D images of the auricle, it has been possible to distinguish additional landmarks on the external ear that are highly useful in indentifying the specific location of different ear acupoints on a structure as small and as convoluted as the ear. In response to reader comments regarding the second and third editions of this manual, the visual images of ear acupoints have been placed in close proximity to the verbal descriptions of the location and function of those same ear acupoints. A consistent format for the naming and numbering of each individual ear acupuncture point according to clinical systems developed in China and in Europe has been further elaborated from previous presentations of this text. The intended purpose of these changes has been to make this book both more informative, yet more user-friendly, than the earlier editions.

My personal exploration of the field of auriculotherapy started with a lecture that I heard while completing my graduate studies at the University of California at Irvine (UCI). The presentation by UCLA professor John Liebeskind focused upon his pioneering research on a concept that was completely new to the field of neuroscience in 1972. His studies had demonstrated that in addition to neurophysiological pathways for the perception of pain, there were separate brain pathways that could inhibit pain. He and his colleagues had demonstrated in rats, then cats and monkeys, that electrical stimulation of the periaqueductal gray of the brainstem could suppress behavioral reflexes to painful stimuli, yet not alter any other aspect of the animal's conscious functions. It was several years later that subsequent studies would lead to the discovery of endorphins, the morphine-like substances that serve as the body's naturally occurring, opiate analgesic. I wrote to Dr. Liebeskind after the lecture, met with him at UCLA, and soon submitted an application for a federally funded post-doctoral scholarship working in his laboratory. As my doctoral dissertation examined the firing patterns of neurons in the somatosensory pathways and auditory pathways of the brain during Pavlovian conditioning, my post-doctoral grant sought to examine neural firing patterns in the brain pathways related to the inhibition of pain sensations.

I began my work in Dr. Liebeskind's laboratory after receiving my PhD in Psychobiology in 1973. It so happened that the neuroscience laboratories at the UCLA Department of Psychology were located in the basement of the building. If one walked down a long, underground hallway, one arrived at the UCLA Acupuncture Research Group. UCLA was the first medical school in the United States that sponsored scientific research on acupuncture. While I conducted animal research experiments during the day on brain research related to the inhibition of pain, I was also able to study the clinical effects of acupuncture for alleviating the pain conditions of human patients. The UCLA pain clinic successfully treated hundreds of chronic pain patients with acupuncture, biofeedback, hypnosis, guided imagery, and nutritional counseling. The Directors of the UCLA clinic, Dr. David Bresler and Dr. Richard Kroening, invited me to their offices one afternoon and asked me to be their Research Director. It was like an invisible energy force pushed me from behind as I leaped at the opportunity. I did not have any acupuncture skills, but as a psychologist, I had extensive training in conducting research. And thus began an amazing journey.

The first research project that we undertook was to examine auricular diagnosis. At that time, and to this very day, most members of the American medical profession have devalued acupuncture as simply a placebo effect. In contrast, a diagnostic study could not be contaminated by a patient's desire to please their practitioner, thus there could be no placebo effect. It took several years to design the research and collect the data, but there was an energizing atmosphere to everyone participating in the project. I was surprised myself when the results were finally analyzed and there was such a strong statistical finding supporting the veracity of auricular diagnosis. By just examining the external ear, yet blind to a patient's diagnosis, a trained physician could identify which parts of the external ear corresponded to specific parts of the body that the patient had reported musculoskeletal pain.

It was only after I presented the results of the auricular diagnosis research to the International Society for the Study of Pain in 1980 that I learned of the whole field of auricular medicine that is practiced in Europe. American doctors seem more impressed by the electrical detection and electrical treatment of acupuncture points than Asian doctors, and several electronic equipment manufacturers sponsored seminars that incorporated the work of European as well as Chinese acupuncturists. I had read about the pioneering auriculotherapy work of Dr. Paul Nogier, but I began studying with physicians who had actually studied with him in France.

Dr. Tsun-Nin Lee sponsored a presentation by Dr. Nogier in San Francisco, and it was then that I first had the opportunity to meet this great man. Dr. Nogier only spoke in French, so Dr. Joseph Helms needed to translate the material into English. As Dr. Nogier had read about my research on auricular diagnosis, he made a special invitation to meet with me. I had three more opportunities to personally interact with him at international symposiums in Europe, and it was always a great honor. I feel very fortunate to have received individual guidance on understanding the underlying mechanisms that can account for the impressive benefits of auriculotherapy.

Dr. Richard Kroening had once told me that in medical school that when one is learning a new medical procedure, the educational motto is as follows: "See one, do one, teach one." While not progressing quite that fast, I have now had the occasion to observe gifted practitioners of auriculotherapy, treat clients with auriculotherapy, and teach courses on auriculotherapy at colleges and universities across the United States. The adage that one learns from one's students continues to apply, even after 30 years of teaching. Students come to me and inform me of patients they have successfully treated with auriculotherapy for unusual conditions that I have only studied in books, thus the spread of this knowledge continues even beyond my experience. I also had the good fortune to connect with Dr. Jim Shores, who co-sponsored the International Consensus Conference on Acupuncture, Auriculotherapy, and Auricular Medicine in 1999 (ICCAAM'99). It was my continued efforts to integrate this unconventional clinical procedure that has led to this most recent edition. It has not seemed either intellectually nor intuitively obvious that stimulation of the external ear could affect medical conditions in other parts of the body. Even after treating hundreds of patients with auriculotherapy, it continues to amaze me that it can work. The purpose of this book is to explain both the theoretical basis and the clinical practice of auriculotherapy so that others may know of its value.

Overview and History of Auriculotherapy

[1.0 | Overview and History of Auriculotherapy

CHAPTER 1 LEARNING OBJECTIVES

1. To describe the applications of auriculotherapy by various health care practitioners.

2. To highlight the historical origins of auricular acupuncture in ancient China.

3. To demonstrate awareness of ear acupuncture procedures in modern China.

4. To summarize the historical origins of auriculotherapy discoveries in the West.

5. To evaluate the discoveries of Dr. Paul Nogier, the Father of Auriculotherapy.

6. To examine research and clinical studies of auriculotherapy in the United States.

7. To compare the similarities and differences between body acupuncture and ear acupuncture.

1.1 Introduction to Auriculotherapy

Auriculotherapy is a health care modality whereby the external surface of the ear, or auricle, is stimulated to alleviate pathological conditions in other parts of the body. The discovery of this therapy is partially based on the ancient Chinese practice of body acupuncture, yet it is also derived from the discoveries by a French physician in the 1950s. Dr. Paul Nogier and colleagues demonstrated that specific areas of the external ear were associated with pathology in specific parts of the body. Many texts on the topic of auriculotherapy tend to focus either on the Chinese approach to auricular acupuncture or on the European practices of auricular medicine. Following my work at the UCLA Pain Management Center in the 1980s, the present text strives to integrate both Chinese and European styles of auriculotherapy.

1.2 Health Care Practitioners Utilizing Auriculotherapy

Acupuncturists: The practice of classical acupuncture and Traditional Chinese Medicine (TCM) includes the insertion of needles into ear acupoints as well as body acupuncture points. Stimulating acupuncture points on the body or on the ear can be done in the same treatment session or in different sessions. Some acupuncturists stimulate ear reflex points as the sole method of their acupuncture practice, whereas other acupuncturists do not include any use of ear acupoints. The majority of American acupuncturists have only been trained in the Chinese localization of ear points, but the integration of Chinese and Western ear reflex acupoints has become a more preferred approach. Many acupuncture schools in the West provide only minimal training in auricular acupuncture or in microsystem models; thus, the present text seeks to demonstrate the considerable value for acupuncturists to take the time to add ear acupuncture points into their treatment plans.

Biofeedback Therapists: Electrophysiological biofeedback equipment facilitates the training of self-control techniques to achieve general relaxation and stress management. Auriculotherapy augments biofeedback procedures by producing more immediate relief of myofascial pain and visceral discomfort as a patient progressively learns to relax.

Chiropractic Doctors: Stimulation of auricular reflex points reduces the mechanical resistance to chiropractic adjustments intended to release muscle spasms and correct misaligned postural positions. Auriculotherapy can be applied before an adjustment or following a manipulative treatment in order to stabilize the chiropractic procedure. Manual therapy techniques more directly balance the biomechanical structure of the body and are a very useful complement to the reductions in muscle tension and the improvement of blood circulation that can be facilitated by auriculotherapy.

Dentists: Auriculotherapy can achieve mild, dental analgesia for the relief of acute pain from dental drilling or for basic teeth cleaning procedures. As many patients experience considerable nervousness prior to certain dental procedures, auriculotherapy can effectively alleviate such anxiety. Treatment of chronic headaches and TMJ dysfunction are both facilitated by the combination of auriculotherapy with trigger point injections, dental splints, and occlusal work.

Medical Doctors: Physicians specializing in anesthesiology, surgery, internal medicine, and family practice have utilized auriculotherapy for the management of chronic pain, the treatment

of acute muscle sprains, and the reduction of unwanted side effects from narcotic medications. Because auriculotherapy treatments can be conducted in a relatively brief period, this type of acupuncture can effectively complement other medical procedures.

Naturopathic Doctors: Naturopathic practitioners include auriculotherapy in the pursuit of homeopathic, nutritional, and preventive aspects of medicine. Auricular diagnosis can determine sources of specific allergies and appropriate herbal recommendations.

Nurses: The standard medical care provided by nurses can be greatly assisted by the application of auriculotherapy for the systematic relief of pain and pathology that is not adequately alleviated by conventional medications or procedures.

Osteopathic Doctors: Auriculotherapy has been utilized to facilitate the correction of misaligned vertebrae, to reduce severe muscle spasms, and to augment pain management procedures.

Physical Therapists: Auriculotherapy is a powerful adjunct to transcutaneous electrical nerve stimulation, traction, ultrasound, and therapeutic exercises for the treatment of acute whiplash injuries, severe muscle spasms, or chronic back pain.

Psychotherapists: Psychiatrists and psychologists have utilized auriculotherapy for the reduction of anxiety, depression, insomnia, alcoholism, and substance abuse.

Reflexologists: Tactile manipulation of reflex points on the ear can be combined with pressure applied to tender regions of the feet and hands to relieve specific body aches and internal organ disorders.

1.3 Historical Overview of Auricular Acupuncture in the Far East

Classical texts on the practice of acupuncture are attributed to the *Yellow Emperor's Classic of Internal Medicine* (Veith, 1972). The Yellow emperor, Huang Di, purportedly came to power in 2698 BCE and reigned until 2598 BCE. The

Haung Di Nei Jing was composed as a dialogue between the emperor and his health ministers. Current scholars, however, suggest that the *Nei Jing* was not written down until the second century BCE. This classic text is probably a collective work by many health care practitioners that was compiled over many centuries, representing a compendium of medical knowledge accumulated in ancient China during a period of 4000 years. According to this text, all six yang meridians connect to the face, whereas the six yin meridians only reach the chest and abdomen. Yin channels connect to the ear indirectly, through their corresponding yang meridian. Those reactive ear acupoints that were tender to palpation were referred to as "*Yang Alarm*" points, which indicated a yang excess pathological disorder. The ancient Chinese ear acupuncture charts, however, were not arranged in any anatomically organized pattern. Rather, they were depicted as acupoints on the ear in a scattered array, with no apparent, logical order.

The historical roots of Chinese medicine have been comprehensively documented in Paul Unschuld's 1943 text, *Medicine in China*. Other excellent texts on this history are found in *Chen's History of Chinese Medical Science* (Hsu and Peacher, 1977), in Peter Eckman's 1996 *In the Footsteps of the Yellow Emperor*, and in Huan and Rose's 1999 *Who Can Ride the Dragon*? As with primitive, medical practice in other areas of the world, Chinese shamans sought to ward off evil demons that they perceived were the source of diseases. The philosophies of Taoism (also spelled Daoism), Confucianism, and Buddhism were incorporated with physical medicine as an integral part of health care practice in China. Metaphorical references to light and dark, sun and moon, fire and earth, hot and cold, dry and damp all contributed to the Chinese understanding of disease. The microcosm of mankind was associated with the macrocosm of the universe, which were said to demonstrate the systematic correspondences between the visible and the invisible worlds.

Human pain and pathology were attributed to disturbances in the flow of "*qi*" (pronounced "chee") along distinct energy channels referred to as meridians or channels. Insertion of fine needles into specific acupuncture points was thought to facilitate the circulation of this invisible energy through acupoint "holes" in the skin. The *Haung Di Nei Jing* text attributed to the Yellow Emperor described 360 such holes as suitable for needling. The earliest records of Chinese medicine have been found on turtle shells and bamboo strips dated to 400 BCE, as paper was not invented in China until 150 CE. Acupuncture needles were first made from bones and stones, and later from bronze metal. In 1027 CE, a full-sized figure of a man was cast in bronze to guide medical practitioners. A replica of this bronze statue is shown in Figure 1.1. Over the surface of this bronze statue was located a series of holes that corresponded to the locations of acupuncture points. Oriental medicine was a complete treatment system based on empirical findings that examined the clinical efficacy of needling acupuncture points.

Dr. Gong Sun Chen (Chen and Lu, 1999), of the Nanjing Medical University, has reported that the *Nei Jing* included numerous references to the unique, healing qualities of the auricle. The ear was not considered an isolated organ, but was intimately connected with all organs of the body, the five viscera (liver, heart, spleen, lungs, and kidneys) and the six bowels (stomach, small intestine, large intestine, gall bladder, bladder, and san jiao or triple warmer). Evaluation of the external ear could predict the onset of specific ailments and the recovery from disease. Ear acupuncture was used to treat a variety of disorders, including headaches, eye disease, asthma, facial nerve paralysis, and stomachaches. According to Huang (1974), the *Nei Jing* stated that "blood and air circulate through the 12 meridians and their 365 accessory points to infiltrate the five sense organs, seven orifices, and brain marrow." Huang further noted that

the meridians of the lesser yang of the hand were said to extend upwards toward the back of the ear. The meridian of the great yang of the foot extended to the upper corner of the ear. The circulation of the six yang meridians passed directly through the ear, while the six yin meridians joined with their corresponding yang meridians.

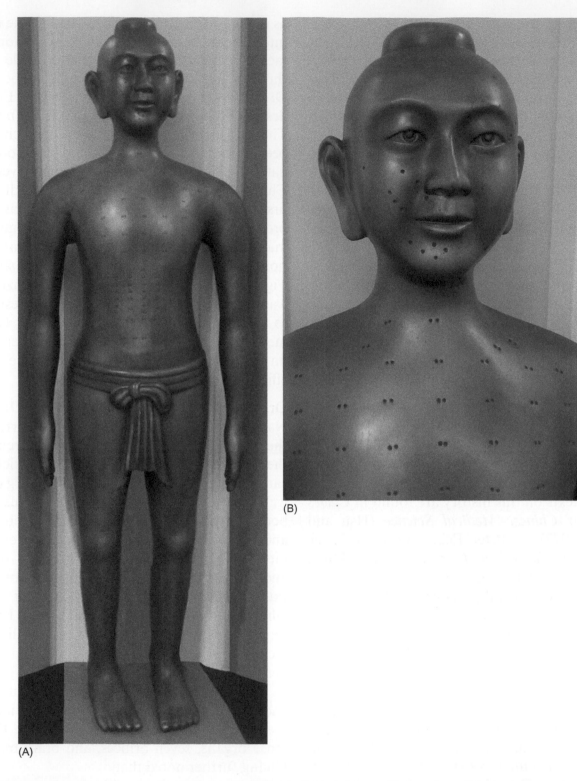

(B)

(A)

⟦**FIGURE 1.1** A replica of an ancient bronze statue that indicated the specific location of acupuncture points by small holes in the surface of the statue. (A) Full view of the statue; (B) close-up of the head of the statue.

Inspection of ancient and modern Chinese acupuncture charts demonstrates that only the Stomach, Small Intestine, Bladder, Gall Bladder, and San Jiao meridian channels circulate around the external ear, with the Large Intestine channel ending nearby. The phrase "meridian channel" is actually redundant, but both words will be used alternatively in the present text. Some meridians are referred to as fu channels that carry yang energy to strengthen the protection of the body from external pathogenic factors and from stress. The zang meridian channels, which carry yin energy, originate or terminate in the internal organs of the chest and abdomen, but they do not project to the head or ear. By forming connections to their corresponding fu meridian when they reach the hand or foot, the zang channels indirectly reach acupuncture points on the ear. The microcosm of the ear was said to have energetic correspondence with the macrocosm of the whole body, and the microcosm of the whole body was said to have cosmic correspondence with the macrocosm of the universe. The Chinese attributed health disorders to some dysfunction in the harmonic balance of these energetic systems.

Huang (1974) traced ear acupuncture treatments for many diseases to the 281 CE Chinese text, *Prescriptions for Emergencies*. In another ancient text written in 581 CE, the *Thousand Gold Remedies* stated that jaundice and a variety of epidemics were cured by applying acupuncture and moxibustion to the upper ridge in the center of the ear. *The Study of Eight Special Meridians*, published in 1572, reported that a network of yang meridians spread from the body to the head and the ear. The external ear was thus said to be the converging place of the main acupuncture meridians. Another text of that time, the *Mystical Gate: Pulse Measurement*, observed that air (qi) from the kidney is connected to the ear. *Criteria in Diagnosis and Treatment* suggested in 1602 that

> *when air in the lungs is insufficient, the ear turns deaf. The lungs control air (qi), which spreads all over the body to converge in the ear. The ear is connected to every part of the body because of the ceaseless circulation of air (qi) and blood through these meridians and vessels. The outer and inner branch vessels serve the function of connecting with the outer limbs to form the harmonious relationship between the ear, the four limbs, and a hundred bones. The ear joins with the body to form the unified, inseparable whole, a theory which forms the basis for diagnosis and treatment.*

The Compendium of Acupuncture and Moxibustion dated to 1602 recorded that cataracts could be cured by applying moxibustion to

the ear apex point. This book also described the use of both hands to pull down the ear lobes to cure headaches. As late as 1888, during the Qing dynasty, the physician Zhang Zhen described in the book *Li Zhen Anmo Yao Shu* that the posterior auricle could be divided into five regions, each region related to one of the five yin organs. The central posterior auricle was said to correspond to the lung, the lateral auricular area to the liver, the middle area to the spleen, the upper area to the heart, and the lower area to the kidney. Massaging the ear lobe was used to treat the common cold, needling the helix rim was used to expel pathogenic wind and relieve backaches, while stimulating the antihelix and antitragus was used to treat headaches due to wind-heat and pathogenic fire.

During the medieval period in Europe, Western physicians cut open major veins on seriously sick patients in order to release the "evil spirits" that were said to cause disease. Chinese doctors conducted a much less brutal form of bloodletting by pricking the skin at acupoints to release just a few droplets of blood. One of the primary loci used for bloodletting was to prick the top of the external ear. Throughout their medicine, Chinese doctors sought to balance the flow of qi and blood. By draining surpluses of spirit, or by supplementing depletions of subtle energies, Oriental medicine provided health care to the Chinese masses throughout the several thousand years of the Han, Sui, Tang, Song, Mongol, Ming, and Manchu dynasties.

However, widespread use of acupuncture in China diminished in the 1800s, when China became dominated by imperialist powers from Europe. In 1822, the minister of health for the Chinese emperor commanded all hospitals to stop practicing acupuncture, but its use nonetheless continued. While the application of Western medical procedures became increasingly prominent in the large cities of China, health care practices in rural China changed much more slowly. The erosion of faith in traditional Oriental medicine followed the defeat of the Chinese military in the Opium Wars of the 1840s. British merchants had purchased large quantities of Chinese tea, porcelain, and silk, but that created a large trade imbalance when the Chinese did not buy European products in return. The European solution was the forced sale of opium to Chinese peasants. Although the emperor of China forbade its importation, smugglers were hired to sneak opium into the Chinese mainland. When Chinese officials burned a warehouse of the British East India Company that was stocked with smuggled opium, the British parliament utilized this "attack on British territory" as justification for the declaration of war. The Chinese should probably have imported European weapons, for they were soundly defeated in the opium wars with England. The Chinese were forced to pay substantial sums of currency for the lost British opium, and they were required to surrender the territory of Hong Kong. Opium houses proliferated, and the Chinese people lost a sense of confidence in uniquely Oriental medical discoveries.

Because the Occidental traders from Europe had more powerful weapons than the Chinese, it came to be believed that Western doctors had more powerful medicine. The official Chinese government attempted to suppress the teaching of Oriental medicine as unscientific, issuing prohibitory edicts in 1914 and again in 1929, yet the practice of acupuncture nonetheless continued. Chinese officials were impressed by Western science and by European, biological discoveries. Antiseptic, surgical interventions that had been introduced from Europe greatly reduced post-surgical infections. The germ theory of Western medicine came to have greater relevance for health than the energetic theory of qi. Jesuit missionaries in China utilized the dissemination of Western medications as a manifestation of the superiority of their Christian faith.

By the 1940s, however, Europe became embroiled in World War II, and Marxism became a more influential Western import to China than Christianity. After the Communist revolution in 1949, Mao Tse Tung (also spelled Mao Zedong) called for a revitalization of ancient Chinese methods for health and healing. Acupuncture had declined in the large cities of China, with large hospitals primarily based on conventional Western medicine. However,

doctors in the rural countryside of China had maintained the ancient ways of healing. It was from these rural routes that Mao derived his military power, and it ultimately led to a renewed interest in classical Oriental practices. Maoist dogma encouraged the development of the scientific *Dialectic of Nature* as the basis for TCM. Nonetheless, the practice of acupuncture still included the energetic concepts of yin and yang, the five elements of fire, earth, wood, water, and metal, and the eight principles for differentiating medical syndromes.

It was fortuitous that the discoveries of the ear reflex charts by Dr. Paul Nogier arrived in China in 1958. This was a time of renewed interest in classical acupuncture approaches to health care. *"Barefoot doctors,"* who were high school graduates given 6 months of medical training, were taught the easily learned techniques of ear acupuncture. With little models of the inverted fetus mapped on the ear, these barefoot doctors brought health care to the large population areas of China. It was relatively simple to train lay healers how to needle just that part of the ear that corresponded to the upside-down, somatotopic map of the body. Although ear acupuncture was used throughout China prior to their learning of Nogier's treatise on the topic, the correspondence of the ear to specific body regions was not shown on ear acupuncture charts prior to 1958. For example, hospitals in Shandong Province reported in 1956 that they had treated acute tonsillitis by stimulating three points on the ear helix chosen according to folk experience. Only later ear charts depicted an upside-down body on the external ear.

After learning about the Nogier ear charts in 1958, a massive study was initiated by the Nanjing Army Ear Acupuncture Research Team. This Chinese medical group verified the clinical effectiveness of the somatotopic approach to auricular acupuncture. This group assessed the conditions of more than 2000 clinical patients, recording which ear points corresponded to specific diseases. As part of the efforts of Mao Tse Tung (Mao Zedong) to de-Westernize Chinese medicine, barefoot doctors were taught the easily learned techniques of ear acupuncture to bring health care to the Chinese masses. Gong Sun Chen (1995) confirmed that it was only after the Chinese learned of Nogier's inverted fetus picture of auricular points that great changes in the practice of ear acupuncture occurred. The Nanjing division of the medical unit of Chinese military enlisted acupuncturists from all over the country to examine and to treat thousands of patients with somatotopic, auricular acupuncture protocols. Their report on the success of ear acupuncture for several thousand different types of patients provided scientific replication of Nogier's work and broad inclusion of this approach in TCM.

Another historian of Chinese medicine, Huang (1974), also stated that it was in 1958 that "there was a massive movement to study and apply ear acupuncture across the nation. As a result, general conclusions were drawn from several hundred clinical cases, and the scope of ear acupuncture was greatly enlarged." Her writings further stated,

Certain individuals began to promote the revisionist line in medicine and health. They spread erroneous ideas, such as Chinese medicine is unscientific and insertion of the needle can only kill pain but not cure disease. Since the Cultural Revolution dispelled these erroneous ideas, ear acupuncture has been again broadly applied all over the country. The method of ear acupuncture is based on the fundamental principle of the unity of opposites. Human being is regarded as a unified, continually moving entity. Disease is the result of struggle between contradictions. By applying Chairman Mao's brilliant philosophical ideas, we can combine the revolutionary spirit of daring to think and daring to do with the scientific method of experimentation in the exploration and application of ear acupuncture.

To modern readers, it might seem unusual that Communist, political rhetoric is integrated within a medical text, but it must be remembered that the Cold War in the 1970s greatly isolated China from Western influences. Huang also included more metaphysical influences in Chinese thought, citing a classic text, *The Mystical Gate: Treatise on Meridians and Vessels*, which indicated that "the ear is connected to every part of the body because of the ceaseless circulation of energy and blood through these meridians and vessels. The ear joins with the body to form the unified, inseparable whole."

Medical research in China has continued since the introduction of the somatotopic relationship of ear acupuncture to classical meridian channels. Chinese acupuncturists have increasingly used small ear seeds held on the skin surface with adhesive tape, rather than inserted needles for the treatment of different diseases. Auricular diagnosis has served as a guide for recommending various Chinese herbal remedies. Three health categories were emphasized that were appropriate for auricular acupuncture:

1. Those conditions that can be cured by auricular acupuncture alone
2. Those conditions whose symptoms can be at least partially alleviated
3. Those conditions where improvement was seen only in individual cases

The auricular points chosen were selected according to five factors:

1. The corresponding body regions where there is pain or pathology
2. The identification of pathological ear points that are tender to touch
3. The basic principles of TCM
4. Physiological understanding derived from modern Western medicine
5. The results of experiments and clinical observations

Having previously used ear acupuncture for postoperative symptoms, the Hong Kong physician H. L. Wen (Wen and Cheung, 1973) observed that opiate-addicted patients no longer felt a craving for their previously preferred drug. The Shen Men and Lung ear points that were used for acupuncture analgesia also alleviated drug detoxification. Wen subsequently studied a larger sample of opium and heroin addicts who were given auricular electroacupuncture. Bilateral, electrical stimulation between the Lung point and the Shen Men point led to complete cessation of drug use in 39 of 40 opiate addicts.

Given that it was Western merchants who enabled widespread opium abuse in China in the 1800s, it is intriguing that a Chinese auriculotherapy treatment for drug addiction is now one of the most widely disseminated applications of acupuncture in the West.

There are distinct discrepancies between Oriental and Occidental ear acupuncture charts. Distortions may have appeared in the transmission of ear maps from France to Germany to Japan to China. Inaccuracies could have been due to mistranslations between European-based languages and Asian-based languages. Moreover, many drawings of the convoluted structures of the auricle were so inaccurate that it has allowed many sources of discrepancies between different ear charts. The Chinese, however, maintain that the ear acupuncture points used in their treatment plans have been verified across thousands of patients. Chinese conferences devoted to research investigations of ear acupuncture were held in 1992, 1995, 2005, and 2010. The Chinese government authorized a committee to standardize the name and location of auricular points. This committee designated the localization of 91 auricular points, standardized along guidelines established by the World Health Organization (WHO) in 1990 and by the World Federation of Acupuncture Societies in 2010.

1.4 Auriculotherapy and Auricular Medicine in the West

Ancient Egypt, Greece, Rome, and Persia: The Egyptologist Alexandre Varille documented that women in ancient Egypt who did not want any more children sometimes had their external ear pricked with a needle or cauterized with heat. Gold earrings were reportedly worn by Mediterranean sailors not just as jewelry but also because they were said to improve vision. Hippocrates, the father of Greek medicine, reported that doctors made small openings in the veins behind the ear to facilitate ejaculation and to reduce impotency problems. The Greek physician Galen introduced Hippocratic medicine to the Roman empire in the second century

CE. Amongst his writings, Galen commented on the healing value of bloodletting at the outer ear and the treatment of sciatic pain by the cutting of veins situated behind the ear. After the fall of Rome, the medical records of Egyptian, Greek, and Roman medicine were best preserved in Middle Eastern Islamic cultures. Included in these Islamic medical records were specific references to medical treatments for sciatica pain produced by cauterization of the external ear.

Modern Europe: The Dutch East India Company actively engaged in trade with China from the 1600s to the 1800s. In addition to the importation of silk, porcelain, tea, and spices, Dutch merchants brought Chinese acupuncture practices back to Europe. The Dutch physician Wilhelm Ten Rhyne was stationed with the Dutch East India Company in Japan and subsequently published *De Acupunctura* in 1683. Dr. Ten Rhyne wrote that the purpose of inserting needles into the skin was to allow "evil wind" to escape from the body. According to the Chinese medical classic *Yellow Emperor's Classic*, this "wind" was at the root of all disease. Knowledge of Chinese acupuncture practices spread to Germany, France, and Great Britain. Intriguingly, little of this knowledge was transmitted to European physicians who came to the United States, nor did such knowledge survive to modern times even in Holland. Discussing this topic in 2010 with practitioners of acupuncture in Amsterdam, very few Dutch doctors were aware of the pioneering work of Dr. Ten Rhyne. Most Dutch schools of acupuncture date back to just the 1970s, approximately the same time when schools of acupuncture began in the United States.

Medical interest in acupuncture waxed and waned throughout Europe for several centuries, from the 1600s to the 1800s. It would elicit great excitement, then be dismissed as unreliable folk medicine and abandoned. Subsequently, a new set of European physicians would rediscover the curative powers of acupuncture as a new way of healing. In the 19th century, the French Academie des Sciences appointed a commission to study acupuncture. Gustaf Landgaren of Sweden conducted acupuncture experiments on animals and on human volunteers at the

University of Uppsala in 1829. Sporadic reports of the use of acupuncture needles were included in European medical writings for the next several decades.

It was in the early 1900s that interest in acupuncture was once again revived in Europe. From 1907 to 1927, Georges Soulié de Morant served as the French consul to China. Stationed in Nanking and Shanghai, he became impressed by the effectiveness of acupuncture in treating a cholera epidemic and many other diseases. Soulié de Morant translated the *Nei Jing* into French and published *L'Acupuncture Chinoise*. He taught Chinese medical procedures to physicians throughout France, German, and Italy. Morant is considered the "Father of Acupuncture in Europe." Of intriguing historical note, the French *Journal des Connaissance Medico-Chirurgicales* had reported in 1850 that 13 different cases of sciatic pain had been treated by cauterization with a hot iron applied to the ear. Only one of the patients failed to dramatically improve. It was not until a century later, however, that the Lyon, France, physician Paul Nogier would rediscover this remarkable ear treatment.

In 1950, Dr. Paul Nogier (1972) was "intrigued by a strange scar which certain of his patients had on their external ear." He found that the scar was due to a treatment for sciatica involving cauterization of the auricular antihelix by a lay practitioner living in Marseille, France. Her name was Mrs. Barrin. The patients were unanimous in stating that they had been successfully relieved of sciatica pain within hours, even minutes, of this ear cauterization. Mrs. Barrin had learned of this auricular procedure from her father, who had learned it from a Chinese Mandarin. As stated by Nogier,

> I then proceeded to carry out some cauterizations myself, which proved effective, then tried some other, less barbarous processes. A simple dry jab with a needle also led to the relief of sciatica if given to the same antihelix area, an area of the ear which was painful to pressure.

Nogier had previous medical experience with the utilization of acupuncture needles, as he had studied the works of the French acupuncturist Soulié de Morant. Another mentor for Nogier was the Swiss homeopathic physician, Dr. Pierre Schmidt, who utilized massage, spinal manipulations, and acupuncture needles in his naturopathic practice. Some critics have contended that Nogier developed his ear maps based on translations of Chinese writings, but as stated previously, the Chinese themselves acknowledge that it was only after they learned of Nogier's findings in 1958 that they develop their own somatotopic ear charts. A quotation attributed to the physiologist Claude Bernard further inspired Nogier:

> It has often been said, that in order to discover things, one must be ignorant. It is better to know nothing than to have certain fixed ideas in one's mind, which are based on theories which one constantly tries to confirm. A discovery is usually an unexpected connection, which is not included in some theory. A discovery is rarely logical and often goes against the conceptions then in fashion.

Nogier discussed his antihelix cauterization experiences with another physician, Dr. René Amathieu, who told him, "the problem of sciatica is a problem of the sacrolumbar hinge." Nogier conjectured that the upper antihelix area used to treat sciatica could correspond to the lumbar–sacral joint, and the whole antihelix could represent the remaining spinal vertebrae, but upside down: "The head would have its correspondence lower on the auricle. The ear could thus roughly resemble an upside down embryo *in utero*."

Nogier subsequently obtained pain relief for other problems. Using electrical microcurrents imperceptible to the patient, Nogier concluded that the pain relief was not due to a nervous reaction to the pain from needle insertion but was in fact caused by the stimulation of a specific area of the ear. Nogier observed, "To discover something is to accomplish one stage of the journey. To push on to the bottom of this discovery is to accomplish another."

In 1955, Nogier mentioned his discoveries to Dr. Jacques Niboyet, the undisputed master of acupuncture in France. Niboyet was struck by this novel, ear reflex zone, which had not

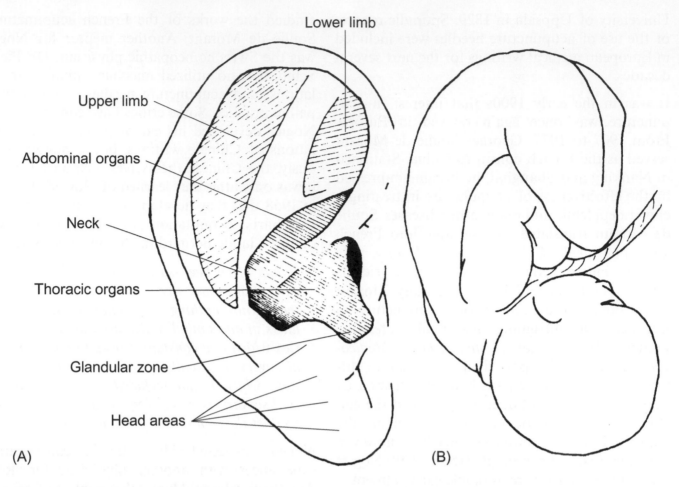

Lower limb

Upper limb

Abdominal organs

Neck

Thoracic organs

Glandular zone

Head areas

(A)   (B)

[**FIGURE 1.2** Early images by Dr. Paul Nogier indicating the correspondences between the physical body and different areas of the ear (A) and an image of the inverted fetus pattern depicted on the external ear (B).
(Reproduced with permission from Nogier, 1972.)

been described in any Chinese text. Niboyet encouraged Nogier to present his findings to the Congress of the Mediterranean Society of Acupuncture in February 1956. Attending this meeting was Dr. Gérard Bachmann of Munich, Germany. Bachmann published Nogier's findings in a 1957 European acupuncture journal, which had worldwide circulation, including distribution to the Far East.

From these translations from French into German, the Nogier's ear reflex system was soon known by acupuncturists in Japan. It was subsequently published in China, where it became incorporated into Chinese ear acupuncture charts. Nogier acknowledged in his own writings that the origins of auriculotherapy might have begun in ancient China or in ancient Persia. The primary change that he brought to auricular

acupuncture in 1957 was that these ear acupoints were not just a scattered array of different points for different conditions, but that there was a somatotopic inverted fetus pattern of auricular points that corresponded to the pattern of the actual physical body. Nogier (1972) devoted his pioneering classic, the *Treatise of Auriculotherapy*, to the musculoskeletal system. Nogier limited his initial writings

to the spinal column and the limbs because the musculoskeletal body is projected onto the external ear in a clear and simple manner. The therapeutic applications are free from ambiguity and ought to allow the beginner to achieve convincing results. It is possible to palpate for tender areas of the ear and readily notice how they correspond to painful areas of the body. The first stages of learning the map of the ear

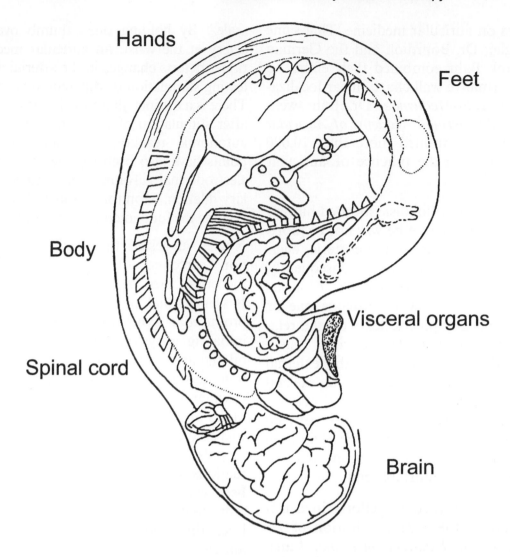

Hands

Feet

Body

Visceral organs

Spinal cord

Brain

[FIGURE 1.3 Ear reflex charts developed by Dr. Paul Nogier that show somatotopic correspondences of the brain, spinal cord, musculoskeletal structures, and internal organs to specific areas of the auricle. *(Reproduced with permission from Nogier, 1972.)*

consist of getting to know the morphology of the external ear, its reflex cartography, and how to treat simple pains of traumatic origin. Each doctor needs to be convinced of the efficacy of this ear reflex method by personal results that he or she is right. They are indeed fortunate people who can convince themselves simply by noting the improvement of a symptom they themselves have experienced.

After he traced the image of the spine and the limbs over different areas of the auricle, Nogier examined thoracic organs, abdominal organs, and central nervous system projections onto the external ear. He needed several more years, however, to understand that the external ear had a

triple innervation, and that each innervation supported the image of an embryological derivative: the endoderm, mesoderm, and ectoderm. These embryological correspondences to the ear were described by Nogier (1968) in another text, *Handbook to Auriculotherapy*, with illustrated anatomical drawings by his friend and colleague, Dr. René Bourdiol.

By 1975, Nogier had created a teaching structure for training in auricular medicine, establishing the organization Group Lyonaise Études Medicales (GLEM), translated into English as the Medical Studies Group of Lyon. The journal *Auriculo-medicine* was also initiated in 1975, providing a professional vehicle for publishing clinical studies on auricular medicine. That same year, Dr. Nogier, Dr. Bourdiol, and the German physician Frank Bahr combined their efforts to publish an informative wall chart on ear localizations, *Loci Auriculo-Medicinae*. Dr. Bahr went on to organize the *German Academy of Auricular Medicine*, which has trained more than 10,000 German physicians in the practice of auricular medicine.

In 1981, Dr. René Bourdiol disassociated himself from Nogier, partly because he was not comfortable with some of Nogier's more esoteric, energetic explanations of healing. Consequently, Bourdiol (1982) wrote his own book, *Elements of Auriculotherapy*. This work remains one of the most anatomically precise texts on the relationship of the auricle to the nervous system and includes detailed pictures of the external ear with representation of the musculoskeletal system, visceral organs, and the central nervous system. The innovative collaborations between Nogier and Bourdiol had lasted from 1965 until 1981, but their collegial association unfortunately came to an uncomfortable end.

Nogier (1983) had turned his efforts in a different direction by the 1981 publication of *De L'auriculothérapie à L'auriculomédecine*, translated into English as *From Auriculotherapy to Auriculomedicine*. In this work, Nogier presented his theory of three somatotopic phases on the ear and he discussed his concepts of electric, magnetic, and reticular energies. The most prominent feature of this auriculomedicine text, however, featured expanded descriptions about Nogier's 1966 discovery of a new pulse, the *réflexe auriculo cardiaque* (RAC). This pulse reaction was later labeled the *vascular autonomic signal* (VAS) because it was related to a more general reactivity of the vascular system.

In honor of its discoverer, this pulse reaction has also been called the *réflexe artériel de Nogier* by Bourdiol and the *Nogier reflex* by Bahr. For the purposes of this text, the Nogier vascular autonomic signal pulse will be abbreviated as "Nogier VAS pulse" so as not to confuse it with a well-known pain assessment measure that uses the letters "V," "A," and "S"—the "visual analogue scale." By holding one's thumb over the radial artery at the wrist, an auricular medicine practitioner detects changes in the arterial waveform following stimulation of different areas of the auricle. There is a distinct alteration in the pulse a few beats after stimulation of the skin over the ear. Similar autonomic reactions to touching sensitive ear points have also been reported for changes in the electrodermal galvanic skin response and in pupillary dilation. Monitoring this radial pulse reaction became the fundamental basis of auriculomedicine.

Nogier suggested that each peripheral stimulation "perceived at the pulse is at first received by the brain, then transmitted by the arterial tree." It seemed that physiological changes in the ear produced a sympathetic nervous system reflex, initiating a systolic cardiac wave that reflected off the arterial wall, followed by a returning, retrograde wave. This reflex established a stationary vascular wave, which could be perceived at the radial artery. Palpation of the Nogier VAS pulse was used to determine changes in pulse amplitude or pulse waveform that were not related to fluctuations in pulse rate. The Nogier VAS pulse has been explained as a general vascular-cutaneous reflex that can be activated by tactile, electrical, or laser stimulation of many body areas, not just the auricle.

Considerable confusion was generated when subsequent books on the Nogier phases on the ear seemed to contradict earlier writings. *Points Réflexes Auriculaires* (Nogier *et al.*, 1987) localized some anatomical structures to different regions of the external ear than had been described in previous publications by Nogier. The most detailed presentation of the three phases was described by Nogier *et al.* (1989) in *Compléments des Points Réflexes Auriculaires*. This text continued to show that in the second phase, the musculoskeletal system shifted from the antihelix to the central concha, whereas in the third phase, musculoskeletal points were located on the tragus, antitragus, and ear lobe. However, Nogier reversed some of the descriptions from his previous writings. In contrast to the presentation of the phases in the 1981 book *De L'auriculothérapie à L'auriculomédecine*, the 1989 *Compléments des Points Réflexes Auriculaires* switched the lateral orientation of the second phase vertebrae and the vertical orientation of the third phase vertebrae. Although Nogier had developed the three-phase explanation as a means of reconciling the differences between his findings and that of the Chinese, it was a drastic departure from the original, inverted fetus picture for the ear. The suggestion of different somatotopic patterns on the same auricular regions bothered many of Nogier's followers as overly confusing and clinically impractical.

Dissention within the European auriculomedicine movement occurred by the 1990s (Nogier, 1999). First, the three-phase theory was not well accepted by many auriculomedicine doctors in France and Germany. Second, Nogier discussed the importance of "reticular energy" without specifically defining what it was. He explored the chakra energy centers of ayurvedic medicine, which seemed to some as a nonscientific endeavor. The energetic theory of Nogier had also been taken by a non-medical school that used Nogier's name to develop more esoteric philosophies of auricular reflexotherapy. These associations threatened the professional credibility of auricular medicine. Many acupuncturists in England, Italy, and Russia preferred to follow the Chinese ear charts, which delineated the localization of ear reflex points in somewhat different arrangements than the ear charts developed by Nogier. A very personal account of the development and progress of auriculomedicine in Europe was presented in the book *The Man in the Ear*, written by Paul Nogier with his son Raphael Nogier (1985). Also a physician, Raphael Nogier has become one of Europe's most prominent figures in the continued training of doctors in the practice of auricular medicine. International symposiums on auricular medicine have been held in France in 1990, 1996, 2006, and 2012.

United States: The long history of acupuncture and moxibustion was generally not known in the United States until after President Richard Nixon's 1972 visit to the People's Republic of China. One of the educational consequences of Nixon's visit was the establishment of the first American acupuncture clinic based within a conventional Western hospital. Dr. David Bresler had studied Oriental medicine with acupuncture masters in the Chinatown region of Los Angeles. He was able to convince hospital administrators at the UCLA School of Medicine to allow him to open a clinical research center to scientifically evaluate the therapeutic efficacy of acupuncture. Dr. Richard Kroening served as the first medical director for the UCLA acupuncture research clinic, and I had the opportunity to serve as their first research director.

At that time, I was a post-doctoral research scholar at the UCLA Brain Research Institute, where I was examining stimulation-produced analgesia in animals under the guidance of Dr. John Liebeskind. His pioneering research in the 1970s had demonstrated that electrical stimulation of the periaqueductal gray (PAG) region of the brainstem could inhibit animal reflexes to aversive stimuli (Oleson and Liebeskind, 1978; Oleson et al., 1980a). What was most surprising at the time was that the opiate antagonist naloxone could block the analgesic effect of this brain stimulation—a finding that ultimately contributed to the discovery of the natural, pain-relieving, endorphin molecules. The UCLA acupuncture clinic was located just down a long hallway from the neuroscience laboratories of Dr. Liebeskind. It seemed like a wonderful opportunity to compare the pain inhibitory patterns observed following brain stimulation in animals to the clinical effects of acupuncture stimulation in human patients. During that time, the first approved course in medical acupuncture for physicians was developed by Dr. Joe Helms under the auspices of the UCLA School of Medicine. When Dr. Paul Nogier visited the United States in 1981, Dr. Helms translated the auriculotherapy lectures of Dr. Nogier to the American audience, as Dr. Helms was one of the few physicians in the United States who was fluent in both French and English and who was also an expert in both Western medicine and Oriental medicine.

The first double blind research of auricular diagnosis was conducted on 40 patients at the UCLA Pain Control Center (Oleson et al., 1980b). The localization of musculoskeletal pain

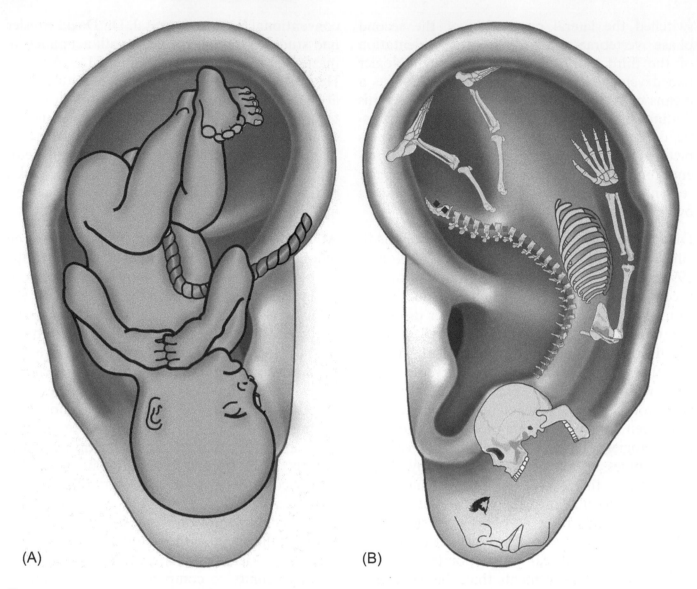

(A)   (B)

FIGURE 1.4 Images of the somatotopic pattern on the external ear developed by Dr. Terry Oleson, showing an inverted fetus perspective (A) and an actual orientation of the somatotopic body (B).

was first established by one investigator, a doctor or nurse. A second physician, Dr. Richard Kroening, then examined the auricle for specific areas of heightened tenderness and increased electrical conductance. The patients were draped with a sheet to conceal any body casts, and this second doctor was not provided any information concerning the location of the patient's pain. Dr. Kroening could only inquire if a particular point on the ear was tender or not, and whether it was electrically conductive or not. Another investigator recorded the digital display of the electrical point finder that Dr. Kroening held on different areas of the patient's auricle. Both the patients and the examining doctor were blind to which

ear points were related to the patient's clinical problem. Reactive ear acupoints that exhibited high tenderness ratings and high skin conductance were associated with specific areas of physical pain or dysfunction in the body, whereas nonreactive points were associated with pain-free areas of the body. These findings are presented in Tables 1.1 and 1.2.

After training with the Hong Kong doctor H. L. Wen, Dr. Michael Smith (1979) brought the utilization of ear acupuncture for the treatment of drug addiction to his clinic at the South Bronx Lincoln Hospital in New York City in 1974. The clinical success of this work led to the

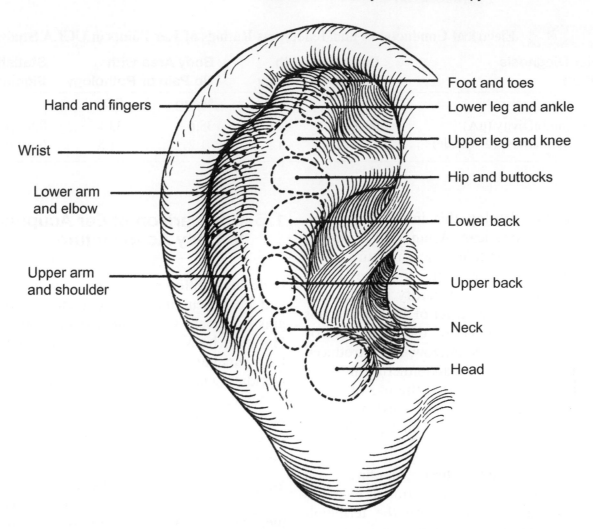

Hand and fingers

Wrist

Lower arm
and elbow

Upper arm
and shoulder

Foot and toes

Lower leg and ankle

Upper leg and knee

Hip and buttocks

Lower back

Upper back

Neck

Head

[**FIGURE 1.5** Drawing of somatotopic regions of the external ear that shows the musculoskeletal ear reflex points examined in the auricular diagnosis study published in 1980.

TABLE 1.1	Findings of 1980 UCLA Auricular Diagnosis Study[a].			
Auricular Diagnosis Evaluation	Body Area with Pain or Pathology		Body Area with No Pain or Pathology	
	N	%	N	%
Reactive ear point[b]	185	38.5	62	12.9
Nonreactive ear point	57	11.9	176	36.7

[a]Established medical diagnosis based on double blind evaluation of 12 areas of the body across 40 patients with musculoskeletal disorders, providing 480 areas of analysis.
[b]Total correct detection of 185 + 176 out of 480 possible comparisons led to total percentage of 75.2% correct detections, which was statistically significant by the chi square test, $\chi^2 = 120$, $df = 1$, $p < .01$.

wider application of auricular acupuncture for assisting drug addicts to recover from a variety of recreational substances, including opiates, cocaine, alcohol, and nicotine. The protocol of using five ear acupuncture points for the treatment of substance abuse led to the formation of the National Acupuncture Detoxification Association (NADA) in 1985 (Smith, 1990).

In 1999, the International Consensus Conference on Acupuncture, Auriculotherapy, and Auricular Medicine (ICCAAAM'09) brought together 40 international experts on auricular acupuncture from Asia, Europe, and America to establish a collective consensus on auricular acupuncture as it is practiced throughout the world. A similar conference was held in the United States in

TABLE 1.2 Electrical Conductance and Tenderness Ratings of Ear Points in UCLA Study.

Auricular Diagnosis Evaluation	Body Area with Pain or Pathology		Body Area with No Pain or Pathology		Statistical Significance
	Mean	SD	Mean	SD	
Auricular conductivity (μA)	60.3	42.6	38.6	33.1	8.81, $p<.01$
Ratings of tenderness (0–4 scale)	1.8	1.3	1.2	1.5	6.47, $p<.01$

2006 to further develop this international collaboration with American, Asian, and European approaches to auricular acupuncture. The Auriculotherapy Certification Institute (ACI) was established in 1999 to certify practitioners who demonstrate a high level of mastery in this field. One of the members of the ACI board of directors, Dr. Richard Niemtzow, has introduced auriculotherapy and body acupuncture into the U.S. military and has initiated the use of auricular acupuncture as a part of battlefield acupuncture procedures that are being provided to American soldiers.

World Health Organization Meetings on Auricular Acupuncture: International meetings of WHO sought to standardize the terminology used for auricular acupuncture nomenclature. Consensus conferences were held in China, Korea, and the Philippines from 1985 to 1989. At the 1990 WHO meeting in Lyon, France, doctors from Asia, Europe, and America agreed to finalize the standardization of names for auricular anatomy. A consensus was arrived at for the identification of ear points according to Chinese and European ear acupuncture charts. Subsequent international conferences were held in China in 1995 and 2010 and in the United States and France in 2006 and 2012. The purpose of these meetings has been to bring together international experts in this field. At a 1994 international congress on auricular medicine held in Lyon, Nogier was honored as the "Father of Auriculotherapy." Nogier died in 1996, leaving an amazing scientific inheritance. He had contributed the unique discovery of somatotopic correspondences to the external ear, developed a new form of pulse diagnosis, and expanded medical appreciation of the complex, subtle energies of the body.

1.5 Comparison of Ear Acupuncture to Body Acupuncture

Historical Differences: Both ear acupuncture and body acupuncture had their historical origins in ancient China more than 2000 year ago. However, body acupuncture has remained essentially unchanged in its perspective of specific meridian channels, whereas Chinese ear acupuncture was greatly modified by the inverted fetus discoveries of the French physician Paul Nogier in the 1950s. Further research has yielded even newer developments in auricular medicine.

Yang Acupuncture Meridians: Body acupuncture is based on a system of 12 meridians, 6 yang meridians and 6 yin meridians, that run along the surface of the body as lines of energy forces. Ear acupuncture is said to directly connect to the yang meridians, but it is not dependent on these yang meridians to function. The ear is a self-contained microsystem that can affect the whole body. In TCM, the head is more associated with yang energy than are lower parts of the body. The Large Intestine, Small Intestine, and San Jiao meridians run from the arm to the head, and the Stomach, Bladder, and Gall Bladder meridians run from the head down the body. Although the yin meridians do not connect directly to the external ear on the head, they do interact with a corresponding yang meridian that does reach the head.

Auricular Correspondence to Pathological Organs: The main principle in auriculotherapy is that there is a correspondence between the cartography of the external ear and pathological conditions in homologous parts of the body. Acupuncture points on the auricle only appear

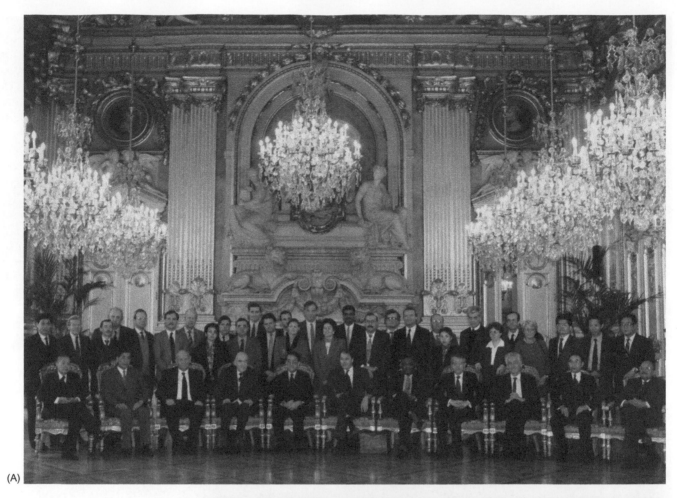

(A)

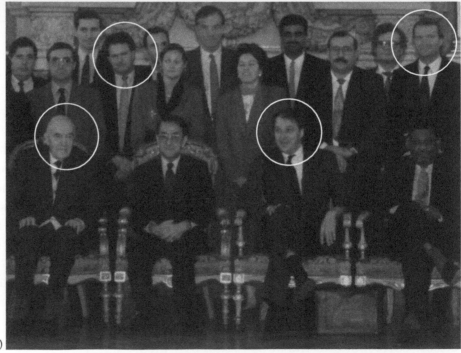

(B)

FIGURE 1.6 Photograph of all participants at the 1990 World Health Organization meeting on auricular acupuncture nomenclature (A) and an enlargement of the photograph (B) with circles surrounding Dr. Paul Nogier and Dr. Raphael Nogier in the front row and Dr. Terry Oleson and Dr. Frank Bahr in the back row.

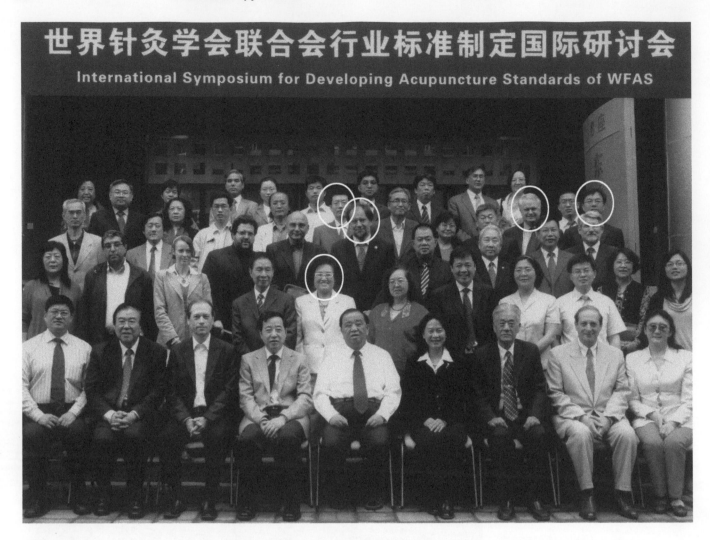

世界针灸学会联合会行业标准制定国际研讨会
International Symposium for Developing Acupuncture Standards of WFAS

FIGURE 1.7 Photograph of participants of the 2010 World Federation of Acupuncture Societies (WFAS) meeting on acupuncture nomenclature with circles surrounding Dr. Li-Chun Huang in the second row and Dr. Liqun Zhou, Dr. Winfried Wojak, Dr. Terry Oleson, and Dr. Baixiao Zhao in the back row.

when there is some physical or functional disorder in the part of the body represented by that region of the ear. There is no evidence of an auricular point if the corresponding part of the body is healthy. Acupuncture points on the body can almost always be detected, whether there is an imbalance in the related meridian channel or not. Moreover, the organ names of different meridian channels found on the body are not necessarily related to any known pathology of that organ, whereas the names of ear acupoints precisely correspond to the body region by which they are labeled.

Somatotopic Inversion: In body acupuncture, the meridian channels run throughout the body, with no apparent anatomical logic regarding the relationship of that channel to the body organ represented by that meridian. Acupoints on the Large Intestine meridians and the Kidney meridians occur in locations far removed from those specific organs. In ear acupuncture, however, there is an orderly, anatomical arrangement of points, based on the inverted fetus perspective of the body. The head areas are represented toward the bottom of the ear, the feet toward the top, and the body in between. As with the somatotopic map in the brain, the auricular homunculus devotes a proportionally larger area to the head and hand than to the other parts of the body. The size of a somatotopic area is related to its functional importance rather than its actual physical size.

Distinct Acupuncture Points: Acupuncture points are anatomically defined areas on the skin relative to certain landmarks on the body. The original Chinese pictographs for acupoints indicated that there were holes in the skin through which qi energy could flow. These acupoints can be reliably detected with electrodermal measurements. A dull, deep, aching feeling called "De Qi" often accompanies the stimulation of body acupuncture points. In ear acupuncture, an acupuncture point can be detected only when there is some pathology in the corresponding part of the body. A sharp, piercing feeling may or may not accompany pressure applied to an active auricular point. Another prominent difference between the two systems is that body acupuncture points lie in the tendon and muscular region deep below the skin surface, whereas ear acupoints reside in the shallow depth of the skin immediately above the cartilage comprising the auricle.

Increased Tenderness to Palpation: Paul Nogier observed that there are some cases of patients with an exceptional sensitivity in which mere palpation of certain parts of the ear provoked a pronounced pain sensation in the corresponding body region. This observation can be repeated several times without the phenomenon diminishing, allowing one to distinctly identify the connection that exists between such ear points and other parts of the body. The tenderness at an ear acupoint tends to increase as the degree of pathology of the corresponding organ worsens, whereas the tenderness on the ear tends to decrease as the health condition improves.

Decreased Skin Resistance: In both body acupuncture and ear acupuncture, the acupuncture points are localized regions of *lowered skin resistance*, small areas of the skin where there is a decrease in opposition to the flow of electricity. Sometimes electrodermal activity is inversely stated as *higher skin conductance*, indicating that there is the equivalent of electrical holes in the skin that allow easy passage of electric current. Electrical resistance and electrical conductance measure the exact same electrodermal phenomena, but they show it as electrical current changes in opposite directions. When pathology in a body organ worsens, the electrodermal conductivity of that ear point rises. As the body organ becomes healthier, the electrodermal conductance of that ear point returns to normal levels. Electrodermal point detection is one of the most reliable methods for diagnosing the location of a reactive auricular point.

Ipsilateral Representation: In both body and ear acupuncture, unilateral, pathological areas of the body are more often represented by acupuncture points on the same side of the body as that body organ than are points on the contralateral side of the body.

Remote Control Sites: Ear points are found at a considerable distance from the area of the body where the symptom is located, such as pain problems in the ankles, the hands, or the lower back. Body acupuncture includes needling of the local body region as well as remote, distal acupoints. Ear points remotely affect the flow of energy in meridian channels rather than exert a direct effect within the channel itself. Auricular acupoints are similar to the way a modern, electronic, remote control unit is used to open a garage door or to switch channels on a television set. Although very small in physical size because of their microchip circuitry, these remote control, electronic devices can produce pronounced changes in much larger machines. Whereas body acupoints lie completely within the meridian channels, ear acupoints seem to remotely control the flood gates to the energetic channel.

Diagnostic Efficacy: Ear acupuncture provides a more scientifically verified means of identifying areas of pain or pathology in the body than do such traditional Chinese medicine approaches as pulse diagnosis and tongue diagnosis. In auricular diagnosis, specific problems in the body are revealed by areas of the external ear that are darker, discolored, or flaky. Pathological ear points are more tender and have higher levels of skin conductance than other areas of the auricle. The subtle changes in auricular reactivity may identify conditions of which the patient is only marginally aware. A new practitioner's confidence in auriculotherapy is often strengthened by the observation of reactive ear points that turn out to correspond to health problems that were not previously reported by a patient.

Therapeutic Verification: Convincing verification of the existence of the correspondence between specific, auricular points and parts of the body is demonstrated by the immediate relief of pain in that area of the body following stimulation of the relevant ear acupoint. Patients demonstrate reactive acupoints at precisely the auricular area predicted by established ear reflex charts. In patients with diffuse regions of pathology, reactive auricular points are found all over the auricle.

Pulse Diagnosis: TCM and European auricular medicine both utilize a form of diagnosis that involves palpation of the radial pulse on the wrist. Classical Chinese acupuncture procedures for examining the pulse require the placement of three middle fingers over the wrist, assessing for subtle qualities in the depth, fullness, and subjective qualities of the pulse. These tactile sensations are utilized to determine conditions of excess, deficiency, stagnation of disorders associated with specific zang-fu organs. The Nogier VAS pulse involves placement of only the thumb over the wrist. Nogier monitored changes in the reaction of the pulse to a stimulus placed on the external ear, whereas Oriental doctors monitor the steady-state qualities of the resting pulse.

Types of Treatment Procedures: Body acupuncture and ear acupuncture are often used together in the same session, or each procedure can be effectively applied separately. Both body acupuncture points and ear acupuncture utilize such procedures as acupressure massage, acupuncture needles, and electroacupuncture. Many patients are afraid of the insertion of needles into their skin, thus they have a strong aversion to any form of needle acupuncture. As an alternative procedure, ear points can be activated by transcutaneous electrical stimulation, laser stimulation, or small pellets taped onto the auricle. It is recommended that because auricular acupuncture can work more quickly than body acupuncture, the ear points should be treated first.

Clinical Efficacy: Stimulation of ear reflex points and body acupoints seem to be equally effective treatments. Each requires only 20 minutes of treatment, yet each can yield clinical benefits that last for days and weeks. Both body and ear acupuncture are utilized for treating a broad variety of clinical disorders, including headaches, back pain, nausea, hypertension, asthma, and dental disorders. Auriculotherapy tends to relieve pain more rapidly than does body acupuncture. Ear acupuncture needling is often the treatment of choice for detoxification from substance abuse rather than body acupuncture, although both can be combined together. Like body acupuncture, ear acupuncture has been used to relieve postoperative pain, inflammations from joint sprains, pain from bone fractures, and the discomfort from gallstones. Since every organ of the body is represented upon the external ear, auriculotherapy can alleviate disorders in all parts of the body. Ear acupuncture is not limited to hearing disorders, or even to problems affecting the head. Nonetheless, auriculotherapy can be very effective for treating inner ear dizziness and for alleviating headaches. Conditions treated by both ear and body acupuncture include appendicitis, tonsillitis, uterine bleeding, dermatitis, allergic rhinitis, gastric ulcers, hepatitis, hypertension, impotency, hypothyroidism, sunburn, heat stroke, frozen shoulder, tennis elbow, torticollis, and low back pain.

Healing, Not Just Pain Relief: Both body acupuncture and ear acupuncture achieve more than just reduction of the experience of pain. Although pain relief is the more immediate effect, both procedures facilitate the internal healing processes of the body. Acupuncture and auriculotherapy treat the deeper, underlying condition, not just the symptomatic representation of the problem. They affect deeper, physiological changes by facilitating the natural, self-regulating homeostatic mechanisms of the body; by reducing muscle tension; and by improving blood circulation. Treatment of a given acupoint can either diminish overactive bodily functions or stimulate deficient physiological processes.

Ease in Mastery of Skills: Because auricular reflex points are organized in the same pattern as the gross anatomy of the body, it is possible to learn the basics of ear acupuncture in just a few days. In contrast, body acupuncture requires several years of intensive didactic training and clinical practice. The points on the ear are labeled with the organ or the condition that they are used to treat. Although there are more than 200 ear acupoints, the few ear points needed for treatment are readily identified by the principle of somatotopic correspondence and by their selective reactivity.

Ease in Treatment Application: Ear acupuncture is often more economical and convenient to use than body acupuncture because there is no disrobing required of a patient. The ear is easily available for diagnosis and treatment while someone is lying down or sitting in a chair in their street clothes. Insertion of needles into superficial ear points is simple to apply compared to the insertion of needles at deeper body acupoints. The skin over the auricle is very thin, and there is little danger of damaging a critical blood vessel when puncturing the skin with a needle.

Possible Side Effects: The primary side effect of auriculotherapy is the piercing sensations that occur when needles are inserted into the external ear or when intense electrical stimulation is applied to an ear acupoint. For sensitive patients, the auricle should be treated more gently, and ear pellets or ear seeds may be preferred to needles. If the stimulation intensity is uncomfortable, the current level should be reduced or the length of stimulation shortened. The ear itself can sometimes become tender and inflamed after the treatment. This post-treatment redness or tenderness usually subsides within a short time. As with body acupuncture, some patients become very drowsy after an auricular acupuncture treatment. They should be offered the opportunity to rest for a while. This sedation effect has been attributable to the systemic release of endorphins.

Electronic Equipment Required: Well-trained acupuncturists can detect body acupuncture points by just their palpation of the surface of the body or by the rotation of an inserted needle. A muscle spasm reflex often seems to "grab" the acupuncture needle and hold it in place when the tip of the needle is on the appropriate acupoint. Auricular diagnosis, however, is best achieved with an electrical point finder. Furthermore, a transcutaneous electrical stimulation device using microcurrent intensities can often achieve profound clinical effects without the unwanted pain that accompanies needle insertion. Since body acupoints typically lie in the muscle region, deep below the skin surface, electrical point finders are usually not practical for detecting body acupuncture points. The auricular skin surface is only a few millimeters deep; thus, it is readily available for diagnostic detection and transcutaneous treatment. Reactive ear reflex points can slightly shift in location from one day to the next; thus, the use of an electrical point finder is imperative for precise determination of point localization. Equipment used for electroacupuncture through inserted needles, or transcutaneous electrical stimulation through metal probes, is typically more effective for pain relief than simple needle insertion.

■ KEY TERMS FOR CHAPTER 1

Key Terms for Auricular Acupuncture History in the Far East

Auriculotherapy: The root words for *auricle* and for *therapy* accurately describe this treatment. The word *auricle* refers to the external ear that first captures sound waves, which are then sent to the middle ear and the inner ear. The term *therapy* refers to any diagnostic procedure or treatment modality for any pathological condition in the body.

Barefoot Doctors: These lay people in China were taught ear acupuncture and basic aspects of Traditional Chinese Medicine to bring health care to the Chinese masses.

Chen, Gong Sun: Chinese doctor who participated in the Nanjing Army Ear Acupuncture Research study, which evaluated the efficacy of auricular acupuncture.

Mao Tse Tung: Also spelled "Mao Dezong," this Chinese military commander served as the first leader of the People's Republic of China in the 1940s and supported the revitalization of ancient ways of Chinese medicine in the 1950s.

Nanjing Army Ear Acupuncture Research Team: This group of Chinese medical doctors evaluated the results for 2000 clinical patients who had received auricular acupuncture according to the inverted fetus map that had been brought to them from Europe.

Opium Wars: The wars between British and Chinese military forces that occurred in the 1800s when Chinese officials tried to prevent British merchants from smuggling forbidden opium sales to the Chinese populace.

Somatotopic Correspondence: The relationship of a specific microsystem area to a specific organ of the body. The root word for *soma* is *body*, and the root word for *topic* is *terrain*, which is a map of a physical area.

Wen, H. L.: The Hong Kong medical doctor who first described the use of ear acupuncture for opiate detoxification in the 1970s.

Yang Alarm: The increased reactivity of ear acupuncture points corresponding to the presence of pathology in the body, like a fire alarm alerting one to a fire. Only the yang meridians directly connect to the external ear, whereas yin meridians indirectly connect to the ear.

Yellow Emperor's Classic of Internal Medicine: The *Haung Di Nei Jing* is the earliest known Chinese text that describes the basic concepts and procedures of classical Chinese medicine, dating back more than 2000 years from modern times.

Key Terms for Auricular Medicine History in the West

Amathieu, René: Physician friend of Paul Nogier who suggested to him that the problem of sciatica is associated with a problem of the sacrolumbar hinge, leading to the inverted fetus map of the ear.

Auriculotherapy Certification Institute: Organization established in 1999 for the training and certification of health care practitioners in auriculotherapy and auricular acupuncture.

Bachmann, Gérard: Physician from Munich, Germany, who published Paul Nogier's findings on the auricular somatotopic pattern that were presented at the 1956 Congress of the Mediterranean Society of Acupuncture. His article in a German acupuncture journal was then distributed to Japan and subsequently to China.

Bahr, Frank: Physician from Munich, Germany, who worked with Paul Nogier and brought his teachings to Germany in the 1970s.

Bourdiol, René: French physician who collaborated with Paul Nogier on many of his early publications and in 1981 wrote the *Elements of Auriculotherapy*, an anatomically precise textbook on the relationship of the auricle to the body.

Bresler, David: California acupuncturist and psychologist who co-founded the first American acupuncture clinic that was based within a conventional Western hospital, the UCLA School of Medicine. Dr. Bresler was a co-investigator on the 1980 UCLA auricular diagnosis study that verified the scientific validity of auricular diagnosis.

Dutch East India Company: Physicians with this Dutch merchant company traded in the Far East and brought acupuncture and classical Chinese medicine to doctors in Europe in the 1600s.

German Academy of Auricular Medicine: A group of German physicians that has trained more than 10,000 German physicians in the practice of auricular medicine.

Group Lyonaise Études Medicales (GLEM): A European organization started in 1975 for training physicians and for publishing clinical studies on auricular medicine.

Helms, Joseph: California physician who initiated the first course in Medical Acupuncture for Physicians at the UCLA School of Medicine and who translated the lectures of Dr. Paul Nogier from French into English when Dr. Nogier visited the United States in 1981.

International Consensus Conference on Acupuncture, Auriculotherapy, and Auricular Medicine (ICCAAAM): An international meeting of scientists and practitioners of auricular acupuncture that was held in the United States in 1999 and 2006 to create an international consensus regarding the location and application of different auricular acupuncture points. Principal organizers for this conference were Dr. Jim Shores and Dr. Terry Oleson.

Kroening, Richard: California physician who served as the first medical director at the UCLA Pain Management Center, which offered acupuncture as one of several complementary and alternative medicine modalities. Dr. Kroening was a co-investigator for the 1980 UCLA auricular diagnosis study.

Liebeskind, John: California scientist who conducted pioneering research in the 1970s that demonstrated that electrical stimulation of the brainstem periaqueductal gray (PAG) could inhibit behavioral reflexes to noxious stimuli.

National Acupuncture Detoxification Association (NADA): This professional acupuncture organization provides clinical trainings for the alleviation of substance abuse by using five ear acupoints: Shen Men, Sympathetic, Lung, Kidney, and Liver.

Niboyet, Jacques: The master of acupuncture in modern France who encouraged Paul Nogier to present his auricular somatotopic charts to a European society of acupuncture.

Niemtzow, Richard: American physician and U.S. Air Force colonel who has introduced auriculotherapy and body acupuncture into the U.S. military and has initiated the use of auricular acupuncture as a part of battlefield acupuncture provided to American soldiers.

Nogier, Paul: Physician who lived in Lyon, France, and is considered the "Father of Auriculotherapy." He developed the concept of the inverted fetus map on the external ear in the 1950s. In 1969, Nogier published the *Treatise of Auriculotherapy*.

Nogier, Raphael: The son of Dr. Paul Nogier, Raphael Nogier is a physician in France who has continued the clinical teachings of auricular medicine through the work of GLEM.

Rhyne, Wilhelm Ten: Dutch physician who worked for the Dutch East India Company in the 1600s and translated Chinese medical texts for the education of European doctors.

Sciatica: A pain problem experienced in the lower back and lower leg that is associated with irritation of the sciatic nerve. Stimulation of points on the ear to treat sciatica pain has been used by physicians in ancient Egypt and in ancient Persia as well as in modern France.

Smith, Michael: New York physician who served as one of the founding fathers of the NADA acupuncture drug detoxification program at Lincoln Hospital in New York City.

Soulié de Morant, Georges: French physician who translated the *Nei Jing* into French in the early 1900s, which served to revitalize the knowledge of acupuncture in Europe.

Vascular Autonomic Signal (VAS): First called the *réflexe auriculo cardiaque* (RAC), in 1981, Paul Nogier developed this form of pulse diagnosis by placing the thumb over the radial artery felt to monitor a diagnostic response to stimulation of the auricle.

■ CHAPTER 1 REVIEW QUESTIONS

1. The term *auricle* refers to_____.
   a. the hearing sensors of the inner ear
   b. the resonating bones of the middle ear
   c. the sensory nerves that connect to the external ear
   d. the anatomical structure of the external ear

2. According to ancient Chinese texts, ear acupuncture points are described as_____.
   a. Qi Balance points
   b. Yang Alarm points
   c. Kidney Yin points
   d. Heart Qi points

3. The earliest reports of the Chinese practice of inserting acupuncture needles into the skin were introduced to European doctors by representatives of the_____.
   a. Dutch East India Company
   b. British East India Company

   c. German Society of Acupuncture
   d. French Society of Acupuncture

4. Dr. Paul Nogier developed the perspective that the auricle seems to correspond to an inverted fetus after he had_____.
   a. trained with Dr. Georges Soulié de Morant, Father of French Acupuncture
   b. studied acupuncture practices in China under Mao Tse Tung
   c. observed scars on the external ear of patients previously treated for sciatica pain
   d. learned of the discoveries of the Nanjing Ear Acupuncture Research Team

5. The Hong Kong physician H. L. Wen was the first modern doctor to demonstrate that ear acupuncture could be effectively used to alleviate_____.
   a. sciatica pain
   b. opiate addiction
   c. eyesight disorders
   d. headaches

6. Nogier's *Treatise of Auriculotherapy* focused on the stimulation of ear reflex points for the treatment of_____.
   a. neurological disorders
   b. addiction disorders
   c. visceral disorders
   d. musculoskeletal disorders

7. Ear acupuncture points show the greatest degree of reactivity to pathologies in the body areas that are located on the_____.

   a. ipsilateral side of the body
   b. contralateral side of the body
   c. inverse side of the body
   d. distal side of the body

8. Reactive points on the ear exhibit a decrease in_____ relative to other areas of the auricle.
   a. electrodermal skin resistance
   b. electrodermal skin conductance
   c. skin temperature
   d. peripheral vasoconstriction

9. A basic distinction that differentiates ear acupuncture from body acupuncture is that the ear acupoints have a_____.
   a. slower response to improvement following treatment
   b. more limited effectiveness following treatment
   c. somatotopic arrangement of acupoints
   d. greater number of side effects

10. One acupuncture procedure that is more frequently used with auriculotherapy than with body acupuncture is the_____.
   a. insertion of acupuncture needles through a guide tube
   b. placement of small pellets on acupoints
   c. electrical stimulation of acupoints through inserted needles
   d. treatment of acupoints by tactile massage

Answers

1 = d; 2 = b; 3 = a; 4 = c; 5 = b; 6 = d; 7 = a; 8 = a; 9 = c; 10 = b

Theoretical Perspectives of Auriculotherapy

2

CONTENTS

[2.0 | Theoretical Perspectives of Auriculotherapy

CHAPTER 2 LEARNING OBJECTIVES

1. To delineate multiple microsystems found on the feet, hands, scalp, and body.

2. To demonstrate awareness of the principal characteristics of microsystems.

3. To describe the theoretical model of the hologram as related to microsystems.

4. To highlight the primary features of Traditional Chinese Medicine utilized in auricular acupuncture.

5. To demonstrate knowledge of neuro-physiological findings related to auriculotherapy.

6. To show the changes in neurochemicals and hormones associated with auriculotherapy.

Although the underlying mechanisms that might explain auricular acupuncture are not fully known, several different theories have been developed that provide a framework and structure to understand the clinical results achieved with this treatment. From a conventional physiological perspective, auriculotherapy may seem illogical. How could treatment of the external ear effectively alleviate pathology in remote parts of the body far from the ear? Even classically trained acupuncturists who have accepted the most esoteric aspects of Traditional Chinese Medicine (TCM) sometimes state that the external ear seems too small and insignificant to accomplish the healing results that can be achieved with body acupuncture. Although it is self-evident that the external ear is an organ for hearing, it is not at all obvious that the ear could relate to any other health condition, such as back pain or addiction. Even when provided repeated clinical examples of patients who have benefitted from auricular acupuncture, most individuals remain skeptical of what they have directly observed. Auriculotherapy may sometimes seem more like magic than medicine. The theories that are presented in this chapter are varied, but they are not mutually exclusive. It may be that the combination of all of these theories can comprehensively account for the clinical observations that follow auriculotherapy treatments. There may develop a previously unknown theoretical model that better accounts for the currently available data, but the viewpoints described here provide a fundamental basis for explaining the clinical benefits seen with auriculotherapy stimulation.

2.1 Micro-Acupuncture Systems

The first theory to be considered is the concept that auricular acupuncture is one of several microsystems throughout the human body, a self-contained system within the whole system. In Oriental philosophy, there is a systematic correspondence of each part to the whole. The microcosm of each person is inter-related to the macrocosm of the world that surrounds them. Even in the West, medieval European philosophers described the relationship between organs of the microcosm of man to the planetary constellations in the macrocosm of the heavens. Modern Western medicine accepts that the micro-organism of each cell within the body is inter-related to the macro-organism of the whole body. Just as each cell has a protective membrane, flowing fluids, and a regulating center, so too does the whole body. For the whole organism to be in balance, each system within that organism must be in balance.

Micro-Acupuncture Systems Versus Macro-Acupuncture Systems: Dr. Ralph Alan Dale (1976, 1985, 1999) of Miami, Florida, was one of the first investigators to suggest that not only the ear but also every part of the gross anatomy can function as a complete system for diagnosis and therapy. Dale spent several decades accumulating clinical evidence from China, Japan, Europe, and America about these multiple microsystems. The term *micro-acupuncture* was introduced by Dale at the 1974 Third World Symposium on Acupuncture and Chinese Medicine. Micro-acupuncture is the expression of the entire body's vital qi energy in each major anatomical region. He labeled them micro-acupuncture systems to distinguish them from the traditional macro-acupuncture systems that connect the acupoints distributed throughout the body. Every micro-acupuncture system contains a distribution of acupoints that replicate the anatomy of the whole organism. Micro-acupuncture systems have been identified by Dale on the ear, foot, hand, scalp, face, nose, iris, teeth, tongue, wrist, abdomen, back, and on every long bone of the body. Each region is a functional microcosm of the traditional energetics of the whole body. Every part of the body exhibits an energetic microcosm through micro-acupoints and micro-channels that reiterate the topology of the body. The accompanying figures depict different microsystems that have been identified on the scalp, the ear, the hand, the metacarpal, and the foot. Dale has identified specific principles regarding these micro-acupuncture systems.

Remote Reflex Response: Every microsystem manifests neurological reflexes that are connected with parts of the body remote from the anatomical location of that microsystem. These reflexes are both diagnostic and therapeutic. When pressure is applied to a reactive microsystem point, a pronounced facial grimace or a behavioral withdrawal reflex is evoked. The locations of these distant tender spots are not due to random chance but, rather, are directly related to a neurological reflex pattern that is centrally mediated.

Somatotopic Reiteration: The microsystem reflex map of the body repeats the anatomical arrangement of the whole body. The term *soma* refers to the word body, and *topography* refers to the mapping of the terrain of an area. Microsystems are similar to the somatotopic responses in the brain, where a picture of a *homunculus*, a "little man," can be identified by brain mapping studies. It is not the actual bone or muscle that is represented on the brain. Rather, it is the movement activity of that area of the body that is monitored by the brain. Such is also the case with microsystem points, which indicate the pathological functioning of an organ, not the anatomical structure of that organ.

Somatotopic Inversion: In some microsystems, the reflex topology directly corresponds to the upright position of the body, whereas in most microsystem maps, the body is configured in an inverse pattern. In the auriculotherapy microsystem, the reflex pattern resembles the inverted fetus in the womb. With the hands pointed downward and the toes stretched out, the hand and foot reflexology systems are also inverted. The scalp microsystem is also represented upside

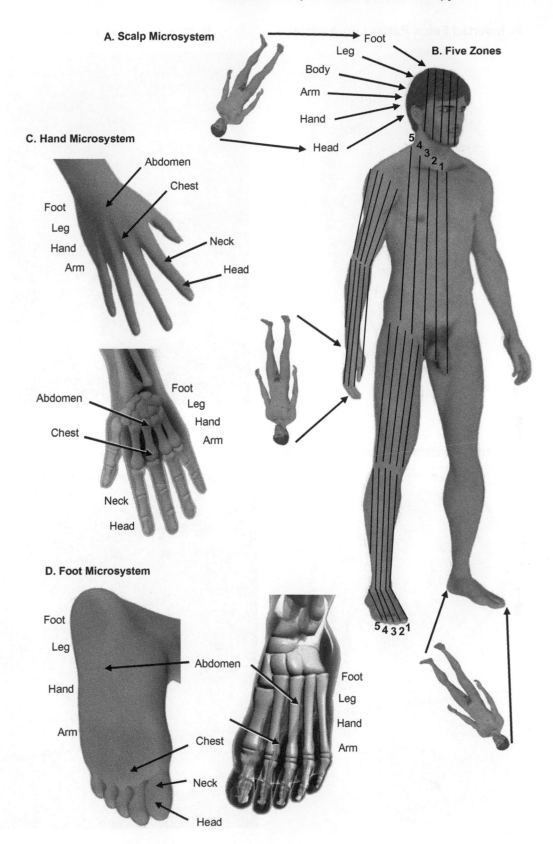

A. Scalp Microsystem

Foot
Leg
B. Five Zones
Body
Arm
Hand
Head

5 4 3 2 1

C. Hand Microsystem

Abdomen
Chest
Foot
Leg
Hand
Arm
Neck
Head

Abdomen
Foot
Leg
Hand
Arm
Chest
Neck
Head

D. Foot Microsystem

Foot
Leg
Hand
Arm
Abdomen
Chest
Neck
Head

Foot
Leg
Hand
Arm
Abdomen
Chest
Neck
Head

5 4 3 2 1

FIGURE 2.1 Microsystems of the whole body that are found in one region of the body have been reported for the scalp, the hand, and the foot. In zone therapy, the vertical length of the body is divided into five continuous zones, with zone 1 running along the midline of the head and body, as well as along the first digit of the hand and the foot, spreading laterally to zones 2, 3, 4, and 5, on the most peripheral regions of the head and body and on the little finger and little toe.

A. Inverted Fetus Pattern on Auricle

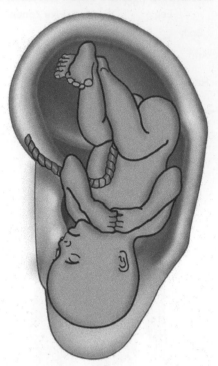

B. Inverted Fetus in Uterus

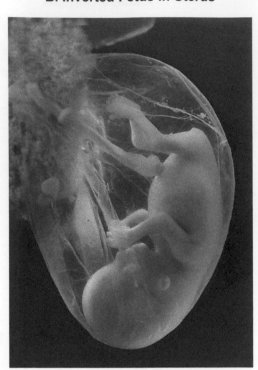

C. Inverted Somatotopic Body on Auricle

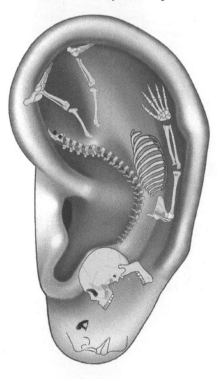

D. Inverted Somatotopic Body Orientation

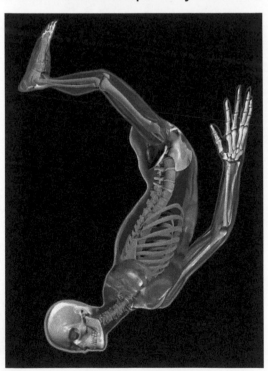

⌈FIGURE 2.2 The original perspective of the somatotopic representation of the body on the external ear (A) was that it was similar in its pattern to that of an inverted fetus within the uterus (B). A more accurate representation of the somatotopic projection of the body onto the auricle (C) is that the spine would be curved in a convex orientation that might only be obtained if one were a gymnast or yogi that tried to touch the bottom of his feet toward the top of his head by bending backwards (D).

down, whereas the more medial microsystems of the abdomen, back, face, nose, and lips are all oriented in an upright pattern. The tongue and teeth microsystems are presented horizontally. The inverted somatotopic pattern is revealed not only in the cerebral cortex of the higher brain but also in the somatosensory thalamus, which sends neural projections to the cortex, and in the brainstem, which sends neural projections from the spinal cord to the thalamus.

Ipsilateral Representation: Microsystems tend to have bilateral effects, but they usually are more reactive when the micro-acupoint and the area of body pathology are ipsilateral to each other, on the same side of the body. Only the scalp microsystem, which corresponds to the underlying somatosensory cerebral cortex, exhibits reactive acupoints on the side of the scalp that is contralateral to the side of body pathology. For the scalp microsystem, the areas on the head are associated with brain functions that are found for the underlying cerebral cortex, which is contralateral to the side of the body controlled by that area of the brain. For the auricular microsystem, a condition on the right side of the body would be represented on the right ear, whereas a problem on the left side of the body would be reflected on the left ear. Actually, each region of the body bilaterally projects to both the right and the left ear. Auricular representation is simply stronger on the ipsilateral ear than the contralateral ear.

Bidirectional Connections: Pathology in a specific organ or part of the body is indicated by distinct changes in the skin at the corresponding microsystem point, whereas stimulating that point can produce changes in the corresponding part of the body.

Organo-Cutaneous Reflexes: In this type of reflex, pathology in an organ of the body produces an alteration in the cutaneous region where that correspondent organ is represented. Localized skin reactions may include changes in skin color, skin roughness, and skin texture. Other alterations include increased tenderness upon palpitation, altered blood flow, elevated temperature, and fluctuations in electrodermal activity. These skin reactions are diagnostically useful for all the microsystems, although the tongue, iris, and pulse microsystems are utilized almost exclusively for diagnosis, not treatment.

Cutaneo-Organic Reflexes: Stimulating the skin at a microsystem acupoint can produce internal, homeostatic changes that lead to the relief of pain and the healing of the corresponding organ. This cutaneous stimulation triggers nervous system messages to the spinal cord and brain, activating physiological changes, biochemical releases, and alterations of the electrical firing in neuronal reflexes.

Interactions with Macrosystems: All of the micro-acupuncture systems interact with the macro-acupuncture systems. Treatment by one system will produce changes in the body's functional patterns as diagnosed by the other systems. Treatment of the overall macrosystem affects the functioning of the microsystems. Conversely, treatment of any of the microsystems affects the functioning of the macrosystem and of the other microsystems. For instance, stimulating an ear reflex point can reduce the intensity of discomfort in a trigger point on the associated acupuncture channel, whereas an electrically reactive point on the ear will become less conductive if the patient positively responds to treatment.

Mu Alarm Points and Shu Transport Points: The first micro-acupuncture systems originated in ancient China, but they were not intentionally developed as such. The *front mu* and the *back shu* channels are diagnostic and therapeutic systems (Dale, 1985). Each of the 12 acupoints on these channels resonates with one of 12 principal organs, including the lung, heart, liver, spleen, stomach, intestines, bladder, and kidney. The front mu points and back shu points are actually surface projections on to the external skin from the visceral organs that are found deeper in the body. These ancient systems may be seen as organ-energy correspondences; acupoint loci on the body surface are able to indicate pathology in the underlying anatomical structures. The mu and shu points for the heart are respectively represented on the

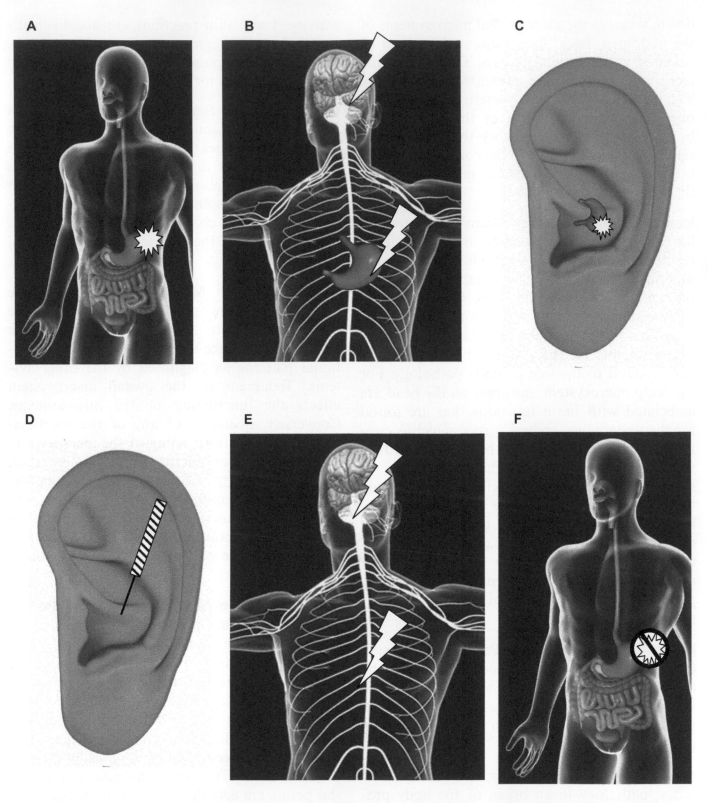

⌈FIGURE 2.3 An organo-cutaneo reflex occurs when there is some pathology in a body organ, such as within the stomach (A) which sends neurological messages to the central nervous system (CNS) spinal cord and brain (B) which then sends neurological messages to the skin surface over the peripheral microsystem point that represents the stomach on the external ear (C). A cutaneo-organo reflex occurs when the skin over a microsystem point representing an organ, such as the stomach (D) is stimulated with a needle or some other device, which then activates neurological messages to the CNS spinal cord and brain (E) which then sends neurological messages to a disturbed organ such as the stomach in order to alleviate any pain or pathology in that organ (F).

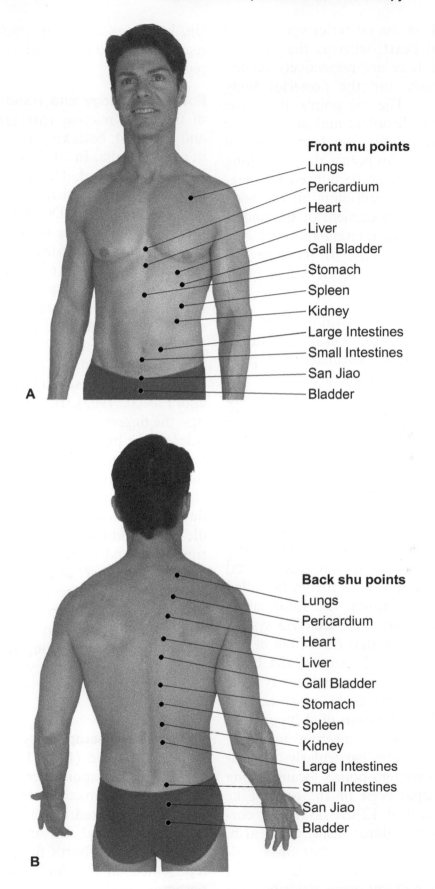

Front mu points
- Lungs
- Pericardium
- Heart
- Liver
- Gall Bladder
- Stomach
- Spleen
- Kidney
- Large Intestines
- Small Intestines
- San Jiao
- Bladder

A

Back shu points
- Lungs
- Pericardium
- Heart
- Liver
- Gall Bladder
- Stomach
- Spleen
- Kidney
- Large Intestines
- Small Intestines
- San Jiao
- Bladder

B

FIGURE 2.4 This photograph shows the classical location of the mu points (A) located underneath specific points on the anterior skin surface of the torso and the shu points (B) located underneath the skin surface on the posterior regions of the back of the body.

anterior chest and on the posterior spine at the level of the actual heart, whereas the mu and shu points for the liver are respectively related to the anterior body and the posterior body near the actual liver. The mu points alarm the body about internal disorders and are sensitive to pain when there is acute or chronic visceral distress. Although the shu points that run along the posterior spine can also be utilized for diagnostic discoveries, these acupoints on the back are more often used for treatment of the underlying organ disorder. Stimulating the back shu points by needles, electricity, or massage can enhance the flow of qi energy to the deeper, internal organs.

Embryo Containing the Information of the Whole Organism: In 1913, Kurakishi Hirata, a Japanese psychologist, postulated the presence of seven micro-acupuncture zones: the head, face, neck, abdomen, back, arms, and legs. Each of the seven zones manifested 12 horizontal subzones of organ-energy function: trachea-bronchi, lungs, heart, liver, gall bladder, spleen-pancreas, stomach, kidney, large intestine, small intestine, urinary bladder, and genitals. The Hirata zones were utilized both for diagnosis and for treatment. Beginning in 1973, Ying-Qing Zhang and colleagues (1992, 1997), from Shandong University in China, published several books and articles proposing a theory he called ECIWO (Embryo Containing the Information of the Whole Organism). This ECIWO system is a microsystem concept that the whole of the body is represented in each part of the body. Zhang delineated micro-acupuncture systems for every long bone of the body, which he presented at the World Federation of Acupuncture Societies and Associations meeting in Paris, France, in 1990. Zhang particularly emphasized a set of microsystem points located along the second metacarpal bone of the hand. Like Hirata, Zhang identified 12 divisions that correspond to 12 body regions: head, neck, arm, lungs and heart, liver, stomach, intestines, kidney, upper abdomen, lower abdomen, leg, and foot. Somatotopic patterns were described for all the primary bones of the body, including the head, spine, upper arm, lower arm, hand, upper leg, lower leg, and foot. Each of these skeletal regions was said to contain the 12 different body regions.

Foot Reflexology and Hand Reflexology: Two of the oldest microsystems are those of the foot and the hand, both known in ancient China and in ancient India. In 1917, William H. Fitzgerald, MD, of Hartford, Connecticut, independently rediscovered the microsystem of the foot as well as the hand. Dr. Fitzgerald referred to these systems as *zone therapy*. The topology of Fitzgerald's microsystem points was derived from the projections of five distinct zones that extended bilaterally up the entire length of the body. Each zone originates from one of the five digits of each hand and each foot. Several other Americans, including White, Bowers, Riley, and Stopfel, developed this procedure as *reflexology*, by which name it is widely known today (Oleson and Flocco, 1993). In hand and foot reflexology, the fingers and toes correspond to the head, whereas the base of the hand and the heel of the foot represent the lower part of the body. The thumb and large toe initiate zone 1 that runs along the midline of the body, whereas the index finger and second toe represent zone 2, the middle finger and third toe are found in zone 3, the ring finger and fourth toe are located in zone 4, and the little finger and little toe demark zone 5. This last zone connects all peripheral regions of the body, including the leg, arm, and ear. The midline of the back is in zone 1, whereas the hips and shoulders occur along zone 5. On the head, the nose is in zone 1, the eyes are in zones 2 and 3, and the ears are in zone 5 of the foot reflexology microsystem.

Koryo Hand Therapy: The Korean acupuncturist Tae Woo Yoo (1993) has described a different set of correspondence points for the hand. In this Korean microsystem, the midline of the body is represented along the middle finger and middle metacarpal, the arms are represented on the second and fourth fingers, and the legs are represented on the thumb and little finger. The posterior head, neck, and back are found on the dorsum of the hand, and the anterior face, throat, chest, and abdomen are represented on

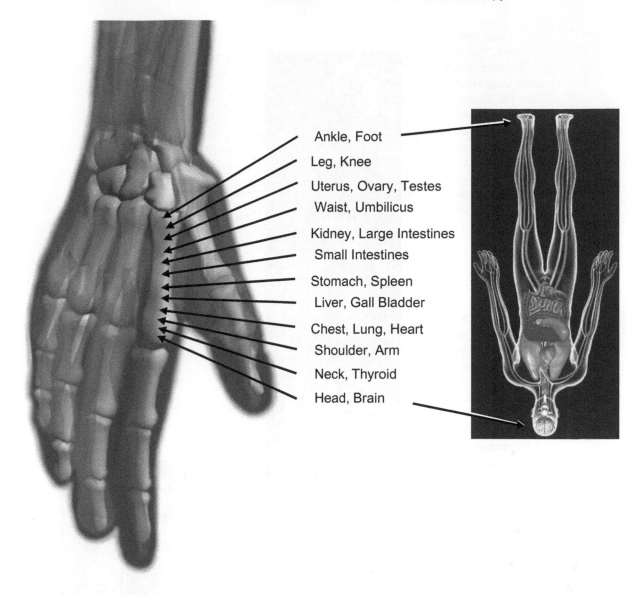

Ankle, Foot
Leg, Knee
Uterus, Ovary, Testes
Waist, Umbilicus
Kidney, Large Intestines
Small Intestines
Stomach, Spleen
Liver, Gall Bladder
Chest, Lung, Heart
Shoulder, Arm
Neck, Thyroid
Head, Brain

[FIGURE 2.5 Chinese doctor Ying-Qing Zhang proposed a microsystem referred to as the ECIWO (Embryo Containing Information of the Whole Organism) that was located on the second metacarpal bone of the hand.

the palmar side. Beyond correspondences to the actual body, Koryo hand therapy also presents points for stimulating each of the meridian acupuncture points that run over the actual body. The macro-acupuncture points of each channel are represented on the micro-acupuncture correspondent regions found on the hand. Acupuncturists insert thin, short needles just beneath the skin surface of these hand points, usually using a special metal device that holds the small needles. That this Korean somatotopic pattern on the hand is so different from the American hand reflexology pattern seems paradoxical, particularly because practitioners of both

systems claim very high rates of clinical success. Because there are also differences in the Chinese and European locations for auricular points, a broader view is that the somatotopic pathways may have multiple microsystem representations. As with auriculotherapy, many practitioners of Koryo hand therapy use this system as their sole method of treatment, whereas other practitioners integrate Koryo therapy with body acupuncture and auricular acupuncture.

Face and Nose Microsystems: Chinese practitioners have identified microsystems on the face and the nose that are oriented in an upright

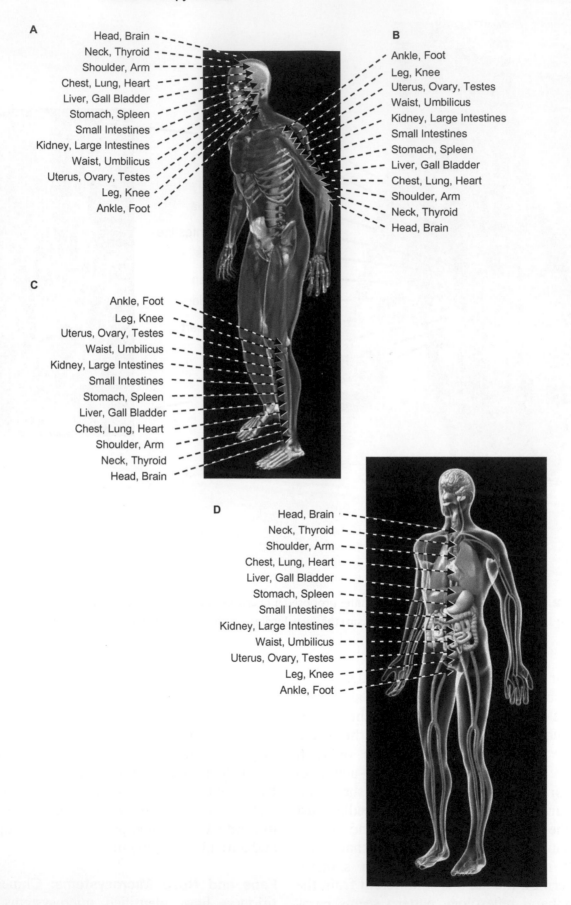

A
Head, Brain
Neck, Thyroid
Shoulder, Arm
Chest, Lung, Heart
Liver, Gall Bladder
Stomach, Spleen
Small Intestines
Kidney, Large Intestines
Waist, Umbilicus
Uterus, Ovary, Testes
Leg, Knee
Ankle, Foot

B
Ankle, Foot
Leg, Knee
Uterus, Ovary, Testes
Waist, Umbilicus
Kidney, Large Intestines
Small Intestines
Stomach, Spleen
Liver, Gall Bladder
Chest, Lung, Heart
Shoulder, Arm
Neck, Thyroid
Head, Brain

C
Ankle, Foot
Leg, Knee
Uterus, Ovary, Testes
Waist, Umbilicus
Kidney, Large Intestines
Small Intestines
Stomach, Spleen
Liver, Gall Bladder
Chest, Lung, Heart
Shoulder, Arm
Neck, Thyroid
Head, Brain

D
Head, Brain
Neck, Thyroid
Shoulder, Arm
Chest, Lung, Heart
Liver, Gall Bladder
Stomach, Spleen
Small Intestines
Kidney, Large Intestines
Waist, Umbilicus
Uterus, Ovary, Testes
Leg, Knee
Ankle, Foot

FIGURE 2.6 Dr. Zhang extended his ECIWO bioholographic theory to every long bone of the body, with a specific orientation of 12 regions of the body found along each major long bone.

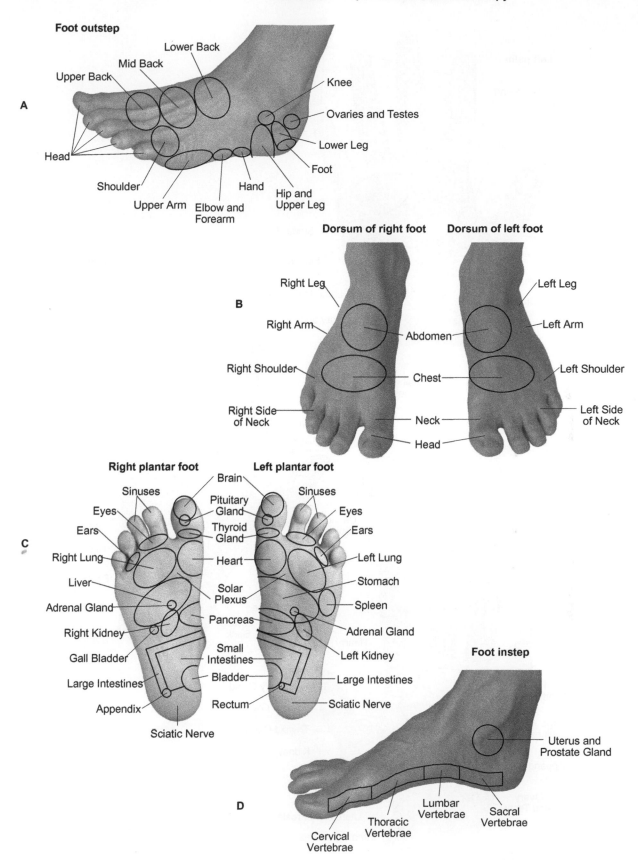

FIGURE 2.7 This photograph shows the location of different regions of the body represented on specific areas of the foot according to the American foot reflexology microsystem. Notice that the Head is found on the tips of the toes, next the Chest, then the Abdomen, and then the Leg and Foot toward the heel. Internal organs are found more on the bottom of the foot than on the top, oriented with the Lung and Heart toward the base of the toes and the Intestines and Bladder toward the heel.

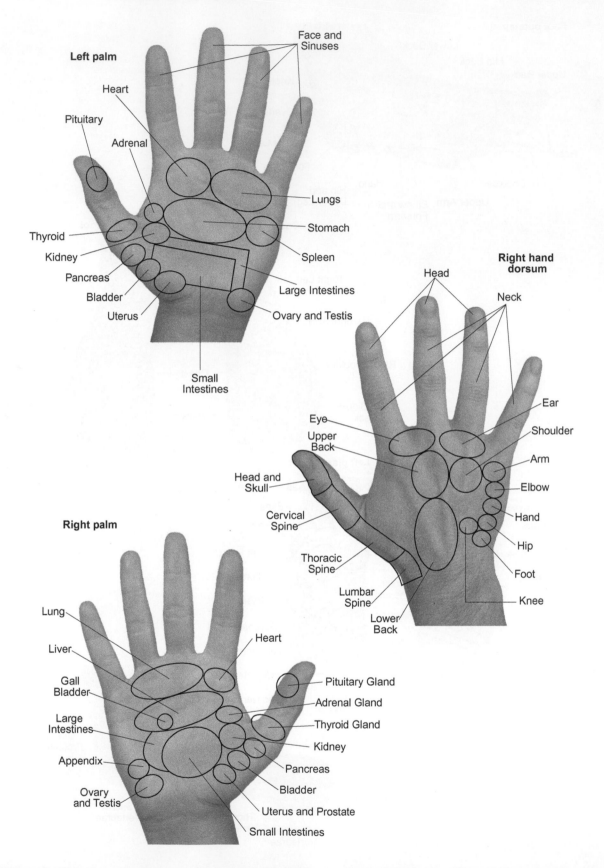

FIGURE 2.8 This photograph shows the location of different regions of the body represented on specific areas of the hand according to the American hand reflexology microsystem. Notice that the Head is found on the tips of the fingers, next the Upper Back, then the Lower Back, and then the Leg and Foot toward the wrist. Internal organs are found more on the palmer side of the hand than on the dorsum, oriented with the Lungs and Heart toward the base of the fingers and the Intestines, Bladder, and Uterus toward the wrist.

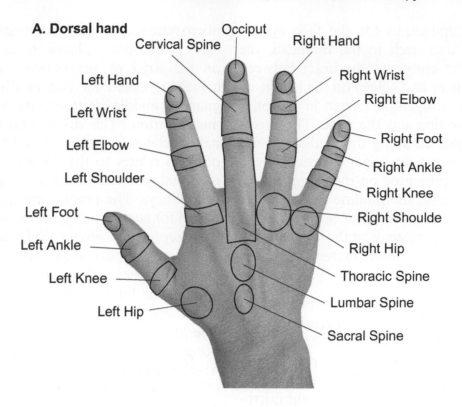

A. Dorsal hand

Occiput
Cervical Spine
Right Hand
Left Hand
Right Wrist
Right Elbow
Left Wrist
Left Elbow
Right Foot
Left Shoulder
Right Ankle
Right Knee
Left Foot
Right Shoulde
Left Ankle
Right Hip
Left Knee
Thoracic Spine
Lumbar Spine
Left Hip
Sacral Spine

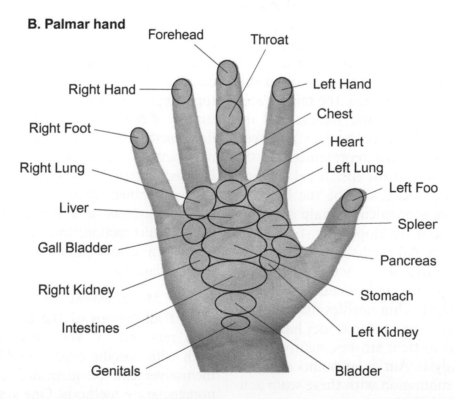

B. Palmar hand

Forehead
Throat
Right Hand
Left Hand
Chest
Right Foot
Heart
Right Lung
Left Lung
Left Foo
Liver
Spleer
Gall Bladder
Pancreas
Right Kidney
Stomach
Intestines
Left Kidney
Genitals
Bladder

FIGURE 2.9 This photograph shows the location of different regions of the body represented on specific areas of the hand according to the Korean hand microsystem. Unlike the American hand reflexology system, both the right side and the left side of the body are represented on each hand. The middle finger and third digit represent the Head and Spinal Vertebrae, the second and fourth digits represent the Arms, and the thumb and little finger represent the Legs. Like the American microsystem, the Head is found toward the tips of the fingers, the Upper Back on the base of the fingers, and the Lumbosacral Vertebrae toward the wrist. Internal organs are found more on the palmer side of the hand than on the dorsum, similarly oriented with the Lungs and Heart toward the base of the fingers and the Intestines, Bladder, and Genitals toward the wrist.

position. The homunculus for the face system places the head and neck in the forehead, the lungs between the eyebrows, the heart between the eyeballs, the liver and spleen on the bridge of the nose, and the urogenital system in the philtrum between the lips and the nose. The digestive organs are located along the medial cheeks, the upper limbs across the upper cheeks, and the lower limbs are represented on the lower jaw. In the nose microsystem, the midline points are at approximately the same location as in the face system, the digestive system is at the wings of the nose, and the upper and lower extremities are in the crease alongside the nose.

Scalp Microsystem: Scalp acupuncture was also known in ancient China, and several modern systems have subsequently evolved. Scalp microacupuncture has been shown to be particularly effective in treating strokes and cerebrovascular conditions. Although there are two scalp microsystems indicated by Dale, the principal system divides the temporal section of the scalp into three parts. A diagonal line is extended laterally from the top of the head to the area of the temples above the ear. The lowest portion of this temporal line relates to the head; the middle area relates to the body, arms, and hands; and the uppermost region represents the legs and feet. This inverted body pattern represented on the scalp activates reflexes in the ipsilateral cerebral cortex to the contralateral side of the body. In recent years, a more sophisticated scalp acupuncture system has been developed by Toshikatsu Yamamoto of Japan. An English language translation of Yamamoto's scalp acupuncture system has been eloquently articulated in a text by Richard Feely (2010). Thin needles inserted into the scalp at specific somatotopic loci have been effectively utilized to treat strokes, neuropathies, aphasia, and paralysis. Auricular points are commonly used in combination with these scalp acupoints for neurological disorders.

Tongue and Pulse Microsystems: Visual observation of the tongue and tactile palpation at the radial artery of the wrist are two of the most commonly used TCM diagnostic systems. Although not initially intended as such, the tongue and pulse can also be viewed as microsystems. For pulse diagnosis, the acupuncture practitioner places three middle fingers on the wrist of the patient. The three placements are called the cun or distal position, the guan or middle position, and the chi or proximal position. The distal position (nearest the hand) relates to the heart and lungs, the middle position relates to the digestive organs, and the proximal position (toward the elbow) relates to the kidneys. The practitioner palpates the pulse to feel for such subtle qualities as superficial versus deep, rapid versus slow, full versus empty, and strong versus weak. In the tongue microsystem, the heart is found at the very tip of the tongue, the lung in the front, the spleen at the center, and the kidney at the back of the tongue. The liver is located on the sides of the tongue. Tongue qualities include observations as to whether its coating is thick versus thin, the color of the coating is white or yellow, and whether the color of the tongue body is pale, red, or purple.

Abdominal Microsystem: Whereas Zhang (1992) focused on the microsystem representations that he identified on the long bones of the body, classical Chinese acupuncturists have identified somatotopic representation of internal organs over the surface of the abdominal muscles. Like other midline microsystems, the organization of abdominal points is oriented in an upright rather than an inverted pattern. The tender points that are detected on the abdomen are more often associated with the energetic aspects of a particular organ than their anatomical function; thus, this system is typically utilized in combination with Chinese pulse and tongue diagnosis.

Dental Microsystem: A complete representation of all regions of the body on the teeth has been reported by Voll, who associated specific teeth with specific organs (Table 2.1). The teeth themselves can be identified by one of several nomenclature methods. One system involves first dividing the teeth into four equal quadrants: right upper jaw, left upper jaw, right lower jaw, and left lower jaw. The individual teeth are then numbered from "1" to "8," beginning with the midline, front incisors at "1," then progressing laterally to the bicuspids, and continuing more posterior toward the molars at "7" or "8." Individuals who have

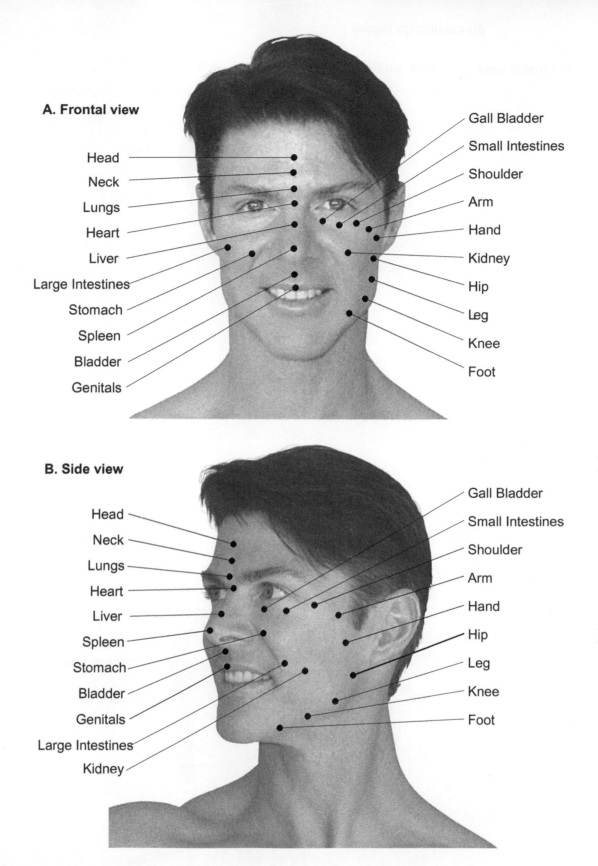

A. Frontal view

Head
Neck
Lungs
Heart
Liver
Large Intestines
Stomach
Spleen
Bladder
Genitals

Gall Bladder
Small Intestines
Shoulder
Arm
Hand
Kidney
Hip
Leg
Knee
Foot

B. Side view

Head
Neck
Lungs
Heart
Liver
Spleen
Stomach
Bladder
Genitals
Large Intestines
Kidney

Gall Bladder
Small Intestines
Shoulder
Arm
Hand
Hip
Leg
Knee
Foot

⟦**FIGURE 2.10** This photograph shows the location of different regions of the body represented on specific areas of the face according to the face and nose microsystems. The midline of the body is shown with the head at the midline of the forehead, below which is found the Neck, and then the Heart and Lungs located on the top ridge of the nose, and next the Liver and Spleen located closer to the lower tip of the nose. As contrasted with the nose microsystem, the face microsystem spreads laterally outward upon the cheeks and jaw of the face, and it includes the Stomach, the Intestines, the Arms, and the Legs in an upright orientation.

A. Frontal view

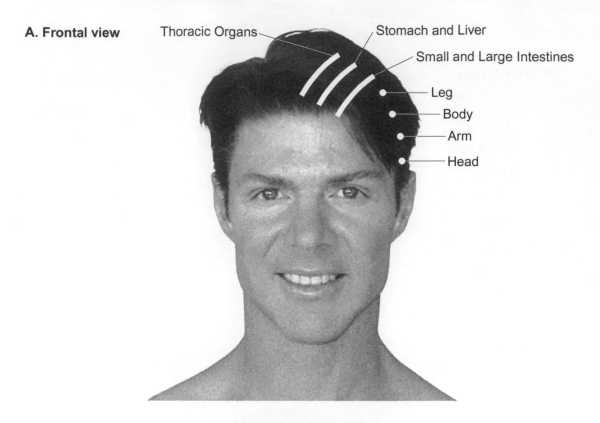

Thoracic Organs

Stomach and Liver

Small and Large Intestines

Leg

Body

Arm

Head

B. Side view

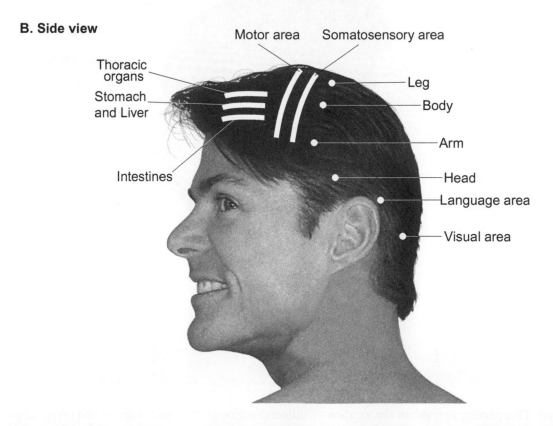

Motor area   Somatosensory area

Thoracic organs

Stomach and Liver

Intestines

Leg

Body

Arm

Head

Language area

Visual area

FIGURE 2.11 This photograph shows the location of different regions of the body represented on specific areas of the frontal and lateral view of the head scalp acupuncture microsystem. Although there are several scalp acupuncture systems, in one representation, the head is located peripherally on the temporal skull, just above the external ear. Proceeding toward the more medial and dorsal regions of the skull, there is shown the Arm, the Body, the Leg, and the Foot, just as they are somatotopically represented on the somatic cerebral cortex beneath the skull.

A . Tongue Microsystem

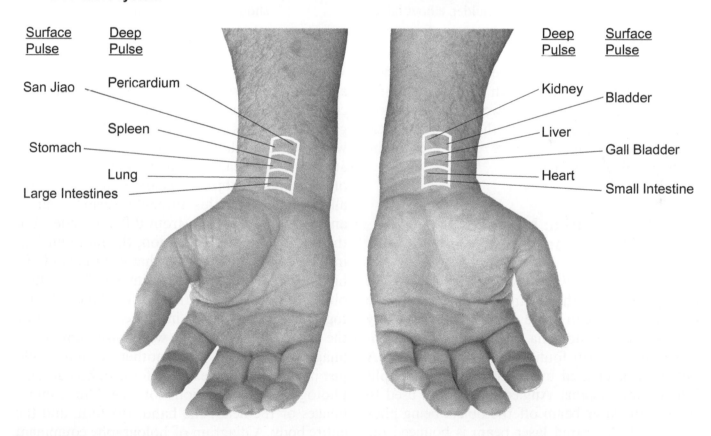

B. Pulse Microsystem

FIGURE 2.12 This photograph shows the location of different regions of the body represented on specific areas of the tongue microsystem and the pulse microsystem. Because these two microsystems are mostly utilized in Chinese medical diagnosis, primary emphasis is placed on the Heart and Lung located on the tip of the tongue and the area of the radial artery closest to the wrist joint. With the Stomach, Liver, and Gall Bladder represented in the middle of the tongue and the radial artery, the Kidney and Bladder are more strongly represented at the back of the tongue and on the more proximal side of the radial artery.

TABLE 2.1	Dental Microsystem Correspondence between Teeth and Body Regions.	
Tooth Position	**Right Upper Jaw and Lower Jaw Quadrants**	**Left Upper Jaw and Lower Jaw Quadrants**
1. Center incisor	Right kidney, bladder, genitals, lumbar vertebrae, knee, ankle, sinus, ear	Left kidney, bladder, genitals, lumbar vertebrae, knee, ankle, sinus, ear
2. Lateral incisor	Right kidney, bladder, genitals, lumbar vertebrae, knee, ankle, sinus, ear	Left kidney, bladder, genitals, lumbar vertebrae, knee, ankle, sinus, ear
3. Canine	Liver, gall bladder, thoracic vertebrae, right hip, right eye	Liver, spleen, thoracic vertebrae, left hip, left eye
4. First bicuspid	Right lung, large intestines, thoracic vertebrae, right foot	Left lung, large intestines, thoracic vertebrae, left foot
5. Second bicuspid	Right lung, large intestines, thoracic vertebrae, right foot	Left lung, large intestines, thoracic vertebrae, left foot
6. First molar	Pancreas, stomach, right jaw, right shoulder, elbow, hand	Spleen, stomach, left jaw, left shoulder, elbow, hand
7. Second molar	Pancreas, stomach, right jaw, right shoulder, elbow, hand	Spleen, stomach, left jaw, left shoulder, elbow, hand
8. Wisdom tooth	Heart, small intestines, inner ear, brainstem, limbic brain, cerebrum, right shoulder, elbow, hand	Heart, small intestines, inner ear, brainstem, limbic brain, cerebrum, left shoulder, elbow, hand

had their wisdom teeth removed on a side of their jaw will only have seven teeth in that quadrant. Urogenital organs and the lower limbs are represented on the more central teeth, and the thoracic organs and the upper limbs are represented on the more peripheral molars.

2.2 Holographic Model of Microsystems

In *The Holographic Universe*, Michael Talbot (1991) described the technological basis of the hologram that can serve as a model for many unexplained phenomena, including the somatotopic microsystem found on the external ear. A hologram is created by a laser light that is split into separate beams. Angled mirrors are used to bounce the laser beam off the object being photographed. A second laser beam is bounced off the reflected light of the first laser beam. The collision of these reflected laser beams generates an interference pattern on the holographic film negative. This interference pattern is the area where the two laser beams interact on the film.

When the film is developed, it initially looks like a meaningless swirl of light and dark images, composed of wavy lines, concentric circles, and geometric shapes similar to snowflakes. However, when the developed film is illuminated by another laser beam, a three-dimensional image of the original object appears. One could actually walk around this three-dimensional image and view the hologram from different sides. For the purpose of this discussion, the more intriguing aspect of holograms is that each part of the holographic film contains an image of the whole object that was photographed. In standard photography of a man, for instance, one section of the photographic negative would just contain the image of the head and another section would just include the image of the foot. In holographic photography, all sections of the film contain images of the head, the hand, the foot, and the entire body. A diagram of holography equipment and the portrayal of such holographic images are presented in the accompanying figures.

The respected Stanford University neurobiologist Karl Pribram (1993) utilized the model of the hologram to explain research experiments demonstrating that memory can be stored in many parts of the brain. Pribram suggested that individual neurons in different parts of the brain have an image of what the whole brain can remember. According to this model, memories are encoded not in neurons, or even in small groupings of neurons, but in patterns of nerve impulses that crisscross the entire brain. This brain map is similar to the way that interference patterns of laser light crisscross the entire area of a piece of holographic film. The holographic theory also explains how the human brain can store so many memories in so little space. It has been estimated that the human brain has the capacity to memorize on the order of 10 billion bits of information during the average human lifetime. Holograms also possess an astounding capacity for information storage. Simply by changing the angle at which the two lasers strike a piece of photographic film, it is possible to record many different images on the same surface. It has been demonstrated that one cubic centimeter of holographic film can hold as many as 10 billion bits of information. One of the most amazing aspects about the human thinking process is that every piece of information seems instantly cross-correlated with every other piece of information, another feature intrinsic to the hologram. Just as a hologram functions as a translating device that is able to convert an apparently meaningless blur of frequencies into a coherent image, Pribram postulates that the brain also utilizes holographic principles to mathematically convert the neurophysiological information it receives from the senses to the inner world of perceptions and thoughts.

The British physicist David Bohm (1980) hypothesized that the energy forces that regulate subatomic particles could also be accounted for by the holographic model. In 1982, a research team led by physicist Alain Aspect, at the University of Paris, discovered that one of two twin photons traveling in opposite directions was able to correlate the angle of its polarization with that of its twin. The two photons seemed to be non-locally connected. The paired particles were able to instantaneously interact with

each other, regardless of the distance separating them. It did not seem to matter whether the photons were 1 millimeter away or 13 meters apart. Somehow, each particle always seemed to know what the other was doing. Bohm suggested that the reason subatomic particles can remain in contact with one another is not because they are sending some sort of mysterious signal back and forth. Rather, he argued that such particles are not individual entities to begin with, but are actually extensions of the same, subatomic substance. The electrons in one atom are connected to the subatomic particles that comprise every other atom. Although human nature may seek to categorize and subdivide the various phenomena of the universe, all such differentiations are ultimately artificial. All of nature may be like a seamless web of energy forces.

Talbot (1991) concluded from the work of these two noted scientists that the cosmos, the world, the human brain, and each subatomic particle are all part of a holographic continuum: "Our brains mathematically construct objective reality by interpreting frequencies that are ultimately projections from another dimension, a deeper order of existence that is beyond both space and time." Just as each part of the holographic negative holds an image of the whole picture, Talbot further suggested that the auricular microsystem could hold an image of the whole body. All microsystems might function like the echo resonance, waveform interference patterns in a hologram, energy signals transmitted from the skin to the corresponding body organs. Similar to photographic hologram plates, each part of the auricle might integrate energetic signals from all the parts of the human body. Ralph Alan Dale (1991, 1993) in America, Ying-Qing Zhang (1992, 1997) in China, and Vilhelm Schjelderup (1982) in Europe have all utilized this holographic paradigm to account for the somatotopic pattern of acupoints found in every micro-acupuncture system.

The holographic model of microsystems is speculative, but it is congruent with the traditional Chinese perspective that every organ in the body is related to specific acupoints on the

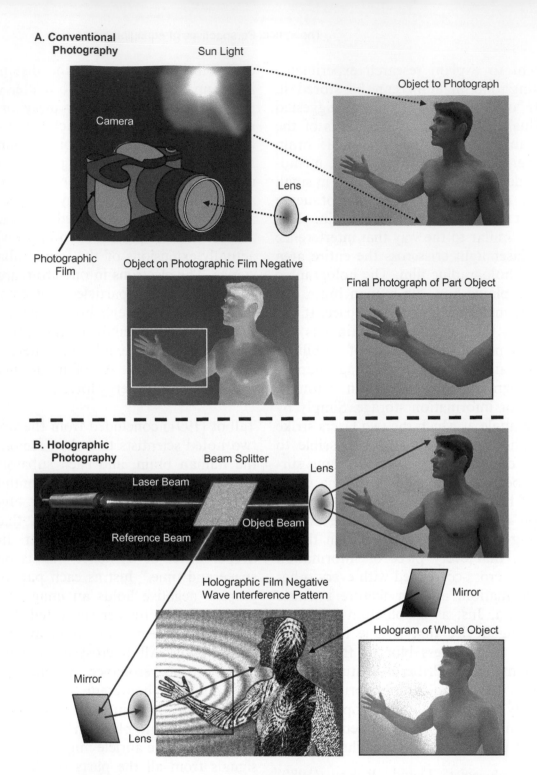

FIGURE 2.13 The images shown in this figure are intended to demonstrate the differences between conventional photography and holographic photography. In conventional photography, the light source is usually sunlight, which sends beams of broad-spectrum light to an object, in this case a person. That light is reflected back onto the lens of a camera, magnified, and recorded as a negative image on photographic film. If only one section of the photographic negative is developed, such as the arm, then only the image of the arm is revealed in the final photograph. In holography, a laser beam generator that creates a single-frequency, coherent light source is sent to a beam splitter, and the laser beam is divided equally into two different directions. One laser beam is sent onto the object being photographed, which is then reflected back onto a mirror and lens. The other coherent laser beam is reflected onto a different mirror and lens, which shines on the holographic film negative plate in a different orientation. The holographic equipment compares the waveform interference patterns from each laser beam source and seemingly creates a bizarre array of wavy images, but when finally developed it looks completely like the original object that was photographed, even though only a portion of the holographic negative was used for development. The whole of the holographic image is contained in each part of the holographic image, which also tends to be more three-dimensional than two-dimensional in perspective.

surface of the body. In his book *The Web That Has No Weaver*, Ted Kaptchuk (1983) states that "the cosmos itself is an integral whole, a web of interrelated things and events. Within this web of relationships and change, any entity can be defined only by its function, and significance only as part of the whole pattern." Another Stanford scientist has also examined this perspective. The physicist William Tiller (1997, 1999) contends that there are non-spatial, non-temporal energy waves functioning in various bands of a vacuum. His research showed that it was possible to focus human intention to alter the physical properties of substances in a simple electronic device. Research participants in a focused meditative state were able to induce either an increase or a decrease in the pH level of water by the simple act of their conscious intention. There was a small but consistent alteration in the pH level of water electromagnetically isolated inside a container within a Faraday cage. The pH level changed in a −1.0 negative direction when the meditators focused on lowering the pH, whereas it changed in a +1.0 positive direction when the meditators focused on raising pH. According to Tiller, the results of these experiments suggest that there is a transfer of unconventional information in previously unknown frequency domains. This unconventional energy could serve as the foundation for auricular medicine and other holographic microsystems. The research investigations by Tiller highlight the role of the healing intention of the practitioner when working with a patient using any health care modality.

Many scientists in the West are not comfortable with the concept of a nebulous, invisible, energy matrix, whether perceived from the orientation of Chinese medicine or from the speculations of quantum physicists. That these energetic viewpoints could be the primary foundation for auriculotherapy is not particularly reassuring to such scientists. A great split in the European auricular medicine community occurred when Paul Nogier expounded on the notion of "reticular energy" as an explanation for the clinical phenomena he observed. Paul Nogier proposed that "reticular energy" was a vital force that

flowed in all living tissue and that it propagated the exchange of cellular information. Any stimulation of the smallest part of the body by this reticular energy was said to be immediately transmitted to all other regions. For practitioners of TCM, the concept of such a vital force has been described as qi.

2.3 Energetic View of Ear Acupuncture in Traditional Chinese Medicine

Although *The Yellow Emperor's Classic of Internal Medicine* (Veith, 1972) and subsequent Chinese medical texts included a variety of acupuncture treatments applied to the external ear, it was not until 1958 that a somatotopic micro-acupuncture system was first described in Chinese acupuncture charts. Some traditionalists even contend that ear acupuncture is not a true part of classical Chinese medicine. A large body of literature, however, has shown that ancient acupuncture practitioners recorded the needling of ear acupoints for the relief of many health disorders. In contrast to many of the European texts based on Paul Nogier's work, Asian acupuncturists emphasize the importance of selecting ear points based on the fundamental principles of TCM. The specific feature of body acupuncture practice that is most relevant to the application of auriculotherapy is the use of distal acupuncture points. Needling acupoints on the tips of the fingers or the toes has long been used for treating conditions in distant parts of the body. There are other practitioners who seek to make auriculotherapy completely divorced from classical acupuncture, suggesting that it is an entirely independent system based on trigger point reflexes. It is my view that without a basic understanding of Oriental medicine, many effective auriculotherapy treatment protocols would not make any sense. The popularity of the five ear points used in the NADA treatment protocol for addictions is only comprehensible from the perspective of TCM principles that are very different from conventional Western thinking.

Influential English language texts on TCM include *The Web That Has No Weaver* by Ted Kaptchuk (1983), *Chinese Acupuncture and Moxibustion* by Cheng Xinnong (1987), *The Foundations of Chinese Medicine* by Giovanni Maciocia (1989), *Between Heaven and Earth* by Beinfeld and Korngold (1991), *Acupuncture Energetics* by Joseph Helms (1995), and *Understanding Acupuncture* by Birch and Felt (1999). All these books describe an energetic system for healing that is rooted in a uniquely Oriental viewpoint of the human body. Although all energy is conceptualized as a form of qi, there are different manifestations of this basic energy substance, including the energy of yin and yang, an energy differentiated by five phases, and an energy distinguished by eight principles for categorizing pathological conditions. Everyday observations of nature, such as the effects of wind, fire, dampness, and cold, are used as metaphors for understanding how this qi energy affects the internal conditions that lead to a particular disease.

The Flow of Qi

The concept of "qi" refers to a vital life force, a primal power, and a subtle essence that sustains all existence. The Chinese pictograph for qi refers to the nutrient-filled steam that appears while cooking rice. Qi is the distilled essence of the finest matter. Similar images for qi include the undulating vapors that rise from boiling tea, the swirling mists of fog that crawl over lowlands, the flowing movement of a gentle stream, or billowing cloud formations appearing over a hill. These ancient, metaphorical pictures were all attempts to describe the circulation of an invisible energy that has many of the attributes described in modern, quantum physics. Different manifestations of qi are shown in the accompanying figures. However, qi was not considered just a metaphor. Acupuncturists view qi as a real phenomenon, as real as widely accepted invisible forces such as gravity and magnetism. Qi is both matter and the energy force that moves matter. Comparable to Western efforts to explain light as understood in

quantum physics, qi is both like a particle and like a wave. Qi permeates everything, occurs everywhere, and is the medium by which all events are linked to each other in an interweaving pattern. There is qi in the sun, in mountains, in rocks, in flowers, in trees, in swords, in clothing, in animals, in people, and in all anatomical organs. Qi is obtained from the digestion of food and is extracted from the air that we breathe. Qi invigorates our consciousness and affects our ability to have willpower to take on a difficult challenge.

As things change in the macrocosm of the heavens, the microcosm of the earth resonates with correspondent vibrations, all related to the movement and interconnectedness of qi. Certain types of qi animate living organisms, with the greatest focus placed on defensive qi and on nutritive qi. Defensive qi is said to be the exterior defense of the human body and is activated when the skin surface and the muscles are invaded by exogenous pathogens. Nutritive qi serves to nourish the internal organs and blood. Prenatal qi is transmitted by parents to their children at conception and affects a child's inherited constitution, similar to modern concepts of DNA, genes, and chromosomes. Rebellious qi occurs when energy flows in conflicting, opposing patterns. Health is the harmonious movement of qi, whereas illness is due to disharmony in the flow of qi.

The original English translations of the zigzagging lines drawn on Chinese acupuncture charts were described by European doctors as meridians, an allusion to the lines of latitude that circle the earth on geographic maps. In acupuncture, the meridians were thought to be invisible lines of energy that allow circulation between specific sets of acupuncture points. Later translations described these acupuncture lines as channels, analogous to the grand canals that allowed boats to carry supplies to different cities in ancient China. Acupoints were thought to be holes (*xue*) in the lining of the body through which qi could flow, like water flowing through a series of holes in a sprinkler system. Water has often been utilized to symbolize invisible energies, and it is still used in the West as a convenient way to convey the properties of electricity traveling along metal

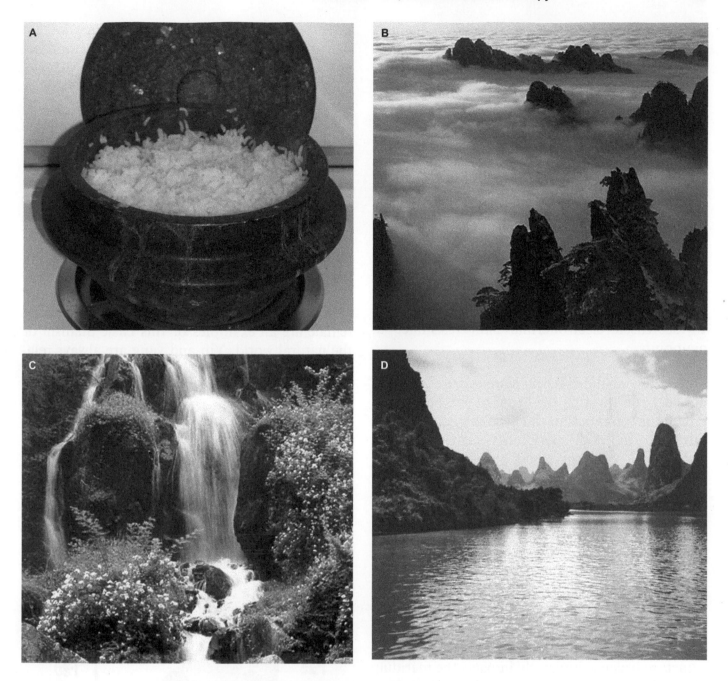

[**FIGURE 2.14** These photographs reflect the multiple ways in which natural phenomena can attempt to represent the invisible qualities of qi. The flowing vitality of qi has been compared to nutrient-enriched steam in cooking rice (A), the flowing mist of clouds over mountaintops (B), the rush of water down a waterfall (C), or the smooth rhythm of a flowing river (D).

wires and the flow of electrical impulses along neurons.

Qi Deficiency: As with channels of water when there is a drought that creates a dry river bed, the flow of qi through acupuncture channels is sometimes abnormally low, such as when there is poor blood circulation in one's extremities,

low blood pressure, or muscle weakness. Needles inserted into specific acupuncture points can improve the circulation of qi and blood so that there is a balance of flow throughout the body.

Qi Excess: After heavy rains, a river channel may flood over its banks, which is comparable to the excessive flow of qi in an acupuncture channel. Physiological effects of qi excess include swelling, heat, high blood pressure, or muscle spasms. Needles inserted into acupuncture points can serve to reduce the excess activity.

Qi Stagnation: At still other times, water becomes backed up in a small region of a channel, not completely dry but not able to move further, developing into a swampy marsh that may become stagnant due to the lack of circulation. Qi stagnation is associated with a lack of flow of qi and blood, which could lead to swelling, heat, and muscle spasms. The subdermal accumulation of toxic chemicals at reactive ear acupoints is considered an example of qi stagnation, leading to heightened tenderness to palpation and to decreased electrodermal skin resistance at acupoints.

Only a few of the classical acupuncture channels actually run through the external ear, but microcirculatory channels in the head may connect the auricle to the body meridian system. The external ear microsystem could best be conceptualized as a remote control station that allows gates within these channels to more fully open when the flow of qi is deficient and to distribute qi to other areas when the flow of qi is in excess or stagnant. The auricular system does not produce qi; rather, it remotely regulates the flow of qi along meridian channels, like a modern, remote control switch for a TV channel or a garage door opener. Some acupuncturists believe that body acupuncture is more effective than auricular acupuncture because it directly impacts the meridian channels that extend over the entire body. It is of important note, however, that a modern microchip computer is quite small yet it has the ability to control major equipment that is a considerable distance away.

Taoism, Yang Qi, and Yin Qi

The philosophy of *Taoism* (also spelled *Daoism*) guides one of the oldest belief systems that originated in ancient China. The black and white teardrop symbols of Taoism are probably the most internationally familiar symbols of Asian

ways of thinking. Taoism's basic tenet is that the whole cosmos is composed of two opposing and complementary qualities, *yin* and *yang*. A Taoist adept is said to follow the way of the Tao, a path that leads to harmony and balance in life. The Taoist symbol shown in the accompanying figures reveals a circle divided into a white teardrop and a black teardrop. A smaller white dot within the black side represents the yang within yin, whereas the small black dot within the white side reflects the yin within yang. The Chinese character for yang referred to the sunny side of a hill that is warmed by bright rays of sunlight, whereas the pictograph character for yin referred to the darker, colder, shady side of a hill. Light and dark, day and night, hot and cold, male and female are all examples of this basic dualism of the natural world. Yin and yang are always relative rather than absolute qualities. The front of the body is said to be yin relative to the back of the body, whereas the upper body is said to be more yang compared to the lower body. The outer skin of the body and the muscles are more yang, and the internal organs are more yin. Disorders related to overactivity are more yang, and diseases of weakness are more yin.

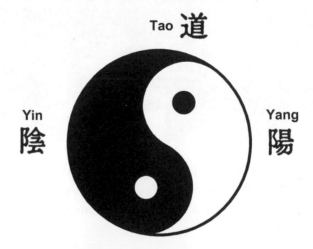

[FIGURE 2.15 The Taoist symbol for the unity of all existence is to show a circle composed of a dark and a light teardrop, with each teardrop containing a circle with the opposite color. The white teardrop represents the Yang forces of sunlight, strength, power, and masculinity, whereas the black teardrop represents the Yin forces of darkness, softness, gentleness, and femininity. Each quality of Yang and Yin contains an element of its opposite, represented by the white and black circles.

The psychologist Carl Jung (1964) and the historian Joseph Campbell (1988) have noted that archetypal images in the ancient cultures of China, India, Egypt, Persia, Europe, and Native Americans have similar themes. In all these societies, the sky, the sun, and fire are typically referred to as masculine qualities, whereas the earth, the moon, and water are associated with feminine qualities. Taoist philosophers described this opposition of dualities in every aspect of nature. There is a tendency in Western culture to place greater value on the masculine qualities of acting in a manner that is strong, forceful, rational, and orderly and to devalue the feminine qualities of being passive, weak, or emotional. Taoism recognized the importance of maintaining the harmonious balance of yin and yang and emphasized the value of feminine qualities of nurturance and intuition as well as the masculine traits of strength and intelligence.

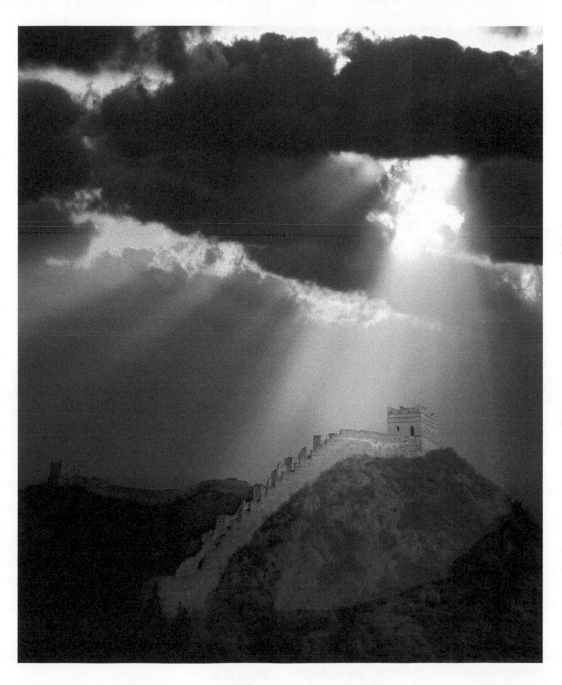

[FIGURE 2.16 This photograph of beams of sunlight shining down one side of a mountain ridge separated by the Great Wall of China symbolizes the Yang forces of light that shine upon the sunny side of a hill and the Yin forces of darkness that shine upon the shaded side of a hill.

TABLE 2.2	Taoist Qualities of Yang and Yin.
Yang Qualities	**Yin Qualities**
Sunny side of hill	Shady side of hill
Light	Dark
Day	Night
Sun	Moon
Sky	Earth
Fire	Water
Hot	Cold
Restless	Passive
Strong	Weak
Rapid	Slow
Aggressive	Nurturing
Rational	Intuitive
Intellectual	Emotional
Head	Heart
Masculine	Feminine
Father	Mother

As shown in Table 2.2, yang qualities include the warm, bright light of the sun during daylight hours when animals are typically more active. Yin qi is like the soft, gentle light of the moon that shines during the darkness of night when the world is more serene, quiet, and restful. Yin calming qualities provide a necessary balance to yang activating qualities. Archetypal, yang, masculine qualities are related to aggressive behaviors, whereas archetypal, yin, feminine qualities are more nurturing behaviors.

Pathological conditions in the human body are often caused by the excess of yang qi, producing symptoms of restlessness, hyperactivity, tremors, anxiety, and insomnia. The stress of overwork frequently involves an overindulgence in yang qi, which often leads to the burnout of yin qi. In addition to the application of acupuncture needles, moxibustion, and herbal remedies, stagnation of yang qi can be corrected by vigorous physical exercise, athletic sports, and the practice of martial arts such as kung fu or karate.

For the most part, the stimulation of ear acupuncture points serves to alleviate pathologies that are attributable to yang excess reactions. Headaches, back pain, addiction, hypertension, and chronic stress can all be perceived as harmful conditions associated with excessive activation of yang qi, sometimes to the point of exhaustion. The ear is located in the head, which tends to be more yang than yin, and only the yang-related meridians ascend to the head. The outer rings of the external ear are functionally associated with neurological impairments, which are also more yang than yin in their impact.

The yin meridians indirectly connect to the auricle through their corresponding yang meridian. Yin qi flows along acupuncture meridians on the front side of body and more frequently affects internal organs and nutritive qi. Symptoms of sleepiness, lethargy, depression, and a desire to be immobile may be due to an excessive focus on craving yin qi. Insufficient yin qi is thought to be at the root of most illness; thus, acupuncture and herbs are used to restore this energy. The flow of yin qi can be enhanced by quiet meditation, by repeating the soothing sounds of a mantra, by visualization of a simple symbol, or by the practice of such physical exercises as qi gong, tai chi, or yoga. The Chinese goddess Kuan Yin (Quan Yin) is said to be the manifestation of the Buddha in feminine form, usually portrayed as a caring, nurturing, ageless woman who is dressed in long, flowing robes but who may be riding a dragon.

Although it has been stated several times that only the yang-related meridians directly connect to the auricle, the internal organs of the body that are represented in the central valley of the external ear are more associated with yin qi than yang qi. The five yin-related organs that are found in the concha of the auricle include the heart, the lungs, the liver, the spleen, and the kidney. Stimulation of these microsystem points can improve the vitality of not only the organs but also the meridian pathways that are named for each organ. For instance, the nutritive value of stimulating the auricular liver point can serve to alleviate liver qi stagnation.

Yang Alarm Reactions and Ashi Points

A reactive ear reflex point is said to show a yang reaction on the ear to signal a stress reaction in the correspondent area of the body. In modern times, an appropriate analogy would be a fire alarm signal in a building, indicating the specific hallway where a fire is burning. An alarm in a car can indicate when a door is ajar or the engine is overheating. Such alarms alert one to the specific location of a problem. Elevation of yang energy manifests in the external ear as a small area where there is localized activation of the sympathetic nervous system. Such sympathetic arousal leads to a localized increase in electrodermal skin conductance that is readily detectable by an electrical point finder. Sympathetic activation also induces localized regions of vasoconstriction of localized blood vessels in the skin covering the auricle. The restricted blood supply causes an accumulation of subdermal, toxic biochemicals, possibly accounting for the perception of tenderness at acupoints or the visible, skin surface reactions seen at ear reflex points. If sympathetic nervous system arousal is viewed as a neurological manifestation of yang excess, the properties used for auricular diagnosis can be explained by known neurophysiological pathways.

In addition to the 12 primary meridian channels that run along the length of the body, the Chinese also described extra-meridian acupoints located outside of these channels. One category of such acupoints was labeled "ashi points," which means the "Ouch!" point. As pressure is applied to a sensitive region of skin or muscle, it is as if the patient is informing the practitioner that "There it is!"—that is the point that you need to treat. The exclamation points in these brief statements highlight the great emotional excitement vocalized at the time pressure is applied to an ashi point, like when a dentist probes a decayed tooth.

Although one's natural inclination is to avoid touching areas of the body that hurt, ancient acupuncturists and modern massage therapists have observed that there is a definite healing value in putting greater pressure on these sensitive regions. The ashi points have been suggested as the origin of the trigger points that have been described by Dr. Janet Travell in her work on myofascial pain (Travell and Simons, 1983). In auricular acupuncture, a tender spot on the external ear is one of the definitive characteristics that indicate that such a point should be stimulated, not avoided.

Five Oriental Elements of Metal, Earth, Fire, Water, and Wood

Also referred to as the five phases or five functions, this Chinese energetic system organizes the universe into five categories: fire, earth, metal, water, and wood. The word "element" is similar to the four elements of nature described in medieval, European texts—the elements of fire, earth, air, and water. The word "phase" is comparable to the phases of the moon, observed as sequential shifts in the pattern of sunlight that is reflected from the moon. It is also related to the phases of the sun as it rises at dawn, crosses overhead from morning to afternoon, sets at dusk, and then hides during the darkness of night. The phases of the seasons in Chinese writings were said to rotate from spring to summer to late summer to fall to winter. These long-ago physicians found observations of natural elements, such as the heat from fire or the dampness of water, to be useful analogies to describe the mysterious, invisible forces that affect health and disease. Many complex metabolic actions in the human body are still not understood by modern Western medicine, even with the latest advances in blood chemical assays and magnetic resonance imaging equipment.

The metaphorical descriptions of five element theory reflect the poetry and rhythm of the Chinese language in their attempts to understand each individual who is seeking relief from some ailment. At the same time, there are certain aspects of the five phases that seem like an arbitrary attempt to assign all things to groups of five. The Western approach of dividing the seasons into the spring equinox, summer solstice, fall equinox, and winter solstice seem more aligned with nature than the Chinese notion to add a fifth season labeled late summer. Moreover, the application of five element theory to the energetic aspects of anatomical organs often contradicts modern understanding of the biological function of those organs. It is difficult for Western minds to accept how the element metal logically relates to the lung organ and the feelings of sadness, whereas the element wood is said to be associated with the liver organ and the emotion of anger. At some point, one can only accept that these five phases are organizing principles to facilitate clinical intuition toward understanding complex diseases. In some respects, it might have been better to have left the names of the meridian channels as Chinese words rather than to translate them into the European names of anatomical organs whose physiological function was already known. The conflicts between the Oriental energetic associations to an organ and the known physiological effects of that organ can lead to confusion rather than comprehension. If one thinks of these zang–fu organs as force fields rather than anatomic structures, their associated function may become more understandable.

Each of the five elements is related to two types of internal organs. The zang organs are more yin, and the fu organs are more yang. The acupuncture channels are the passages by which the zang–fu organs connect with each other. The zang meridians tend to run along the inner side of the arms and legs and up the front of the body. The fu meridians run along the outer side of the limbs and down the back of the body. The zang organs store vital substances, such as qi, blood, essence, and body fluids, whereas the fu organs are constantly filled and then emptied. The Chinese character for zang alluded to a depot storage facility, whereas the pictograph for fu depicted ancient Chinese grain collection centers that were called palaces. Although Confucian principles forbade official dissections of the human body, anatomical investigations probably still occurred in ancient China, as did examinations of animals. Physical observations of gross internal anatomy revealed that the fu organs were hollow, tube-like structures that either carried food, as in the stomach, small intestines, and large intestines, or carried fluid, as in the urinary bladder and gall bladder. In contrast, the zang organs seemed essentially solid structures, particularly the liver, spleen, and kidneys. Although the heart and lungs have respective passages for blood and air, one would not describe these two organs as hollow tubes but, rather, as having interconnecting chambers.

The specific characteristics of each zang–fu channel are presented in Table 2.3, which indicates the internal organ for which each channel

TABLE 2.3	Anatomical Location of Yang and Yin Meridian Channels.				
Yang Channel	Location	Reflex Zones	Corresponding Yin Channel	Direction of Energy Flow	Reflex Zones
Large Intestine	External hand to arm to shoulder and face	1–2	Lung	Inner chest to inner arm and hand	1
San Jiao	External hand to external arm and head	3–4	Pericardium	Inner chest to inner arm and hand	3
Small Intestine	External hand to arm to shoulder and face	5	Heart	Inner chest to inner arm and hand	5
Stomach	Face to anterior body to anterior leg	2–3	Spleen	Foot to inner leg to anterior body	1–2
Gall Bladder	External head to external body and foot	5	Liver	Foot to inner leg to anterior body	1–2
Bladder	Posterior head to back to posterior leg	1–2	Kidney	Foot to inner leg to anterior body	1–2
Governing Vessel (Du Mai)	Midline of buttocks to midline back to midline head	1	Conception Vessel (Ren Mai)	Midline abdomen to midline chest to midline face	1

is named, the international abbreviation for that channel according to the World Health Organization (WHO), alternative abbreviations that have been used in various clinical texts, the differentiation of each channel, and designation of the primary element associated with that channel. The acupoints that are most frequently used in acupuncture treatments are also presented. The sequential order of the channels presented in Table 2.3 indicates the circulation pattern in which energy is said to flow throughout the day. The channels are differentiated into three yin meridians and three yang meridians on the hand and three yin meridians and three yang meridians on the foot. In Table 2.4, the zang–fu channels are regrouped according to those meridians that are more yang and the corresponding channels that are more yin. This table also describes the relationship of the anatomical location of each meridian that is shown on acupuncture charts compared to the zone regions of the body that are used in foot and hand reflexology. The zang channels tend to run along the inside of the arms or legs, whereas the corresponding fu channels typically run along the external side of the arms or legs.

As seen in the accompanying figures, when the arms are raised upward toward the sun, yang energy descends down the posterior side of the body along fu channels, whereas yin energy ascends the anterior side of the body along zang channels. Only the fu Stomach channel descends along the anterior side of the body. Because the fu channels have acupuncture points located on the surface of the head, these yang meridians are said to be more directly connected to the ear. The Large Intestine channel crosses from the neck to the contralateral face, the Stomach channel branches across the medial cheeks and in front of the ear, the Small Intestine channel projects across the lateral cheek, the Bladder meridian goes over the midline of the head, and both the San Jiao channel and the Gall Bladder channel circle around the ear at the side of the head. Acupuncture points on the zang channels only reach as high as the chest; thus, they have no physical means to connect to the ear. Another set of acupuncture channels, the Conception Vessel meridian (Ren Mai) on the front of the body and the Governing Vessel meridian (Du Mai) on the back of the body, both ascend the midline of the body to reach the head.

TABLE 2.4	**Differentiation of Zang–Fu Meridian Channels.**[a]					
Organ Channels	**WHO Code**	**Other Codes**	**Channel Differentiation**	**Element**	**Zang–Fu**	**Primary Acupoints**
Lung	LU		Hand Tai Yin	Metal	Zang	LU 1, LU 7, LU9
Large Intestine	LI		Hand Yang Ming	Metal	Fu	LI 4, LI 11
Stomach	ST		Foot Yang Ming	Earth	Fu	ST 36, ST 44
Spleen	SP		Foot Tai Yin	Earth	Zang	SP 6, SP 9
Heart	HT	H, HE	Hand Shao Yin	Fire	Zang	HT 7
Small Intestine	SI		Hand Tai Yang	Fire	Fu	SI 3, SI 18
Urinary Bladder	BL	B, UB	Foot Tai Yang	Water	Fu	BL 23, BL 40
Kidney	KI	K, Kid	Foot Shao Yin	Water	Zang	KI 3, KI 7
Pericardium	PC	P	Hand Jue Yin	Fire	Zang	PC 6
San Jiao	SJ	TW, TE	Hand Shao Yang	Fire	Fu	SJ 5
Gall Bladder	GB		Foot Shao Yang	Wood	Fu	GB 20, GB 40
Liver	LR	Liv	Foot Jue Yin	Wood	Zang	LR 3, LR 14
Conception Vessel	CV	Ren Mai	Front—Mu Yin			CV 6, CV 17
Governing Vessel	GV	Du Mai	Back—Shu Yang			GV 4, GV 20

[a]Energy is said to circulate through these zang-fu channels in the order presented, from Lung to Large Intestine to Stomach to Spleen to Heart to Small Intestine to Bladder to Kidney to Pericardium to San Jiao to Gall Bladder to Liver and back to Lung.

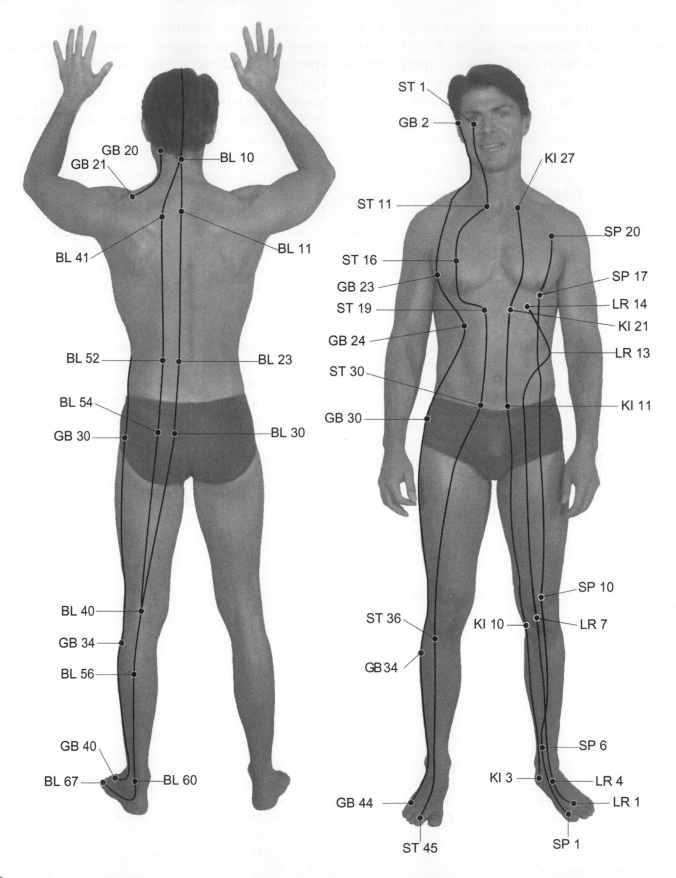

FIGURE 2.17 This photograph shows on an actual person the location of the primary acupuncture points found along Yang meridian points of the Bladder (BL), Gall Bladder (GB), and Stomach (ST) and the corresponding Yin meridian points of the Kidney (KI), Liver (LR), and Spleen (SP).

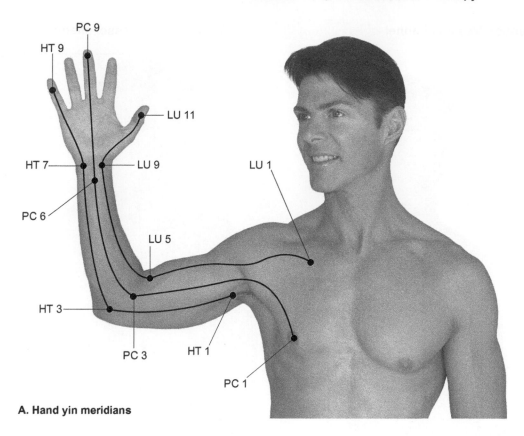

A. Hand yin meridians

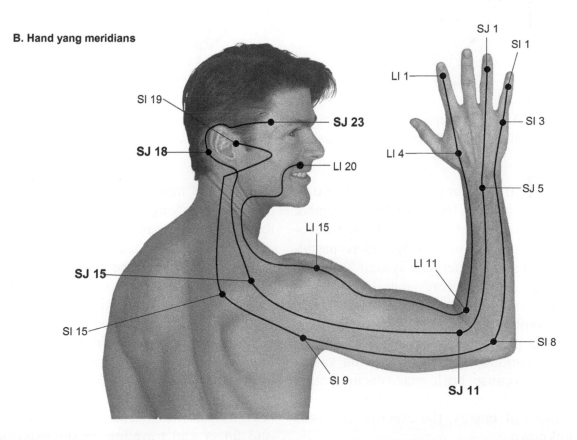

B. Hand yang meridians

FIGURE 2.18 This photograph shows on an actual person the location of the primary acupuncture points found along Yang meridian points of the Large Intestine (LI), Small Intestine (SI), and San Jiao (SJ) and the corresponding Yin meridian points of the Lung (LU), Heart (HT), and Pericardium (PC).

A. Conception Vessel channel

B. Governing Vessel channel

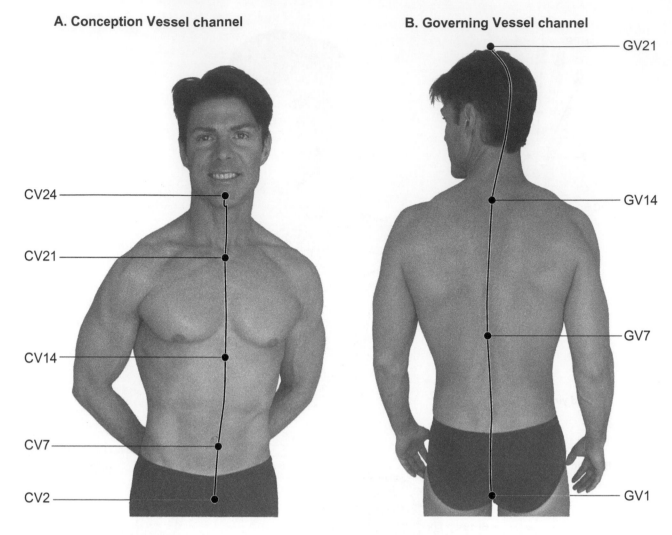

CV24

CV21

CV14

CV7

CV2

GV21

GV14

GV7

GV1

FIGURE 2.19 This photograph shows on an actual person the location of the primary acupuncture points found along the Conception Vessel (CV) and the Governing Vessel (GV) meridians along the midline of the body.

The Chinese charts do not show how the external ear directly connects to the six zang channels. Dale (1999) hypothesized that all micro-acupuncture systems function through micro-meridians, just as the macro-energetic system functions through macro-acupuncture meridians. It is further postulated that the entire macro–micro channel complex forms an extensive energetic network, perhaps similar to the way veins, arteries, and capillaries characterize the vascular network. Because both macro-acupuncture channels and micro-acupuncture meridians carry invisible forces of energy, the exact mechanisms remain unknown.

Metal: The metaphor of metal is related to the Bronze Age development of heating the minerals of the earth to a *white* hot intensity with fire,

shaping the malleable object while it is warm, and then allowing it to cool and contract into a fixed shape. The yin nourishing aspects of metal are represented by the ability to cook rice in a metal pot, whereas the yang aggressive aspects of metal are demonstrated by the creation of the sword and protective suits of armor. The acupuncture meridians related to metal are the Lung channel that descends from the chest distally down the inner arm and ends on the palm side of the thumb, whereas the Large Intestine channel is found on the opposing side of the hand, beginning at the external, dorsum side of the second finger and traveling up the external side of the arm toward the head.

Earth: The *yellow* earth is the stable foundation on which crops are grown and cities are created.

The late summer qualities of earth allow one to be solid and grounded and accompany the autumn harvest of many food crops. The acupuncture meridians related to earth are the Spleen channel that begins on the large toe and travels up the inner leg and the Stomach channel that travels down the external body and external leg to end on the second toe.

Fire: The *red* flames of a fire bring warmth and comfort to a cold day, allowing one to move about and function with greater ease and speed. The summer qualities of fire accompany a time when there is great activity and a gathering of crops. The acupuncture meridians related to fire include the Heart channel that descends from the chest distally down the inner arm and ends on the little finger, whereas the Small Intestine channel begins on the little finger and travels up the external arm toward the head. Two other channels also related to fire are the Pericardium channel that travels distally down the inner arm and the San Jiao channel that travels up the outer arm from the hand to the head.

Water: The refreshing coolness of *blue* waters quenches one's thirst and provides the body with one of its most necessary elements. Associated with winter, the qualities of water are stillness, quietness, and a time for reflective meditation. The acupuncture meridians related to water are the Kidney channel that begins on the little toe and travels up the inner leg to the abdomen, whereas the Bladder channel begins on the forehead, crosses over the top of the head to the back of the head, runs down the back of the neck, down the spine, and down the back of the leg to the foot. Both the kidney and the bladder organs are involved in regulating body fluids.

Wood: The image of wood is best thought of as the initial spring growth of new branches on a tree, each limb sprouting bright *green* leaves. Wood is associated with new beginnings, new growth, and changing temperaments. The acupuncture meridians related to wood include the Liver channel that begins on the large toe and travels up the inside of the leg to the chest, whereas the Gall Bladder channel descends along the external side of the head and body and down the external leg to the little toe.

Zang Organ Meridians

Although all the internal organs are more yin than yang, a predominant focus in Chinese medicine is given to the clinical importance of the zang organs. The five principal zang organs are the Lung, Heart, Liver, Spleen, and Kidney. The energetic functions of zang organs are utilized in classical acupuncture more often than the physiological functions of that organ. Western language translations of the acupuncture meridians might have been better left as Chinese pinyin terms. The discrepancies between the anatomical function of these organs in conventional medicine as contrasted with their clinical use in Oriental medicine has sometimes led to confusion rather than understanding by Western medical doctors.

Lung: The thoracic organ of the lung, in the Upper Jiao, dominates the qi of respiration, inhaling pure qi and exhaling toxic qi. If Lung Qi is weak, defensive qi will not reach the skin, thus the body will be more easily invaded by pathogenic factors, particularly cold. Besides its inclusion in the treatment of respiratory disorders, the Lung point on the auricle is one of the most frequently used ear points for detoxification from addictive substances, such as opium, cocaine, and alcohol. The skin also connects to respiration and to the release of internal toxic substances through the process of sweating. Consequently, the auricular Lung point is also used for the treatment of skin disorders.

Heart: This thoracic organ promotes blood circulation and supports vigorous heart qi. Heart Qi is said to be essential for forming blood and is associated with the mind and the spirit. In addition to its application for coronary dysfunctions, the auricular Heart point is stimulated to relieve nervous disorders, memory problems, sleep impairment, and disturbing dreams.

Liver: In Chinese thought, Liver Qi helps to store blood and to increase blood circulation. It is needed for vigorous movements by nourishing the sinews, ligaments, and tendons that attach muscles to bones. Liver Qi is responsible for unrestrained, harmonious activity of all organs and maintains the free flow of qi. Stagnation

**A. Surface view
of zang organs**

**B. Posterior view
of zang organs**

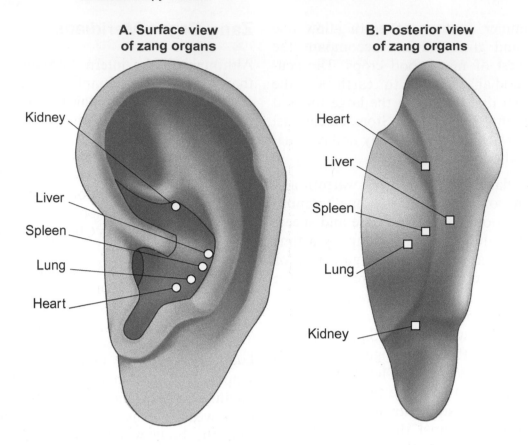

[**FIGURE 2.20** This image of the anterior and posterior sides of the auricle depicts the location of the five zang organs of traditional Oriental medicine that are represented on the external ear, which are commonly used in many auricular treatment plans.

of Liver Qi is associated with resentment, bitterness, irritability, repressed anger, and mental depression, whereas excessive Liver Qi may cause headaches and insomnia. The auricular Liver point is used for myofascial pain, muscle tension, and repressed rage.

Spleen: Of all the zang organs, the Chinese conceptualization of the spleen is probably the most different from Western understanding of this organ. In TCM, this abdominal organ governs the transportation of blood and nourishes the muscles and the four limbs. If Spleen Qi is weak, the muscles will be weak. Excessive mental work or worried thinking is said to weaken Spleen Qi. In Western anatomical texts, the spleen is considered a part of the lymphatic drainage system and has little effect on muscles or on mental worry. Some of the digestive functions that the Chinese assigned to the spleen seem like they would be more appropriately delegated to the

nearby abdominal organs of the stomach and the pancreas. Nonetheless, the Chinese Spleen point on the ear is effectively used for the treatment of muscle tension and general nourishment.

Kidney: Lower in the abdomen, Kidney Qi is related to the congenital essence of the physical body that a person inherits from one's parents. The Chinese concept of the kidney qi affects growth, development, and reproduction. The kidney organs dominate water metabolism and regulate the distribution of body fluids. According to TCM, Kidney Qi also nourishes the spinal cord and brain, strengthens one's will power, enhances vitality, and affects the hearing functions of the inner ear.

Pericardium: A sixth zang organ is the Pericardium (PC), which refers to the protective membranes that surround the heart. This acupuncture channel has also been labeled the

Master of the Heart or the Circulation–Sex channel. The Pericardium meridian functions very similar to the Heart channel and runs along an adjacent region of the inside of the arm as it travels distally toward the hand.

Fu Organ Meridians and Pathogenic Factors

The fu organs include the Stomach, the Small Intestine, the Large Intestine, the Urinary Bladder, and the Gall Bladder. These organs are not as prominently discussed in Oriental medicine as the zang organs, but the acupuncture channels associated with each fu organ are very important in acupuncture treatment plans. Two of the most commonly used acupoints in all of Oriental medicine are LI 4 (Hegu or Hoku) on the Large Intestine meridian and ST 36 (Zusanli) on the Stomach meridian. Stimulation of acupoints on the Large Intestine channel can relieve pain in the index finger, wrist, elbow, shoulder, neck, or jaw—anatomical structures that occur along the Large Intestine channel. Needling acupoints on the Stomach channel can alleviate conditions in the face, neck, chest, abdomen, leg, knee, or foot—all skeletal structures found along the Stomach meridian.

San Jiao: This term has been translated as Triple Warmer (TW), Triple Heater (TH), Triple Burner (TB), and Triple Energizer (TE). Members of an international nomenclature committee of WHO ultimately decided to keep the Chinese term for this meridian because San Jiao (SJ) really has no correspondence in Western anatomical thinking. The classical division of the body was distinguished as three regions: the Upper Jiao (the chest region that regulates circulatory and respiratory functions), the Middle Jiao (the upper abdominal region that affects digestive functions), and the Lower Jiao (the lower abdominal region that affects sexual and excretory functions). These three warmers might be conceptualized as three different pots containing boiling water. San Jiao refines the subtle essences of qi in a manner similar to the distillation process by which a brewery creates alcohol from a warm mash of grains. First, the creamy mash of soaked grains is brought to a boil. The steam of that mixture is allowed to rise and then cool into a second container of water mixed with alcohol. Finally, the heated mist of the second container is allowed to rise, then cooled and condensed, then descend in a tube and be collected in a final container of pure alcohol. The Upper Jiao is like a vaporous mist in the region of the heart and lungs, the Middle Jiao is like foam in the region of the stomach and spleen, and the Lower Jiao is like a dense swamp in the region of the kidneys, intestines, and bladder. The physiological effects of San Jiao could be physiologically related to the arousal actions of the sympathetic nervous system or to the release of circulating hormones in the endocrine system.

Shen (Spirit): This ethereal substance is the vitality behind the processes related to one's spiritual essence. Shen is associated with a particular personality style and it affects one's general well-being. One of the most widely used points in all of auriculotherapy is the Shen Men point in the triangular fossa.

Wind: The nature of an ill wind is used in TCM to identify one of the basic pathogenic factors that affect health and disease. This Chinese concept of Wind may be the vehicle through which other climatic factors, such as cold or dampness, invade the body and can injure blood, yin, or defensive qi. Wind tends to first affect the lungs, then the skin, and may manifest as neurological convulsions or muscle paralysis. A frequently used Chinese auricular acupoint is located on the internal helix where it meets the upper scaphoid fossa. This ear acupoint is known as the Windstream point, and it practically serves as a master point for allergies and immune system disorders.

2.4 Neurophysiological Perspectives of Auricular Acupuncture

Classical Chinese medicine did not highlight the role of the nervous system as currently conceived in Western medical science. Even recent Chinese ear acupuncture charts contain just a few auricular localizations for the brain. In contrast, the auriculotherapy texts by Paul Nogier (1972) and Rene Bourdiol (1982) predominantly focused on neurological reflex systems as an explanation for the auricular microsystem they investigated. There have been many advances in the field of neuroscience in the past several decades that have substantially altered basic understanding of brain pathways. It is now known that there are mechanisms by which the nervous system not only perceives pain but also has the capacity to suppress the pain experience. Neurophysiological research has examined the role of both ear acupuncture and body acupuncture in altering the neurobiological processes of pain perception and pain modulation. Some scientists contend that all of the energetic qualities described in Chinese medicine can ultimately be accounted for by observable electrophysiological and biochemical phenomena in the brain and nervous system. See the texts *Understanding Acupuncture* by Birch and Felt (1999), *Neuro-Acupuncture* by Cho *et al.* (2001), and *Clinical Acupuncture: Scientific Basis* edited by Stux and Hammerschlag (2001), all describing numerous research studies demonstrating the neurobiological basis of acupuncture analgesia. The accumulated research studies on neurobiology have demonstrated that the different regions of the brain significantly affect the basic mechanisms of acupuncture, but they do not necessarily refute the energetic concepts of acupuncture.

Higher Brain Processing Centers

The overall organization of the brain is divided into a lower brain, an intermediate or border brain, and the higher brain. Spinal cord pathways connect to the brainstem at the medulla oblongata, ascend to the pons, and then the midbrain. The reticular formation extends throughout the core of the lower brain, receiving sensory signals from the spinal cord below and sending output messages to higher brain centers above, thus activating neurons throughout the cerebral cortex that can lead to general arousal. The serotonergic raphe nuclei that facilitate sleep and

sedation are also found in the medulla, pons, and midbrain, running along the midline of the brainstem. The intermediate, border brain consists of the thalamus, the hypothalamus, the limbic system, and the striatum or basal ganglia. The thalamus projects somatosensory messages to the cortex and modulates sensory information that ascends to consciousness. The hypothalamus affects autonomic arousal and endocrine hormones, whereas the limbic system modulates emotional reactions and long-term memory storage. The higher brain centers consist of the four lobes of the neocortex: the somatosensory parietal lobe that processes body awareness and spatial relations, the occipital lobe that processes visual recognition, the temporal lobe that processes auditory recognition and thought associations, and the movement control centers in the frontal lobe. The prefrontal lobe has come to be known as the "executive brain." It controls the intentional decisions made by a conscious individual. The cerebellum is an offshoot of the pons, which has higher brain functions that interact with both the frontal lobe and the basal ganglia to regulate well-learned habits. Although the higher cortical centers in human brain are the most evolved portions of the nervous system, it is the lower limbic brain, the hypothalamus, and the brainstem that play a more active role in acupuncture analgesia.

Brain Computer Model

A common analogy for understanding the brain is to cite the example of modern computers. If the brain is compared to a computer, then the external ear can be viewed as a computer terminal that has peripheral access to the body's central microprocessor unit. Needle insertion or electrical stimulation of ear acupoints would be like typing a message on a computer keyboard, whereas the computer screen would be like the appearance of specific diagnostic signs on the auricle. Losing or damaging the ear would not necessarily be destructive to the brain computer, any more than losing one keyboard would necessarily affect a physical computer that has multiple inputs from other terminals. The peripheral

A. Frontal View of Brain and Spinal Cord

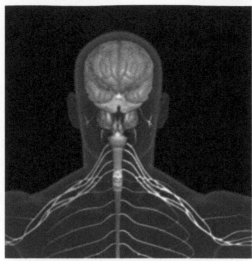

B. Side View of Brain and Spinal Cord

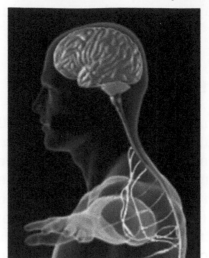

C. Side View of Brain and External Ear

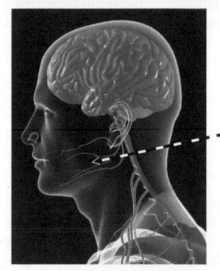

— Trigeminal Nerve

D. Mid-Saggital View of Triune Brain

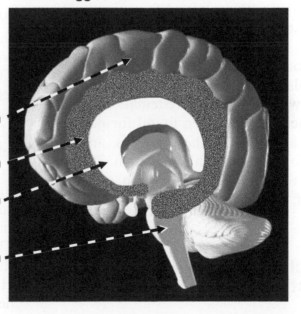

Higher Primate Brain

Middle Limbic Brain

Corpus Callosum

Lower Reptilian Brain

FIGURE 2.21 This series of images depicts the higher brain, brainstem, spinal cord, and peripheral nerves as seen from a frontal (A) and a sagittal or side (B) perspective. Indicated in image C is the relationship of the external ear to the location of the temporal cortex, cerebellum, and brainstem inside of the nearby skull, in addition to the spread of the trigeminal nerve to various regions of the face and the auricle. The concept of the triune brain is represented in image D, which depicts the higher primate brain that can make conscious decisions, the lower reptilian brain that regulates primitive reflexes, and the middle limbic brain that impacts social bonding in mammalian species.

terminal on the external ear allows ready access to the central brain computer that is encased in the skull.

Somatotopic Brain Map

Research by Pennfield and Rasmussen (1950) demonstrated that when the brain of a human patient undergoing neurosurgery was electrically excited, stimulation of specific cortical areas evoked verbal reports of sensations in specific parts of the patient's body. Stimulation of the most superior and medial region of the somatosensory cortex elicited sensations from the feet, whereas stimulation of the more inferior and peripheral region of the cortex produced the perception of fuzziness in the head. The rest of the body was represented in an anatomically logical pattern. If the right cortex was stimulated, the patient reported that his or her perceived sensation was on the left side of the body, whereas if the left cortex was stimulated, the patient felt a sensation on his or her right side. Parallel research by Mountcastle and Henneman (1952) and Woolsey (1958) showed that a similar pattern existed for animals. When electrical stimulation was applied to the foot of an animal, neurons on the contralateral, somatosensory cortex began firing; when the lower leg was stimulated, a different but nearby region of the brain was activated. A systematic representation of the body has been found for neurons in the cerebral cortex, in the thalamus, and in the reticular formation of the brainstem. This brain map has the same overall pattern as the map on the ear, representing the body in an inverted orientation.

Cerebral Laterality and Contralateral Connections to the Auricle

The higher brain processing centers are split into a left cerebral cortex and a right cerebral cortex, each side with a frontal lobe, a parietal lobe, a temporal lobe, and an occipital lobe. A broad band of neurons called the corpus callosum bridges the chasm between these two sides of the brain. The left side of the higher brain receives signals from and sends messages out to control the right side of the body, whereas the right side of the higher brain receives signals from and sends messages out to the left side of the body. Besides controlling the ability to write with the right hand, the left neocortex dominates one's ability to understand language, to verbally articulate words, to solve math problems, to analyze details, and to report on one's state of consciousness. Even left-handed individuals tend to exhibit dominance for language on the left side of their brain. The right side of the cerebral cortex regulates a different set of psychological functions. Besides controlling the left hand, the right side of the brain is superior to the left side of the brain in recognizing facial features, in perceiving inflections and intonations, and in understanding the rhythms that distinguish different songs. Our recognition of negative emotional feelings is more highly processed by the relationship-oriented right brain than by the more logically oriented left brain. Table 2.5 presents the different qualities of the left and right cerebral hemispheres in dualistic perspective of Taoism.

What is important to right brain perception is the overall relationship of the parts to the whole, which is also the predominant perspective of TCM. Although information processed by the left hemisphere is necessary to remember someone's name, the right brain is essential to recall his or her face. Dominance for language in the left cerebral cortex is found in 95% of the whole population, with only a few left-handers exhibiting language dominance in the right cerebral cortex. Note that both the left side and the right side of the brain are actively used by everyone. The two hemispheres constantly cross-reference their respective information with each other. However, there can be certain learning disorders in which the communication between the left cerebral cortex and the right cerebral cortex leads to confusion rather than order. An example is dyslexia, in which someone perceives a sequence of numbers, letters, or words in a reversed or even random order. This condition is 10 times more likely to be found in someone

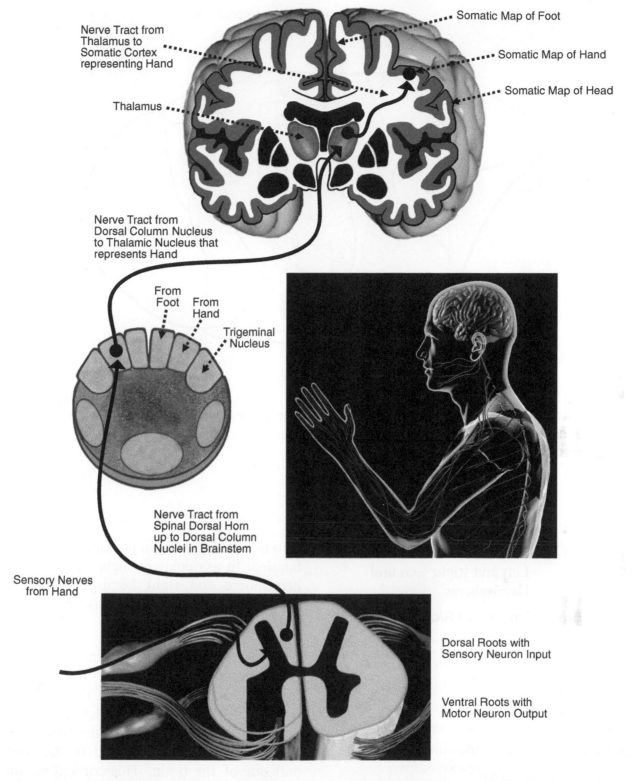

FIGURE 2.22 This series of images demonstrates the neural connections between somatic sensory messages about the body entering spinal nerves through the dorsal roots of the spinal cord. From there, electrical messages are sent up the dorsal column of the spinal cord to the dorsal column nucleus at the base of the brainstem. After synapsing there, neurophysiological messages next travel up to the somatosensory thalamus, synapse again, and then travel to the somatotopic somatic sensory cortex. Neurons representing sensory input from the head are found in the more peripheral portion of the parietal lobe that is above the auricle, whereas neurons representing sensory input from the feet are found in the more central and dorsal portion of the parietal lobe, with the rest of the body represented in between.

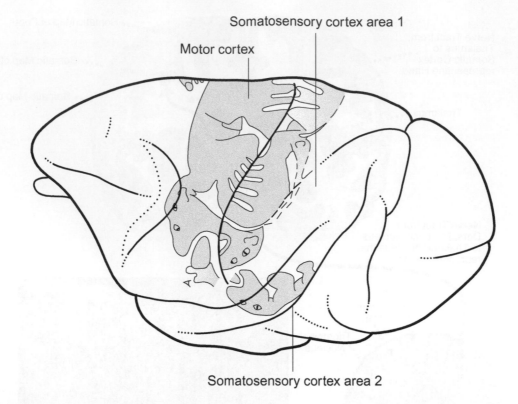

Motor cortex

Somatosensory cortex area 1

Somatosensory cortex area 2

FIGURE 2.23 The somatotopic organization of the human brain is also represented in lower animal species, which demonstrates that multiple representations of sets of neurons arranged in the same inverted fetus as found on the auricle are also found in other animals.

TABLE 2.5	Taoist Dualities in the Left and Right Cerebral Hemispheres.
Yang Left Brain Activity	**Yin Right Brain Activity**
Logical	Relational
Linguistic	Artistic
Linear	Circular
Literal	Symbolic
Sequential	Simultaneous
Word recognition	Identifies spatial relationships
Understands verbal meaning	Senses intonations and inflections
Name recognition	Facial recognition
Mathematical calculations	Musical rhythms
Analyzes details	Forms global impressions
Rational thinking	Emotional feeling
Abstract constructs	Metaphorical images

who is left-handed than in someone who is right-handed. In auricular medicine, problems of left hemisphere and right hemisphere interactions are referred to as laterality disorders or oscillation problems.

It sometimes confuses beginning practitioners of auriculotherapy that different body regions are represented contralaterally in the brain but are represented ipsilaterally on the ear. The explanation is that nerves originating from ear reflex points are centrally projected to the contralateral side of the brain. This cortical region then sends descending projections to the contralateral organ. Signals from the left ear cross to the right side of the brain and then cross back to the left side of the body. Conversely, a point on the right ear projects to the left brain, which then processes the information and activates homeostatic regulating mechanisms sent to the right side of the physical body.

A. Frontal View of Thalamus to Cortex

B. Angled View of Thalamus to Cortex

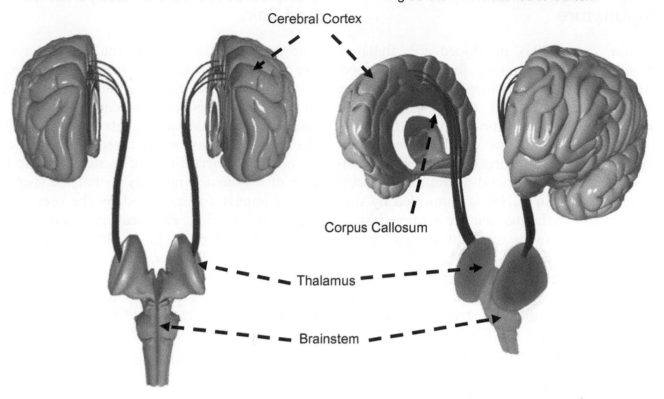

Cerebral Cortex

Corpus Callosum

Thalamus

Brainstem

C. Frontal View of Corpus Callosum

D. Angled View of Corpus Callosum

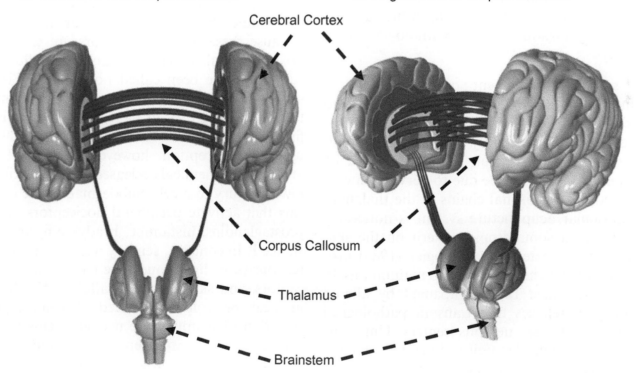

Cerebral Cortex

Corpus Callosum

Thalamus

Brainstem

FIGURE 2.24 This series of brain images depicts the different levels of the triune brain if it were pulled apart. The reptilian lower brain is at the base, the mammalian middle brain is immediately above it, and then long axon fibers connect the thalamus up to the cerebral cortex higher brain. The right and left sides of the cerebral hemispheres are connected by a band of fibers known as the corpus callosum.

Thalamic Neuron Theory of Acupuncture

Tsun-nin Lee (1994) developed the thalamic neuron theory to account for reflex connections between acupuncture points and the brain. According to this theory, pathological changes in peripheral tissue lead to malfunctioning firing patterns in the correspondent brain pathways. The natural organization of the connections between peripheral nerves and the central nervous system (CNS) is controlled by sites in the sensory thalamus that are arranged like a homunculus, an image of a "little man" within the functional patterning of thalamic neurons. The CNS institutes corrective measures intended to normalize the pathological neural circuits, but strong environmental stressors or intense emotions may cause the CNS circuitry to misfire. If the neurophysiological programs in the neural circuits are impaired, the peripheral disease becomes chronic. Pain and disease are thus attributed to maladaptive, dysfunctional patterns that are learned programs in these neural circuits. Stimulation of acupuncture points on the body or the ear can serve to induce a functional reorganization of these pathological brain pathways.

The spatial arrangement of these neuronal chains within the thalamic homunculus is said to account for the arrangement of acupuncture meridians in the periphery. The invisible meridians that purportedly run over the surface of the body may actually be due to nerve pathways projected onto neuronal chains in the thalamus. The auricular acupuncture system is noticeably arranged in a somatotopic pattern on the skin surface of the external ear. Nogier (1983) proposed that for a chronic illness to maintain itself, the disorder must be accompanied by altered neurological reflexes that transmit pathological messages to higher nervous centers. Until this dysfunctional neural circuit is corrected, somatic reflexes controlled by the brain will remain dysfunctional. Stimulation of correspondent somatotopic points on the ear sends messages to the brain that facilitate the correction of this pathological brain activity.

Peripheral Nerve Pathways for Touch and Pain

The fundamental units of the nervous system are the individual neurons, long slender threads of nerve fibers. Neurons are one of the few types of biological cells that can carry electrical signals. Body acupuncture points occur at regions underneath the skin where there is a nerve plexus or nervous innervations of a muscle. One feature of myelinated neurons is that the speed of neural impulses is increased by the presence of segments of high electrical resistance myelin separated by gaps of lower electrical resistance at the nodes of Ranvier. This aspect of neurons corresponds to the electrodermal feature of acupuncture points, a series of low skin resistance gaps separated by regions of high skin resistance non-acupuncture points.

Although it is the cause of much unwanted suffering, pain is nonetheless a biological necessity. Pain sensations trigger protective withdrawal reflexes essential for survival. The initiation of pain signals begins with the activation of microscopic neuron endings in the skin, the muscles, the joints, the blood vessels, or the viscera. Because these sensory receptors are excited by noxious stimuli, capable of damaging cellular tissue, they have been called nociceptors. Electric shock, intense heat, intense cold, or pinching of the skin all lead to an increase in the neuronal firing rate of these nociceptors. The natural stimulus for nociception, however, seems to be an array of biochemicals released into the skin following injury to a cell. Subdermal, acidic chemicals that activate peripheral nociceptors include prostaglandins, histamine, bradykinin, and substance P. In contrast, sensory neurons specifically responsive to light touch are called mechanoreceptors, and skin receptors affected by changes in heat or cold are called thermoreceptors. Insertion of acupuncture needles seems to activate nociceptors in deep muscles under body acupuncture points, whereas in ear acupuncture the nociceptors are located in the superficial skin surface.

Afferent sensory neuron fibers travel in bundles of nerves that project from the peripheral skin surface or from deep lying muscles to the CNS at the midline of the body. Each neuron is capable of rapidly carrying electrical neural impulses over long, anatomical distances, such as from the foot to the lower back or from the finger tips to the spinal cord in the neck. The neurons from mechanoreceptors, thermoreceptors, and nociceptors all travel along together, like the individual copper wires in an extension cord. However, the type of neuron carrying each type of message is different. The categories of neurons are distinguished by the size and the presence of myelin coating. The thinnest neurons, which have no myelin coating, are called type C fibers and tend to carry information about nociceptive pain. The next larger neurons are called type B fibers, which are larger and have some myelin coating. They typically carry information about skin temperature or internal organ activity.

Neurons that have the thickest diameter are called type A fibers. These type A neurons are myelinated and large in size, making them much faster than the type B and the type C fibers. They are further subdivided into myelinated type A beta fibers and type A delta fibers. The type A beta neurons carry information about light touch stimuli that activate mechanoreceptors, whereas the type A delta fibers, which are not as large nor as fast as the type A beta fibers, carry information about immediate, nociceptive pain. The type A delta fibers are still faster than the type C fibers, which also are activated by nociceptors. When one is hurt, there is the perception of first pain from rapid information carried by A delta fibers and the delayed perception of second pain that is carried by the slower type C fibers. First pain is immediate, sharp, and brief, like a pin prick, whereas second pain is more throbbing, aching, and enduring, such as when one is burned or hits one's hand with a hammer. Chronic pain sensations seem more related to type C fiber activity than type A delta fiber activity because type C fiber firing can summate over time rather than habituate. The fastest neurons are type A alpha fibers. These motor neurons carry electrical impulses from the spinal cord to the peripheral muscles, thus completing a sensorimotor reflex arc. Type A gamma motor neurons are affected by proprioceptive feedback in order to regulate muscle tone, which seems to be the source of the maintained muscle contractions that often cause myofascial pain.

Gate Control Theory of Descending Pain Inhibitory Systems

The spinal cord is divided into a more central gray matter core that is surrounded by white matter, so designated because the neurons in white matter are coated with white myelin. When cut into cross sections, the spinal cord gray matter looks like a butterfly, with a left and a right dorsal horn (posterior horn) and a left and a right ventral horn (anterior horn). Sensory neurons carrying nociceptive signals form synapses in the first and fifth layers of the ipsilateral, dorsal horn of the spinal cord. Messages concerning light touch form synapses in the fourth layer of the dorsal horn. The sensory messages about touch versus pain are then sent by long, myelinated axons up to the brain in two separate sections of the spinal cord white matter. Information about touch is carried in the long axon fibers of the dorsal column spinal cord, whereas information about nociceptive pain is carried in the long axon fibers of the anterolateral (ventrolateral) spinal cord. Impulses from the spinal cord travel up these respective regions of the white matter telegraph lines to carry differential information about touch and pain to higher brain centers.

In 1965, Ronald Melzack and Patrick Wall proposed that inhibitory interneurons in the dorsal horn of the spinal cord are differentially affected by input from type A fiber and type C fiber neurons. The fast-conducting type A beta axon fibers, which carry information about light touch, excite inhibitory interneurons that suppress the experience of pain. The slow-conducting type C axon fibers, which carry information about pain, inhibit these same inhibitory interneurons. The consequence of inhibiting a neuron that is itself inhibitory results in a further increase in neural discharges that ascend toward

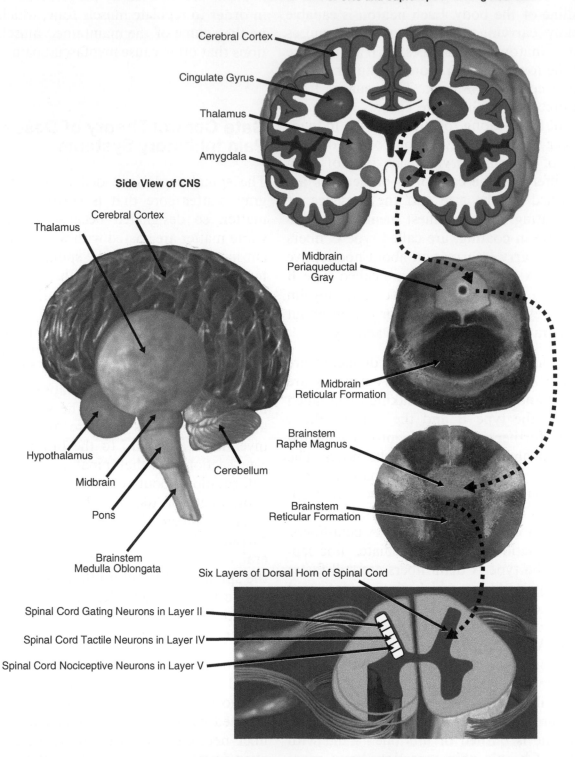

Cross View of CNS and Supra-Spinal Gating Neurons

Cerebral Cortex

Cingulate Gyrus

Thalamus

Amygdala

Side View of CNS

Cerebral Cortex

Thalamus

Midbrain
Periaqueductal
Gray

Midbrain
Reticular Formation

Brainstem
Raphe Magnus

Hypothalamus

Cerebellum

Midbrain

Brainstem
Reticular Formation

Pons

Brainstem
Medulla Oblongata

Six Layers of Dorsal Horn of Spinal Cord

Spinal Cord Gating Neurons in Layer II

Spinal Cord Tactile Neurons in Layer IV

Spinal Cord Nociceptive Neurons in Layer V

FIGURE 2.25 Since the 1970s, neuroscientists have discovered that the brain not only contains specific regions that can sense painful signals but also contains a pain inhibitory pathway. The cerebral cortex seems to play only a minimal part of this pathway. Other regions of the brain that do contribute to this descending neural pathway that can inhibit the ascending pain message include the cingulate gyrus, the amygdala, the thalamus, the midbrain periaqueductal gray, and the brainstem reticular formation. Neurons in layer IV of the spinal cord dorsal horn seem to exclusively respond to nonpainful light touch, whereas neurons in layer V of the spinal cord dorsal horn predominantly respond to painful, noxious stimuli. Interneurons in layers II and III of the spinal cord have the ability to turn off the pain-related neurons in layer V; thus, they are called pain gating neurons.

the brain. The dorsal horn gating cells allow only a brief burst of neural firing going up to the brain following their excitation by tactile type A beta neurons. When they are activated by nociceptive type C neurons, these same spinal gating cells lead to very prolonged neural firing going up to the brain. The increased brain activation by the lack of inhibition of type C neuron signals thus sustains the pain experience. The occurrence of brief versus prolonged bursts of neuronal firing accounts for differences in the perception of touch versus pain. Melzack and Wall also theorized that there were supraspinal gating systems in the brain. Specific areas of the brain send descending input to the spinal inhibitory neurons, which thus allow the brain to suppress the incoming pain messages.

Empirical support for the existence of descending pain inhibitory pathways was obtained in the 1970s with the pioneering research investigations at UCLA by Dr. John Liebeskind and Dr. David Mayer (Liebeskind *et al.*, 1974; Mayer *et al.*, 1971; Mayer and Liebeskind, 1974). Electrical stimulation of the midbrain periaqueductal gray (PAG) was found to suppress behavioral responses to noxious heat. One of the most surprising findings was that this stimulation-produced analgesia could be reversed by the opiate antagonist, naloxone. Although the PAG was the most potent region to produce analgesia in rats and cats, brain stimulation research in monkeys (Oleson and Liebeskind, 1978; Oleson *et al.*, 1980b) demonstrated that the thalamus was the most potent primate site to yield stimulation-produced analgesia. Examination of deep brain stimulation in human patients has shown similar findings (Hosobuchi *et al.*, 1979). Human research has confirmed that nociceptive pain messages activate positron emission tomography scan activity in the PAG, thalamus, hypothalamus, somatosensory cortex, and prefrontal cortex (Hseih *et al.*, 1995). These are the same brainstem and thalamic areas that are able to suppress pain messages. Although direct connections between auricular acupuncture points and these anti-nociceptive brain pathways have not yet been investigated, neurophysiological investigations of body acupuncture points suggest that

the regions of the brain related to pain inhibition are also affected by the stimulation of acupoints (Kho and Robertson, 1997).

The midbrain PAG was one of the first brain regions from which stimulation-produced analgesia was obtained. This descending system could also be activated by microinjections of morphine, which binds to opiate receptors that otherwise respond to endorphin neurotransmitters. Neurons in the dorsal raphe nuclei and raphe magnus can be excited by PAG stimulation. These serotonergic raphe neurons then descend the spinal cord in the dorsal lateral funiculus and synapse on gating cells in layer II of the dorsal horn. Basbaum and Fields (1984) showed that lesions in the descending, dorsolateral funiculus tract in the spinal cord blocked behavioral analgesia from deep brain stimulation. The raphe neurons release serotonin to excite the spinal gating cells, which then release the endorphin neurotransmitter enkephalin to inhibit nociceptive sensory neurons. A different descending pathway carries impulses from the reticular formation, releasing the neurotransmitter norepinephrine to activate the inhibitory gating cells in layer III of the dorsal horn. There is also a descending system in the CNS that makes pain sensations more intense. Wei *et al.* (1999) showed that destruction of descending, serotonergic pathways from the raphe magnus and the descending noradrenergic pathways from the locus coeruleus both lead to an increase in the Fos protein activity of nociceptive spinal neurons. Conversely, destruction of descending reticular gigantocellular pathways leads to a decrease in the Fos protein activity of nociceptive spinal neurons. The pain inhibition system was selectively damaged by the raphe and locus coeruleus lesions, whereas the pain facilitation system was disconnected by the reticular lesion. It is these same descending spinal pathways that affect acupuncture analgesia.

Afferent and Efferent Pathways for Acupuncture Analgesia

Two major CNS pathways lead to acupuncture analgesia—an afferent sensory pathway and an efferent motor pathway. Stimulation of acupuncture points activates the afferent pathway that travels from peripheral nerves into the spinal cord and then to the brain. Neurons in the afferent pathway connect to the efferent pathway, which then sends descending neurons down the spinal cord to inhibit nociceptive behavioral reflexes (Takeshige *et al.*, 1992). Two brain circuits related to acupuncture have been revealed by a series of experiments conducted by Takeshige (2001) in Japan and Han (2001) in the United States.

Afferent Acupuncture Pathway: This afferent pathway begins with stimulation of an acupuncture point in the skin that sends neural impulses to the spinal cord. These signals then ascend through the contralateral, ventrolateral tract of the spinal cord to the reticular gigantocellular nucleus and the raphe magnus in the medulla. The signal next goes to the dorsal PAG. Low-frequency (2 Hz) electrical stimulation of the acupoints LI 4 and ST 36 leads to behavioral analgesia, an elevation of tail flick latency, or an increase in the threshold for aversive reactions to foot shock. The intensity of electrical stimulation at an acupoint must be sufficient to cause muscle contraction. Stimulation of other muscle regions does not produce this increase in the tail flick latency associated with pain perception. Brain potentials can be evoked specifically in the PAG by stimulation of the muscles underlying the LI 4 and ST 36 acupoints, but not by stimulation of other muscles. These evoked potentials in the PAG were blocked by contralateral lesions of the anterolateral tract, by administration of an antiserum to endorphinergic molecule enkephalin, by the opiate antagonist naloxone, but not by the administration of antagonists to dynorphin. Moreover, lesions of the PAG abolished acupuncture analgesia, indicating that the anatomical integrity of the PAG is necessary for producing pain relief from acupuncture stimulation. This afferent pathway projects from the PAG to the posterior hypothalamus, the lateral hypothalamus, and the central, median nucleus of the thalamus. These neurons project through the hypothalamic preoptic area to the pituitary gland, from which beta-endorphins are secreted into the blood.

Efferent Acupuncture Pathway: The descending pain inhibitory system begins in a different area of the midbrain PAG than the afferent pathway. These efferent neurons project from the PAG to dopaminergic neurons in the posterior hypothalamic area and the ventromedian nucleus of the hypothalamus. This path then splits into a serotonergic system and a noradrenergic system, which descend down the spinal cord. The pathway for the efferent acupuncture system originates at non-acupoints and ends in the anterior part of the hypothalamic arcuate nucleus. Neurons from the ventral PAG synapse in the raphe magnus, which then travels down the spinal cord to release the neurotransmitter serotonin on to spinal gating cells. An alternative efferent pathway travels from the reticular paragigantocellularis nucleus down to spinal gating cells. Spinal interneurons produce either presynaptic inhibition or post-synaptic inhibition on the neuron that transmits pain messages to the brain, thus blocking the pain message.

Electroacupuncture Stimulation Frequencies

The opiate peptides enkephalin and dynorphin, two subfractions of the larger polypeptide molecule known as beta-endorphin, are activated by different frequencies of electroacupuncture. Analgesia produced by low-frequency (2 Hz) stimulation versus high-frequency (100 Hz) electroacupuncture was evaluated by Han (2001). Analgesia following low-frequency (2 Hz) electroacupuncture was selectively attenuated by enkephalin antibodies but not by dynorphin antibodies. In comparison, analgesia obtained by high-frequency (100 Hz) electroacupuncture was reduced by antibodies to dynorphin but not by antibodies to enkephalin. Han concluded that 2 Hz electroacupuncture activates enkephalin synapses, whereas 100 Hz electroacupuncture activates dynorphin synapses. Both forms of electroacupuncture produced more pronounced analgesia than needle insertion alone. In general, electrical stimulation of acupoints is almost always more effective than the simple insertion of acupuncture needles because the electroacupuncture repeatedly stimulates the acupoints, whereas the primary effect of needle acupuncture alone is the initial penetration of the skin.

Cranial Nerve Connections to the External Ear

There are four principal peripheral nerves that innervate the human ear. The distribution of nerves to different auricular regions is presented as follows.

Somatic Trigeminal Nerve: The auriculotemporal branch of the fifth cranial nerve is part of the somatic nervous system pathway that processes sensations from the face and controls some facial movements. The mandibular division of the trigeminal nerve is distributed across the antihelix and the surrounding auricular areas of the antitragus, scaphoid fossa, triangular fossa, and helix. This auricular region represents nervous tissue associated with musculoskeletal mesodermal organs.

Somatic Facial Nerve: The seventh cranial nerve is an exclusively motor division of the somatic nervous system, controlling most facial movements. It predominantly affects the posterior regions of the auricle that represent motor nerve control of mesodermal tissue.

Autonomic Vagus Nerve: The auricular branch of the tenth cranial nerve is the only instance in which the parasympathetic vagus nerve rises to the surface of the skin. The vagus nerve processes sensations from visceral organs in the head, the thorax, and the abdomen, and it controls the smooth muscle activity of the internal viscera. The vagus nerve extends throughout the concha of the ear and represents internal organs derived from visceral endodermal tissue.

Cerebral Cervical Plexus Nerves: A specific set of cervical nerves affect neuronal supply to the head, neck, and shoulder. The minor occipital nerve and the greater auricular nerve of the cervical plexus supply the ear lobe, tragus, and helix tail regions of the auricle. These auricular regions correspond to neurological ectodermal tissue.

Somatic and Autonomic Control of Physiological Functions

Somatic Control of Muscle Tension: There are two main divisions of the peripheral nervous system—the somatic nervous system and the autonomic nervous system. Myofascial pain is typically produced by the activation of somatic nerves exciting the contraction of muscle fibers to create muscle spasms. These muscle contractions become fixated, no matter what conscious efforts are exerted. Myofascial tension is the most common type of chronic pain, including back pain, headaches, shoulder pain, and joint aches. A muscle will not initiate a movement or maintain any action by itself. The muscle must first be stimulated by a motor neuron to cause it to contract. If one has rigidity and stiffness in a limb, neural reflexes are maintaining that postural pattern. The question becomes what factor would cause the brain to tell spinal motor neurons to sustain muscle contraction in a pathological state. The thalamic neuron theory of Lee and the writings by Nogier suggest that such chronic pain is due to a learned pathological reflex circuit established in the brain; it is that maladaptive brain circuit which unconsciously

TABLE 2.6	Taoist Dualities of Sympathetic and Parasympathetic Nerves.
Yang Sympathetic Arousal	**Yin Parasympathetic Sedation**
Utilization of energy	Conservation of energy
Rapid, shallow breathing	Slow, deep breathing
Rapid heart rate	Slow heart rate
Increased blood pressure	Lowered blood pressure
Peripheral vasoconstriction	Peripheral vasodilation
Cold hands	Warm hands
Sweaty hands	Dry hands
Increased skin conductance	Reduced skin conductance
Pupillary dilation	Pupillary constriction
Dry mouth	Increased salivation
Impaired digestion	Improved digestion
Diarrhea	Constipation
Muscle tension	Muscle relaxation

maintains chronic pain. Auriculotherapy can promote homeostatic balancing of that pathological brain–somatic nerve circuit.

Sympathetic Control of Blood Flow: Blood circulation and control of other visceral organs is regulated by the autonomic nervous system. Sympathetic arousal leads to peripheral vasoconstriction and a reduction of blood flow to that area. The localized skin surface reactions can be detected with auricular diagnosis. Symptoms such as white, flaky skin can be attributable to lack of blood because of micro-vasoconstriction. Auriculotherapy stimulation produces peripheral vasodilation, which patients often feel as a sensation of heat in the part of the body that corresponds to the points being treated. This treatment can therefore be used for Raynaud's disease, arthritis, and muscle cramps that are due to restricted blood circulation.

Sympathetic Control of Sweat Glands: The sympathetic control of sweat glands is also controlled by the autonomic nervous system (Hsieh, 1998; Young and McCarthy, 1998). Sweat is released when it is hot outside or when one is anxious. An electrodermal discharge from sweat glands can be recorded from skin surface electrodes. Selective changes in the electrical activity of the skin surface can be detected by an electrical point finder held over the auricle. Such devices reflect localized increases in skin conductance that are produced by the sympathetic nervous system, which innervates the sweat glands. Paradoxically, histological investigations of the skin overlying the auricle do not reveal the presence of any sweat glands, indicating that some other process must account for spatial differences in skin resistance at reactive ear reflex points.

Brain Activity Associated with Auricular Acupuncture

Direct evidence of the neurological effect of acupuncture stimulation on the human brain initially came from Z. H. Cho (Cho and Wong, 1998; Cho et al., 2001) at the University of California at Irvine. Recording functional magnetic resonance imaging (fMRI) of the human cerebral cortex, these investigators showed that needles inserted into a distal acupuncture point on the leg used for visual disorders could activate increased fMRI activity in the visual, occipital cortex, whereas needling a different acupuncture point activated the auditory, temporal lobe. If only tactile nerves were relevant to stimulation of acupuncture points in the skin, an increase in fMRI activity should have only been observed in the somatosensory, parietal cortex. More recent work by Cho has shown that experimentally induced pain leads to increased fMRI activity in the cingulate gyrus of the limbic brain, in the thalamus, and in the PAG. After the volunteer subjects were given acupuncture stimulation, this elevation of fMRI activity in each of these three brain regions was dramatically reduced, suggesting that body acupuncture inhibits the neurons in the brain that respond to pain.

Specificity of fMRI brain activity to auricular stimulation has been shown by Dr. David Alimi of France (Alimi, 2000; Alimi et al., 2002). Stimulation of the hand area of the auricle selectively altered fMRI activity in the hand region of the somatosensory cortex, whereas stimulation of a different area of the external ear did not produce this response. Similar correspondent changes were obtained in brain fMRI activity from stimulation of the elbow, knee, and foot regions of the auricle. Stimulation of specific areas of the auricle led to selective changes in the fMRI responses in the brain.

The areas of the brain that have been classically related to weight control include two regions of the hypothalamus. The ventromedial hypothalamus (VMH) has been referred to as a satiety center. When the VMH is lesioned, animals fail to restrict their food intake. In contrast, the lateral hypothalamus (LH) is referred to as a feeding center because stimulation of the LH induces animals to start eating food. Asamoto and Takeshige (1992) studied selective activation of the hypothalamic satiety center by auricular acupuncture in rats. Electrical stimulation of inner regions of the rat ear, which corresponds to auricular representation of the gastrointestinal tract, produced evoked potentials in the VMH satiety center but not in the LH feeding center. Stimulation of more peripheral regions of the rabbit ear did not activate hypothalamic evoked potentials, indicating the selectivity of auricular acupoint stimulation. Only the somatotopic auricular areas near the region representing the stomach caused these specific brain responses. The same auricular acupuncture sites that led to hypothalamic activity associated with satiety led to behavioral changes in food intake. Auricular acupuncture had no effect on weight in a different set of rats that had received bilateral lesions of the VMH. These results provide a compelling connection between auricular acupuncture and a part of the brain associated with neurophysiological regulation of feeding behavior.

In support of this evoked potential research, Shiraishi *et al.* (1995) recorded single-unit, neuronal discharge rates in the VMH and LH of rats. Neurons were recorded in the hypothalamus following electrical stimulation of low-resistance regions of the inferior concha Stomach point. Auricular stimulation tended to facilitate neuronal discharges in the VMH and inhibit neural responses in the LH. Out of 162 neurons recorded in the VMH, 44.4% exhibited increased neuronal discharge rates in response to auricular stimulation, 3.7% of VMH neurons exhibited inhibition, and 51.9% showed no change. Of 224 neurons recorded in the LH feeding center of 21 rats, 22.8% were inhibited by auricular stimulation, 7.1% were excited, and 70.1% were unaffected. When the analysis was limited to 12 rats

A. Frontal View of Limbic Brain

B. Angled View of Frontal View of Limbic Brain

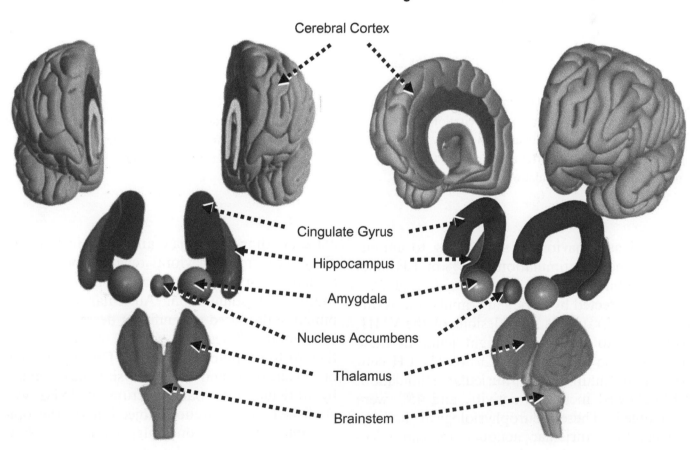

Cerebral Cortex

Cingulate Gyrus

Hippocampus

Amygdala

Nucleus Accumbens

Thalamus

Brainstem

FIGURE 2.26 This series of brain images depicts different subsections of the limbic brain, which collectively affects emotions, memory, and the perception of pain. Located both below and within the cerebral cortex, but above and outside of the thalamus and the brainstem, the limbic brain contains the following specific nuclei: the cingulate gyrus, the hippocampus, the amygdala, and the nucleus accumbens. fMRI studies in human volunteers have demonstrated significant changes in activity following stimulation with acupuncture.

A. Pre-Acupuncture fMRI Brain Activity to Pain

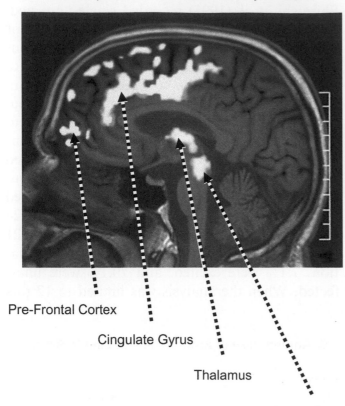

Pre-Frontal Cortex

Cingulate Gyrus

Thalamus

Periaqueductal Gray

B. Post-Acupuncture fMRI Brain Activity to Pain

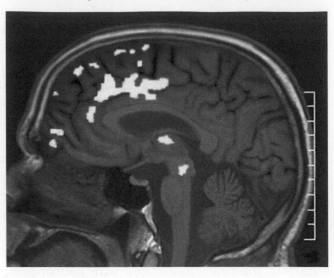

FIGURE 2.27 This fMRI image of the human brain is from a series of studies by Dr. Z. H. Cho. The lighter areas of the image indicate stronger neural excitation in that part of the brain. The images of the brain taken before acupuncture stimulation show much higher brain activity in the cingulate gyrus, the thalamus, and the periaqueductal gray than the fMRI images taken after acupuncture stimulation, suggesting that the acupuncture stimulation led to a reduced response to painful stimulation.

classified as behaviorally responding to auricular acupuncture stimulation, 49.5% of LH units were inhibited, 15.5% were excited, and 35% were not affected by auricular stimulation. A different set of rats was given lesions of the VMH, which led to significant weight gain. In these hypothalamic obese rats, 53.2% of 111 LH neurons were inhibited by auricular stimulation, 1.8% showed increased activity, and 45% were unchanged. These neurophysiological findings suggest that auricular acupuncture can selectively alter hypothalamic brain activity and is more likely to produce sensations of VMH satiety than reduction of LH appetite.

Fedoseeva *et al*. (1990) applied electrostimulation to the ear lobe of rabbits, on an area corresponding to the jaw and teeth in humans. They measured behavioral reflexes and cortical somatosensory evoked potentials in response to tooth pulp stimulation. Auricular electroacupuncture produced a significant decrease in both behavioral reflexes and cortical evoked potentials to tooth pulp stimulation. The suppression of behavioral and neurophysiological effects by auricular electroacupuncture at 15 Hz was abolished by intravenous injection of the opiate antagonist naloxone, suggesting endorphinergic mechanisms. Naloxone did not diminish the analgesic effect of 100 Hz stimulation frequencies. Conversely, injection of saralasin, an antagonist for angiotensin II, blocked the analgesic effect of 100 Hz auricular acupuncture but not 15 Hz stimulation. The amplitude of cortical potentials evoked by electrical stimulation of the hind limb was not attenuated by stimulation of the auricular area for the trigeminal nerve.

2.5 Endorphin and Neurochemical Changes Following Auricular Acupuncture

The natural pain-relieving biochemicals known as endorphins are identified as endogenous morphine substances. Enkephalin is a subfraction of the larger endorphin molecule, similar to a strand of 5 pearls in a necklace of more than 40 pearls. Enkephalin is a neurotransmitter occurring in the brain at the same sites where opiate receptors have been found. Both body acupuncture and ear acupuncture have been found to raise blood serum and cerebrospinal fluid (CSF) levels of endorphins and enkephalins (Pomeranz and Chiu, 1976; Sjolund *et al.*, 1977, 1996; Clemente-Jones *et al.*, 1979, 1980; Ng *et al.*, 1975, 1981; Ho *et al.*, 1978; Ho and Wen, 1989; Chen, 1993; Gao *et al.*, 2008, 2011, 2012). As stated in the previous section, naloxone is the opiate antagonist that blocks morphine, blocks endorphins, and also blocks the analgesia produced by the stimulation of auricular reflex points and body acupuncture points. The discovery by H. L. Wen and Cheung (1973) that auricular acupuncture facilitates withdrawal from narcotic drugs has led to a plethora of studies demonstrating the clinical use of this technique for substance abuse (Wen, 1977; Smith, 1988; Dale, 1993). Auricular electroacupuncture has also been shown to raise met-enkephalin levels in humans (Sjolund *et al.*, 1977; Clement-Jones *et al.*, 1979) and beta-endorphin levels in mice withdrawn from morphine (Ho *et al.*, 1978). Pomeranz (2001) reviewed the extensive research on the endorphinergic basis of acupuncture analgesia. He substantiated 17 arguments to justify the conclusion that endorphins have a scientifically verifiable role in explaining the pain-relieving effects of acupuncture.

Mayer *et al.* (1977) were the first investigators to provide scientific evidence that there is a neurophysiological and neurochemical basis for acupuncture in human subjects. Stimulation of the body acupuncture point LI 4 produced a significant increase in dental pain threshold. Acupuncture treatment raised dental pain threshold by 27.1%, whereas a no-treatment control group showed only a 6.9% increase in dental pain threshold. A total of 20 out of 35 acupuncture subjects reported that their pain thresholds increased by more than 20%, whereas only 5 out of 40 subjects in the control condition exhibited a 20% elevation of pain threshold. Statistically significant reversal of this elevated pain threshold was achieved by intravenous administration of 0.8 mg of intravenous naloxone, reducing the subject's pain threshold to the same level as that of a control group given saline. A double blind study by Ernst and Lee (1987) similarly found that there was a 27% increase in pain threshold after 30 minutes of electroacupuncture at LI 4. The analgesic effect induced by acupuncture in the Ernst and Lee study was also blocked by the intravenous injection of 0.8 mg of naloxone.

Contradictory findings with regard to the naloxone reversibility of acupuncture analgesia have been presented by Chapman *et al.* (1983). Differences in experimental design could account for some of the discrepancies, but a more probable explanation for the contrasting findings may be the low sample size employed in Chapman *et al.*'s research. Their study examined only 7 subjects in the experimental group given naloxone and 7 individuals in the control group given saline. Although all 14 subjects did exhibit significant analgesia with acupuncture stimulation at LI 4, they failed to obtain a statistically significant reversal in pain threshold by 1.2 mg of intravenous naloxone. The mean decrease in the electrical current levels needed to evoke pain was 4.8 microamps following naloxone administration, but it was only 0.4 microamps for the control group given saline administration. Although the mean change in pain threshold difference between groups was small, it might have reached statistical significance with a much larger sample size.

The aforementioned studies all obtained acupuncture analgesia with acupoint LI 4 located on the hand. Simmons and Oleson (1993) examined naloxone reversibility of auricular acupuncture analgesia to dental pain induced in human subjects. Utilizing a Stim Flex 400 transcutaneous electrical stimulation unit, 40 subjects were randomly assigned to be treated at either eight auricular points specific for dental pain or eight placebo points—ear regions that have not been associated with dental pain. All subjects were assessed for tooth pain threshold by a dental pulp tester at baseline, after auriculotherapy, and then again after double blind injection of 0.8 mg of naloxone or placebo saline. Four treatment groups consisted of true auricular electrical stimulation (AES) followed by an injection of naloxone, true AES followed by an injection of saline, placebo stimulation of the auricle followed by an injection of naloxone, or placebo stimulation of the auricle followed by an injection of saline. Dental pain thresholds were significantly increased by AES conducted at appropriate auricular points for dental pain, but they were not altered by sham stimulation at inappropriate auricular points. Naloxone produced a slight reduction in dental pain threshold in the subjects given true AES, whereas the true AES subjects then given saline showed a further increase in pain threshold. The minimal changes in dental pain threshold shown by the sham auriculotherapy group were not significantly affected by saline or by naloxone. Research by Oliveri et al. (1986) and Krause et al. (1987) has also demonstrated statistically significant elevation of pain threshold by transcutaneous auricular stimulation, whereas Kitade and Hyodo (1979) and Lin (1984) found increased pain relief by needles inserted into the auricle. These earlier investigations of auricular analgesia did not test for the effects of naloxone.

Direct evidence of the endorphinergic basis of auriculotherapy was first provided by Sjolund and Eriksson (1976) and by Abbate et al. (1980). Assaying plasma beta-endorphin concentrations in subjects undergoing surgery, they observed a significant increase in beta-endorphins after acupuncture stimulation was combined with nitrous oxide inhalation, whereas control subjects given nitrous oxide without acupuncture showed no such elevation of endorphins. Pert et al. (1981) demonstrated that 7 Hz electrical

stimulation through needles inserted into the concha of the rat produced an elevation of hot plate threshold, an analgesic effect that was reversed by naloxone. The behavioral analgesia to auricular electroacupuncture was accompanied by a 60% increase in radioreceptor activity in CSF levels of endorphins. This auricular-induced elevation in endorphin level was significantly greater than was found in a control group of rats. Concomitant with these CSF changes, auricular electroacupuncture produced depletion in beta-endorphin radioreceptor activity in the VMH and the medial thalamus but not in the PAG. Supportive findings in human back pain patients were obtained by Clement-Jones et al. (1980). Low-frequency electrical stimulation of the concha led to relief of pain within 20 minutes of the onset of electroacupuncture and an accompanying elevation of radioassays for CSF beta-endorphin activity in all 10 subjects. Abbate et al. (1980) examined endorphin levels in six patients undergoing thoracic surgery with 50% nitrous oxide and 50 Hz auricular electroacupuncture. They were compared to six control patients who underwent surgery with 70% nitrous oxide but no acupuncture. The auricular acupuncture patients needed less nitrous oxide than the control participants. Moreover, acupuncture led to a significant increase in beta-endorphin immunoreactivity.

Extending the pioneering work of H. L. Wen and Michael Smith on the benefits of the auricular acupuncture for opiate addicts, Kroening and Oleson (1985) examined auricular electroacupuncture in chronic pain patients. Fourteen subjects were first switched from their original analgesic medication to an equivalent dose of oral methadone, typically 80 mg per day. An electrodermal point finder was used to determine areas of low skin resistance for the Lung point and the Shen Men point. Needles were bilaterally inserted into these two ear points and electrical stimulation was initiated between two pairs of needles. After 45 minutes of electroacupuncture, the patients were given periodic injections of small doses of naloxone (0.04 mg every 15 minutes). All 14 patients were withdrawn from methadone within 2–7 days, yielding a mean of

4.5 days. Only a few patients reported minimal side effects, such as mild nausea or slight agitation. It was proposed that occupation of opiate receptor sites by narcotic drugs leads to the inhibition of the activity of natural endorphins, whereas auricular acupuncture facilitates withdrawal from these drugs by activating the release of previously suppressed endorphins.

Other biochemical changes also accompany auricular acupuncture. Debreceni (1991) examined changes in plasma adrenocorticotropic hormone (ACTH) and growth hormone (GH) levels after 20 Hz electrical stimulation through needles inserted into the Chinese Adrenal Gland point on the tragus of the ears of 20 healthy females. Whereas GH secretions increased after electroacupuncture, ACTH levels remained the same. Jaung-Geng *et al.* (1995) evaluated lactic acid levels from pressure applied to ear vaccaria seeds positioned over the Liver, Lung, San Jiao, Endocrine, and Thalamus (Subcortex) points. The authors used a within-subjects design, wherein an individual's response to a stimulus was compared to that same person's response to a different stimulus—pressure applied to ear points. Acupressure at the appropriate auricular acupoints produced significantly lower levels of lactic acid following physical exercise on a treadmill test than when ear seeds were placed over the same auricular points but not pressed. Stimulation of auricular acupressure points reduced the toxic buildup of lactic acid to a greater degree than the control condition. The reduced lactic acid accumulation was attributed to improved peripheral blood circulation.

As indicated in Table 2.7, the dualistic principles of Taoism can be used to distinguish the arousing and sedating qualities of different hormones and different neurotransmitters. The pituitary and tropic hormones related to adrenalin, cortisol, thyroxin, and testosterone all induce general arousal and energy activation, whereas the contrasting hormones endorphin, GH, parathormone, estrogen, and progesterone all promote a quieting response or metabolic nurturance. The neurotransmitter glutamate produces excitatory post-synaptic potentials throughout the brain,

TABLE 2.7	Taoist Dualities of Hormones and Neurotransmitters.
Yang Arousing Neurochemicals	**Yin Sedating Neurochemicals**
Adrenalin for general arousal	Endorphin for pain relief
ACTH and cortisol for stress arousal	Melatonin for sleep cycles
TSH and thyroxin for metabolism	Parathormone for calcium
FSH and testosterone for sexual arousal	Estrogen and progesterone for seduction
Glutamate excitation of synapses	GABA inhibition of synapses
Sympathetic norepinephrine	Parasympathetic acetylcholine
Dopamine for pleasure arousal	Serotonin for calming comfort

whereas the neurotransmitter gamma-aminobutyric acid (GABA) produces inhibitory post-synaptic potentials throughout the brain. Glutamate thus excites brain neurons into greater firing rates and increased cortical arousal, whereas GABA reduces the firing activity of brain neurons and thus leads to slower brain activity. Norepinephrine is released by post-ganglionic axon fibers in the adrenergic, sympathetic nervous system to activate general arousal, whereas acetylcholine is released by postganglionic axon fibers in the cholinergic, parasympathetic nervous system to facilitate physiological relaxation. In the brain, dopamine tends to increase motor excitation and intensely pleasurable feelings, whereas enkephalin activates opiate receptors to both reduce pain and induce a calming sense of bliss.

Opiate Activity in Acupuncture Analgesia

The afferent acupuncture pathway produces a type of analgesia that is naloxone-reversible, disappears after hypophysectomy, persists long after stimulation of the acupoint is terminated, and exhibits individual variation in effectiveness. In this first pathway, electrical brain potentials are evoked by stimulation of acupoints in the same areas that produce analgesia. In contrast, stimulation of brain areas associated with the efferent acupuncture pathway produce analgesia that is not naloxone-reversible, is not affected by hypophysectomy, and is found only during the period of electrical stimulation. Because hypophysectomy only disrupts the activity of the first pathway, the second pathway can function without the presence of endorphin. Microinjection of either beta-endorphin or morphine into the hypothalamus produces analgesia in a dose-dependent manner, whereas microinjections of naloxone to the hypothalamic arcuate nucleus tends to antagonize acupuncture analgesia in a dose-dependent manner.

Adrenal Activity and Acupuncture Analgesia

Acupuncture analgesia and stimulation-produced analgesia are both abolished after removal of the adrenal glands. Electroacupuncture produces significant increases of beta-endorphin and ACTH released by the pituitary gland into the peripheral bloodstream. There is a steady release of both peptides for more than 80 minutes after termination of acupuncture stimulation; this increase in peptides gradually diminishes thereafter. Electroacupuncture applied to a donor rat was able to induce behavioral analgesia in a crossed-circulated recipient rat. An increase of endorphins in the CSF after electroacupuncture suggests that there may be a correlation between cerebral and peripheral beta-endorphin levels. Beta-endorphin and ACTH are co-released from the pituitary gland after an animal is stressed. Endorphins are most renowned for their pain-relieving qualities, whereas ACTH and cortisol are more associated with neurobiological responses to stress. They can reach levels high enough to activate long periods of stimulation of the acupuncture analgesia pathways.

Neurotransmitters in Acupuncture Analgesia

Acupuncture's pain-relieving effects can be abolished by concurrent lesions of the raphe nucleus and the reticular paragigantocellular nucleus. These are the known origins of the serotonergic and the noradrenergic descending pain-inhibitory systems. Synaptic transmission from the arcuate hypothalamus to the VMH is facilitated by dopamine agonists and is blocked by dopamine antagonists. Neurons in the VMH that respond to acupoint stimulation also respond to microinjections of dopamine into that part of the brain. Conversely, neurons in the arcuate hypothalamus that do not respond to acupoint stimulation also do not respond to iontophoretically administered dopamine.

Neurochemicals in the brain that tend to exhibit more yang arousing properties are shown in Table 2.7, where they are contrasted with complementary neurochemicals that tend to exhibit more yin sedating properties. Adrenalin accompanies sympathetic arousal responses, such as increased heart palpations and sweating, whereas the release of endorphins leads to a sense of calm relaxation and a reduction in pain perception. Cortisol and its pituitary trigger ACTH are released during times of great stress, whereas the highest levels of the hormone melatonin are found during the middle of the night when we are asleep. Thyroxin and its pituitary trigger thyroid-stimulating hormone (TSH) are released in high amounts when metabolic rates are high, whereas the parathyroid gland that is located nearby in the neck conserves body resources for calcium. The classical distinction between males and females is that when male testosterone levels are high, there is an increase in masculine aggressiveness and sexuality (whether in a male or in a female), whereas female estrogen levels are associated with feminine receptivity for sex and more passive tendencies. The two most frequent neurochemicals throughout the brain are glutamate and GABA. Most synapses have both neurotransmitters, but with opposing effects. Activation of glutamate receptors leads to increased electrical excitation of that neuron, whereas activation of GABA receptors leads to decreased electrical excitation of that neuron. Direct application of norepinephrine leads to increased heart rate and to increased neuronal firing throughout the brain, particularly the prefrontal cortex and reticular formation. Acetylcholine produces a slowing of the heart and has more selective effects in the brain. The neurotransmitter dopamine is associated with pleasurable arousal, whereas the substance serotonin is most associated with the ability to fall asleep and reduce pain.

2.6 Integrating Energetic and Physiological Views of Auriculotherapy

There has been great interest by some investigators of alternative and complementary medicine that suggests that continued neurophysiological research will ultimately provide a more scientific basis for acupuncture and auriculotherapy. The discovery of endorphins in the 1970s provided a biochemical mechanism that could account for the amazing observation that injecting the blood or CSF from one laboratory animal to another could also transfer the analgesic benefits of acupuncture to the second animal. The neuroanatomical pathways that comprise the descending pain inhibitory systems can biologically account for the pain-relieving effects of both opiate analgesia and acupuncture analgesia. The fMRI studies of the human brain have demonstrated neural changes in the brain that are related to stimulation of a particular acupoint on the body or on the ear. At the same time, many practitioners of the field of traditional Oriental medicine maintain a deep belief in the energetic principles that were developed in ancient times. Whether viewed as a self-contained micro-acupuncture system, a conduit to macro-acupuncture meridians, ashi points, or the quantum physics of holograms, there is sufficient reason to suggest that an unconventional energy profoundly affects the healing benefits of auricular acupuncture and body acupuncture. Western scientists seem to prefer the neurophysiological perspective, whereas individuals trained in Oriental medicine more readily accept an energetic viewpoint. Both may be correct when all the details are ultimately known.

After Nogier first discovered the inverted fetus map on the ear in the 1950s, the subsequent investigations of the inverted auricular cartography took somewhat divergent paths in Europe and China. Although there is great overlap in the correspondent points shown in the Chinese and European auricular maps, there are also specific differences. There is a tendency by many individuals to feel the need to choose one system over the other. In my discussions on the subject, I have promoted the acceptance and integration of both systems as clinically valid and therapeutically useful. It seems paradoxical that opposite observations could both be correct, but such is the nature in many parts of life. At the 1999 meeting of the International Consensus Conference on Acupuncture, Auriculotherapy, and Auricular Medicine, I cited the work of Rudyard Kipling's classic poem, *The Ballad of East and West*. The first line of the following phrase is well-known to many, yet it is the rest of the poem that gives this work even greater relevance to the understanding of the different theoretical views of auriculotherapy:

Oh, East is East, and West is West, and never the twain shall meet

Till earth and sky stand presently at god's great judgment seat;

But there is neither East nor West, nor border, nor breed, nor birth,

When two strong men stand face to face, tho' they come from the ends of the earth.

—Rudyard Kipling

■ KEY TERMS FOR CHAPTER 2

Key Terms for Microsystem Theories

Abdominal Microsystem: Similar to the midline systems of the face, nose, and tongue, an additional microsystem can be perceived by palpating areas of tenderness on specific areas of the abdomen, with the correspondence between inner organs and the body surface reflecting an upright representation rather than an inverted representation. The most tender spots on the abdomen can be needled or warmed with moxa.

Cutaneo-Organic Reflexes: Stimulating the skin at a microsystem acupoint produces homeostatic internal changes that lead to the relief of pain and the healing of the corresponding organ.

Dental Microsystem: A complete representation of all regions of the body on the teeth has been reported by German investigator, Voll. He correlated specific teeth with specific organs. The teeth are first divided into four equal quadrants: right upper jaw, left upper jaw, right lower jaw, and left lower jaw. Urogenital organs and the lower limbs are represented on the more central teeth, whereas thoracic organs and the upper limbs are represented on the more peripheral molars.

Embryo Containing the Information of the Whole Organism (ECIWO): The Chinese doctor Ying-Qing Zhang described several microsystems that are found along all long bones of the body. Each region on these bones was said to represent 12 different body regions in a somatotopic pattern.

Face and Nose Microsystems: Chinese microsystems on the face and nose are oriented in an upright position, with the head and neck on the forehead, the lungs between the eyebrows, the heart between the eyeballs, the liver and spleen on the nose, the digestive organs over the cheeks, the upper limbs across the upper jaw, and the lower limbs over the lower jaw. The nose microsystem is very similar, except that representations of all body organs are compressed onto the ridges of the nose.

Foot Reflexology: This somatotopic system represents specific areas of the body upon the feet.

Hand Reflexology: The American hand reflexology system corresponds to the somatotopic pattern that was first described on the foot. The tips of the fingers represent the head, the second digit the neck, and the metacarpals reflect the body and internal organs.

Hirata Microsystems: The Japanese clinician Kurakishi Hirata postulated that there were seven micro-acupuncture zones on the body surface—the head, face, neck, abdomen, back, arms, and legs—that manifested dysfunctions of 12 internal organs.

Ipsilateral Representation: Most microsystem points are more reactive over the microsystem area that is ipsilateral (on the same side) to the side of the body that is the source of pathology.

Koryo Hand Therapy: The Korean acupuncturist Tae Woo Yoo described a set of correspondence points on the hand that are somewhat different than the hand reflexology charts. In the Korean microsystem, the whole body is contained on each hand. The spine is represented along the middle finger, the arms are represented on the second and fourth fingers, and the legs are represented on the thumb and little finger of each hand.

Macro-Acupuncture Systems: The traditional macro-acupuncture meridians that are most commonly referred to in Traditional Chinese Medicine.

Micro-Acupuncture Systems: A self-contained system within the whole acupuncture system of meridian channels that stretch out over the whole body.

Mu Alarm Points and Shu Transport Points: The front mu and the back shu channels consist of 12 acupoints that resonate with one of 12 principal organs—the lung, heart, liver, spleen, stomach, intestines, bladder, and kidney.

Organo-Cutaneous Reflexes: Pathology in an organ of the body produces an alteration in the cutaneous microsystem region where that correspondent organ is represented.

Reflexology: The systematic arrangement of areas on the foot and on the hand that correspond to specific areas of the body.

Remote Reflex Response: Neurological reflexes connect to remote areas of the body that are located at a considerable distance from the site of stimulation.

Scalp Microsystem: Scalp acupuncture was known in ancient China and several modern systems have subsequently evolved. Scalp micro-acupuncture has been shown to be particularly effective in treating strokes and cerebral–vascular conditions. The inverted body pattern represented on the scalp reportedly activates reflexes in the ipsilateral, cerebral cortex that lies just underneath the area of the skull where the scalp acupuncture point is needled.

Somatotopic Inversion: The microsystem body map is configured in an inverse pattern.

Somatotopic Reiteration: A reflex map of the body that repeats the anatomical arrangement of the whole body. The term *soma* refers to the word "body," whereas *topography* refers to the mapping of the terrain of an area.

Tongue and Pulse Microsystems: The tongue and pulse diagnostic systems used in classical Chinese medicine can also be viewed as microsystems. The distal position of the radial pulse correlates to the heart and lungs, the middle position correlates to the digestive organs, and the proximal position correlates to the kidneys. In the tongue microsystem, the heart is at the tip of the tongue, the lung in the front, the spleen at the center, the kidney at the back of the tongue, and the liver along the sides.

Key Terms for Holographic Images

Holographic Model of the Brain: The neurobiologist Karl Pribram utilized the model of the hologram to explain the enormous memory capacity stored in many parts of the brain. Individual neurons in different parts of the brain can create interference pattern images of what the whole brain can remember.

Holographic Perspective of Subatomic Particles: The British physicist David Bohm suggested that subatomic particles can remain in contact with one another. He argued that such particles are not individual entities to begin with but are actually extensions of the same subatomic dimension.

Holographic Photography: A hologram is created when uniform, laser light is split into separate beams and bounced off the object being photographed. The collision of reflected laser beams generates an interference pattern on holographic film. Each part of the holographic film negative contains an image of the whole object that was photographed.

The Holographic Universe: Michael Talbot proposed that the human brain and subatomic particles are all part of a holographic continuum. Human brains seem to mathematically construct objective reality by resonating with frequencies that are projections from another dimension.

Key Terms for Traditional Chinese Medicine

Ashi Points: This term literally means the word "Ouch!" when a tender area of the body is touched. There is a strong grimace or facial flinch reaction when a reactive microsystem region of an auricular acupoint is palpated.

Five Oriental Elements: This Chinese energetic system organizes the universe into five essential categories or forces: wood, fire, earth, metal, and water. The metaphorical descriptions of these five elements reflect the poetry and rhythm of the Chinese language in their attempts to understand the complexities of different health conditions.

Meridian Channels: The invisible lines of energy that allow the circulation of qi and blood along an array of acupuncture points. Acupuncture meridians are also called channels.

Qi: An invisible energy that refers to a vital life force, a primal power, and a subtle essence that sustains all existence. Qi is both matter and the energy force that moves matter. Both auricular acupoints and body acupuncture points can facilitate the flow of qi.

Qi Deficiency: Occurs when the flow of qi or blood is abnormally low, such as when there is poor blood circulation in one's extremities, low blood pressure, muscle weakness, or a lack of energy. Clinical manifestations include tiredness, breathlessness, a weak voice, a pale tongue, and a slow or empty pulse.

Qi Excess: Occurs when the flow of qi or blood is abnormally high, such as when there is swelling, heat, high blood pressure, or muscle spasms. Clinical manifestations include fever, agitation, anger, insomnia, a red tongue, and a rapid, full pulse.

Qi Stagnation: Occurs when qi and blood stay in one place for too long, becoming abnormally congested, such as with lung congestion or with muscle spasms that will not release their contraction. Clinical manifestations include feeling distension, fluid accumulation, mood swings, irritability, a purple tongue, and a wiry or tight pulse. These symptoms are often related to a cold environment or to blocked emotions.

San Jiao: This term has been translated as Triple Warmer, Triple Heater, Triple Burner, and Triple Energizer. The torso of the body is distinguished by three regions: the upper jiao (the chest region that regulates circulatory and respiratory functions), the middle jiao (the upper abdominal region that affects digestive functions), and the lower jiao (the lower abdominal region that affects sexual and excretory functions).

Shen: The Chinese term for the human spirit is Shen. The Shen Men point (Gateway to the Spirit) is one of the most widely used points in all of auriculotherapy.

Tao: The philosophy of Taoism (Daoism) proposes that the cosmos is composed of two opposing and complementary qualities, yin and yang. Both auricular and body acupuncture are utilized to achieve a harmonious balance of yin and yang.

Wind: A pathogenic factor that affects health and disease, such as when wind invades the body due to cold or dampness, impacting blood, yin, and defensive qi.

Yang Alarm Reactions: Reactive ear reflex points exhibit increased electrical conductance and heightened tenderness when there is pathology in the corresponding body organ.

Yang Qi: Like the warm, bright light of the sun, yang qi is said to be strong, forceful, vigorous, exciting, and active. Yang meridian channels have direct connections to the ear.

Yin Qi: Like the soft, gentle light of the moon, yin qi is said to be serene, quiet, restful, and nurturing. The yin meridians connect to the auricle through corresponding yang meridians.

Zang–Fu Organs: Each of the five elements is related to two types of internal organs, zang and fu. Acupuncture channels reportedly connect the zang–fu organs with each other. The zang meridians tend to run along the inner side of the arms and legs and up the front of the body. The fu meridians run along the outer side of the limbs and down the back of the body. It is these fu meridians that rise to the head which have direct connections to the auricle. The six fu meridians include the Small Intestine, Large Intestine, Stomach, Urinary Bladder, and Gall Bladder channels. The six zang meridians are the Lung, Heart, Liver, Spleen, Kidney, and Pericardium channels, which only indirectly connect to the ear.

Key Terms for Neurophysiological Areas Related to Auriculotherapy

A Beta Fibers: Large-diameter, myelinated neurons carry rapid information about tactile stimuli from the skin or muscles to the spinal cord and brain.

A Delta Fibers: Moderate-diameter, myelinated neurons carry rapid information about superficial tissue pain messages from the skin or muscles to the spinal cord and brain.

Afferent Acupuncture Pathway: The afferent pathway for acupuncture begins with stimulation of an acupuncture point in the skin that sends neural impulses to the spinal cord. These signals then ascend through the contralateral, ventrolateral tract of the spinal cord to the reticular formation and the raphe nuclei in the brainstem. The signal next goes to the PAG and then projects from the PAG to the thalamus and hypothalamus. Hypothalamic neurons project to the pituitary gland, from which endorphin hormones can be secreted into the blood.

Autonomic Vagus Nerve: The tenth cranial nerve is a branch of the parasympathetic division of the autonomic nervous system. The vagus nerve carries sensations from visceral, internal organs and controls the smooth muscle activity of the internal viscera. Vagus nerve fibers spread throughout the concha of the ear.

Brain Computer Model: If the brain is compared to a master, central computer, then the auricle and all other microsystem centers can be viewed as different computer terminals, each with their own access to the central brain computer and from there to other parts of the body.

Brain Imaging and Acupuncture Stimulation: fMRI of the human cerebral cortex has shown that needles inserted into a distal acupuncture point on the leg could selectively activate fMRI activity in the visual, occipital cortex or the auditory, temporal cortex.

Brain Processing Centers: The overall organization of the brain is divided into a lower brainstem, a middle border brain, and the higher cerebral cortex. Spinal pathways connect peripheral nerves to the brainstem at the medulla, pons, and then the midbrain. Brainstem projections are sent to the thalamus and finally to the cerebral cortex.

C Fibers: Thin-diameter neurons, with no myelin coating, carry information about deeper destructive pain messages from the skin or muscles to the spinal cord and brain.

Central Nervous System: The brain and the spinal cord, which receive sensory messages from the eyes, ears, skin, and internal organs, internally assess and process that information and then send out commands through motor neurons to activate some behavior.

Cerebral Cervical Plexus Nerves: This set of cervical nerves affects neuronal supply to the head, neck, and shoulder. The lesser occipital nerve and the greater auricular nerve of the cervical plexus supply the ear lobe, tragus, and helix tail regions of the auricle.

Cerebral Laterality: A broad band of neuronal axon fibers that are called the corpus callosum serve to bridge the space between the two sides of the brain. The left side of the neocortex controls the right side of the body, which understands logic, language, and math, whereas the right side of the higher brain monitors the left side of the body and recognizes facial features.

Contralateral Crossing in the Brain: Sensory messages from different regions of the body are sent to the contralateral brain and behavioral messages from the motor cortex cross over at the brainstem and control the opposite side of the body. Ipsilateral representation on the auricle suggests that the messages cross from the body to the opposite brain area but then cross again back to the original side of the body where there is pathology.

Descending Pain Inhibitory Systems: Activation of supraspinal gating cells in the brain can send neuronal messages to spinal gating cells in the spinal cord, which can thus suppress incoming pain messages, preventing them from reaching the brain.

Efferent Acupuncture Pathway: The descending pain inhibitory system for acupuncture begins in the midbrain PAG, which then projects to neurons in the posterior hypothalamus and the ventromedial hypothalamus. The hypothalamus subsequently activates a serotonin system and a norepinephrine system that descend the spinal cord, blocking pain messages through the activation of spinal gating cells.

Gate Control Theory: Inhibitory interneurons in the dorsal horn of the spinal cord are differentially affected by input from type A axon fibers and type C axon fibers. The fast-conducting type A beta axon fibers carry information about light touch and excite inhibitory interneurons that suppress the experience of pain. The type A delta axon fibers carry information about acute pain, such as from a needle prick. Slow-conducting type C neurons carry information about prolonged pain. These type C neurons inhibit the inhibitory interneurons, which thus leads to prolonged neural firing in the spinal cord pain pathways to the brain.

Neurons: The fundamental units of the nervous system are the individual neurons, which are long slender threads of nerve tissue that can carry electrical signals along axon fibers. Ear acupoints are associated with neurons found in the skin covering the auricle, not in the cartilage.

Nociceptors: Pain sensations trigger protective withdrawal reflexes essential for survival. Because these sensory receptors are excited by noxious stimuli (stimuli capable of damaging cellular tissue), they have been called nociceptors. The natural stimulus for nociception seems to be an array of acidic biochemicals released into the skin following an injury.

Peripheral Nerve Pathways: Sensory neuron fibers travel in bundles of nerves that project from the peripheral skin surface toward the spinal cord and central nervous system.

Somatic Facial Nerve: The seventh cranial nerve is an exclusively motor division of the somatic nervous system, controlling most facial movements. It supplies the posterior regions of the auricle that represent motor nerve control of musculoskeletal tissue.

Somatic Trigeminal Nerve: The fifth cranial nerve is part of the somatic nervous system pathway that processes sensations from the face and controls some facial movements. It innervates the antihelix and anatomical regions on surrounding areas of the auricle.

Somatotopic Brain Map: When the brain of a patient undergoing neurosurgery is electrically excited, stimulation of specific cortical areas is evoked in specific parts of the patient's body.

Spinal Cord Pathways: Sensory neurons carrying nociceptive pain signals synapse in the first and fifth layers of the dorsal horn of the spinal cord, whereas messages responding to light touch lead to synapses in the fourth layer of the dorsal horn. Touch signals are carried in the dorsal columns of the spinal cord, whereas nociceptive pain is carried in the ventrolateral tract of the spinal cord.

Stimulation-Produced Analgesia: Electrical stimulation of the midbrain PAG suppresses behavioral responses to noxious stimuli. Such analgesia can be reversed by the chemical opiate antagonist, naloxone.

Key Terms for Neurochemicals Associated with Auricular Acupuncture

Acetylcholine: The neurotransmitter that is utilized in the parasympathetic nervous system that is associated with rest, relaxation, and improved digestion and greater circulation. At synapses in the brain, acetylcholine is involved with memory and with dream activity.

Adrenal Glands: Acupuncture analgesia and stimulation-produced analgesia are both abolished after removal of the adrenal glands. These glands release either adrenalin or cortisol, thus they are related to aroused actions in response to emergencies or to prolonged stress.

Adrenocorticotropic Hormone (ACTH): Hormone released by the pituitary gland that stimulates the release of cortisol from the adrenal gland in response to stress.

Dopamine: The primary neurotransmitter in the brain that is related to pleasurable feelings and substance abuse. All addictive substances that are used as recreational drugs by humans have the ability to activate synaptic receptors for dopamine.

Endorphins: The endogenous pain-relieving biochemicals that form a natural substance similar to morphine and are found in the pituitary gland and the central nervous system. Acupuncture and physical exercise can lead to the release of endorphins into the blood.

Enkephalin: A subfraction of the larger endorphin molecule. Both body acupuncture and ear acupuncture have been found to raise blood serum and cerebrospinal fluid levels of endorphins and enkephalins.

GABA (Gamma-Aminobutyric Acid): The primary inhibitory neurotransmitter in the brain that opens the synaptic gates for negatively charged chloride ions, thus causing neurons to fire less frequently. Alcohol, barbiturates, and benzodiazepines are external substances that activate GABA receptors, which therefore lead to the reduction in neural firing rates in certain brain regions and ultimately lead to sleep.

Glutamate: The primary excitatory neurotransmitter in the brain opens the synaptic gates for positively charged sodium ions, which causes neurons to fire more frequently.

Naloxone: The opiate antagonist substance that can block acupuncture analgesia in addition to its ability to block the analgesic action of opiate medications and brain stimulation-produced analgesia.

Norepinephrine: A neurotransmitter found in the brainstem and the sympathetic nervous systems, which has arousing qualities and is part of the acupuncture efferent pathway.

Serotonin: A neurotransmitter found in the raphe nucleus, which has sedating qualities and is part of the acupuncture efferent pathway.

■ CHAPTER 2 REVIEW QUESTIONS

1. The term *somatotopic* refers to the observation that_____.
   a. activation of a microsystem leads to somatizing of body symptoms
   b. two-way connections occur between the body and the microsystems
   c. the organization of all microsystem maps is found in an inverted orientation
   d. the representation of body areas on a microsystem map conforms to the arrangement of the topography of the body

2. An organo-cutaneous reflex is a neural circuit that connects_____.
   a. a microsystem point to a specific brain region
   b. a microsystem point to the body region that it represents
   c. an internal organ to the skin over the corresponding microsystem point
   d. an area of the brain to the body region that it controls

3. The Korean hand reflexology system is distinctive from the American hand reflexology system in that in Koryo hand therapy, the_____.

   a. right arm, right leg, left arm, and left leg are all represented on each hand
   b. right arm and right leg are represented on the right hand, whereas the left arm and left leg are represented on the left hand
   c. right arm and right leg are represented on the left hand, whereas the left arm and left leg are represented on the right hand
   d. internal organs are represented on the back of the hand, whereas the physical body is represented on the palm of the hand

4. A hologram serves as a theoretical model for microsystems in that_____.
   a. microsystem points resonate at frequencies that are similar to holographic beams
   b. interference patterns of brain waves match the resonant frequencies of holograms
   c. holograms reveal three-dimensional photographic images of the body
   d. each part of the holographic film negative contains an image of all parts of the whole holographic picture

5. Which one of the following microsystems is used for the diagnosis of a reactive somatotopic point but is not typically used for treatment of a pathological problem in the corresponding body area?
   a. Scalp microsystem
   b. Tongue microsystem
   c. Face microsystem
   d. Foot microsystem

6. Which of the following meridians is associated with a fu acupuncture channel that travels from the hand to the head?
   a. Large Intestine meridian
   b. Spleen meridian
   c. Liver meridian
   d. Kidney meridian

7. Most microsystem points are more strongly represented on the_____ where there is pain or pathology.
   a. ipsilateral side of the brain
   b. ipsilateral side of the body
   c. contralateral side of the body
   d. oscillating side of the brain

8. A yang alarm reaction on a micro-system point is related to an increase in_____.

    a. peripheral muscle paralysis
    b. serum liver enzymes
    c. electrodermal skin conductance
    d. kidney metabolism

9. The gate control theory contends that pain messages can be blocked by the_____.

    a. excitation of inhibitory interneurons located in the spinal cord
    b. excitation of excitatory interneurons located in the spinal cord
    c. direct inhibition of spinal nerves before they reach the spinal cord
    d. direct excitation of spinal nerves before they reach the spinal cord

10. Scientific demonstration that the periaque-ductal gray (PAG) is part of the acupuncture pathway in the brain has been shown by the finding that_____.

    a. PAG neurons show increased firing rates following the termination of acupuncture
    b. endorphin levels decrease following the stimulation of the PAG and ear acupoints
    c. acupuncture analgesia is reduced after brain lesions of the PAG
    d. GABA synapses are blocked by either acupuncture stimulation or PAG stimulation

Answers

1 = d; 2 = c; 3 = a; 4 = d; 5 = b; 6 = a; 7 = b; 8 = c; 9 = a; 10 = c

Overview of the Anatomy of the Auricle

3

[CONTENTS]

[3.0 | Overview of the Anatomy of the Auricle

CHAPTER 3 LEARNING OBJECTIVES

1. To understand the different embryological and nerve innervations of the auricle.
2. To demonstrate awareness of the curving contours of the auricle.
3. To identify the specific anatomical nomenclature associated with specific regions of the auricle.
4. To differentiate the nomenclature of the posterior auricle from that of the anterior surface of the external ear.
5. To identify specific auricular landmarks that distinguish the boundaries of different regions of the external ear.

3.1 Biological Variations in Auricular Function

As with other areas of human anatomy, there are specific terms for identifying different positions on the external ear and for indicating alternative perspectives in viewing the ear. Because other texts on the topic of auricular acupuncture have used various terminologies to describe distinct regions of the ear, this chapter provides the specific definitions of anatomical terms that are used in this manual. Taking the time to learn the Latin or Greek origins for the anatomical terms that describe the convoluted structures of the auricle greatly facilitates one's comprehension of auriculotherapy. By first familiarizing oneself with these anatomical structures, an individual can more readily appreciate the somatotopic connections between distinct regions of the external ear and specific organs of the body.

Although it seems a matter of common sense that the auricle is part of the auditory sensory pathway, examination of different animal species

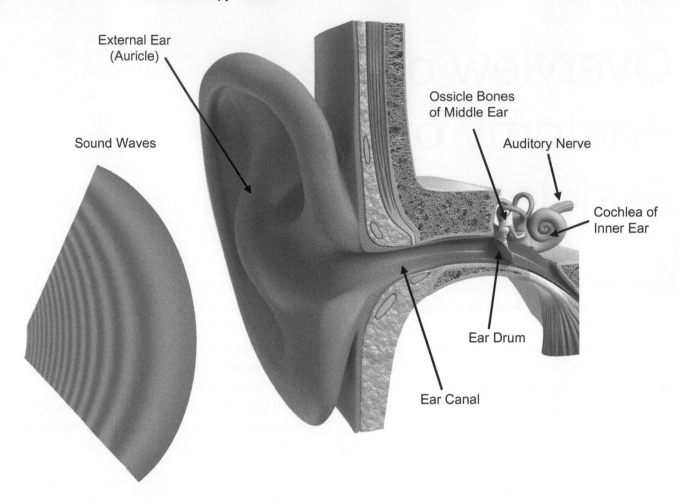

FIGURE 3.1 This anatomical view of the ear shows the curving structures of the external ear, or auricle, that collect resonating sound waves. The tubular ear canal allows the sound wave oscillations to be funneled toward the ear drum, which then vibrates the ossicle bones of the middle ear. The amplified vibrations of these bones send traveling waves to the coiled cochlea of the inner ear, which then converts the original signal into electrical neural impulses that are transmitted through the auditory nerve to the brain.

shows that the external ear is not only used for the function of hearing. The established purpose of this auricular appendage is to facilitate the transmission of oscillating sound waves from the environment to meaningful messages that are ultimately interpreted by the brain. As presented in Figure 3.1, a wave of compression of air molecules that are first gathered by the external ear are then funneled into the ear canal and travel toward the ear drum, which beats against the ossicle bones of the middle ear like a musical drum. From the middle ear, auditory signals are amplified fourfold and then transmitted to the cochlea of the inner ear. The selective bending of fine hair cells within the spiraling tube of the cochlea converts the sound wave signals into neurological messages that are sent to the brain in the

auditory nerve. Bats have relatively large external ears compared to similarly sized rodent species because of their need for echolocation, providing bats with hearing abilities far in excess of most land animals. Other species, though, have evolved to develop alternative applications of the auricle.

The external ears of some animals in the wild are used for non-auditory, adaptive purposes, as was first noted by Bossy (2000). Elephants do have excellent hearing abilities, but their large external ears are utilized for other purposes as well. African elephants living in the dry, hot plains of the African savannah have evolved significantly larger external ears than Indian elephants found in the moist jungles of Asia. As seen in Figure 3.2, the desert hare and desert

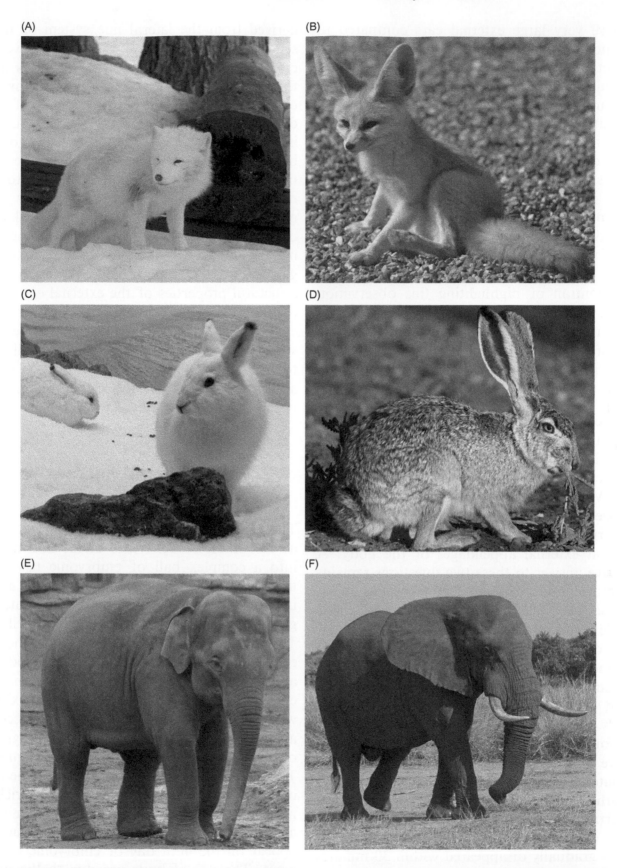

[FIGURE 3.2 This series of photographs exemplifies the finding that the arctic fox (A), arctic hare (C), and Asian elephant (E) all have much smaller ears than the desert fox (B), the desert hare (D), and the African elephant (F). The larger ears of the desert animals of the same species is not for the purpose of better hearing abilities but, rather, for the purpose of thermoregulation by increased blood circulation to the ears, allowing greater release of internal body heat.

fox have very large external ears compared to their non-desert relatives, the arctic hare and the arctic fox. The purpose of this difference in external ear size in elephants, foxes, and hares is the need for differential thermoregulation in different climates. The thin skin of the highly vascularized external ears provides an important source of heat loss. Greater vascular supply to the ears of desert animals allows for more rapid release of internal heat to provide thermoregulation of homeostatic body temperature on hot desert days. In contrast, the arctic hare and the arctic fox need to conserve internal body heat to protect them from freezing cold temperatures. The intention of highlighting this observation by Bossy is that biological development can lead to the use of a particular anatomical structure for more than one adaptive purpose, including the purpose of pain control as well as thermal homeostasis.

A logical, Darwinian question regarding the somatotopic system that has been attributed to the auricle would be to ask what natural selection factors led to the evolution of such a system? What biological mechanisms could have produced the lines of acupuncture points over the surface of the body or the microsystem points at external appendages of the body? A definitive answer to these two questions remains conjectural, but previously cited investigations of the bioelectric properties of acupuncture points provide some possible explanations. Chiou *et al.* (1998) observed that the topography of low skin resistance points (LSRPs) was found to be distributed symmetrically and bilaterally over the shaved skin of rats. The arrangement of these LSRPs corresponded to the acupuncture meridians found in humans. These electrically conductive points on the surface of the body were attributed to the neural and vascular elements beneath these LSRPs. Interestingly, the electrical properties of these specific skin areas required living physiological mechanisms because the LSRPs gradually disappeared within 30 minutes after the animal's death.

One interpretation of this observation of LSRPs on the skin of animals is that the occurrence of body acupoints and ear acupoints could be

derived from the lateral line system of fish. A school of fish can sense the subtle movements of water by neighboring fish, and this allows them to act as a group against any invading object. This collective, sensory ability of fish is due to their lateral line detection system, which is located in their skin along the length of their body. Such a system could serve as the evolutionary foundation for the ear's ability to sense remote sounds that became the auditory system of land animals, and it could also explain the occurrence of acupuncture points on the external ear and the body that can sense subtle energies surrounding humans and other animals. The structural properties of the external ear allow it to funnel vibrating air molecules into the inner ear, which then resonates to the frequency of sound waves. The auricle can additionally serve to regulate body temperature and thus provide a basic reflex system for regulating pain and pathology in other parts of the body.

3.2 Embryological Representations on the External Ear

The biological life of the human embryo begins as the union of cells that divide and multiply into a complex ball of embryonic tissue. The union of a single sperm and egg creates a fertilized original cell, which then divides into progressively more balls of accumulated cell mass. This ball of cells ultimately becomes the more embryologic layers of endodermal, mesodermal, and ectodermal tissue. Further evolution of the embryo differentiates into the complex fetus, which subsequently takes on the more recognizable shape of a human baby. This progression of cellular development is shown in Figure 3.3. The portions of the fetus that lead to the development of different sections of the auricle are revealed in Figure 3.4. The external ear is created from the coalescence of six fetal buds that appear on the 40th day of embryonic development. These fetal buds are due to the mesenchymal proliferation of the first two branchial arches, which then develop into the cranial nerves that ultimately innervate the auricle and connect it to the central nervous system.

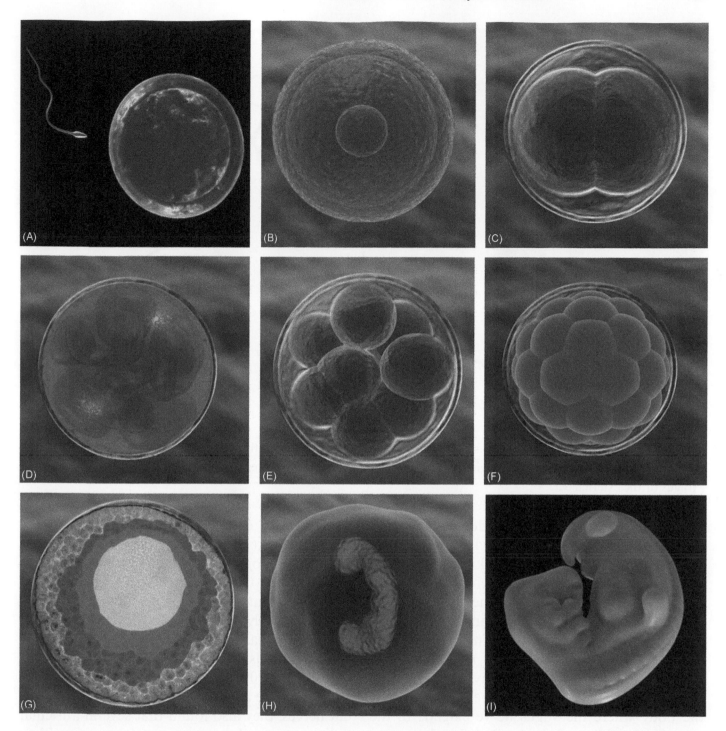

FIGURE 3.3 The developmental progression of a simple cell to a multicellular tissue to an embryological tissue to a fetus. A single sperm unites with the egg (A), the egg becomes fertilized with the sperm (B) and then begins to divide into two cells (C), forming a ball of tissue with increasingly more individual cells (D–F), until it ultimately becomes the embryo (G) that has three concentric layers. This embryo further differentiates in a primitive fetus (H) and then a more developed fetus (I) that begins to appear like a human baby.

Bossy (1979) summarized a range of basic anatomy studies which suggested that there are three primary territories of the auricle. His work is represented in Figure 3.5. The outer ridges of the auricle were found to be primarily innervated by the auriculotemporal branch of the mandibular trigeminal nerve, which represents a somesthetic region associated with somatic muscles. The lower mandibular branch or the middle maxillary branch of the trigeminal nerve is

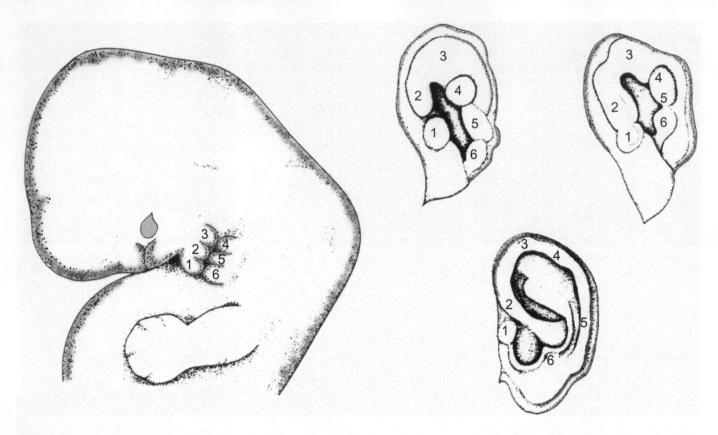

[FIGURE 3.4 This series of diagrams of the developing human fetus shows that from six original buds on the primitive fetus there develops the curving cartilaginous structures of the different sections of the helix, antihelix, and tragus of the external ear.

anesthetized with Novocain by doctors performing dental procedures. The third branch of the trigeminal nerve supplies the skin and muscles of the face and forehead, which could lead to facial twitches if damaged. The central valley of the external ear is highly innervated by the auricular branch of the parasympathetic vagus nerve. This tenth cranial nerve regulates all of the internal organs of the body. Of particular note, the auricle of the ear is the only region of the body where the vagus nerve extends to the superficial surface of the body. It has been suggested that many of the clinical effects found with auricular acupuncture are primarily due to the autonomic nerve connections to the concha region of the external ear. The third primary region of the auricle is the lobular and tragal areas that are innervated by the superficial cervical plexus. There is no simple explanation for all of the biological reflexes related to the cervical plexus, but the function of these nerves tends to be more neurological than either somatic or autonomic.

The external ears of dogs were examined by Chien *et al.* (1996) for retrograde horseradish peroxidase projections to the auricle. The auricular branch of the trigeminal nerve was observed to demonstrate somatotopic organization of nervous supply to terminal fields on the external ear, whereas the vagus nerve innervated more central regions of the auricle. Although Peuker and Filler (2002) reported that the anteriolateral surface of the auricle is supplied by three different nerves, they also found that several auricular regions received innervations from more than one nerve. Close inspection of seven human cadavers revealed that the auricular branch of the autonomic vagus nerve predominately innervated the cymba concha and cavum concha, but the antihelix and the tragus also received projections from the vagus nerve. The auriculotemporal nerve primarily supplied the helix rim, whereas the greater auricular nerve provided nervous innervation to the helix tail, scaphoid fossa, antihelix crura, antitragus, and lobule. The tragus, cavum concha, and antihelix received dual

Nerve Connections to the Auricle

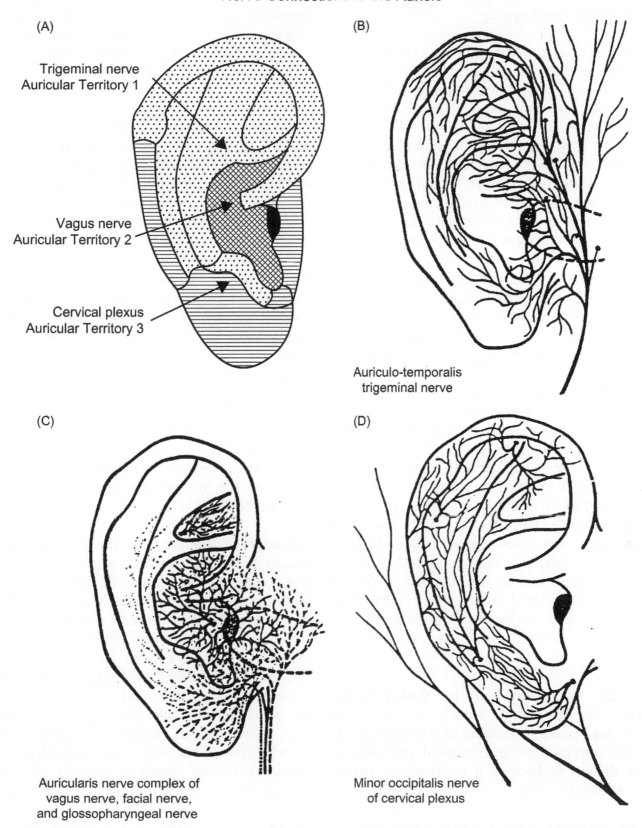

(A)

Trigeminal nerve
Auricular Territory 1

Vagus nerve
Auricular Territory 2

Cervical plexus
Auricular Territory 3

(B)

Auriculo-temporalis
trigeminal nerve

(C)

Auricularis nerve complex of
vagus nerve, facial nerve,
and glossopharyngeal nerve

(D)

Minor occipitalis nerve
of cervical plexus

FIGURE 3.5 This series of drawings of the external ear shows the broad projection of three cranial nerves to three different territories of auricle (A). (B) The auriculo-temporalis division of the trigeminal nerve projecting to parts of the helix, antihelix, and antitragus. (C) The auricularis nerve primarily projects to the concha and the triangular fossa. (D) The minor occipitalis nerve of the cervical plexus primarily projects to the ear lobe, helix tail, and scaphoid fossa.

innervations from the greater auricular nerve and from the vagus nerve.

The differential projection of cranial nerves to different regions of the auricle provides both a neurological and an embryological basis for somatotopic divisions of the external ear. These findings serve as a biological foundation that allows the theory that specific auricular regions can represent different parts of the gross anatomy. The somatosensory trigeminal nerve innervates cutaneous and muscular regions of the actual face and also supplies the region of the auricle that corresponds to musculoskeletal functions. The autonomic vagus nerve innervates thoracic and abdominal visceral organs, which supply the central region of the auricle that is associated with most internal organs. A third region of the auricle is supplied by the minor occipital nerve and the greater auricular nerve, both branches of the cervical plexus. The cervical plexus nerves regulate blood supply to the brain and are associated with cerebral cortex functions represented on the ear lobe. The facial nerve connections to the posterior side of the auricle were associated with somatic nervous system control of facial muscles. Dr. Sebastian Leib (1999) of Germany has referred to Nogier's embryological perspective as three functional layers, with each layer representing a different homeostatic system in the organism. Most health disorders are related to disturbances in one of these three functional layers, and this has been used as one explanation for Paul Nogier's concept of different phases that are represented on the auricle.

Auricular Representation of Embryological Tissue: As previously stated, all vertebrate organisms begin as the union of a single egg and a single sperm. This one original cell progressively divides to become a multicellular organism. A circular ball of cells ultimately folds in on itself, appearing more like a bowl than a sphere, and then further differentiates into the three different layers of embryological tissue. It is from these three basic types of tissue that all other body organs are formed. In a similar organization, the different anatomical organs derived from these three embryological layers are projected onto different regions of the auricle (Figure 3.6). Table 3.1 outlines these embryological divisions and the corresponding auricular territories associated with each embryological division.

Endodermal Tissue: The inner endodermal tissues of the embryo become the internal organs of the body, including the gastrointestinal digestive tract, the respiratory system, and abdominal organs such as the liver, pancreas, urethra, and bladder. This portion of the embryo also generates parts of the endocrine system, including the thyroid gland, parathyroid gland, and thymus gland. Most of these deep embryological tissues are somatotopically represented in the concha, the central valley of the ear. Stimulating this area of the ear affects metabolic activities and nutritive disorders of the internal organs that originate from the endoderm layer of the embryo. Disturbances in internal organs create an obstacle to the success of many medical treatments; thus, these metabolic disorders must be corrected before complete healing can occur. In traditional Oriental medicine, maintaining the health of the internal organs is vital to overall physical health.

Mesodermal Tissue: The middle mesodermal tissues of the embryo become the skeletal muscles, cardiac muscles, smooth muscles, connective tissue, joints, and bones. Mesodermal tissue creates blood cells from bone marrow, the blood vessels of the circulatory system and lymphatic systems, hormones created by the adrenal cortex, and the tubules that comprise the urogenital organs. Musculoskeletal balance is regulated by negative feedback control of somatosensory reflexes, which prevent overcontraction of muscles that could lead to damaged tissue but provide sufficient muscular strength when it is needed. The medially located embryological tissue of the mesoderm is represented on the middle ridges and valleys of the auricle, including the antihelix, scaphoid fossa, triangular fossa, and portions of the helix. Mobilization of body defense mechanisms is only possible if the region of this middle mesodermal layer is working

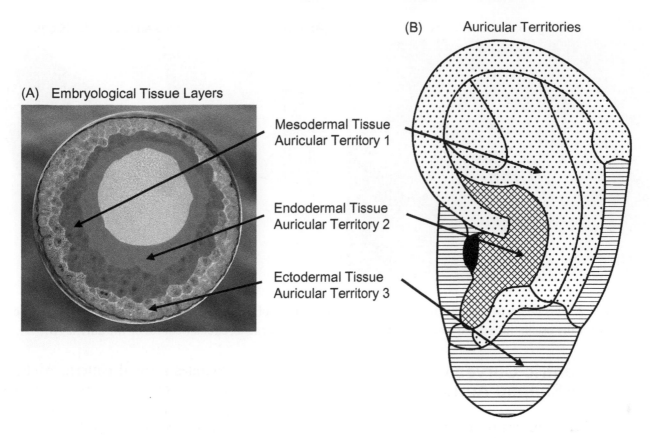

(A) Embryological Tissue Layers

Mesodermal Tissue
Auricular Territory 1

Endodermal Tissue
Auricular Territory 2

Ectodermal Tissue
Auricular Territory 3

(B)   Auricular Territories

FIGURE 3.6 The ball of primal tissue that develops into the human embryo contains three concentric tissue layers—the inner endoderm layer, the middle mesoderm layer, and the outer ectoderm layer (A). These three embryological layers ultimately connect to three different territories on the auricle (B).

TABLE 3.1	Auricular Representation of Embryological Tissue Layers.	
Endodermal Tissue	**Mesodermal Tissue**	**Ectodermal Tissue**
Inner Layer	Middle Layer	Outer Layer
Viscera	Skeletal bones	Skin
Stomach	Striate muscles	Hair
Intestines	Fascia	Sweat glands
	Tendons	Nerves
Lungs		Spinal cord
Tonsils	Heart	Brainstem
Liver	Blood cells	Thalamus
	Blood vessels	Hypothalamus
Pancreas	Lymph vessels	Limbic Brain
		Striatum
Bladder	Spleen	Cerebrum
Thyroid	Kidneys	Pineal
Parathyroid	Gonads	Pituitary
Thymus	Adrenal cortex	Adrenal medulla
Concha	Antihelix	Lobe
Vagus nerve	Trigeminal nerve	Cervical plexus

functionally, for both conscious and unconscious muscular movements require a musculoskeletal system that is optimally ready to react to the stressors of life.

Ectodermal Tissue: The outer ectodermal tissues of the embryo become the outer skin, cornea, eyeball, lens, nose epithelium, teeth, peripheral nerves, spinal cord, brain, and the endocrine glands of the pituitary, pineal, and adrenal medulla. This embryological tissue is represented on the ear lobe, tragus, and helix tail. The surface embryological layer affects the capacity for adaptation to and contact with the external environment. The neurological structures created from ectodermal tissue are impacted not just by physical challenges but also by internal psychological reactions from the conscious mind and from deeper, unconscious, psychic levels. Both the outer skin and the internal central nervous system integrate inborn, instinctive information with individual, learned experiences.

(A)   Rings of Water Waves

(B) Oscillating Sound Waves and Auricular Ridges

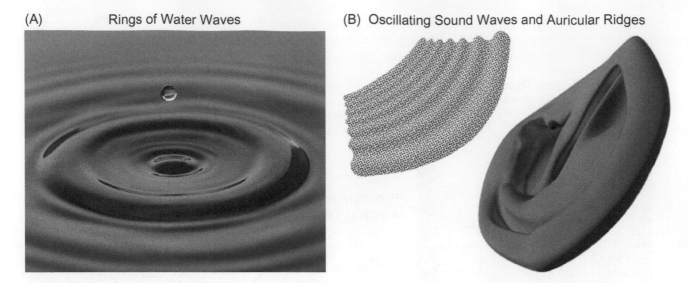

[FIGURE 3.7 This image of a single drop of water creating a series of concentric rings of water waves (A) is used as an analogy for the oscillating sound waves that resonate with the concentric, circular curves of the auricle (B).

3.3 Concentric Curves of Spiral-Shaped Auricle

The external ear consists of a series of concentric circles that radiate from the center of the auricle, like a series of curving ridges and deep valleys that spread outward from a central source. This configuration is similar to the undulating waves of water that spread over the surface of a pond after the splash from a pebble. Sound waves are similar to the waves of water, consisting of oscillating increases and then decreases in the compression of air molecules as the sound travels through the air (Figure 3.7). The external ear is shaped somewhat like a ring and somewhat like a funnel. The purpose of this shape is to direct the subtle motions of vibrating air molecules into the ear canal. These sound waves then vibrate against the eardrum, like a baton pounding against a musical drum. After being amplified by the serial activation of the ossicle bones of the middle ear, the sound signals then generate a traveling wave in the cochlea that produces deflections of hair cell sensors within the snail-shaped inner ear. The arrangement of cochlear hair cells is similar to the arrangement of the strings of a harp, with the activation of different strings leading to the experience of different sounds.

The basic shape of both the cochlea of the inner ear and the curving ridges of the external ear repeats and reiterates a spiral pattern. Archetypal representations of a spiral pattern are shown in Figure 3.8. Spiraling, circular shapes are exhibited by astronomical images of the solar system, the swirling clouds of a hurricane, the double helix shape of the DNA molecule, the coiled shell of the cochlear portion of the inner ear, the fossilized shell of a prehistoric snail, and the circular horn of a mountain goat. The Latin word for a spiral shape is *helix*. Just as there are two spiraling helices that form the basic structure of DNA, there are two helices comprising the auricle—an outer helix rim and an opposing antihelix ridge within it. The other common pattern that is represented on the ear is that of a spiraling seashell. The Latin term for the deep, central valley of the auricle is *concha*, which means shell shaped. Several examples of conch shells and other types of shells are shown in Figure 3.9. Several grooves that separate one ridge of the auricle from another are referred to as "fossa," which is similar to the English word "fissure," meaning a crack in the surface of the earth, and is also the term used for the crevices that separate different sections of the cerebral cortex of the brain. One region of the upper auricle has been identified as the "triangular fossa," a somewhat triangularly shaped valley. Actually, the true shape of this auricular region is more similar to an arch than a triangle. The arched Gateway to the West, located near the Mississippi River in the city of Saint Louis, Missouri, is shown in Figure 3.10.

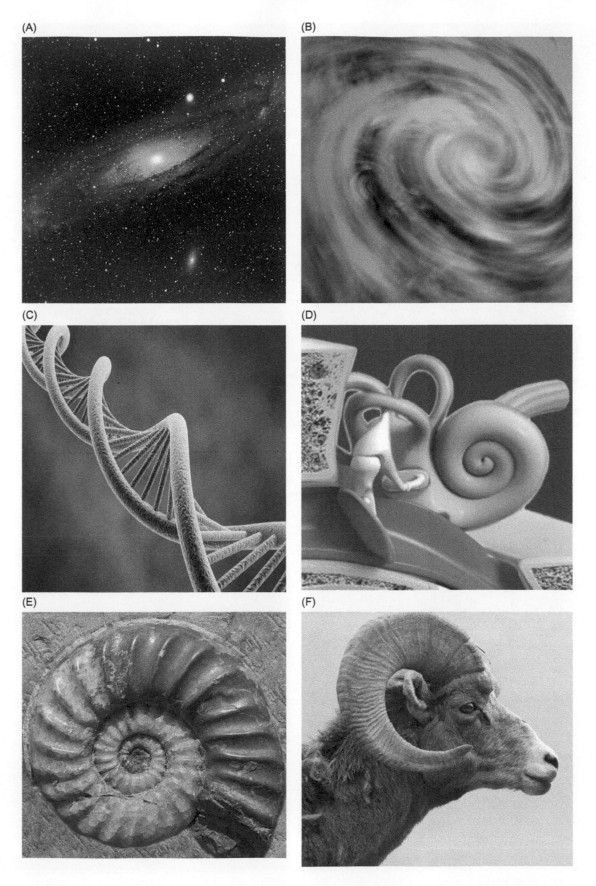

FIGURE 3.8 The anatomical terminology for the curving shape of the circular ridges of the helix of the ear is compared to the spiral patterns of the solar system (A), hurricanes (B), the double helix of DNA (C), the coiled cochlear of the inner ear (D), fossils of coiled seashells (E), and the horn of a mountain goat (F).

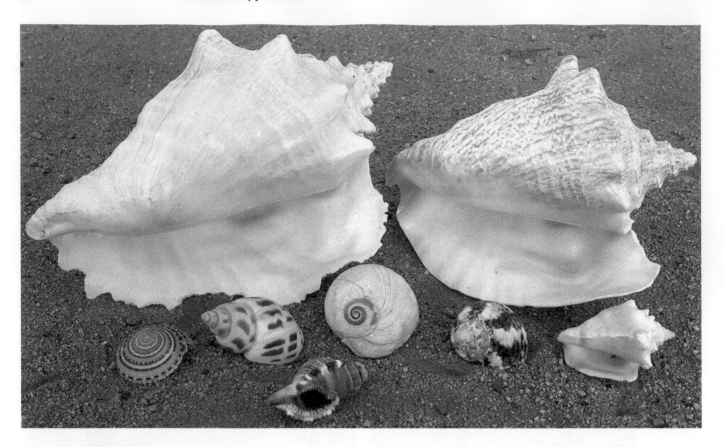

FIGURE 3.9 Several images of conch shells demonstrate both the classical spiral shape of the helix of the external ear and the inner curve of central core of a shell, which are similar to the coiled curvature of the inner ear.

(A)   (B)

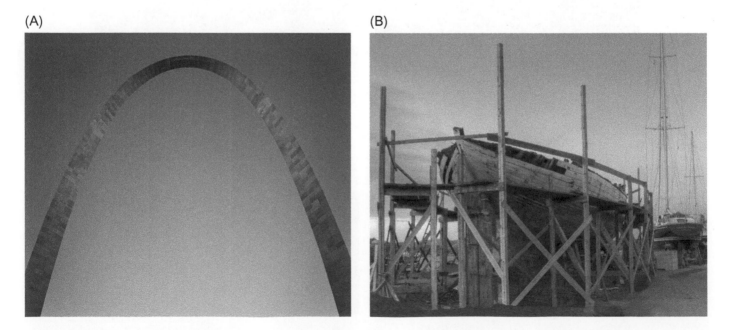

FIGURE 3.10 The shape of the triangular fossa of the auricle is closer to the shape of an arch, such as the St. Louis Gateway Arch (A). The terminology for the scaphoid fossa comes from a boat-like shape, based on the use of scaffolding that has been used to build boats (B).

Separating the outer rim of the external ear from the ridge that lies alongside it is the auricular area known as the scaphoid fossa, which literally means scaffolding-shaped fissure. The reasoning behind the naming of this grooved region of the auricle can be better understood from the ancient process of building large boats by first creating a scaffolding structure within which the boat will be constructed. The term scaphoid fossa is thus better interpreted as "boat-shaped," similar to the crescent-shaped boats used in ancient Egypt, Greece, and Rome.

3.4 Anatomical Views Differentiating Auricular Topography

Reference to any object in three-dimensional space is designated by points of comparison. The complex, convoluted structure of the auricle must be viewed from different angles and from different depths. Specific terms are used in this text to indicate these different perspectives of the ear that are indicated in Figure 3.11. As is always true in the science of anatomy, the purpose of developing specific terminology for certain anatomical structures is to better understand the structure and function of that anatomical region.

Surface View: The front side of the external ear is easily available to view. The auricle is diagonally angled from the side of the skull such that it extends from both the anterior aspects of the face and the lateral sides of the head. The auricle is thus oriented in an anterolateral position, but many texts state that the external ear is on the lateral side of the skull, thus only the term lateral is used.

Hidden View: Vertical or underlying surfaces of the external ear are not easy to view, but the auricle can be pulled back by retractors to reveal the hidden regions.

Posterior View: The back side of the external ear faces the mastoid bone behind the ear and can best be viewed by flipping the ear forward toward the face.

External Surface: The visible, external ear forms the external surface view.

Internal Surface: The underlying surface of the ear forms the hidden view.

Superior Side: The top of the ear is directed toward the upper or dorsal position.

Inferior Side: The bottom of the ear is directed toward the lower or ventral position.

Central Side: The medial, proximal side of the ear is directed inward toward the head.

Peripheral Side: The lateral, distal side of the ear is directed outward, away from the head.

(A) Anatomical Directions for Anterior Front Surface of Auricle

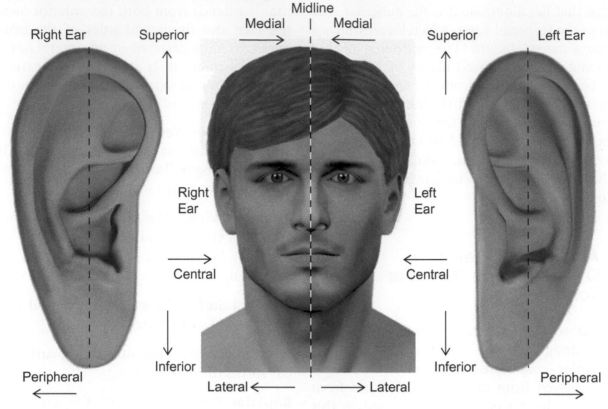

(B) Anatomical Directions for Posterior Back Surface of Auricle

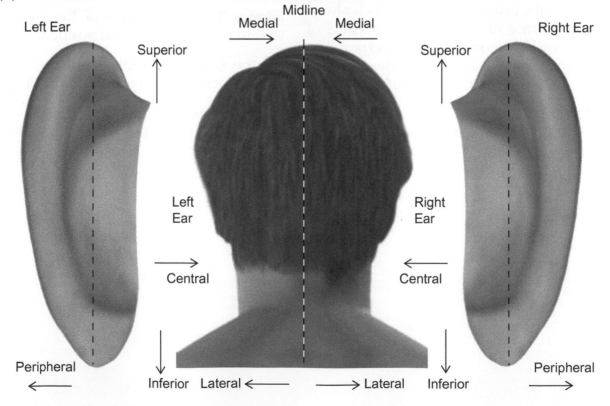

[FIGURE 3.11 Anatomical terms used for different perspectives of the head and the external ears, indicating both anterior and posterior views of the head and the auricles. Superior refers to the top of the auricle, inferior refers to the bottom, central refers to more regions of the ear, and peripheral refers to more lateral areas of the auricle.

3.5 Symbols to Represent Depth of Ear Points

As shown in the photographs of Figures 3.12 and 3.13, the external ear can be viewed from different angles. In both of these sets of photographs, the side view of the face is followed by a closer photograph of the external ear from a more anterior lateral view, then a lateral ear view that is more perpendicular to the surface structures of the ear, and then progressive views of the auricle from more posterior lateral

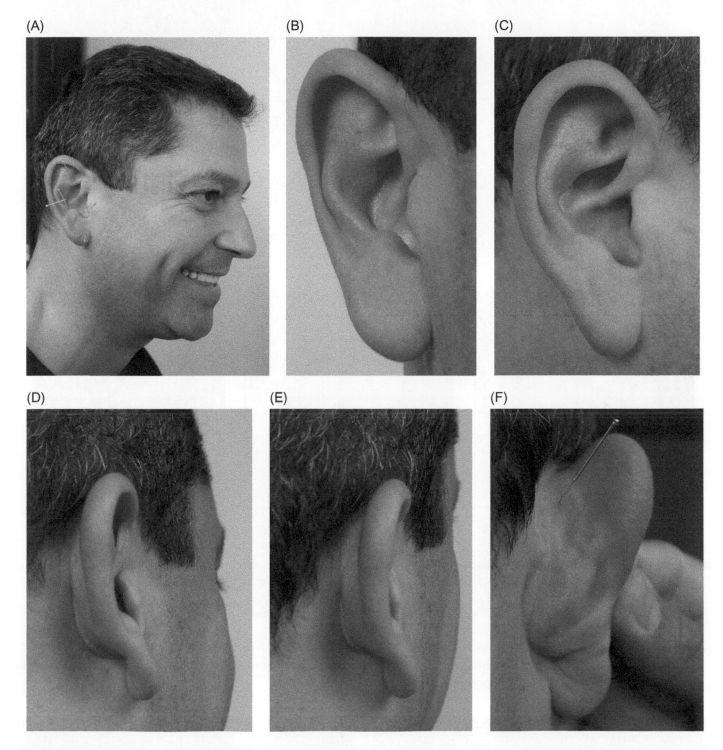

(A)   **(B)**   **(C)**

(D)   **(E)**   **(F)**

⎡**FIGURE 3.12** These photographs of the external ear of an Hispanic male (A) are seen from different angles of the surface view of the auricle (B and C) and other angles that reveal the more hidden areas of the posterior auricle (D and E). One must pull back the ear with one's fingers in order to view these posterior ear points (F).

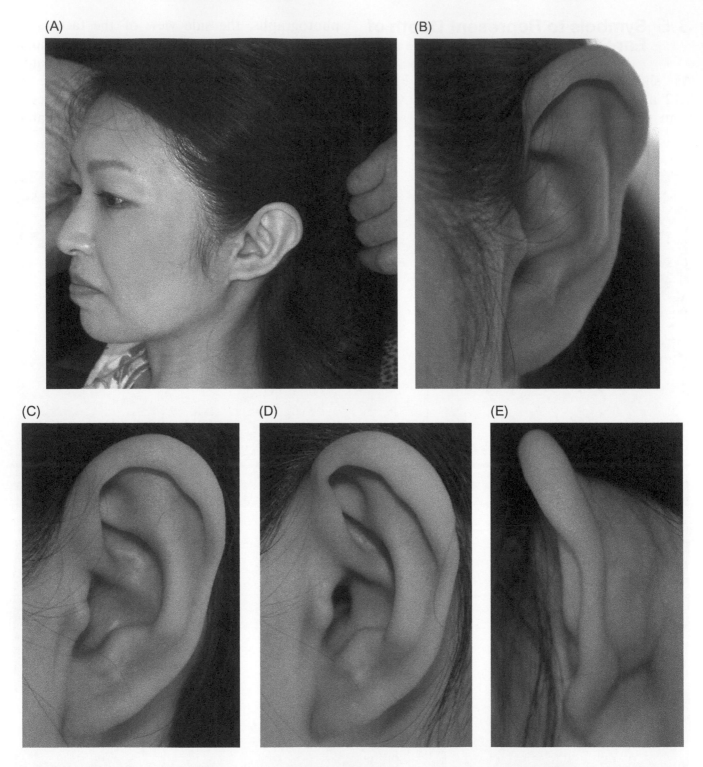

(A) (B) (C) (D) (E)

[FIGURE 3.13 These photographs of the external ear of an Asian female (A) are seen from different angles of the surface view of the auricle. A more anterior view is seen in B, a perpendicular side view is seen in C, a more posterior side angle is shown in D, and a fully posterior view is revealed in E.

angles. Different structural perspectives and deeper depths of the auricle can be observed from some angles but not from other viewpoints. In both the pictures of an example male and an example female external ear, the basic regions of the auricle are essentially the same, although most females have smaller external ears than most males. Textbooks on auricular acupuncture typically use just one basic diagram of the external ear to represent all of these perspectives.

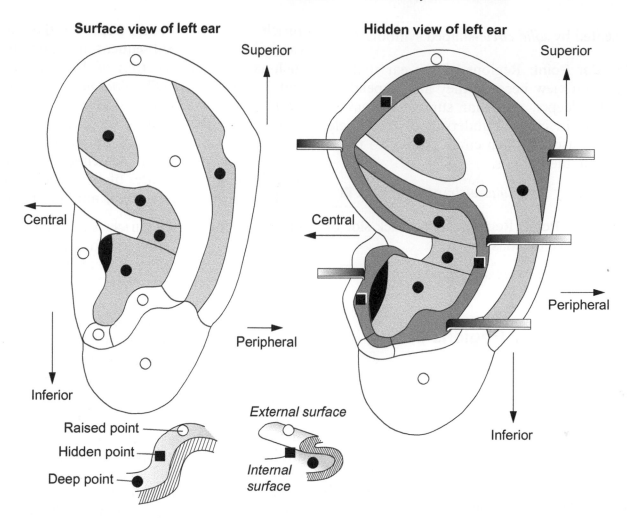

Surface view of left ear

Superior

Central

Peripheral

Inferior

Hidden view of left ear

Superior

Central

Peripheral

Inferior

Raised point
Hidden point
Deep point

External surface

Internal surface

[**FIGURE 3.14** Symbols used to indicate different depths of the ear consist of open circles to represent higher ridges of the auricle, solid circles to represent lower valleys in the auricle, and squares to show vertical walls of the auricle that are often hidden from a surface view. Retractors are utilized in views of hidden areas of the auricle that better indicate ear points represented by solid squares.

That approach has definite limitations in accurately representing the variety of views that photographs of the ear can show. However, the problem with close-up photography is that the different depths of the auricle often leave one auricular area out of focus as one zooms in on any specific region of the auricle. This chapter presents several artistic representations of different features of the auricle to indicate the different depths and different viewpoints of the external ear.

Because two-dimensional paper cannot adequately represent the three-dimensional depth of the auricle, certain symbols have been developed to represent differences in auricular depth. If one were to think of the rising and falling swells of a wave, or the ridges of a hill contrasted with a valley below, the top of the peak is the highest position, indicated by an open circle, the descending slope is indicated by a square, and the lowest depths are shown as filled circles. In this manual, the deeper, central concha is indicated by auricular areas represented by filled circles, the surrounding wall of the concha is represented by squares, and the peaks of the antihelix and antitragus are shown with open circles (Figure 3.14).

Raised Ear Point: Regions of the ear that are elevated ridges or protrusions.

Represented by *open circle*-shaped symbols. ○

Deeper Ear Point: Regions that are lower in the ear, like a groove or depression.

Represented by *solid circle*-shaped symbols. ●

Hidden Ear Point: Regions of the ear that are hidden from view because they are perpendicular to the deeper, auricular surface regions or they are on the internal underside of the auricle. Some texts use a broken circle symbol to represent these hidden points.

Represented by *solid square*-shaped symbols. ■

Posterior Ear Point: Regions of the back side of the ear that face the mastoid bone.

Represented by *open square*-shaped symbols. ❑

3.6 Anatomical Regions of the External Ear

Classic anatomical texts have presented specific anatomical terms for certain regions of the external ear. This auricular appendage for auditory sensation is also known as the pinna. Latin phrases have traditionally been utilized to describe designated regions of the external ear. Additional terms were developed at the meetings of the 1990 World Health Organization on acupuncture nomenclature. Some regions of the external ear are described in auricular acupuncture texts but are not discussed in conventional anatomy books. The official terms for the external ear are described in the *Nomina Anatomica*. Whereas there are 112 different terms listed by this text under the section on the auris interna and 97 terms listed for the parts of the auris media, *Nomina Anatomica* presents only 30 phrases for different regions of the auris externa. Woerdeman's (1955) classic text on human anatomy refers to just nine primary auricular structures: the helix, antihelix, tragus, antitragus, scapha, fossa triangularis, lobule, concha, and Darwin's tubercle. There are two additional subdivisions for the limbs of the antihelix, the superior crus and the inferior crus, and two subdivisions of the concha—a superior, cymba concha and an inferior, cavum concha. Delineation of the antitrago–helicine fissure, which separates the antitragus from the antihelix, brings the total to 14 auricular terms for the lateral view of the

auricle and 12 additional terms for the mastoid view of the ear. Subsequent anatomy books, such as Hild's (1974) *Atlas of Human Anatomy* and Clemente's (1997) *Anatomy: A Regional Atlas of the Human Body*, basically concur with these earlier designations for the external ear. Anatomists interested in auricular acupuncture have proposed supplemental terminology to delineate the structures of the auricle that are used in the clinical practice of auriculotherapy.

The outer ridge of the auricle is referred to as the helix, which is the Latin term for a spiral pattern. A middle ridge within this outer ridge is called the antihelix. The prefix "anti" refers to an object that is opposite in position to another object. The helix is subdivided into a central helix root, an arching superior helix, and the outermost helix tail. The cauda, or tail, refers to a long, trailing hind portion, like the tail of a comet. The subsections of the antihelix include an antihelix tail at the bottom of the middle ridge, an antihelix body in the center, and two limbs that extend from the antihelix body—the superior crus and the inferior crus. A fossa in Latin refers to a fissure or groove. Between the two arms of the antihelix lies a deep sloping valley known as the triangular fossa, whereas the scaphoid fossa is a long, slender groove that separates the middle ridge of the antihelix from the outer ridge of the helix tail.

Adjacent to the face and overlying the auditory canal is a flat section of the ear known as the tragus. Opposite to the tragus is another flap, labeled the antitragus. The latter is a curving continuation of the antihelix, forming a circular antihelix–antitragus ridge that surrounds the whole central valley of the ear. A prominent crease separates the antihelix from the antitragus. Below the antitragus is the soft, fleshy ear lobe, and between the antitragus and the tragus is a "U"-shaped curved known as the intertragic notch. The deepest region of the ear is called the concha, indicating it is shell-shaped in its structure. The concha is further divided into an inferior concha below and a superior concha above. Although most anatomical texts respectively refer to these two areas as the *cymba conchae* and the *cavum conchae*, the 1990 nomenclature committee of the World Health Organization concluded that superior concha and inferior concha were more useful designations. These two major divisions of the concha are separated by a slight mound. This prolongation of the helix onto the concha floor is identified in this text as the concha ridge. A vertical elevation that surrounds the whole concha floor has been designated as the concha wall. This hidden wall area of the auricle is not specifically identified in most anatomical texts. Two other hidden areas of the external ear include the subtragus underneath the tragus and the internal helix beneath the helix root and superior helix.

On the back side of the ear is a whole surface referred to as the posterior side of the auricle. It lies across from the mastoid bone of the skull. This region is subdivided into a posterior groove behind the antihelix ridge, a posterior lobe behind the ear lobe, a posterior concha behind the central concha, a posterior triangle behind the triangular fossa, and the posterior periphery behind the scaphoid fossa and helix tail. Taking the time to both visually recognize and tactilely palpate these different contours of the ear greatly assists beginning practitioners of auriculotherapy in understanding the somatotopic correspondences between the external ear and specific anatomical structures.

Anatomical Regions of Auricular Surface View

Ear Canal (Auditory Meatus): This funnel-shaped orifice leads from the external ear to the middle ear and then the inner ear. The opening to this elliptical tube is surrounded by the inferior concha next to it and the subtragus above it.

Helix (Outer Ridge): This circular, cartilaginous ridge spirals around the outermost rim of the external ear and is shaped somewhat like a question mark symbol (?) (Shown in Figure 3.15).

Helix Root: The initial segment of the helix ascends from the center of the ear upward toward the face.

Helix Arch: The highest section of the helix is shaped like a broad arch.

Helix Tail: The final region of the helix descends vertically downward along the most peripheral aspect of the ear.

Antihelix (Middle Ridge): This "Y"-shaped ridge is "anti" or opposite to the helix ridge, forming a concentric series of ridges that surround the central concha of the auricle.

Antihelix Tail: A narrow ridge at the inferior third of the antihelix.

Antihelix Body: A broad sloping ridge at the central third of the antihelix.

Superior Crus of the Antihelix: The upper arm and vertical extension of the antihelix.

Inferior Crus of the Antihelix: The lower arm and horizontal extension of the antihelix. This flat-edged ridge overhangs the superior concha below it.

Tragus (Facial Ridge): The tragus of the auricle is a vertical, trapezoid-shaped area joining the ear to the face. It projects over the ear canal, and pressing down on the tragus would limit one's ability to hear from that ear.

Antitragus (Lobe Ridge): This angled ridge is "anti" opposite to the tragus. It rises like a mountain range over the lowest portion of the inferior concha and then joins the ear lobe below it. The antitragus ridge is a curved continuation of the antihelix ridge, with a distinct groove that separates the antitragus from the antihelix tail.

Intertragic Notch (Notch Ridge): This "U"-shaped curve lies immediately superior to the ear lobe region that joins to the face and it separates the tragus from the antitragus.

Lobe: This soft, fleshy tissue is found at the most inferior part of the external ear.

Scaphoid Fossa (Outer Valley): This crescent-shaped, shallow valley separates the helix from the antihelix. "Fossa" refers to a fissure, groove, or crevice, whereas "scaphoid" refers to the scaffolding used to form the outer structure of a boat or building during construction. The word "scapha" refers to boat shape.

Triangular Fossa (Triangular Valley): This triangular groove separates the superior crus and the

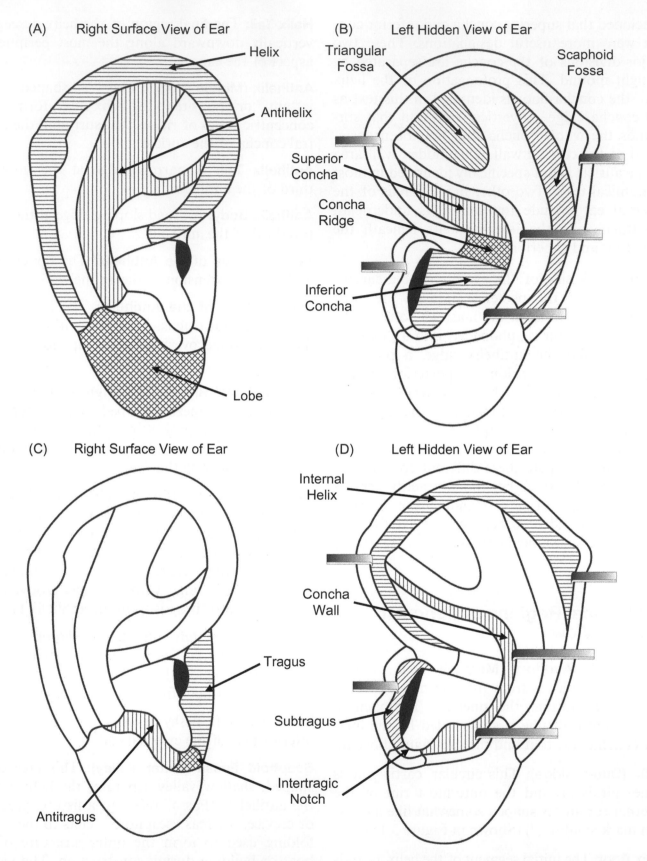

(A)   Right Surface View of Ear

Helix

Antihelix

Lobe

(B)   Left Hidden View of Ear

Triangular Fossa

Scaphoid Fossa

Superior Concha

Concha Ridge

Inferior Concha

(C)   Right Surface View of Ear

Tragus

Antitragus

Intertragic Notch

(D)   Left Hidden View of Ear

Internal Helix

Concha Wall

Subtragus

Intertragic Notch

FIGURE 3.15 Anatomical terms that characterize specific regions of the auricule show the different sections of outer rim helix, different sections of the middle ridge antihelix, and the ear lobe below (A). The other ear diagrams indicate the deeper valleys of the auricle, which include the concha, scaphoid fossa, and triangular fossa (B); the tragus, antitragus, and intertragic notch (C); and hidden areas of the internal helix, concha wall, and subtragus (D).

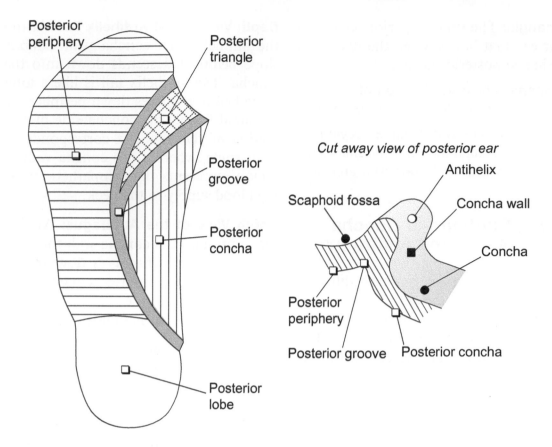

FIGURE 3.16 Anatomical terms that characterize specific regions of the posterior auricle include the posterior lobe, posterior concha, posterior periphery, posterior triangle, and posterior groove.

inferior crus of the antihelix. It is shaped like an arch on the window of a Gothic cathedral.

Concha (Central Valley): This shell-shaped valley is found at the very center of the ear. The term concha refers to the shape of a conch seashell.

Superior Concha (Upper Valley): Identified as the *cymba concha* in classical anatomical texts, the upper hemiconcha is found immediately below the inferior crus of the antihelix.

Inferior Concha (Lower Valley): Officially known as the *cavum concha* in classical anatomical texts, the lower hemiconcha is found immediately peripheral to the ear canal.

Concha Ridge (Inner Ridge): This raised ridge divides the superior concha from the inferior concha. It is the anatomical prolongation of the helix root onto the concha floor.

Concha Wall (Valley Wall): The hidden, vertical region between the concha floor and the surrounding antihelix and antitragus. The concha wall curves vertically upward from the concha floor to meet the higher ridges of the antihelix and the antitragus.

Subtragus: This underside of the tragus lies above the ear canal.

Internal Helix: This hidden, underside portion of the brim of the helix spirals from the center of the helix to the top of the ear and around to the helix tail.

Anatomy of Posterior Ear

Posterior Lobe: This soft, fleshy region behind the lobe occurs at the bottom of the posterior ear.

Posterior Groove: This long, vertical depression along the whole back of the posterior ear lies immediately behind the "Y"-shaped antihelix ridge that is on the front side of the auricle.

Posterior Triangle: The small superior region on the posterior ear that lies between the two arms of the "Y"-shaped posterior groove.

Posterior Concha: The central region of the posterior ear is found immediately behind the concha.

Posterior Periphery: The outer, curved region of the posterior ear lies behind the helix and the scaphoid fossa. It lies peripheral to the posterior groove.

3.7 Curving Contours of Concha Wall, Antihelix, and Antitragus

The contours of the external ear have different shapes at different levels of the antihelix and antitragus as the concha wall rises up to meet them. These differences in contour are useful in distinguishing different anatomical features on the ear that relate to different correspondences to body regions.

Depth View of the Inferior Crus of Antihelix: At this level of the antihelix, the concha wall exhibits a sharp overhang before it curves back underneath and then descends down into the superior concha. The inferior crus itself is somewhat flat, before gradually descending into the triangular fossa. The top surface of this section of the antihelix corresponds to the lumbosacral vertebrae, whereas the concha wall below it represents the sympathetic nerves affecting blood supply to the lower spine.

Depth View of the Antihelix Body: At this level of the antihelix, the concha wall exhibits a gradual slope before it descends down into the superior concha. The antihelix body is like a broad, gentle mound before it curves down peripherally into the scaphoid fossa. The concha side of this section of the antihelix corresponds to the thoracic spine, whereas the concha wall below this region represents the sympathetic nerves affecting blood supply to the upper back.

Depth View of the Antihelix Tail: At this level of the antihelix, the concha wall exhibits a steep slope before it descends down into the inferior concha. The antihelix tail is like a long, narrow ridge before it curves down peripherally into the scaphoid fossa. The concha side of this inferior section of the antihelix corresponds to the cervical spine, whereas the concha wall below this region represents the sympathetic nerves affecting blood supply to the neck.

Depth View of the Antitragus: At this level of the antitragus, the concha wall forms an angled, vertical wall, which curves downward from the antitragus to the inferior concha. The antitragus corresponds to the skull, whereas the concha wall represents the thalamus of the brain.

The images in Figure 3.17 reveal the changes in the slope of the concha wall as it descends from the higher auricular ridges to the lower valleys of the concha. It is optimal for a new practitioner of auriculotherapy to verify for himself or herself the reality of these structural differences by actually touching the different sections of the antihelix and tactilely feeling the changes in the slope of the curving descent from different regions of the antihelix. Another procedure for indicating the different shapes and depths of different auricular areas is by the use of different auricular charts. In Figure 3.18, photographs of actual ears show retractors that are used to reveal the hidden regions of the external ear. Without such devices, one can also pull or stretch the external ear with one's fingers in order to examine portions of the auricle that are not readily visible from a simple surface view. The different regions of the auricle are depicted from a surface view, a posterior view, and a hidden view in Figure 3.19. Photographs of the different regions of the auricle are presented in Figures 3.20 and 3.21.

Contours of the antihelix and antitragus

Depth view of auricle

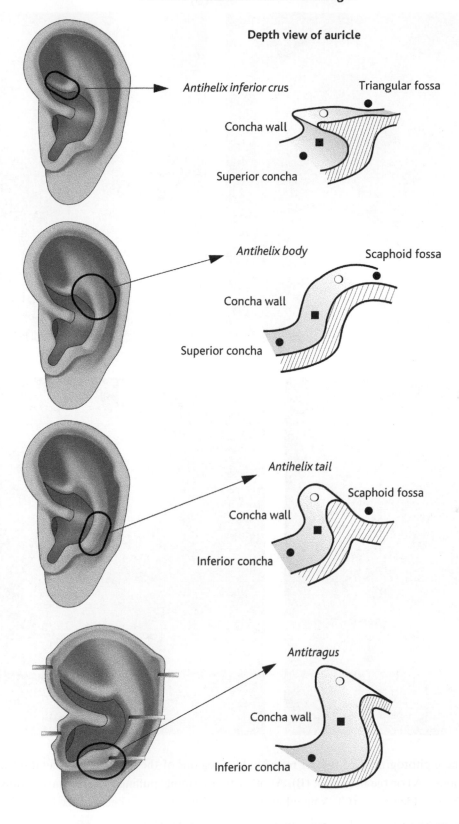

Antihelix inferior crus

Triangular fossa

Concha wall

Superior concha

Antihelix body

Scaphoid fossa

Concha wall

Superior concha

Antihelix tail

Scaphoid fossa

Concha wall

Inferior concha

Antitragus

Concha wall

Inferior concha

[**FIGURE 3.17** A depth view of the auricle that highlights the sloping contours of the external ear from the concha floor to the concha wall to the middle ridge of the auricle. At the more superior inferior crus, the antihelix flat ledge forms a sharp edge before curving under the inferior crus to the concha wall. Whereas the antihelix body is noted by a gradual slope into the deeper superior concha, the antihelix body is shaped more like a steep ridge. The concha wall behind the antitragus curves vertically downward toward the inferior concha floor.

(A)

(B)

(C)

(D)

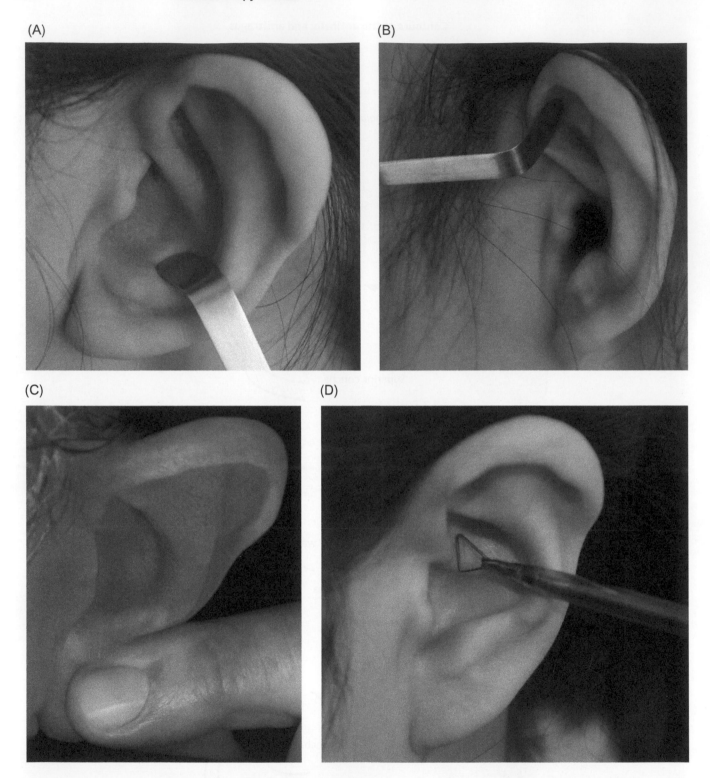

FIGURE 3.18 These photographs of the ear reveal hidden regions of the auricle when metal retractors are used to pull back the antitragus (A) or the helix root (B). At other times, simply pulling the external ear downward with one's fingers can reveal these hidden areas (C). A metal probe with a flat ending has been utilized to indicate notches in the skin surface that are associated with different landmarks on the auricle (D).

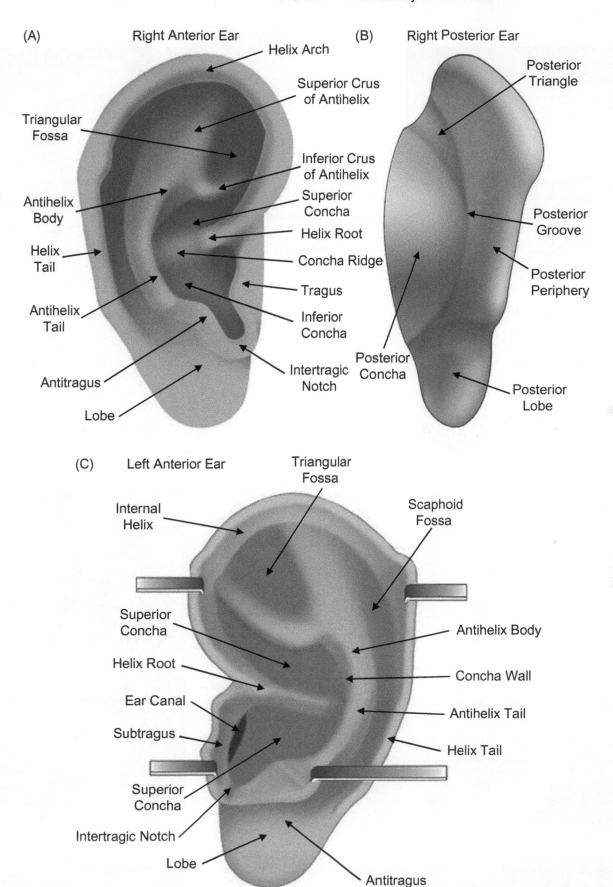

(A)   Right Anterior Ear

Helix Arch

Superior Crus
of Antihelix

Triangular
Fossa

Inferior Crus
of Antihelix

Antihelix
Body

Superior
Concha

Helix
Tail

Helix Root

Concha Ridge

Antihelix
Tail

Tragus

Antitragus

Inferior
Concha

Intertragic
Notch

Lobe

(B)   Right Posterior Ear

Posterior
Triangle

Posterior
Groove

Posterior
Periphery

Posterior
Concha

Posterior
Lobe

(C)   Left Anterior Ear

Triangular
Fossa

Internal
Helix

Scaphoid
Fossa

Superior
Concha

Antihelix Body

Helix Root

Concha Wall

Ear Canal

Antihelix Tail

Subtragus

Helix Tail

Superior
Concha

Intertragic Notch

Lobe

Antitragus

FIGURE 3.19 These illustrations of the right anterior ear (A), right posterior ear (B), and a hidden view of the left anterior ear (C) are labeled to indicate the anatomical terminology used for different regions of the auricle.

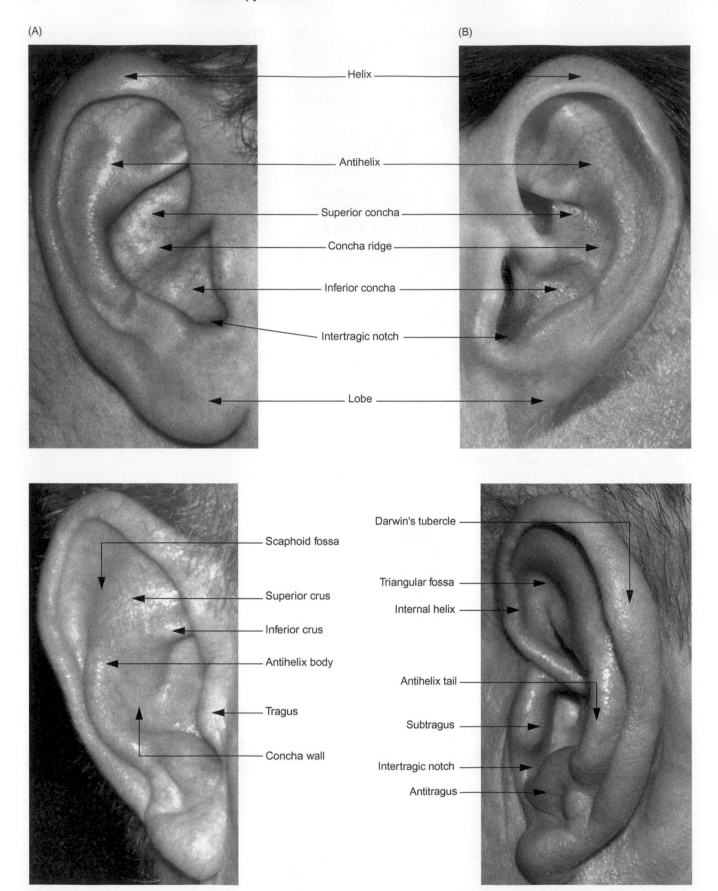

FIGURE 3.20 These photographs of the anterior auricle indicate specific anatomical regions that are found on a surface view of the external ear.

(A)   (B)   (C)

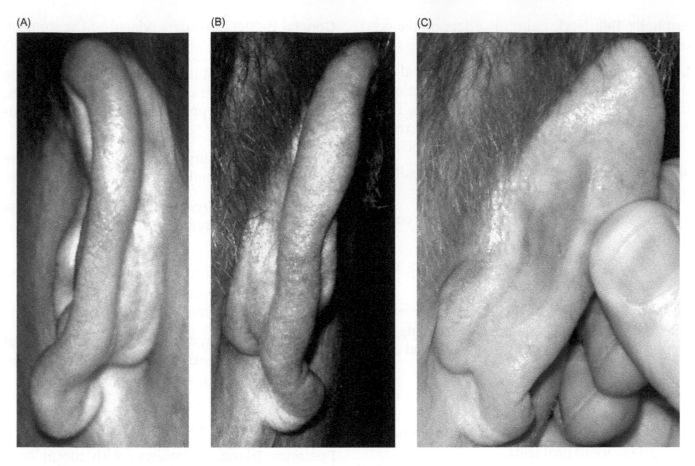

FIGURE 3.21 These photographs of the posterior auricle indicate specific anatomical regions that are found on a posterior view of the external ear.

3.8 Somatotopic Correspondences to Specific Auricular Regions

In auriculotherapy, an active reflex point is only detected when there is some pathology, pain, or dysfunction in the corresponding part of the body. If there is no bodily problem, there is no ear reflex point. An active reflex point is identified as an area of the ear that exhibits increased sensitivity to applied pressure and increased electrodermal skin conductivity. The health disorders that are commonly associated with each part of the auricle when there is pathology in a particular anatomical organ are presented next.

Helix: Anti-inflammatory points and treatment of allergies and neuralgias.

Helix Root: Dysfunctions of one's external genitals, sexual disorders, urinary dysfunctions, and diaphragmatic problems such as hiccups.

Helix Arch: Allergies, arthritis, tonsillitis, and anti-inflammatory processes.

Helix Tail: Representing the dorsal horn, sensory neurons of the spinal cord, and the preganglionic sympathetic nervous system, this region is used for the treatment of peripheral neuropathies and neuralgias.

Antihelix: Treatment of problems related to the main torso of the body that are related to pain and tension associated with the musculoskeletal system.

Superior Crus: Disorders of the lower extremities of the leg and foot.

Inferior Crus: Low back pain, lumbosacral disorders, buttocks spasms, and sciatica.

Antihelix Body: Thoracic spine back problems, chest pain, shingles, and problems with the abdominal muscles.

Antihelix Tail: Neck pain, disorders of the cervical spine, and throat problems.

Lobe: Dysfunctions related to the cerebral cortex of the brain, uncomfortable facial sensation, eye disorders, jaw pain, and dental analgesia. The ear lobe further represents conditioned reflexes, psychological resistances, and emotional blocks.

Tragus: Problems with the corpus callosum, appetite control, and adrenal glands.

Antitragus: Frontal, temporal, and occipital headaches.

Intertragic Notch: Hormonal disorders of the pituitary gland control of other glands.

Scaphoid Fossa: Problems in the upper extremities, such as frozen shoulder, stiff arm, tennis elbow, sprained wrist, hand tremors, and aching fingers.

Triangular Fossa: Problems in the lower extremities, such as hip pain, knee injuries, sprained ankle, foot pain, cold feet, uterus dysfunctions, and pelvic organ problems.

Concha: Visceral organ disorders.

Superior Concha: Disorders related to abdominal organs, such as the dysfunctions of the pancreas, gall bladder, kidney, and urinary bladder.

Inferior Concha: Disorders related to thoracic organs, such as heart problems and lung disease. It is also used for the treatment of substance abuse.

Concha Ridge: Disorders related to the stomach and liver.

Concha Wall: Dysfunctions associated with the thalamus of the brain, including general pain, sympathetic nerve problems, and vascular circulation disorders.

Subtragus: Laterality problems, auditory nerve deafness, and internal nose and throat disorders.

Internal Helix: Dysfunctions related to the internal genital organs, kidney disorders, and allergies.

Posterior Ear: Disorders related to motor activity and problems with the musculoskeletal body, such as muscle spasms and motor paralysis.

Posterior Lobe: Dysfunctions of the pyramidal motor cortex, the extrapyramidal striatal system, cerebellar tremors, and eye twitches.

Posterior Groove: Pain and muscle spasms of paravertebral muscles.

Posterior Triangle: Problems with motor control of leg movement, leg muscle spasms, and leg motor weakness.

Posterior Concha: Problems with motor control of internal organs.

Posterior Periphery: Problems with motor neurons of spinal cord, including tremors in arm and hand movements.

3.9 Three-Dimensional Model of the External Ear

Most pictorial representations of the external ear display only surface views of the auricle, which just reveal the more easily visible structures on the ear. Hidden views of the convoluted curves of the auricle are less easily represented. Previous texts by myself and others have shown hidden views of internal regions of the ear by the use of retractors that pull back overhanging auricular areas. However, many beginning students of auricular acupuncture find these retractor renderings difficult to conceptualize. The two-dimensional (2-D) perspectives that have classically been used to represent the external ear have failed to adequately represent the complexities of the curving contours and rolling depths of the auricle. It was thus decided to develop a three-dimensional (3-D) graphic model of the external ear that could more accurately reveal hidden points on the auricle than can be indicated by 2-D images used to standardize auricular nomenclature.

A 2-D ear diagram was first created which matched the dimensions of a standardized ear that was based on the mean measurements obtained from hundreds of clinical subjects. Photographs of the external ear of different individuals were also obtained using different camera angles. A graphic artist then utilized a commercially available Internet source to provide a basic 3-D representation of human anatomy. This process turned out to take far greater time than had been anticipated because the available 3-D images of the external ear were grossly insufficient for the detailed requirements for auricular acupuncture charts. The basic 3-D ear model was then restructured to more accurately depict the configurations that had been determined by the observations of the actual ears of human participants.

The specific 3-D computer graphics software used to create 3-D computer-generated imagery of the human auricle was developed from the Autodesk software Maya. The curving contours of the auricle of a computerized image of the external ear were customized by adjusting different layers and different dimensions of stylized graphic shapes. These basic 3-D images were then rendered to conform to a more anatomically recognizable view of the ear. A primary advantage of the 3-D ear models was that they could be viewed from a variety of angles, with the ability to be rotated in multiple planes that connect vertices points according to an x-axis, y-axis, and z-axis. The final Maya software version was then rendered as a wire mesh image of the ear that appears as multidimensional polygon segments that conform to the different contours of the 3-D ear. Figure 3.22 presents several examples of these wire mesh images. This Maya software image was then exported to an Adobe Photoshop program for further artistic delineation of the topographic contours and deeper structures of the auricle. The 3-D model was able to indicate arching curves and vertical walls of the auricle that have not been previously seen in 2-D auricular images. Final presentation of the 3-D ear model and the relative location of different auricular regions are revealed in Figure 3.23. With the ability to view this 3-D model of the auricle from multiple perspectives, a variety of 3-D auricular images are utilized to represent auricular acupuncture points in the remainder of this text.

(A)

(B)

(C)

(D)

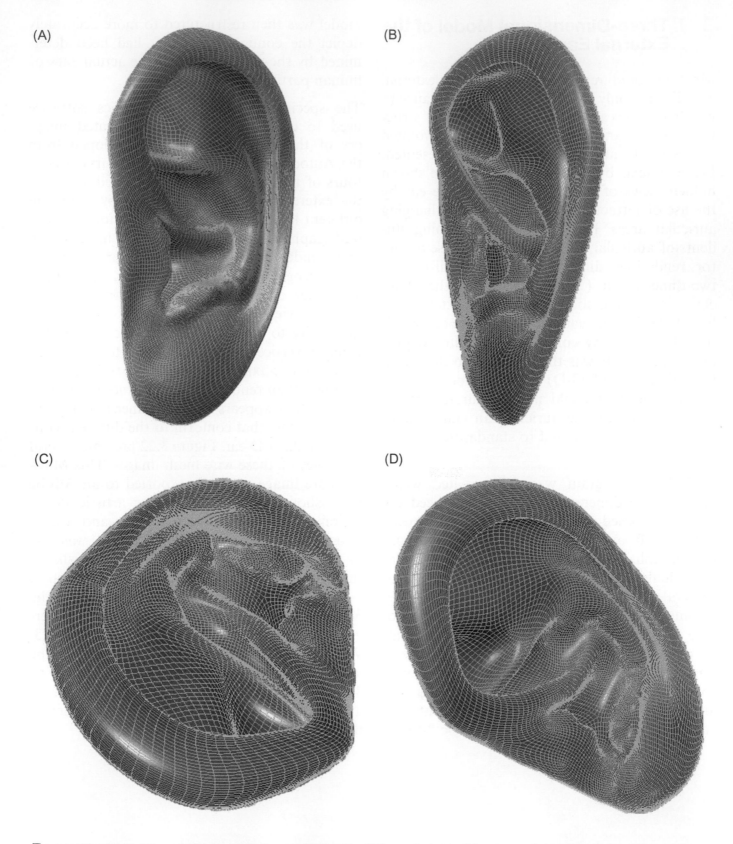

⟦**FIGURE 3.22** These 3-D wire mesh images indicating different holographic perspectives of the external ear were developed from the 3-D software program Maya.

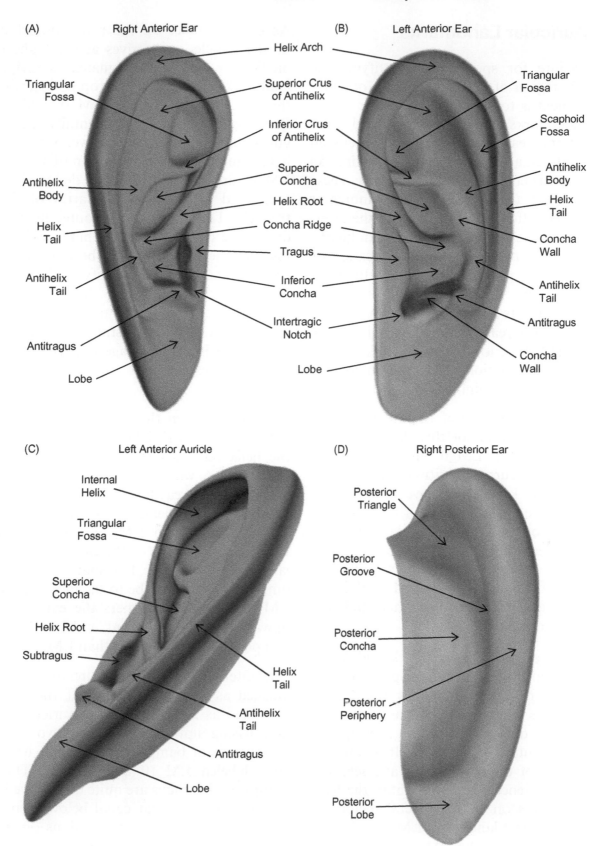

FIGURE 3.23 The 3-D wire mesh images that were shown in Figure 3.22 were then converted to more realistic 3-D images of the auricle. Anatomical terminology that indicates different structural regions of the auricle is shown for a surface view of the right ear (A), the left ear (B), a hidden view of the left anterior auricle (C), and an image of the posterior ear (D).

3.10 Auricular Landmarks

One procedure for specifically identifying the comparable region of the auricle from one person to the next is to examine the ear for distinguishing landmarks. Although the size and shape of the external ear may vary greatly between different individuals, these auricular landmarks are fairly consistent across most patients. These landmarks are distinguished by the beginning or the end of the different subsections of the external ear. The utilization of anatomical landmarks is very common in determining the location of body acupuncture points. For instance, the body acupoint Stomach 36 (ST 36) on the lower leg is determined by its specific position relative to the knee joint, whereas the body acupoint Large Intestine 4 (LI 4) is located at the base of the thumb in specific relationship to the anatomical location of the second digit of the hand.

The name and numbering of the different landmarks in earlier editions of this *Auriculotherapy Manual* began with LM_0 and ended with LM_17. In the current edition, these original 18 auricular landmarks have been supplemented with six additional landmarks, LM_18 to LM_23. Most of these additional landmarks lie in hidden or deeper regions of the auricle. In the accompanying figures, all auricular landmarks are shown within a hexagon-shaped symbol and a number is used to distinguish that landmark from other landmarks.

The most central auricular landmark is identified as LM_0. It is located at the master point referred to as Point Zero. Also known as Ear Center, this landmark is distinguished by a pronounced notch where the diagonal helix root rises upward from the horizontal concha ridge. It is found at the very center of the external ear and serves as the primary reference point to identify the location of acupoints on the peripheral regions of the auricle. The next landmark, LM_1, is located on the helix root where the external ear separates from the face. It lies immediately below the region between the auricle and the head, on the region of skin where the frames of eyeglasses rest upon top of the junction of the auricle with the skull.

As one continues up the helix toward the top of the auricle, one arrives at the highest point on the ear, which is designated as LM_2. This landmark is located at the top of a straight line that can connect LM_2, LM_0, and LM_13. Bending the auricle horizontally can distinguish this landmark from lower regions of the helix rim. The next two landmarks, LM_3 and LM_4, are two notches that define the uppermost and lowermost boundaries of Darwin's tubercle. This bulge on the outer helix is quite distinctive in some persons, but it is barely visible in others; thus, it can be one of the least reliable landmarks to identify. LM_3 is located along the central edge of the peripheral helix arch, whereas LM_4 is found more peripherally on the helix. LM_4 is distinguished by a prominent break in the cartilage underneath the skin that separates the helix arch from the helix tail below it.

Progressing down the helix tail toward the ear lobe, the landmark labeled LM_5 occurs where the helix takes a curving turn, below which is found LM_6, where the cartilaginous helix meets the soft, fleshy, ear lobe. The bottom of the ear lobe at LM_7 is identified by a straight line from LM_2, LM_0, and LM_13 and then ends at LM_7. The junction of the ear lobe to the lower jaw is labeled LM_8. For some individuals, the junction of the ear lobe to the face occurs below LM_7, whereas for others the ear lobe curves upward as it joins the head, and LM_8 is located at a position that is higher than LM_7.

The intertragic notch has already been distinguished as a separate region of the ear and is identified as LM_9 where the auricle meets the jaw. Rising upward, there are two prominent protrusions or bumps on the tragus, which have been labeled LM_10 and LM_11. These two bumps on the tragus are quite distinctive because they overhang the ear canal below them. There are two less prominent protrusions on the antitragus, which have been labeled LM_12 and LM_13. The landmark LM_12 occurs near the junction of the antitragus and the intertragic notch, whereas landmark LM_13 occurs at the tip or apex of the antitragus.

A. Right Ear Auricular Landmarks

B. Left Ear Auricular Landmarks

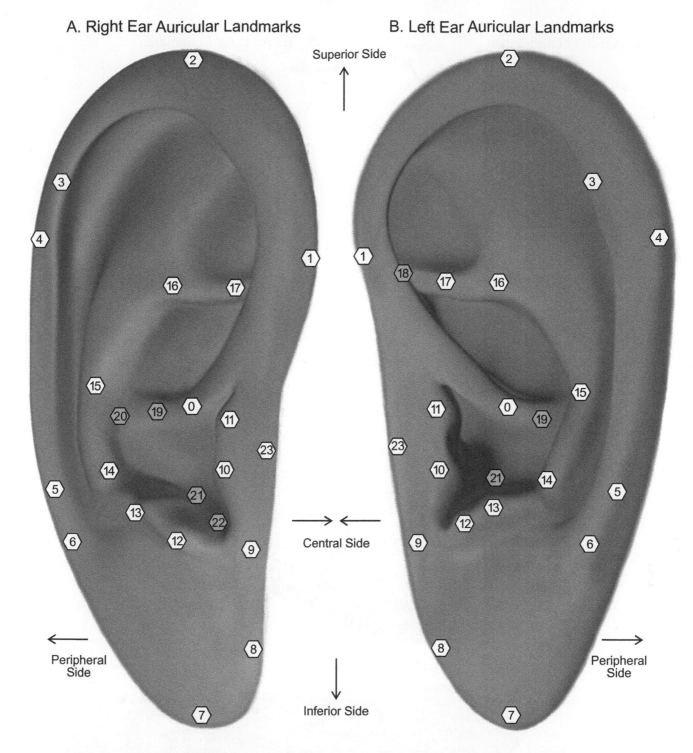

Superior Side

Central Side

Inferior Side

Peripheral Side

Peripheral Side

FIGURE 3.24 The specific locations of the 23 auricular landmarks indicated on the 3-D model of the external ear are shown for the right auricle (A) and the left auricle (B).

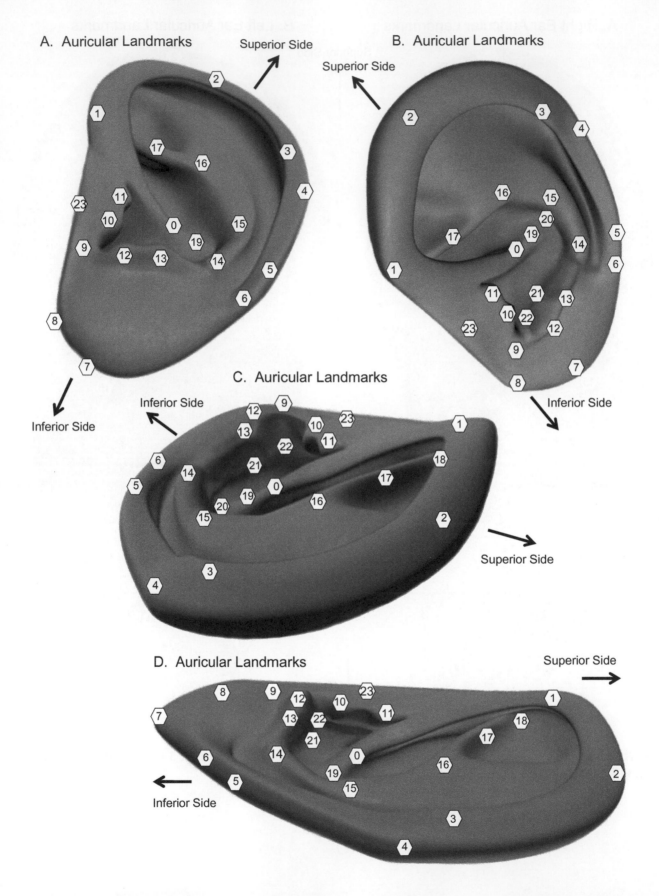

[FIGURE 3.25 Different perspectives of the 3-D model of the ear show the locations of auricular landmarks as seen from these different viewpoints.

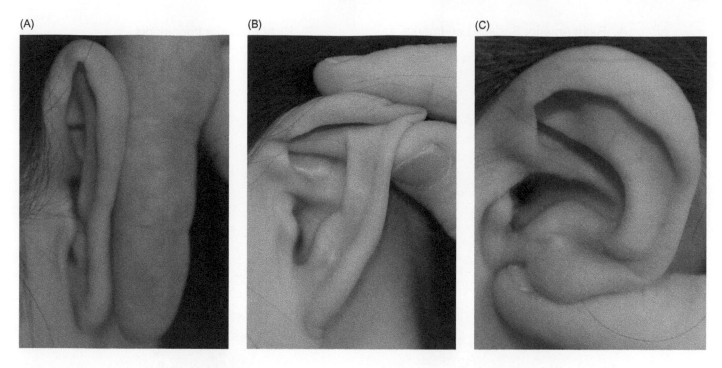

FIGURE 3.26 The identification of auricular landmarks on an actual person can be facilitated by bending the ear in different directions. Folding the external ear lengthwise (A) shows the location of LM_2 at the top of the ear and LM_7 at the bottom of the ear lobe. Folding the top of the ear in a horizontal manner (B) shows landmarks LM_1 toward the head and LM_4 at Darwin's tubercle. The crease that divides the antitragus and ear lobe respectively from the antihelix and helix can be better indicated by bending the ear diagonally above the ear lobe (C).

Above a distinct groove that separates the ridges of the antitragus from the antihelix, there is a protruding bump that is found on the base of the antihelix tail and has been identified as LM_14. From this landmark LM_14, one can use a flat-edged probe to follow the antihelix tail upwards toward the antihelix body. At an abrupt angle, the antihelix curves in a different direction at landmark LM_15. This notch divides the antihelix tail below from the antihelix body above. In addition, LM_15 lies horizontally across from LM_0 and directly above the concha ridge. If one continues with a flat-edged probe to feel the concha side of the antihelix body, it curves around the superior concha until one reaches a distinct notch at LM_16. This distinctive landmark separates the gradually sloping antihelix body from the flat-edged ridge of the inferior crus of the antihelix. The next landmark, LM_17, occurs at a notch that divides the peripheral and central halves of the antihelix inferior crus, halfway between LM_16 and LM_1. This notch somatotopically

corresponds to the sciatic nerve and is particularly noteworthy as the auricular point first discovered by Dr. Paul Nogier for the treatment of sciatica pain.

The first of the six additional landmarks is a continuation of the inferior crus of the antihelix from the notch at LM_17 toward the end of the inferior crus, where it meets the internal helix. Labeled LM_18, this new landmark lies directly underneath LM_1. It is found where the arching internal helix connects to the flat inferior crus of the antihelix. Because it is mostly hidden by the helix rim above it, LM_18 is difficult to observe. However, because it corresponds to the auricular master point known as the Sympathetic Point or Autonomic Point, it is important to learn. The next additional auricular landmark is LM_19, which lies peripheral to LM_0 on the concha ridge. It is located in a notch at the midpoint of the concha ridge, halfway between LM_0 and the concha wall. LM_19

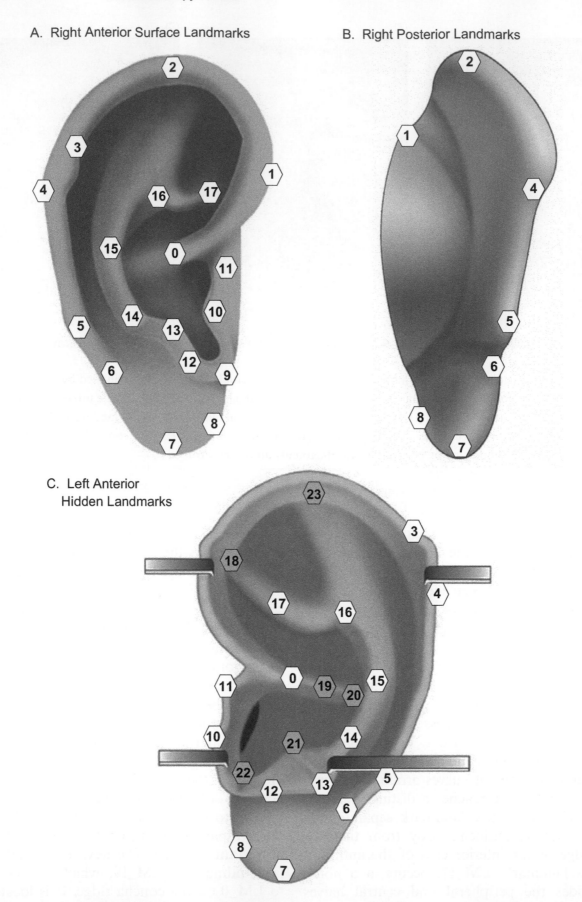

FIGURE 3.27 The 23 auricular landmarks are identified in these illustrations of the auricle from the perspective of a surface view of the ear (A), a posterior view of the ear (B), and a hidden view of the auricle (C).

indicates the boundary between the ear reflex points for the more central Stomach point and the more peripheral Liver point. Continuing more peripherally on the concha ridge toward the concha wall is LM_20, where the horizontal concha ridge meets the vertical concha wall. LM_20 lies directly below LM_15 on the antihelix ridge above it.

If one progresses downward, around the peripheral border of the inferior concha, one arrives at a newly labeled landmark, LM_21. This landmark LM_21 occurs at the junction of the inferior concha floor with the vertical concha wall below the antitragus apex. There is actually a prominent ridge that descends down the concha wall from LM_13, at the apex of the antitragus, to a deep notch where the concha wall joins the inferior concha. This landmark LM_21 corresponds to the location of another important master point, the Thalamus point or Subcortex point. A nearby auricular landmark is found at the bottom of the vertical wall of the intertragic notch. Designated LM_22, this landmark is located where the vertical intertragic wall becomes perpendicular to the concha floor. As with several other of these additionally identified auricular landmarks, LM_22 corresponds to the location of a master point, the Master Endocrine point. The final additional landmark that has been recognized is referred to as LM_23. It is found at the midpoint of the tragus, halfway between the top and bottom of the tragal flap that joins the external ear to the face. For the most part, landmark LM_23 lies between LM_10 and LM_11 on the tragus, but it has been specifically recognized in European auricular medicine charts as Point Zero Prime. According to these European charts, LM_23 lies exactly halfway along a line that connects LM_1 down to LM_8. That is, it is the midpoint between that point on the external ear where the helix root leaves the head and that point where the ear lobe rejoins the jaw. Taking the time to learn the specific location of all of these auricular landmarks greatly facilitates the recognition of which regions of the somatotopic auricle correspond to which regions of the physical body.

Locations of Original Auricular Landmarks

LM_0: Ear Center: A distinct notch is found at the central most position of the ear. It is found where the horizontal concha ridge meets the vertically rising helix root. It can be easily detected when one feels for this notch with a fingernail or a flat metal probe. LM_0 is the most common landmark to reference other anatomical regions of the auricle. Reactive ear points on the peripheral helix rim are often found at 30° angles from a diagonal line connecting LM_0 to the peripheral auricular point that corresponds to an area of body pathology. This region of the helix root represents the autonomic solar plexus and the umbilical cord, bringing body dysfunctions toward a more balanced state.

LM_1: Helix Insertion: This region of the ear occurs where the helix root separates from the face and where the helix brim crosses over the inferior crus of the antihelix below it. The external genitalia are found on the external surface of the helix root at LM_1, and internal genital organs are found on the internal helix root near LM_0.

LM_2: Apex of Helix: The most superior point of the ear is also called the apex of the auricle. It lies along a line that is vertical to LM_0 and LM_13. This ear point represents functional control of allergies and is the point pricked for bloodletting to dispel toxic energy.

LM_3: Superior Darwin's Tubercle: This notch along the central side of the helix lies immediately superior to Darwin's tubercle. This region corresponds to ear points that are used for the treatment of inflammatory reactions and tonsillitis.

LM_4: Inferior Darwin's Tubercle: This landmark is located more peripherally on the helix, above a crack in the cartilage where the helix arch is separated from the helix tail. The region of the helix tail below LM_4 corresponds to the lumbosacral spinal cord.

LM_5: Helix Curve: The helix tail angles centrally toward the ear lobe at this landmark. This auricular area represents the cervical spinal cord.

LM_6: Lobular-Helix Notch: A subtle notch where cartilaginous tissue of the inferior helix tail meets the soft, fleshy tissue of the ear lobe. This auricular area represents the medulla oblongata of the brainstem.

LM_7: Base of Lobe: The most inferior point of the ear lobe lies vertically below a straight line connecting LM_2 to LM_0 to LM_13 to LM_7. It corresponds to ear points used to treat inflammatory problems and facial spasms.

LM_8: Lobular Insertion: This landmark indicates where the ear lobe attaches to the jaw. The position of this landmark may vary considerably. For some individuals, LM_8 is located inferior to LM_7, whereas in other individuals, LM_8 is found superior to LM_7. This landmark corresponds to ear points that represent the inflammatory prostaglandin neurochemicals.

LM_9: Intertragic Notch: The curving notch that divides the tragus from the antitragus represents pituitary gland control of hormones from other endocrine glands.

LM_10: Tragus Inferior Protrusion: This protruding bump on the lower tragus represents endocrine control of the adrenal glands and is used for the treatment of various stress-related disorders.

LM_11: Tragus Superior Protrusion: This protruding bump on the upper tragus affects vitality, thirst, and water regulation.

LM_12: Antitragus Protrusion: This protruding bump on the lower antitragus lies near the intertragic notch. It corresponds to the forehead of the skull.

LM_13: Antitragus Apex: This protruding bump at the top of the antitragus represents the temples of the skull and is used for the treatment of migraine headaches and for asthma.

LM_14: Antihelix Base: This bump at the bottom of the antihelix tail lies above the antitragal–antihelix groove that divides the antitragus from the antihelix tail. The auricular region central to LM_14 represents the upper cervical vertebrae. The antihelix tail, which extends from LM_14 up to LM_15, corresponds to all seven cervical vertebrae and is used for the treatment of neck pain.

LM_15: Antihelix Curve: A slight notch divides the antihelix body above from the antihelix tail below. This landmark is located above the concha ridge and lies along a horizontal line across from LM_0. Ear points found at this landmark correspond to the junction of the lower cervical vertebrae with the upper thoracic vertebrae. The antihelix body, which extends from LM_15 up to LM_16, represents all 12 thoracic vertebrae and is used to alleviate back pain.

LM_16: Antihelix Notch: A distinct notch divides the flat ledge of the antihelix inferior crus from the sloping antihelix body. This landmark corresponds to the somatotopic representation of the lower thoracic vertebrae that lie next to the upper lumbar vertebrae. The antihelix inferior crus is used for the treatment of low back pain.

LM_17: Inferior Crus Midpoint: This notch on the top surface of the inferior crus of the antihelix divides the inferior crus into two halves, lying halfway between LM_16 and LM_18. This notch separates the lower lumbar vertebrae from the upper sacral vertebrae and was first identified by Dr. Paul Nogier as the Sciatica point, which led to the discovery of the inverted fetus map of the rest of the ear.

Locations of Additional Auricular Landmarks

LM_18: Internal Helix Insertion: This additional landmark is found at the region of the auricle that lies below LM_1, where the internal helix root meets the inferior crus of the antihelix.

LM_19: Concha Ridge Midpoint: This additional landmark is found at a notch peripheral to LM_0, located at the midpoint of the concha ridge, halfway between LM_0 on the helix root and LM_20 on the concha wall.

LM_20: Concha Ridge—Antihelix: This additional landmark is found at the junction of the concha ridge with the concha wall that lies immediately below the antihelix curve, LM_15.

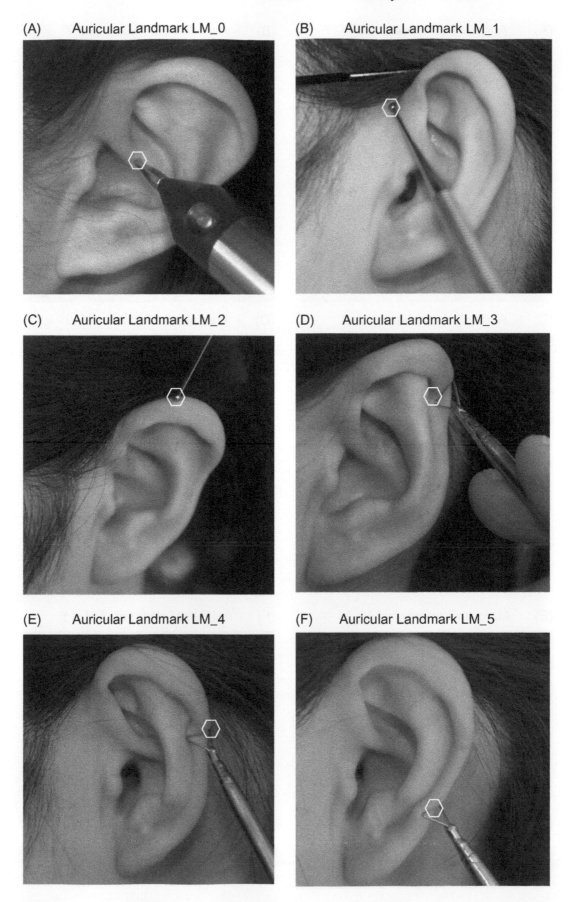

(A)   Auricular Landmark LM_0

(B)   Auricular Landmark LM_1

(C)   Auricular Landmark LM_2

(D)   Auricular Landmark LM_3

(E)   Auricular Landmark LM_4

(F)   Auricular Landmark LM_5

FIGURE 3.28 These six photographs of the ear show a pointer or probe that identifies the specific locations of auricular landmarks LM_0–LM_5.

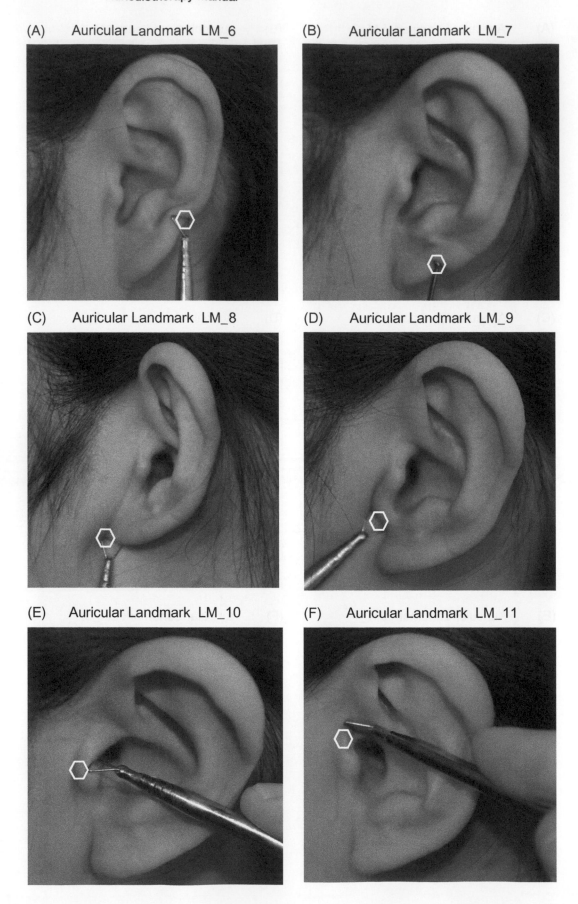

(A)   Auricular Landmark LM_6

(B)   Auricular Landmark LM_7

(C)   Auricular Landmark LM_8

(D)   Auricular Landmark LM_9

(E)   Auricular Landmark LM_10

(F)   Auricular Landmark LM_11

FIGURE 3.29 These six photographs of the ear show a pointer or probe that identifies the specific locations of auricular landmarks LM_6–LM_11.

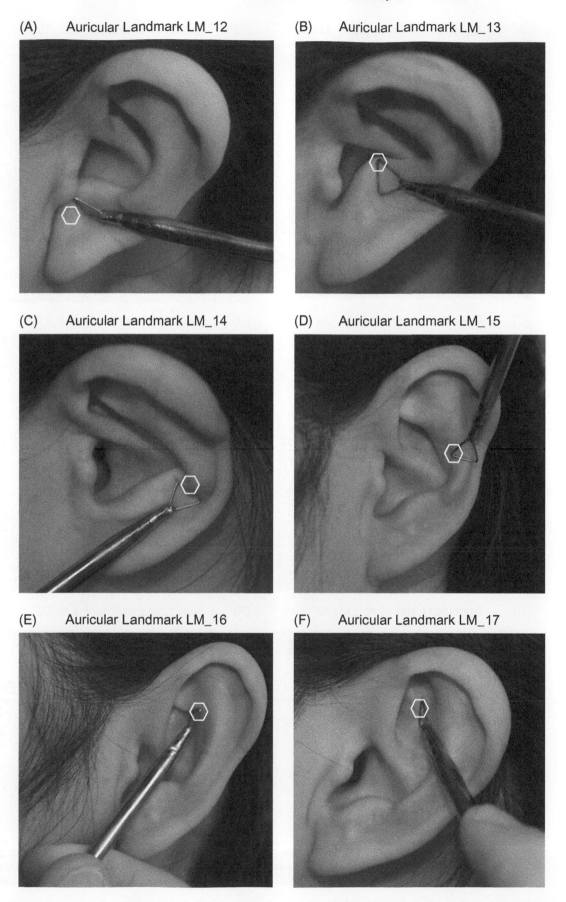

(A)   Auricular Landmark LM_12

(B)   Auricular Landmark LM_13

(C)   Auricular Landmark LM_14

(D)   Auricular Landmark LM_15

(E)   Auricular Landmark LM_16

(F)   Auricular Landmark LM_17

FIGURE 3.30 These six photographs of the ear show a pointer or probe that identifies the specific locations of auricular landmarks LM_12–LM_17.

(A) Auricular Landmark LM_18

(B) Auricular Landmark LM_19

(C) Auricular Landmark LM_20

(D) Auricular Landmark LM_21

(E) Auricular Landmark LM_22

(F) Auricular Landmark LM_23

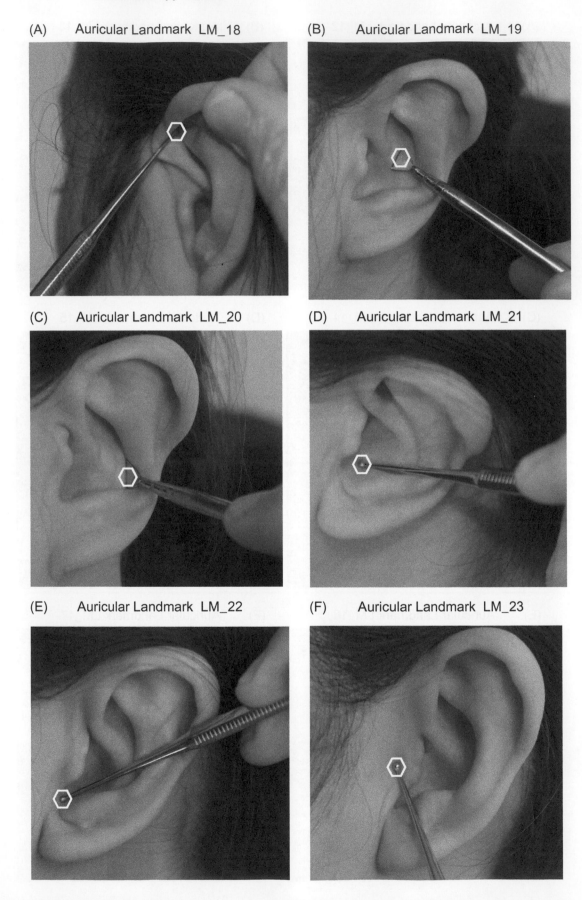

FIGURE 3.31 These six photographs of the ear show a pointer or probe that identifies the specific locations of auricular landmarks LM_18–LM_23.

LM_21: Concha Base—Antitragus: This additional landmark is found at the deepest point in the inferior concha, in a notch at the bottom of a ridge that runs vertically behind the antitragus at LM_13.

LM_22: Concha—Intertragic Notch: This additional landmark is found at the region of the inferior concha that lies immediately below the intertragic notch near LM_9.

LM_23: Midpoint of Tragus: This additional landmark is found midway along the tragus, halfway between LM_1, where the ear leaves the head, and LM_8, where the ear lobe rejoins to the jaw. It also lies approximately halfway between LM_10 and LM_11, where the tragus joins the face.

Relationship of Auricular Landmarks to Each Other

Auricular Quadrants: Two interconnecting straight lines can be drawn that form a cross dividing the ear into four equal quadrants, with LM_0 at its center. A vertical line runs along landmarks LM_2, LM_0, LM_13, and LM_7. A horizontal line can connect the landmarks LM_11, LM_0, and LM_15. The actual horizontal level of the external ear depends on the vertical orientation of the person's head, which can be held either slightly forward or bent slightly back. For the purposes of these ear diagrams, the horizontal level is set relative to its perpendicular relationship to the vertical line that runs from LM_2 to LM_7.

Auricular Grid Coordinates: Squares of approximately equal proportions can be formed by a grid pattern composed of five vertical columns and eight horizontal rows, with LM_0 at the center. The length of each square is approximately equal to the distance between the landmarks LM_0 and LM_15—approximately 10 mm. Figure 3.32 shows the grid coordinates and the lines of measurement obtained for different landmarks.

Standard Dimensions of Auricular Landmarks

To substantiate the relative proportions of the standardized ear chart used in this work, the landmark locations on the external ears of 154 volunteers were measured for the relative distances between landmarks. Volunteers were recruited by students at two different acupuncture schools in Southern California. Auricular landmark points were marked with a felt pen, and multiple measurements were made of the distances between two sets of landmarks. The means, standard deviations, and ranges of the measurements were computed for specific sets of landmarks. In addition, measurements of the width and length of the head, hand, and foot were recorded. The height of the head was measured from the chin to the top of the forehead, whereas the width of the head was designated as the distance between the ears. The length of the hand was computed between the wrist and the middle finger, whereas the width of the hand was measured between the thumb and the little finger. The length of the foot was assessed between the heel and the longest toe, and the width of the foot was measured between the big toe and the little toe. All of these measurements were used to determine the consistency of using the auricular zone system described in this chapter with actual persons.

Across the sample of 154 volunteers, there were an equal number of male and female subjects, with a mean average age of 39.7 years (SD = 14). The ethnic frequency of these participants consisted of 105 Caucasians (68.2%), 30 Asians (19.5%), 11 Hispanics (7.1%), and 8 blacks (5.2%). The larger representation of Caucasians and Asians in this sample probably reflected the social network of students attending acupuncture colleges in the Los Angeles area, from whom volunteers for this study were recruited. It was not intended that the external ears measured in this study were representative of the general population, only that there be a large cross-sampling of the external ears of different individuals.

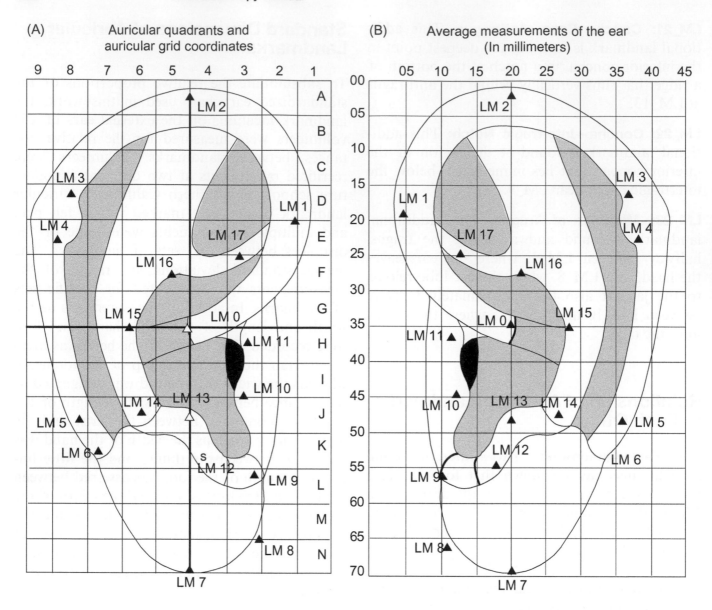

(A)   Auricular quadrants and
        auricular grid coordinates

(B)   Average measurements of the ear
        (In millimeters)

FIGURE 3.32 Diagrams of the external ear on the ear are divided into a rectilinear grid system with numbers "1" to "9" indicating horizontal sections and letters "A" to "N" indicating vertical sections. A thick vertical line between columns "4" and "5" and a thick horizontal line between rows "G" and "H" meet at Landmark 0, dividing the auricle into four quadrants. This same auricular grid system is placed on the ear diagram on the right side of the figure, with each section divided by 5-mm segments.

The accumulated mean data from the multiple observations of different auricles are presented in Table 3.2. This table indicates the relative mean distances between each landmark and the central landmark LM_0 and between each landmark and other landmarks. This set of measurements provides an overall indication of the shape and size of different ears. Acupuncture practitioners and students asked to identify the auricular landmarks on these 154 participants were readily able to distinguish each landmark on each subject.

The relatively low standard deviation data across these measurements suggests that examining the landmarks on many different ears is a reliable procedure for recognizing the specific areas of the auricle. A series of analyses of variance compared auricular measurements between male and female participants. Correlation coefficients were also obtained across all subjects for all measurements.

In *Treatise of Auriculotherapy*, Paul Nogier reported that the vertical axis of the auricle

TABLE 3.2	Measurements between Auricular Landmarks (LM).				
Landmarks	Mean (mm)	SD (mm)	Landmarks	Mean (mm)	SD (mm)
LM_2–LM_7	70.8	9.8	LM_0–LM_12	18.3	3.6
LM_1–LM_4	38.8	6.5	LM_0–LM_13	11.6	2.5
LM_0–LM_1	23.6	5.1	LM_0–LM_14	11.2	2.8
LM_0–LM_2	34.5	5.5	LM_0–LM_15	10.0	2.6
LM_0–LM_3	28.9	4.9	LM_0–LM_16	10.2	2.8
LM_0–LM_4	26.1	5.2	LM_0–LM_17	11.8	3.9
LM_0–LM_5	24.0	4.3			
LM_0–LM_6	26.5	5.0	Head height	195.1	22.7
LM_0–LM_7	36.3	5.6	Head width	165.2	28.4
LM_0–LM_8	34.4	5.3	Hand length	172.2	27.9
LM_0–LM_9	24.8	4.8	Hand width	102.1	16.7
LM_0–LM_10	14.9	2.5	Foot length	234.7	30.8
LM_0–LM_11	11.6	3.2	Foot width	95.3	14.5

varied from 60 to 65 mm and that the horizontal axis varied between 30 and 35 mm. Slightly larger measurements were found in the present study. For the 154 individuals examined in the present investigation, the mean height of the auricle, measured between the top of the ear apex at LM_2 and the bottom of the ear lobe at LM_7, was 70.8 mm. The mean width of the auricle, measured between the helix root as it leaves the face at LM_1 and the most peripheral part of Darwin's tubercle at LM_4, was 38.8 mm. In the assessment of the length and width of the head, hand, and foot, significantly larger measurements were found for males than females, at the $p < 0.05$ level. This result was not surprising because men are typically larger than women. Men had significantly larger external ears than women with regard to vertical length, a mean of 72.3 versus 68.4 mm, but there was no significant gender difference with regard to the horizontal width of the external ears.

Correlation coefficients for these measurements that were greater than $r = 0.40$ were considered statistically significant. The length of the foot was significantly correlated with the length of the hand ($r = 0.44$) and the width of the hand ($r = 0.42$) but only moderately with the width of the foot ($r = 0.39$). Curiously, there was only a small correlation between the height and width of the head ($r = 0.22$). Of all the auricular measurements, the only significant correlation ($r = 0.41$) with the foot,

hand, or head was between the width of the head and the distance between LM_0 on the helix root and LM_12 on the superior tragus.

The auricular measurements that most correlated with each other were for the distances between the ear center, LM_0, and the more peripheral regions of the ear. Significant correlations that ranged from $r = 0.44$ to $r = 0.89$ were found for the measurements of LM_0 to all of the landmarks that are arranged in a radial circle on the helix and tragus. The distances from LM_0 to more central landmarks on the antitragus and antihelix had fewer significant correlations, probably because they were smaller in length and did not vary as much from one person to the next. The purpose of obtaining these auricular measurements was primarily to demonstrate that these specific landmarks on the external ear can be reliably observed on many individuals. These measurements are consistently found on the auricle and are as useful for conducting auriculotherapy as the skeletal landmarks used for locating acupoints on the hand and the foot. Although the absolute size of the external ears does vary from one person to the next, specific cartilaginous structures on the auricle are found in relatively similar patterns on each individual.

A rectangular grid pattern was developed whereby a vertical linear axis was created from LM_2 at the top of the external ear down to LM_0 at the center of the ear and down to LM_7 at the bottom of the

TABLE 3.3	Horizontal and Vertical Coordinates for Landmarks (LM).			
Auricular Landmark	Vertical Axis		Horizontal Axis	
	Mean (mm)	SD (mm)	Mean (mm)	SD (mm)
LM_0	0.0	0.0	0.0	0.2
LM_1	17.7	2.1	−16.2	1.2
LM_2	34.5	2.9	0.0	0.0
LM_3	17.8	2.1	15.7	3.3
LM_4	15.7	2.6	22.6	1.8
LM_5	−14.2	3.0	18.2	2.8
LM_6	−20.3	1.5	14.6	2.4
LM_7	−36.3	2.0	0.0	0.0
LM_8	−30.4	2.2	−10.0	2.0
LM_9	−21.0	2.7	−11.7	1.4
LM_10	−9.7	1.4	−13.7	2.0
LM_11	4.3	1.4	−11.6	1.3
LM_12	−18.1	3.3	−3.0	2.9
LM_13	−11.6	1.8	0.0	0.0
LM_14	−10.2	1.8	6.4	1.0
LM_15	0.0	0.0	10.0	1.2
LM_16	8.1	1.1	2.4	0.7
LM_17	11.0	2.1	−6.4	1.6

ear lobe. A horizontal linear axis was created that crossed this vertical axis at auricular landmark LM_0 and also connected to the auricular landmarks LM_11 and LM_15 to form a straight line perpendicular to the vertical axis. Table 3.3 shows the mean average values for the vertical and horizontal coordinates for each auricular landmark relative to these vertical and horizontal primary axes. The average distance between LM_0 at the ear center and LM_15 horizontally peripheral to it on the antihelix was 10 mm, whereas LM_8 where the ear lobe joined the face was typically 10 mm medial to LM_0 and 30 mm inferior to LM_0.

■ KEY TERMS FOR CHAPTER 3

Key Terms for Embryological Perspectives of Auriculotherapy

Ectodermal Tissue: Ectodermal layers of the middle division of the embryo form the outer skin, cornea, teeth, peripheral nerves, spinal cord, brain, and the endocrine glands of the pituitary, pineal, and adrenal medulla. This embryological tissue is represented on the ear lobe and helix tail. This layer integrates inborn, instinctive information with individual learned experiences.

Embryological Tissue Layers: The embryo that develops from the initial fertilization of an egg and sperm then forms three layers of tissue: the ectoderm, mesoderm, and endoderm.

Endodermal Tissue: Endodermal layers of the inner division of the embryo form the gastrointestinal digestive tract, the respiratory system, and abdominal organs such as the liver, pancreas, urethra, and bladder. Auricular points related to this type of embryological tissue are represented in the central concha of the ear.

Mesodermal Tissue: Mesodermal layers of the middle division of the embryo form skeletal muscles, cardiac muscles, smooth muscles, connective tissue, joints, bones, the circulatory system, the lymphatic system, the adrenal cortex, and urogenital organs. Auricular representations of musculoskeletal tissues are found on the antihelix, the scaphoid fossa, the triangular fossa, and portions of the helix.

Key Terms for Auricular Anatomy

Antihelix (Middle Ridge): This "Y"-shaped ridge is "anti," or opposite, to the helix ridge.

Antihelix Body: A broad sloping ridge at the central third of the antihelix.

Antihelix Inferior Crus: The lower arm and horizontal extension of the antihelix.

Antihelix Superior Crus: The upper arm and vertical extension of the antihelix.

Antihelix Tail: A narrow ridge at the inferior third of the antihelix.

Antitragus (Lobe Ridge): "Anti" opposite to the position of the tragus.

Auricular Landmark: Prominent structural feature on the external ear that facilitates the distinction between one auricular area and another.

Cavum Concha (Inferior Concha): The classical name for the auricular area also known as the inferior concha that is the deep valley found peripheral to the ear canal.

Central Side: The medial, proximal side of the ear is directed inward toward the head.

Concha (Central Valley): A shell-shaped valley at the very center of the ear; concha refers to the conch seashell.

Concha Ridge (Inner Ridge): This ridge divides the superior concha from the inferior concha. It is the anatomical prolongation of the helix root onto the concha floor.

Concha Wall (Valley Wall): The hidden, vertical region of the ear rises up from the concha floor to the surrounding antihelix and antitragus.

Cymba Concha (Superior Concha): The classical name for the auricular area also known as the superior concha that is found below the inferior crus of the antihelix.

Ear Canal (Auditory Meatus): The funnel-shaped orifice that leads from the external ear to the middle ear and inner ear.

External Surface: The visible, external ear.

Helix (Outer Ridge): The outermost, circular ridge on the external ear.

Helix Arch: The highest section of the helix is shaped like a broad arch.

Helix Root: The initial segment of the helix ascends from the center of the ear.

Helix Tail: The final region of the helix descends vertically down the peripheral ear.

Hidden View: Vertical or underlying surfaces of the external ear are not easy to view.

Inferior Concha (Lower Valley): Formally known as the cavum concha in classical anatomical texts, the lower hemiconcha is found peripheral to the ear canal.

Inferior Side: The bottom side of the ear is toward the lower or ventral position.

Internal Helix: This hidden, underside portion of the brim of the helix spirals from the center of the helix to the top of the ear and around to the helix tail.

Internal Surface: The underlying surface of the ear.

Intertragic Notch (Notch Ridge): This "U"-shaped curve superior to the ear lobe separates the tragus from the antitragus.

Lobe: This soft, fleshy tissue is found at the most inferior part of the external ear.

Peripheral Side: The lateral, distal side of the ear is directed outward from the head.

Posterior Concha: The central region of the posterior ear is found behind the concha.

Posterior Groove: This long, vertical depression along the whole back of the posterior ear lies immediately behind the "Y"-shaped antihelix ridge.

Posterior Lobe: Soft, fleshy region behind the ear lobe.

Posterior Periphery: The outer, curved region of the posterior ear behind the helix.

Posterior Triangle: The small superior region on the posterior ear that lies between the two arms of the "Y"-shaped posterior groove.

Posterior View: The back side of the external ear faces the mastoid bone behind the ear.

Scaphoid Fossa (Outer Valley): This crescent-shaped, shallow valley separates the helix and the antihelix.

Subtragus: This underside of the tragus overlies the ear canal.

Superior Concha (Upper Valley): Identified as the cymba concha in classical anatomical texts, the upper hemiconcha is found below the inferior crus of the antihelix.

Superior Side: The top side of the ear is toward the upper or dorsal position.

Surface View: The front side of the external ear is easily available to view.

Tragus (Facial Ridge): The tragus of the auricle is a vertical, trapezoid-shaped area joining the ear to the face, projecting over the ear canal.

Triangular Fossa (Triangular Valley): This triangular groove separates the superior crus and the inferior crus of the antihelix.

■ CHAPTER 3 REVIEW QUESTIONS

1. The cartilaginous, outer rim of the auricle that ends in the soft, fleshy ear lobe is referred to as the_____.
   a. concha ridge
   b. antihelix tail
   c. helix tail
   d. helix root

2. The region of the auricle that hangs over the ear canal, adjacent to the face, is the_____.
   a. tragus
   b. superior concha
   c. internal helix
   d. antitragus

3. The narrow, flat ridge that forms the lower arm of the "Y"-shaped antihelix is called the_____.
   a. superior crus
   b. inferior crus

   c. helix arch
   d. intertragic notch

4. The extension of the helix root onto the floor of the concha has been labeled the_____.
   a. concha ridge
   b. concha wall
   c. inferior concha
   d. superior concha

5. The long, narrow groove that lies peripheral to the antihelix and alongside the helix tail is called the_____.
   a. tragus
   b. antitragus
   c. triangular fossa
   d. scaphoid fossa

6. The cavum concha deep valley of the auricle, which is found just peripheral to the ear canal, is referred to as the_____.
   a. superior crus
   b. inferior crus
   c. superior concha
   d. inferior concha

7. The deep crevice that is found on the back of the auricle, immediately behind the antihelix ridge, is called the_____.
   a. posterior groove
   b. posterior triangle
   c. posterior concha
   d. posterior lobe

8. The antihelix body shows somatotopic correspondence to the_____.
   a. thoracic spinal cord
   b. thoracic spinal vertebrae
   c. thoracic organs of the heart and lungs
   d. internal organs of the kidneys and bladder

9. Headaches are typically treated by the stimulation of auricular microsystem points located on the_____.
   a. tragus
   b. triangular fossa
   c. antitragus
   d. superior concha

10. The auricular landmark that is found at the same site where Dr. Paul Nogier first identified a reactive, auricular point for the treatment of sciatica pain is found on the_____.
    a. intertragic notch
    b. antihelix tail
    c. scaphoid fossa
    d. inferior crus of the antihelix

Answers

1 = c; 2 = a; 3 = b; 4 = a; 5 = d; 6 = d; 7 = a; 8 = b; 9 = c; 10 = d

Overview of the Auricular Zone System

CONTENTS

4.0 | Overview of the Auricular Zone System

CHAPTER 4 LEARNING OBJECTIVES

1. To demonstrate knowledge of the history of anatomical nomenclature systems.
2. To understand the alphanumeric code system developed for auricular zones based on proportional subsections of different auricular regions.
3. To identify specific auricular zones that correspond to particular anatomical organs.

4.1 Review of Auricular Zone Systems

In order to provide a systematic method for locating the precise position of a point on the ear, a zone system was developed that utilizes the proportional subdivision of major anatomical regions of the auricle. A set of two letters and a number represent each ear zone, in concurrence with guidelines established by the World Health Organization (WHO) Acupuncture Nomenclature Committee (Akerele, 1991; WHO, 1990b). This zone system was modified from the auricular zone system first developed in 1983 at the UCLA Pain Management Center (Oleson and Kroening, 1983b). The original zone system developed at UCLA utilized a single letter to designate each area of the auricular anatomy, and a number designated each subdivision of that area (Figure 4.1). A different zone system was originally suggested by Paul Nogier (1983) (Figure 4.2).

The 1983 Nogier zone system divided the whole auricle into a rectangular grid pattern of rows and columns. The capitol letters "A"–"O" identified the horizontal axis, whereas the lower-case letters "a"–"z" indicated the vertical axis. Although such a grid pattern is simple to use on flat, two-dimensional (2-D) paper, it is not as easily adaptable to the 3-D depths of the auricle. A similar, yet different, grid pattern has been more recently proposed by Winfried Wojak (2004) of Germany. This auricular nomenclature system is discussed in greater depth later in this chapter.

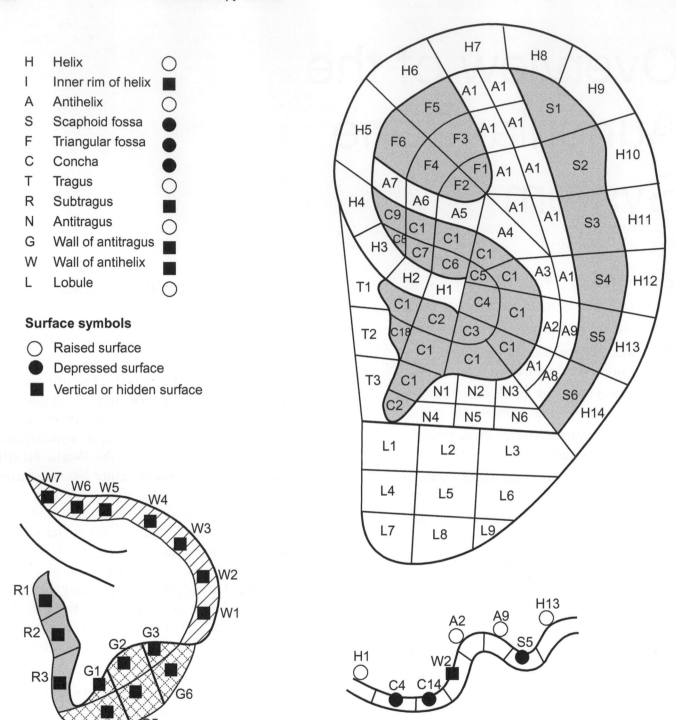

[FIGURE 4.1 The original auricular zone system developed in the 1980s at the UCLA Pain Management Center that shows specific subdivisions of each anatomical region of the external ear as represented by a single letter and a number.

The curving contours and depths of the external ear, however, do not easily conform to the configuration of rectangular rows and columns. The Nogier auricular system did not provide any method for indicating hidden or posterior regions of the auricle. Moreover, as the ear measurement presented in Chapter 3 indicated, there is a marked variance in the size of different areas of the auricle, even though the relative proportions remain the same. The distance from the ear apex at LM_2 to the base of the lobe at LM_7 ranged from 40 to 80 mm,

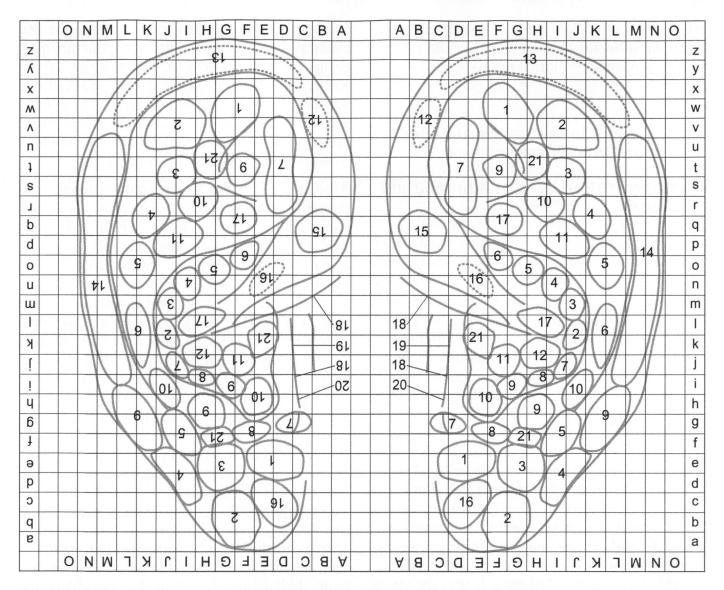

[**FIGURE 4.2** The auricular zone system first proposed by Dr. Paul Nogier shows a rectangular grid system distinguished by capital letters for each column and by small letters for each row. The numbers refer to the somatotopic organ represented by that section of the ear. (*Reproduced from Nogier (1983), with permission.*)

typically larger in men than women. Just the measured lengths of the ear lobes in these participants ranged from 15 to 45 mm, with some people exhibiting very large ear lobes, whereas the ear lobes of others were very small. A gridwork of rows and columns that are fixed in length does not allow for the correction of these variances in size.

The auricular zone system originally developed at UCLA designated each section of the external ear based on the proportional size of the auricular region of the individual, not the absolute size of the whole ear. This UCLA nomenclature system utilized a logical order for the numbering of each anatomical subdivision of the external ear. The lowest numbers begin at the most inferior and most central zone of that anatomical part of the external ear. The numbers ascend from 1 to 2 to 3, etc., while progressing from inferior to superior zones of that anatomical area and while progressing from central to peripheral zones. International communications about the location of ear acupoints can be referred to by their specific anatomical zone designation rather than the body organ to which it corresponds. Most publications on ear acupuncture identify different auricular acupuncture points by the name of the body area, such as the knee or the kidney, which does not allow for the anatomical differences in auricular location between the Chinese and European auriculotherapy systems.

4.2 International Standardization of Auricular Nomenclature

Standardization of Terms for Human Anatomy

The first concerted effort to create a standard terminology for human anatomy was developed by a group of German scientists in 1895 (International Congress of Anatomists, 1977). The *Basle Nomina Anatomica* (*BNA*) was first adopted in Germany, Italy, and the United States and later in Great Britain. In 1950, an International Congress of Anatomists met in Oxford, England, to discuss revisions to the earlier anatomical nomenclature system. A new *Nomina Anatomica* was accepted by the Sixth International Congress of Anatomists at a meeting in Paris in 1955. Most phrases were adopted from the original *BNA*, with all anatomical terms derived from Latin, utilizing words that were simple, informative, and descriptive. Changes to *Nomina Anatomica* were made by subsequent nomenclature committees in an attempt to simplify unnecessarily complex or unfamiliar terms. Although it was the strong opinion of the international nomenclature committee that only official Latin terms should be employed in scientific publications, it was also recognized that many scientific data-retrieval systems accept vernacular anatomical terms. English words in particular are commonly used in computer searches because English is currently the most widely used scientific language at international meetings and on the Internet.

WHO sought to bring an international consensus to the terminology used for acupuncture points by holding a series of international meetings of distinguished acupuncturists. Dr. Olayiwola Akerele (1991) presented the findings by the WHO working group that had been convened to specify the criteria for the standardization of acupuncture nomenclature. The first WHO working group meeting on this topic was held in Manila, Philippines, in 1982. There was general acceptance of a standard nomenclature for 361 classical acupuncture points. Acupuncture programs in Australia, China, Hong Kong, Japan, Korea, New Zealand, Philippines, and Vietnam adopted this meridian acupuncture system. The conclusions of the WHO regional working group were published in 1984 as the *Standard Acupuncture Nomenclature* (Wang, 1984).

Alphanumeric codes to designate different acupuncture points were labeled with two-letter abbreviations (Helms, 1990). Thus, "LU" was used for the Lung meridian and "LI" for the Large Intestine meridian. Some authors had used only one letter to represent a meridian, such as using "P" for the Pericardium meridian instead of "PC" or using "H" for Heart meridian instead of "HT." The least agreed upon English designation was the term Triple Energizer and its abbreviation "TE." The Han character for this meridian is often translated as Triple Warmer or Triple Heater, but some members of the nomenclature committee believed that this meridian should have been left with its original Chinese Han name, San Jiao. Consequently, this meridian channel is sometimes abbreviated "SJ." Representatives from each country who were at this meeting were encouraged to communicate to journals, textbook publishers, and universities in their country to only use the official WHO two-letter designations for Zang–Fu meridians and for acupuncture points.

The second WHO working group was held in Hong Kong in 1985 (WHO, 1985). Representatives reported general acceptance of the Standard Acupuncture Nomenclature from nine Asian countries. Revisions were suggested for standardization of extra meridian points and for new points. Two documents were presented at this WHO meeting to guide standardization ear acupuncture—the text *Ear Acupuncture* by Helen Huang (1974) and a journal article written by myself and Dr. Richard Kroening (Oleson and Kroening, 1983b). However, all decisions about auricular acupuncture nomenclature were deferred to a later meeting. The third WHO working group met in Seoul, Korea (WHO, 1987). Having already arrived at a consensus regarding classical meridian points, the final area of discord was with the nomenclature for auricular points. Because the meeting was organized by the WHO Regional Office for the Western Pacific, most of the representatives were from Asia. Only Dr. Raphael Nogier of France represented a European perspective.

Standard nomenclature was adopted for 43 auricular points, with each point designated by one or two letters and by a number. In addition to the standard nomenclature accepted for 43 auricular points identified as Category 1 points, another 36 ear points were identified as Category 2 points that needed further study for verification. All ear points were preceded by the letters "MA" to designate "Microsystem Auricular." For example, "MA-HX 1" indicated the location for the ear center point on the helix and "MA-TF 1" indicated the location for the shen men point in the triangular fossa. The only other approved designation for a microsystem was the designation "MS" for "Microsystem Scalp." No agreement was obtained for the two main schools of auricular points, the one initiated by Dr. Paul Nogier of France and the other one utilized by Chinese practitioners of ear acupuncture.

1990 Meeting of the World Health Organization

The final WHO General Working Group on Auricular Acupuncture Nomenclature met in Lyon, France (WHO, 1990a). The meeting was led by Dr. Raphael Nogier and Dr. Jean Bossy of France, Dr. C. T. Tsiang of Australia, and Dr. Olayiwola Akerele representing WHO. International participants at this meeting included representatives from Europe, Asia, America, and the Middle East, including the following countries: Australia, Austria, China (P.R.), Columbia, Egypt, Finland, France, Germany, Italy, Japan, Korea (D.P.R.), New Zealand, Norway, Spain, Switzerland, Venezuela, and the United States. Dr. Hiroshi Nakajima, Director-General of WHO, proclaimed to the gathering that "auricular acupuncture is probably the most developed and best documented, scientifically, of all the microsystems of acupuncture and is the most practical and widely used." He further acknowledged that

"unlike classical acupuncture, which is almost entirely derived from ancient China, auricular acupuncture is, to a large extent, a more recent development that has received considerable contributions from the West."

In his personal address to the audience, Dr. Paul Nogier observed that

the studies by Dr. Niboyet have proved that the ear points, like the body acupuncture points, can be detected electrically. We also know from the studies by Professor Durinian of the USSR that the auricle, by virtue of its short nerve links with the brain, permits rapid therapeutic action that cannot otherwise be explained. The time has come to identify each major reflex site in the auricle, and I know that some of you are busy on this. This identification seems to me to be essential so that there can be a common language in all countries for the recognition of the ear points.

Three qualities were emphasized:

1. Ear points that have international and common names in use
2. Ear points that have proven clinical efficacy
3. Ear points whose localization in the auricular area is generally accepted

The group agreed that each anatomical area of the ear should be designated by two letters, not one, to conform to the body acupuncture nomenclature. The abbreviation for Helix became "HX" rather than "H," and the designation for Lobe became "LO" rather than "L." Terminology was also added for points on the back of the ear, with each area to begin with the initial letter "P," as in "PP" for "Posterior Periphery" and "PL" for "Posterior Lobe."

The primary difficulty for this WHO nomenclature conference was dealing with the discrepancy between the Chinese and European locations for some ear points. For example, the Knee point is localized on the superior crus of the antihelix in the Chinese system but in the triangular fossa in the European system. No concurrent agreement on this issue was determined. The group did adopt a standardized nomenclature for 39 auricular points, but it decided that another

TABLE 4.1	WHO 1990 Standard Nomenclature for Accepted Auricular Points.

Anatomical Area	Numeric Code	English Name	Pinyin Name
Helix	MA-HX 1	Ear Center	Erzhong
	MA-HX 2	Urethra	Niaodao
	MA-HX 3	External Genitals	Waishengzhiqi
	MA-HX 4	Anus	Ganmen
	MA-HX 5	Ear apex	Erjian
Antihelix	MA-AH 1	Heel	Gen
	MA-AH 2	Ankle	Huai
	MA-AH 3	Knee	Xi
	MA-AH 4	Pelvic Girdle	Tun Kuan
	MA-AH 5	Sciatic Nerve	Zuogu shenjing
	MA-AH 6	Autonomic Point	Jiaogan
	MA-AH 7	Cervical Vertebrae	Jingzhui
	MA-AH 8	Thoracic Vertebrae	Xiongzhui
	MA-AH 9	Neck	Jing
	MA-AH 10	Thorax	Xiong
Scaphoid fossa	MA-SF 1	Fingers	Zhi
	MA-SF 2	Wrist	Wan
	MA-SF 3	Elbow	Zhou
	MA-SF 4	Shoulder Girdle	Jian
Triangular fossa	MA-TF 1	Ear Shen Men	Ershenmen
Tragus	MA-TG 1	External Nose	Waibi
	MA-TG 2	Apex of Tragus	Pingjian
	MA-TG 3	Pharynx and Larynx	Yanhou
Antitragus	MA-AT 1	Head	Zhen
Intertragic notch	MA-IT 1	Pituitary Gland	Nao Chui Ti
Inferior concha	MA-IC 1	Lung	Fei
	MA-IC 2	Trachea	Qiguan
	MA-IC 3	HPA axis	Neifenmi
	MA-IC 4	Triple Energizer	San Jiao
	MA-IC 5	Mouth	Kou
	MA-IC 6	Esophagus	Shidao
	MA-IC 7	Cardia	Bennen
Superior concha	MA-SC 1	Duodenum	Shi erzhichang
	MA-SC 2	Small Intestine	Xiaochang
	MA-SC 3	Appendix	Lanwei
	MA-SC 4	Large intestine	Dachang
	MA-SC 5	Liver	Gan
	MA-SC 6	Pancreas–gall bladder	Yidan
	MA-SC 7	Ureter	Shunianoguan
	MA-SC 8	Bladder	Pangguang
Lobe	MA-LO 1	Eye	Mu

36 ear points did not as yet meet the three working criteria. The Category 1 and Category 2 ear points described by the 1987 working group from the Western Pacific Division of WHO were similar to the "Agreed Upon" and "Not Agreed Upon" or "Additional" auricular points listed by the 1990 WHO meeting. The two lists of ear points are respectively presented in Tables 4.1 and 4.2. During the course of discussions, many divergent points of view emerged concerning

TABLE 4.2	WHO 1990 Standard Nomenclature for Additional Auricular Points.		
Anatomical Area	**Numeric Code**	**English Name**	**Pinyin Name**
Helix	MA-HX 6	Internal Genitals	Neishengzhiqi
	MA-HX 7	Upper Ear Root	Shangergen
	MA-HX 8	Lower Ear Root	Xiaergen
	MA-HX 9	Root of Ear Vagus	Ermigen
Antihelix	MA-AH 11	Toe	Zuzhi
	MA-AH 12	Lumbosacral Spine	Yaodizhui
	MA-AH 13	Abdomen	Fu
	MA-AH 14	Pelvis	Penqiang
Scaphoid fossa	MA-SF 5	Wind Stream	Fengxi
Triangular fossa	MA-TF 2	Middle Triangular Fossa	Jiaowozhong
	MA-TF 3	Superior Triangular Fossa	Jiaowoshang
Tragus	MA-TG 4	Adrenal Gland	Shenshangxian
Antitragus	MA-AT 2	Subcortex or Thalamus Point	Pizhixia
	MA-AT 3	Apex of Antitragus	Duipingjian
	MA-AT 4	Central Rim or Brain	Yuanzhong
	MA-AT 5	Occiput	Zhen
	MA-AT 6	Temple	Nie
	MA-AT 7	Forehead	E
Inferior concha	MA-IC 4	Heart	Xin
	MA-IC 5	Spleen	Pi
	MA-IC 6	Stomach	Wei
Superior concha	MA-SC 9	Kidney	Shen
	MA-SC 10	Angle of Superior Concha	Tingjiao
Lobe	MA-LO 2	Tooth	Ya
	MA-LO 3	Tongue	She
	MA-LO 4	Jaw	He
	MA-LO 5	Eye	Yan
	MA-LO 6	Internal Ear	Nei'er
	MA-LO 7	Cheek	Mianjia
	MA-LO 8	Tonsil	Biantaoui
	MA-LO 9	Anterior Ear Lobe	Chuiqian
Posterior lobe	MA-PL 1	Eye	Yan
Posterior peripheral	MA-PP 1	Hypertension	Goo Xue Ya Dian
Posterior intermediate	MA-PI 1	Groove of Posterior Surface	Erbeigou
Posterior central	MA-PC 1	Heart of Posterior Surface	Erbeixin
	MA-PC 2	Spleen of Posterior Surface	Erbeipi
	MA-PC 3	Liver of Posterior Surface	Erbeigan
	MA-PC 4	Lung of Posterior Surface	Erbeifei
	MA-PC 5	Kidney of Posterior Surface	Erbeishen

both the localization and the terminology of auricular points. After a free exchange of ideas and opinions, the WHO working group agreed that a priority of future activity should be the development of a standard reference chart of the ear. This chart should provide a correct anatomical illustration of the ear, an appropriate anatomical mapping of topographical areas, consultation with experts in anatomy and auricular acupuncture, illustrations of correct zones in relation to auricular acupuncture, and the actual delineation and localization of ear points.

A subsequent committee directed by Dr. O. Akerele (WHO, 1990b) developed specific anatomical drawings of the ear and specific terminology for the auricle.

4.3 World Meetings on Standardization of Auricular Acupuncture Points

Since the publication of the third edition of *Auriculotherapy Manual* in 2001, the World Federation of Acupuncture–Moxibustion Societies (WFAS) has held several working group meetings on the international standardization of auricular acupuncture. Recent international meetings that held panels which examined auricular acupuncture nomenclature systems were held in Beijing, China, in May 2010 and in Lyon, France, in June 2012.

Objectives of Meetings on Acupuncture Standardization

1. To review and summarize previous procedures for developing an auricular nomenclature system

2. To develop an integrated nomenclature system for the external ear that incorporates the best features of previous nomenclature systems

3. To provide specific guidelines for using an alphanumeric system to describe the location of an area of the external ear that corresponds to pathology in a specific part of the whole body

4. To develop a simplified auricular nomenclature system that is both scientifically accurate in the presentation of the anatomy of the external ear and is user-friendly for beginning students and advanced practitioners of auriculotherapy and auricular diagnosis

5. To discuss the merits and limitations of different auricular nomenclature systems and to support the findings of a consensus of international experts in this field regarding the most optimal, auricular, nomenclature system to be utilized throughout the world

Chinese Auricular Nomenclature System

Dr. Liqun Zhou (1995) utilized the official findings from the 1990 WHO international meeting to develop updated ear acupuncture charts that were distributed throughout the Chinese medicine community (Figure 4.3). This Chinese ear acupuncture format incorporated an alphanumeric code of two letters and a number, with some differences in nomenclature from the system proposed by Oleson (1996). In the auricular zone system developed by Oleson, the lowest numbers for each auricular area began at the most inferior and most central zones of each anatomical region. The numbers then ascended to higher digits as one progressed to more superior and more lateral sections of that anatomical region. The auricular zone system developed by Zhou typically assigned sequential numbers in a descending, rather than ascending, pattern. The anatomical areas of the auricle and all ear points were represented in English and with Han script.

There were no further professional reports to evaluate the international standardization of auricular acupuncture points from 1990 to 2008. In 2009, Liqun Zhou and Baixiao Zhao of the Beijing University of Chinese Medicine finished their literature research of auricular nomenclature and the location of auricular acupuncture points (AAP). They proposed a new national standard of nomenclature to identify the location of AAP as part of an international project by WFAS. Sponsored by the State Administration of TCM and the China Academy of Acupuncture and Moxibustion, an international conference of the working group of nomenclature and location of auricular acupuncture points was held in Beijing, China, on May 18, 2010. From this gathering of professionals from different nations was developed the International Standard of Auricular Acupuncture Points (ISAAP). The working group presented three observations:

• The nomenclature and location of Chinese AAP is mainly based on the specific therapeutic effectiveness of the acupoint as a part of Traditional Chinese Medicine (TCM).

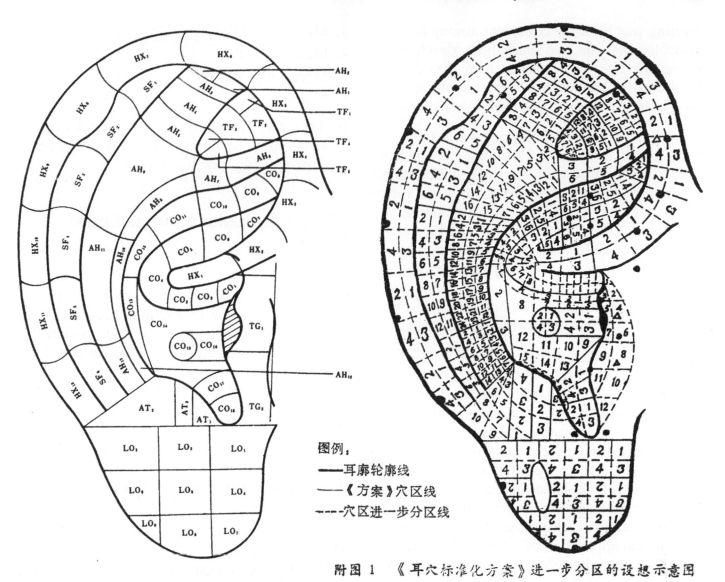

附图 1 《耳穴标准化方案》进一步分区的设想示意图

[**FIGURE 4.3** The ear acupuncture nomenclature system developed in China after the WHO international conference in 1990. The English version of this chart shows the same two letters for representing each region of the ear as was proposed at the WHO conference, with smaller districts within each region represented by numbers. The numbering system developed by Chinese doctors is different from the numbering system developed at UCLA, and the whole concha region of the ear is represented by the letters "CO." The ear diagram on the right shows each district subdivided into even smaller areas of the ear, with numbers ranging from "1" to "4."

- American studies of auricular acupoints have been chiefly based on numerical codes of AAP with specific nomenclature and specific point location.

- European reports of auricular medicine are mostly based on the theoretic system of Western medicine and reflex point on the auricle of all systems of the body to be nominated and located.

Based on the previous 20 years of acupuncture research and the collective efforts of WHO, the draft document proposed by WFAS for the ISAAP was comprehensive, systematic, and normative, which is a great improvement. Through overall discussion and consultation with an international panel of experts in the field, the standardization of nomenclature and location of auricular points was evaluated for consistency and international consensus. The delegates suggested that an Internet network forum be established in order to cooperate and communicate with regard to further developments of this system. The ISAAP system presented at this 2010 Beijing meeting was basically consistent among the three auricular systems that have been developed in China, Europe, and America with regard to the location of ear reflex points corresponding to the face, head, trunk, arm, and most internal organs.

However, it was nonetheless noted that there were still significant differences in the nomenclature and location of certain auricular reflex points, specifically differences in the location of auricular points that represented spinal vertebrae, leg, foot, heart, kidney, and most parts of the nervous systems. The differences in auricular systems for different countries are partially a reflection of the differences in the medical culture of Chinese medicine and Western medicine, both in clinical practice and in fundamental theories of medicine.

The different wall charts of AAP of different countries and schools are the result of ethnic culture, medical thinking models, and neuroanatomical knowledge at certain times in history. The Chinese auricular system utilizes the concepts of holistic medicine and the thinking of traditional Chinese medicine as a product of the theoretical integration of Chinese medicine and modern Western medicine. The auriculotherapy systems of France and America are guided by the theories and clinical application of modern Western medicine. They are relatively less influenced by TCM.

There are both differences and similarities in the nomenclature and location of AAP throughout the world. Therefore, differences and similarities should be made known clearly in order to promote the process of the international standardization of AAP. The draft report of the ISAAP is based on the scientific research and published literature of several thousands of years. Moreover, it is based on a large-scale investigation of clinical observations and fundamental research and on the collective wisdom of the group of experts in the field of auricular medicine organized by national governments.

According to the findings of the 2010 working group, the ISAAP has the following advantages over other nomenclature systems:

1. More normative
2. More comprehensive
3. More compatible
4. More applicable
5. More authoritative
6. More popular

In this sense, the international standard of AAP is a milestone summary of the knowledge of AAP of auricular acupuncturists.

Oleson Auricular Nomenclature System

My presentations to the international nomenclature meetings at the Beijing conference in 2010 and at the Lyon symposium in 2012 were derived from revisions of the auricular zone system that I originally advanced at the 1990 international WHO gathering. I described how photographic pictures of actual ears were used by graphic artists to render different drawings of the external ear to serve as a representative auricle. These images of the external ear were then used to differentiate specific subdivisions of the anatomy of the external ear to develop, which was then further distinguished by a 3-D model of these auricular regions.

The auricular zone system developed at the UCLA Pain Management Center was published in the *Auriculotherapy Manual: Chinese and Western Systems of Ear Acupuncture* (Oleson, 1990) (Figures 4.4 and 4.5). Both the second edition (Oleson, 1996) and the third edition (Oleson, 2003) of *Auriculotherapy Manual* utilized the nomenclature information developed at the 1990 WHO meeting. Two-letter abbreviations for each region of the auricle were accompanied by a one- or two-digit number for different subdivisions of each auricular zone.

Similar to the cun measurements that are used to locate the position of body acupuncture points, the landmarks identified on the auricle are useful for distinguishing where one zone ends and the next one begins. It is the proportional representation of the distance between adjacent landmarks that most readily facilitates the distinction of a particular area of the auricle in someone with large ears as opposed

Surface, hidden, and posterior auricular zones

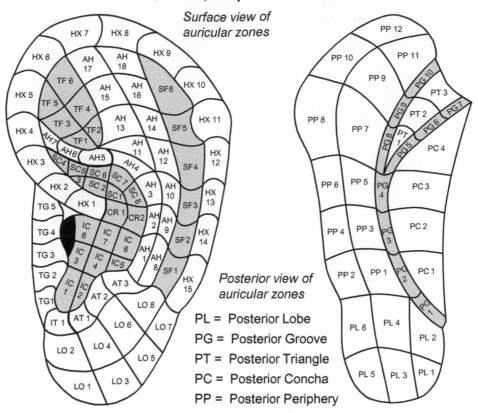

Surface view of auricular zones

Posterior view of auricular zones

PL = Posterior Lobe
PG = Posterior Groove
PT = Posterior Triangle
PC = Posterior Concha
PP = Posterior Periphery

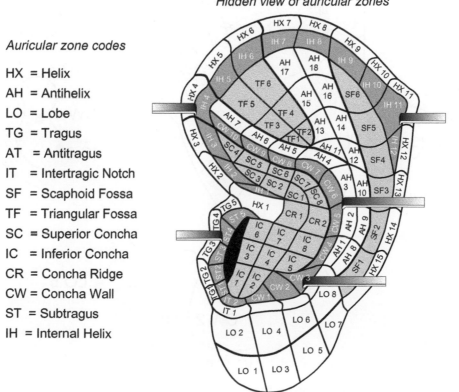

Hidden view of auricular zones

Auricular zone codes

HX = Helix
AH = Antihelix
LO = Lobe
TG = Tragus
AT = Antitragus
IT = Intertragic Notch
SF = Scaphoid Fossa
TF = Triangular Fossa
SC = Superior Concha
IC = Inferior Concha
CR = Concha Ridge
CW = Concha Wall
ST = Subtragus
IH = Internal Helix

[FIGURE 4.4 The updated auricular nomenclature system originally developed by Dr. Terry Oleson at UCLA with revisions based on the WHO international conference in 1990. In this newer version, each subsection of an auricular region is indicated by two letters and a number, with the progression of numbers beginning from the bottom of the ear toward the top and from the more central regions of the ear toward the periphery.

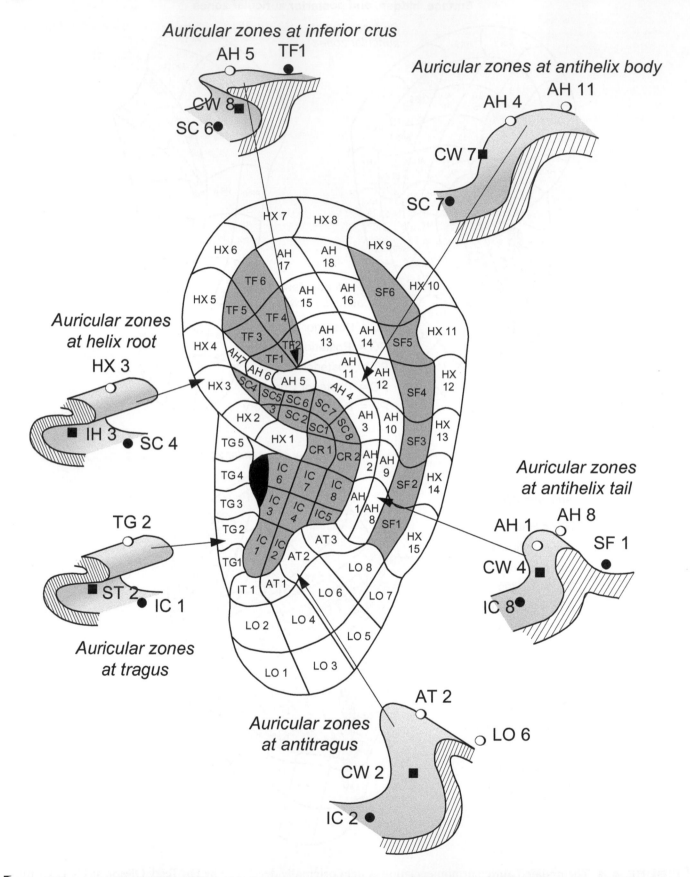

FIGURE 4.5 A depth view of the auricular zone system developed by Dr. Oleson which indicates the location of specific auricular regions showing deeper zones in the concha represented by solid circles, adjacent zones on the concha wall represented by black squares, and the higher zones on adjacent ridges represented by open circles.

to someone with small ears. The location of auricular points within these auricular zones is denoted by the letter ".c" or the superscript [C] for Chinese ear charts and by the letter ".e" or the superscript [E] when it conforms to the charts developed by European practitioners of auricular medicine.

The concept of an auricular zone to differentiate auricular subsections is similar to the use of ZIP codes (Zone Improvement Plan) by the U.S. Postal Service. The five decimal, numerical digits used for ZIP codes were developed in 1963 to improve mail delivery to specific postal regions. Many years earlier, the city of Paris, France, was divided into 20 administrative districts referred to as *arrondissements* to facilitate mail delivery. The 20 arrondissements of Paris are arranged in the form of a clockwise spiral, starting in the middle of the city, with the first on the north bank of the Seine River. Different sections of the city of Los Angeles, California, are also subdivided in this way. Chinese representatives at the 2010 nomenclature meeting were more familiar with the term "district" than the term "zone" because different areas of the city of Beijing are referred to as districts.

Wojak Auricular Nomenclature System

A linear grid system that uses only numbers and not letters has been proposed by Dr. Winfried Wojak (2004) of Germany to abbreviate different areas of the auricle. This German system first designates different auricular territories on the anterior side of the external ear with the numbers 1–7, whereas the numbers 8, 9, and 0 are used for specific regions of the back of the auricle. Two additional digits are then used to subdivide the horizontal and vertical axes of the auricle, with the second of three numbers representing the "x-axis" and the third of three numbers representing the "y-axis."

Dr. Wojak has proposed that the advantage of using only numbers (as with a postal code) is that they can be read throughout the world. The first digit of the auricular zone system refers to the following auricular regions: Zone 1 = lobe and antitragus, Zone 2 = tragus, Zone 3 = inferior concha, Zone 4 = superior concha, Zone 5 = triangular fossa, Zone 6 = helix ascending, Zone 7 = helix descending, Zone 8 = posterior concha, Zone 9 = posterior helix, and Zone 0 = posterior lobe. Wojak noted that although ears may differ in the dimensions of the described zones, these 10 zones can be found on everyone's external ear. Figure 4.6 presents several examples of Wojak's zone system.

For the two other numbers in the Wojak auricular zones, it was easiest to use "x" and "y" coordinates known from classical mathematics. Every auricular zone has nine vertical columns and nine or six horizontal rows. Following the principle of the classical Chinese system of cun and fen, these zones allow the numerical codes to individualize the system for everyone's ears. In those zones in which nine lines would have led to very small square fields, it was decided to use only six lines. For example, the triangularis fossa and the posterior lobules zones only required six horizontal rows.

The localization of any ear acupuncture point can thus be described in the Wojak nomenclature system with three Arabic numbers:

First number = auricular zone

Second number = x coordinate

Third number = y coordinate

The Wojak nomenclature for ear acupuncture points was introduced during the 2004 Second World Congress of TCM in Nanjing, China, and was presented again in Beijing in 2010. The numerical descriptions of the auricular points shown on the auricle are presented in Figure 4.6. In my own discussions with Dr. Wojak, there were several differences of opinion that became known. Although I concurred with him that there are some useful features of a purely numeric system that is similar to telephone area codes and ZIP codes in the United States, the use of English letters for abbreviations of terms is widely used

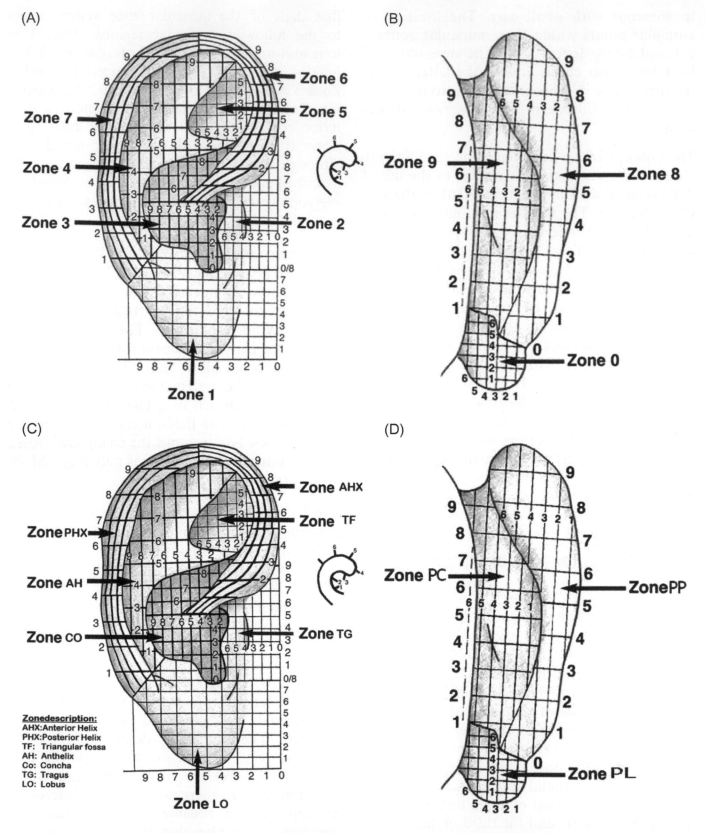

(A)

Zone 6
Zone 5
Zone 7
Zone 4
Zone 3
Zone 2
Zone 1

(B)

Zone 9
Zone 8
Zone 0

(C)

Zone AHX
Zone TF
Zone PHX
Zone AH
Zone CO
Zone TG
Zone LO

Zonedescription:
AHX: Anterior Helix
PHX: Posterior Helix
TF: Triangular fossa
AH: Anthelix
Co: Concha
TG: Tragus
LO: Lobus

(D)

Zone PC
Zone PP
Zone PL

FIGURE 4.6 The auricular zone system developed by Dr. Winfried Wojak of Germany shows 10 different regions of the external ear indicated by the first digit of a three digit number. The zones are numbered from "0" to "9". The second digit refers to the horizontal *x*-axis of rectangular zones from the medial to the central region of a given zone region, and the third digit refers to the vertical *y*-axis of a specific subsection within a given zone. In a subsequent version of this system, Dr. Wojak replaced the first digit with a two-letter abbreviation of each region of the auricle.

for international communication. For instance, two or three letters designating different nations are commonly used for website extensions and for Olympic IOC codes events. The letters CN or CHN are well-known abbreviations for the nation of China, US or USA for the United States, FR or FRA for France, and DE or DEU for Germany (Deutsch).

Romoli Auricular Nomenclature System

Still another format for indicating the location of different regions of the external ear has been suggested by Marco Romoli of Italy (1982, 2009). A classification system was developed for the right and left auricle that was based on the circular radiation of specific lines that were like the spokes of a bicycle wheel. Each radiation line began at Paul Nogier's Point Zero at the center of the ear. The 40 radiation lines that spread from this central source were referred to as *auricular sectograms* (SA) by

Romoli. The distribution of skin alterations was observed on the external ears of 354 medical patients and the locations of reactive ear points were transcribed onto sectogram maps utilizing the Romoli zone system. As shown in Figures 4.7 and 4.8, reliable transcription of specific auricular acupoints on different regions of the sectogram charts revealed that selective regions of the external ear were associated with some medical conditions more than others. The format of dividing the ear by radiating lines has also been proposed by David Alimi of Paris, France. A primary difference between the Romoli and the Alimi mapping systems is that Alimi centered the source point for the radiating lines of subdivisions on the Point Zero Prime region on the tragus rather than the original Point Zero on the helix root.

To provide further validation of his sectogram system, Romoli conducted extensive research on auricular diagnosis studies that utilized his mapping system. The 3-D representation of the Oleson auricular zone system is shown in Figure 4.9.

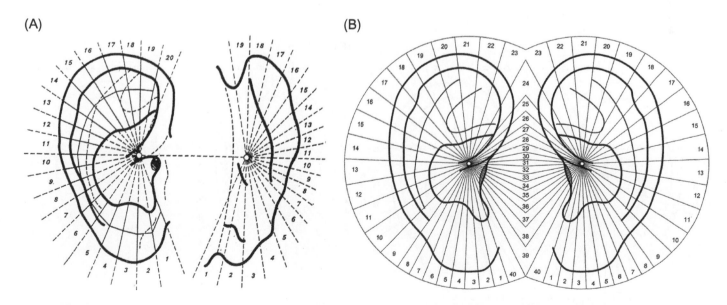

FIGURE 4.7 The auricular zone system developed by Dr. Marco Romoli of Italy shows 20 diagonal lines that radiate outward from Point Zero at the center of the auricle (A). The same radial lines found on the front surface of the auricle are also found on the posterior surface. In a further refinement of this Romoli system shown in panel B, there are 40 radial lines that divide the medial and the peripheral regions of the auricle into pie-shaped zones.

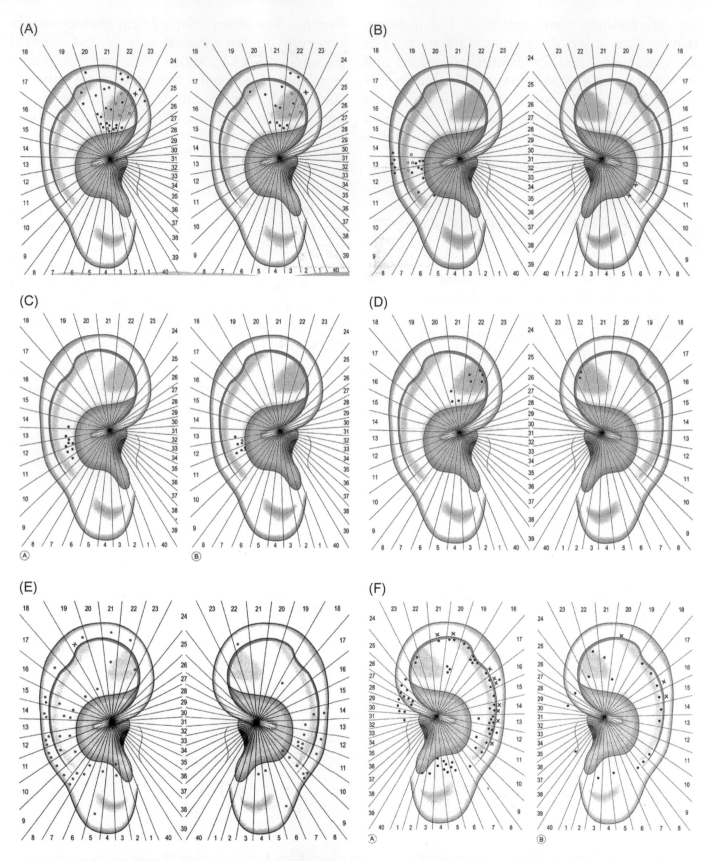

FIGURE 4.8 The results from observational research studies by Dr. Romoli show the spread of reactive ear points indicated in his radial zone charts for patients diagnosed with lumbago (A), cervical disk pain (B), shoulder pain (C), menstrual bleeding (D), breast and thyroid disorders (E), and fibromyalgia (F). The sectograms for patients with different health problems show an array of reactive ear points over different somatotopic regions of the auricle.

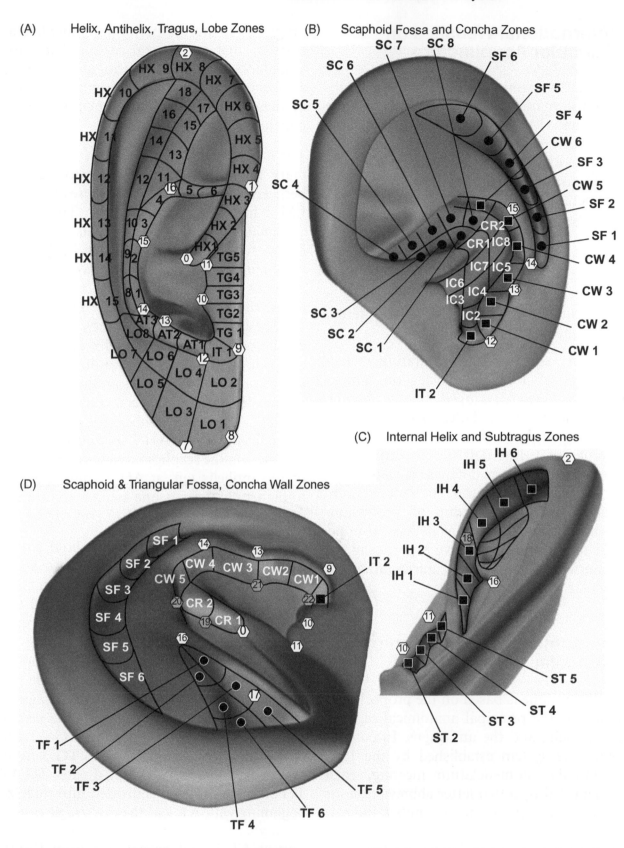

FIGURE 4.9 The different auricular zones in the Oleson nomenclature system are shown in 3-D images of the external ear. The different subsections of the helix, antihelix, tragus, antitragus, and lobe zones are indicated in panel A. The different subsections of the scaphoid fossa, superior concha, inferior concha, concha ridge, and concha wall zones are indicated in panel B. The different subsections of the internal helix and subtragus zones are indicated in panel C. The different subsections of the triangular fossa, scaphoid fossa, concha ridge, and concha wall zones are indicated in a different view of the auricle in panel D.

4.4 International Websites on Auricular Acupuncture

The May 2010 meeting of the WFAS established an International Auricular Acupuncture Nomenclature (IAAN) committee, an online forum for further discussions of the standardization of acupuncture nomenclature and for further discussion of the location of auricular acupuncture points. The publications of the 2010 meeting in Beijing concurred with many of the conclusions of the 1990 WHO meeting held in Lyon, France, but predominantly focused on the Chinese system of ear acupuncture. The website http://www.earchina.com was developed in order to facilitate further discussions of different auricular nomenclature systems.

An Internet source for integrating scientific abstracts of research articles on auriculotherapy has been developed by the French physician André Lentz. Titled *Your Auricular Acupuncture Database*, the website address for this international Internet site is http://www. auriculo.fr. This literature database is maintained by the International Auricular Acupuncture Bibliography (IAAB), a group of professionals from many different nations in Asia, Europe, and the United States who have expertise in the field of auricular acupuncture, auriculotherapy, and auricular medicine.

4.5 Anatomical Identification of Auricular Zones

Each auricular zone is based on the proportional subdivision of the principal anatomical regions, such as the helix and the antitragus. In concurrence with the system established by the 1990 WHO auricular nomenclature meeting, each zone is identified by a two-letter abbreviation for each anatomical region and a number indicating that particular subsection of that anatomical area. The revised auricular zones on the anteriolateral and the posterior sides of the ear are shown in Figures 4.10–4.16. The lowest numbers for each auricular area begin at the most inferior and most central zone of that anatomical region. The numbers then ascend to higher digits as one progresses to more superior and more lateral sections of that anatomical region. The auricular landmarks are useful in distinguishing where one zone ends and the next one begins. A depth view of these auricular zones is shown in the accompanying figures.

The first zone of the helix, HX 1, begins at landmark LM_0 and then proceeds to higher numbers, HX 2 and HX 3, as one rises to landmark LM_1 higher on the helix root. These numbers continue from HX 4 to HX 7 as one rises even higher to the apex of the auricle, LM_2. The helix numbers progress higher as the helix arch descends toward Darwin's Tubercle, finally ending at the bottom of the helix tail in zone HX 15. The first zone of the antihelix, AH 1, begins on the bottom of the antihelix tail, on the concha side of LM_14. The antihelix zones then rise toward LM_15, as the antihelix body curves around the superior concha to meet the inferior crus at LM_16; the numbers for the inferior crus range from AH 5 to AH 7. The antihelix numbers continue on the scaphoid fossa side of the bottom of the antihelix tail, at AH 8, and then progress to higher numbers as one ascends toward the top of the superior crus, at AH 17 and AH 18.

The deeper valleys of the scaphoid fossa and the triangular fossa are divided into six equal parts. The zones for the scaphoid fossa rise from SF 1 near the ear lobe to SF 6 toward the top of the ear, whereas the zones for the triangular fossa increase from TF 1 at the lower tip of the triangular fossa to TF 6 toward the top of the ear. A series of five vertical zones divide the tragus, rising from TG 1 near the intertragic notch to TG 5, where the tragus meets the helix root. The landmark LM_10 separates TG 2 from TG 3, the landmark LM_23 divides TG 3 from TG 4, and the landmark LM_11 divides TG 4 from TG 5. The antitragus is divided into three zones, beginning with AT 1 at the intertragic notch, rising higher in number and more superior in location at AT 2, and progressing from LM_13 to LM_14 for zone AT 3. There are two zones for the intertragic notch. The zone IT 1 is found higher toward the surface of the auricle, whereas the zone IT 2 occurs on the vertical wall of the intertragic notch, between LM_9 and LM_22.

The zones for the inferior concha begin at IC 1 and IC 2 at the intertragic notch near LM_22. The zone numbers then rise on a second concha row that begins with IC 3 near the ear canal, then continue peripherally on the concha floor to IC 5 near the concha wall. Subsequent inferior concha sections are found on a third row that begins at IC 6 below the helix root and then progress peripherally below the concha ridge to IC 8 at the concha wall. The zones for the superior concha begin with SC 1, immediately above the central concha ridge, and ascend to higher concha regions at SC 4. These values for the superior concha zones then circle back peripherally to SC 8, found above the more peripheral concha ridge and LM_20. The concha ridge itself is divided into two zones—the central zone CR 1, between LM_0 and LM_19, and the peripheral zone CR 2, between LM_18 and LM_20.

The different auricular zones of the posterior auricle each begin with the letter "P." They ascend from lower to higher numbers as anatomical subdivisions progress from a central to peripheral direction and from an inferior to superior direction. There are different zones for the posterior lobe (PL), the posterior concha (PC), and the posterior periphery (PP), behind the helix rim and the scaphoid fossa. The most prominent crevice that is found behind the external ear zones is the posterior groove (PG), which is the deep valley behind the antihelix ridge.

The intention in providing such a detailed and complex auricular zone system is to identify specific auricular reflex points by the actual area of the external ear on which an auricular point is found during clinical detection. Both Chinese and European ear charts designate the auricular acupoints by the somatotopic body organ that is represented. The standardization of zone terminology for verbally designating different anatomical regions of the ear provides a universal system to facilitate international communication based on ear anatomy, not somatotopic correspondences related to that point on the auricle. Photographs and illustrations of the auricle are quite useful in depicting various regions of the external ear, but verbal descriptions of these images are not adequate to precisely depict the auricular area represented. Table 4.3 shows the auricular locations of the principal reflex points used in ear acupuncture by this zone coding system. Also indicated in this table are the differences between the location of auricular points as described by Chinese auricular acupuncturists, denoted by the suffix ".c" or the superscript [C], and the auricular zones delineated by European practitioners of auricular medicine, indicated by the suffix ".e" or the superscript [E].

To further specify the exact location of an ear point within a larger auricular zone, each region designated by two letters and a number can be further subdivided into nine smaller regions indicated by a decimal number from ".1" to ".9" added to the larger number. These nine subdivisions are derived from taking each rectangular-shaped auricular zone and dividing it into three rows and three columns, forming nine individual cells.

4.6 Somatotopic Correspondences to Auricular Zones

The somatotopic representation of the cervical spinal vertebrae is shown in zones AH 1 and AH 2 in European charts but in the more peripheral zone AH 8 in many Chinese ear charts. The Chinese further report that the Lumbar Spinal Vertebrae ear points are found on the antihelix body, in zones AH 11 and AH 12, whereas the European charts indicate that ear points for the Lumbar Spine are located on the inferior crus, in zones AH 5 and AH 6. A primary difference between the European and Chinese auricular charts is the location of acupoints for the Leg. The Knee ear point is found on the superior crus zone AH 15 in Chinese ear charts, but it is represented in the triangular fossa zone TF 4 in European ear charts. Internal organs are also found in different auricular regions in these two systems. For example, the Uterus ear point is found in the triangular fossa zone TF 6 in the Chinese system, but it is found underneath the helix root in the European system, in zone IH 3.

TABLE 4.3	Primary Auricular Points Represented in Different Auricular Zones.

Zone	Auricular Point	Zone	Auricular Point	Zone	Auricular Point
AH 1–2	Cervical Vertebrae	LO 1	Master Cerebral	IC 1	Pituitary Gland
AH 3–4	Thoracic Vertebrae	LO 2	Irritability Point {E}	IC 2	Lung 2
AH 5–6	Lumbar Vertebrae	LO 3	Master Sensorial Point	IC 3	Trachea, Larynx {E}
AH 7	Sacral Vertebrae	LO 5	Trigeminal Nerve	IC 4	Heart {C}
AH 8	Thyroid Glands {C}	LO 6	Anti-Depressant Point	IC 5	Lung 1
AH 9–10	Chest, Breast	LO 7	Teeth, Lower Jaw	IC 6	Mouth, Throat
AH 11–12	Abdomen	LO 8	TMJ, Upper Jaw	IC 7	Esophagus, Stomach
AH 13	Hip {C}	HX 1	Point Zero	IC 8	Spleen {C}
AH 15	Knee {C}	HX 2	Diaphragm {C}, Genitals {E}	CR 1	Stomach
AH 17	Ankle {C}, Foot {C}	HX 3	Rectum {C}	CR 2	Liver
TF 1	Hip {E}	HX 4	Genitals {C}	SC 1	Duodenum
TF 2	Shen Men	HX 7	Apex of Ear	SC 2	Small Intestines
TF 3–4	Knee {E}, Leg {E}	HX 12	Lumbar Nerves	SC 3	Large Intestines
TF 5–6	Ankle {E}, Foot {E}, Uterus {C}	HX 13	Thoracic Nerves, Helix Points	SC 4	Prostate {C}, Urethra {E}
SF 1–2	Shoulder	HX 14	Cervical Nerves	SC 5	Bladder
SF 3–4	Elbow, Arm	HX 15	Medulla Oblongata	SC 6	Kidney {C}
SF 5	Wrist, Hand	IH 1	Ovary / Testes {E}	SC 7	Pancreas
SF 6	Fingers	IH 2	Prostate / Vagina {E}	SC 8	Spleen {E}
AT 1	Forehead	IH 3	Uterus {E}	IT 2	Endocrine Point
AT 2	Temples, Asthma	IH 4	Autonomic Point	CW 2	Thalamus Point
AT 3	Occiput	IH 5–6	Kidney {E}, Ureter {E}	CW 3	Brain {C}
TG 1	Pineal Gland	IH 7	Allergy Point	CW 4	Brainstem {C}
TG 2	Tranquilizer Point	IH 11	Windstream {C}	CW 5	Thyroid Glands {E}
TG 3	Appetite Control {C}	ST 2	Master Oscillation	CW 6	Thymus Gland {E}
TG 4	Vitality Point {E}	ST 3	Larynx {C}, Throat {C}	CW 7	Adrenal Glands {E}

Many ear points are more easily identified on the actual ear of a patient's body once one knows this auricular zone system. Depicting the location of the Sympathetic Autonomic point or the Thalamus Subcortex point is often confusing because these two auricular points are hidden from a conventional view of the ear. The Sympathetic point is shown in zone IH 4, which is underneath the helix near the triangular fossa, whereas the Thalamus point is found in zone CW 2, which lies on the concha wall behind the antitragus, adjacent to the inferior concha, at LM_21. These zone identifications reveal the distinct localization of these two ear points more clearly than many pictures of these points. It is also possible to show the differential location of other points found on the concha wall. The Chinese Brain ear point is found in zone CW 3, and the European auricular locations for the endocrine glands are represented on the concha wall. Ear points for the Thyroid Glands are found on zone CW 4, the Thymus Gland on CW 6, and the Adrenal Glands on zone CW 7. Understanding how the contours and landmarks on the external ear can facilitate the identification of specific ear points provides additional information for localization of somatotopic correspondences.

4.7 Specific Microsystem Ear Points Represented in Auricular Zones

Each anatomical part of the human body and each health condition are represented in the auricular microsystem code system by an ear reflex point, with each body organ designated by a number and a letter extension. The numbers continue from 0.0 to over 200.0, with each number related to a different part of human anatomy. The letter extensions that follow a decimal point indicate whether that ear reflex point is part of the Chinese ear acupuncture microsystem (".c" or "{C}"), part of the European auriculotherapy microsystem (".e" or "{E}"), or included in both Chinese and European auriculotherapy systems (".0"). In some cases, there is more than one Chinese or European ear reflex point for a given body area. In these instances, there can be several extensions, such as ".c^1," ".c^2," and ".c^3." In the Nogier phase system of auriculotherapy, the different phases for representation of auricular microsystem points are indicated by ".F1" for the primary phase of the French system, ".F2" for the second French phase, ".F3" for the third French phase, and ".F4" for the fourth French phase on the posterior side of the ear. The Phase IV auricular points conform to the inverted fetus somatotopic orientation as Phase I ear points, only they are found in auricular zones on the posterior side of the ear. The localization of specific ear points related to the different phases is presented in a subsequent chapter.

The specific locations and functions of more than 200 auricular acupoints are presented in Chapter 7, and specific ear points that are used in auriculotherapy protocols for different health conditions are presented in Chapter 9. However, sometimes when one conducts auricular diagnosis on a particular patient, a reactive ear point may be discovered that is not expected based on the descriptions in Chapters 7 and 9. By consulting the anatomical auricular areas presented next, one may identify a particular ear point that may best explain the function of the ear point that was discovered.

Auricular Microsystem Codes

0	=	Universal Ear Reflex Point
.c	=	Chinese {C} Ear Reflex Point
.e	=	European {E} Ear Reflex Point
HX	=	Helix zones
IH	=	Internal Helix zones
AH	=	Antihelix zones
LO	=	Lobe zones
TF	=	Triangular Fossa zones
SF	=	Scaphoid Fossa zones
TG	=	Tragus zones
AT	=	Antitragus zones
IT	=	Intertragic zones
ST	=	Subtragus zones
SC	=	Superior Concha zones
IC	=	Inferior Concha zones
CR	=	Concha Ridge zones
CW	=	Concha Wall zones
PC	=	Posterior Concha zones
PG	=	Posterior Groove zones
PP	=	Posterior Periphery zones
PL	=	Posterior Lobe zones

Ear Points in Helix Zones

HX 1   0.0_Point 0 (Point of Support), 112.e_Solar Plexus

HX 2   76.c_Diaphragm [C], 90.e_Genitals [E], 184.e_Sexual Desire [E]

HX 3   67.c_Rectum [C], 87.c_Urethra [C], 198.e_Weather Point [E]

HX 4   90.c_Genitals [C], 183.e_Psychosomatic Point [E]

HX 5

HX 6   188.e_Omega 2 [E]

HX 7   3.c_Allergy Point 1, 179.c_Apex of Auricle (Ear Apex)

HX 9   75.c^1_Tonsil 1

HX 10 80.c^1_Liver Yang 1

HX 11 80.c^2_Liver Yang 2, 180.c^1_Helix 1, 200.e_Darwin's Point [E]

HX 12 124.c_Lumbosacral Spinal Cord, 53.e_Dermatitis [E], 194.e_Alertness [E]

HX 13 125.e_Thoracic Spinal Cord, 53.e_Dermatitis [E], 180.c^2_Helix 2

HX 14 126.e_Cervical Spinal Cord, 75.c^2_Tonsil 2, 180.c^3_Helix 3, 171.c_Nephritis [C]

HX 15 127.e_Medulla Oblongata, 75.c^3_Tonsil 3, 180.c^4_Helix 4, 185.e_Sexual Compulsion [E]

Ear Points on Internal Helix Zones

IH 1   91.e_Ovaries [E]/Testes [E]

IH 2   88.e_Vagina [E]/Prostate [E], 67.e_Rectum [E]

IH 3   89.e_Uterus [E]

IH 4   2.0_Sympathetic Autonomic Point, 85.e_Ureter [E]

IH 5   84.e_Kidney [E], 174.c^1_Hemorrhoids 1

IH 6   202.e_Progesterone

IH 7   3.e_Allergy Point 2

IH 10 53.c_Dermatitis [C] (Urticaria)

IH 11 175.c_Windstream [C], 123.c_Minor Occipital Nerve [C]

IH 12 108.e_ Sympathetic Preganglionic Nerves, 208.e_Beta-1 Receptor [E]

4.7.01. Ear Points in Helix Zones

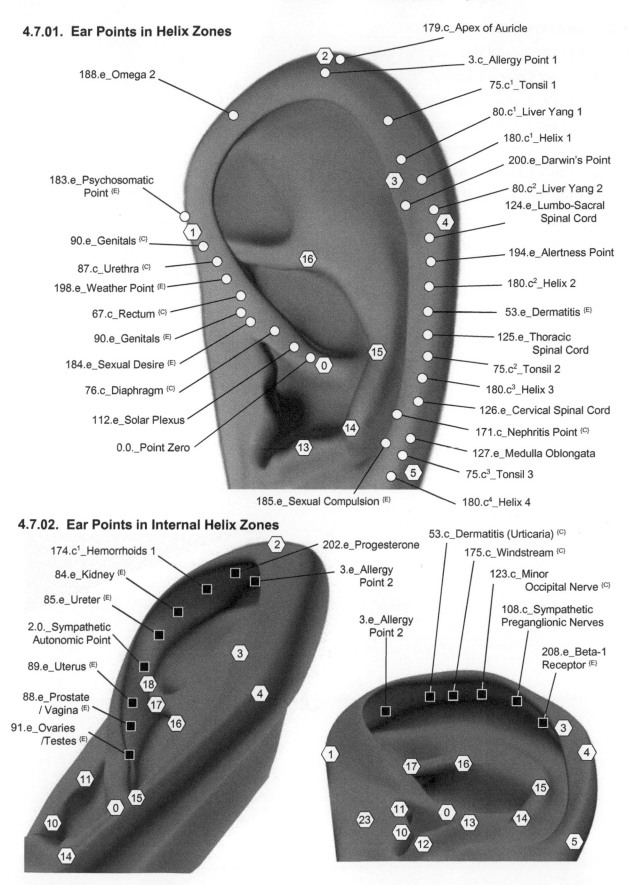

179.c_Apex of Auricle

3.c_Allergy Point 1

75.c¹_Tonsil 1

80.c¹_Liver Yang 1

180.c¹_Helix 1

200.e_Darwin's Point

80.c²_Liver Yang 2

124.e_Lumbo-Sacral Spinal Cord

194.e_Alertness Point

180.c²_Helix 2

53.e_Dermatitis {E}

125.e_Thoracic Spinal Cord

75.c²_Tonsil 2

180.c³_Helix 3

126.e_Cervical Spinal Cord

171.c_Nephritis Point {C}

127.e_Medulla Oblongata

75.c³_Tonsil 3

180.c⁴_Helix 4

185.e_Sexual Compulsion {E}

188.e_Omega 2

183.e_Psychosomatic Point {E}

90.e_Genitals {C}

87.c_Urethra {C}

198.e_Weather Point {E}

67.c_Rectum {C}

90.e_Genitals {E}

184.e_Sexual Desire {E}

76.c_Diaphragm {C}

112.e_Solar Plexus

0.0._Point Zero

4.7.02. Ear Points in Internal Helix Zones

174.c¹_Hemorrhoids 1

84.e_Kidney {E}

85.e_Ureter {E}

2.0._Sympathetic Autonomic Point

89.e_Uterus {E}

88.e_Prostate / Vagina {E}

91.e_Ovaries /Testes {E}

202.e_Progesterone

3.e_Allergy Point 2

3.e_Allergy Point 2

53.c_Dermatitis (Urticaria) {C}

175.c_Windstream {C}

123.c_Minor Occipital Nerve {C}

108.c_Sympathetic Preganglionic Nerves

208.e_Beta-1 Receptor {E}

FIGURE 4.10 The somatotopic organs that are represented in helix zones and internal helix zones are shown from different perspectives of 3-D ear images.

Ear Points on Antihelix Zones

AH 1	10.e_Upper Cervical Vertebrae [E], 145.e_Cerebellum
AH 2	10.e_Lower Cervical Vertebrae [E]
AH 3	11.e_Upper Thoracic Vertebrae [E], 69.e_Heart [E], 95.c_Mammary Glands [C]
AH 4	11.e_Lower Thoracic Vertebrae [E], 12.c_Lumbar Vertebrae [C]
AH 5	12.e_Upper Lumbar Vertebrae [E], 14.0_Buttocks
AH 6	12.e_Lower Lumbar Vertebrae [E], 107.0_Sciatic Nerve (Sciatica)
AH 7	13.e_Sacral Vertebrae [E] (Coccyx)
AH 8	15.0_Throat (Neck Muscles), 10.c_Cervical Vertebrae [C], 96.c_Thyroid Glands [C]
AH 9	15.0_Throat (Neck Muscles), 16.e_Clavicle [E], 11.c_Thoracic Vertebrae [C]
AH 10	17.0_Breast, 18.0_Chest, 95.c_Mammary Glands [C], 11.c_Thoracic Vertebrae [C]
AH 11	19.0_Abdomen, 12.c_Lumbar Vertebrae [C], 158.c_Lumbago [C], 168.c_Heat Point [C]
AH 12	19.0_ Abdomen
AH 13	21.c_Hip [C]
AH 14	
AH 15	23.c_Knee [C]
AH 16	29.0_Thumb
AH 17	27.c_Foot [C], 25.c_Ankle [C], 26.c_Heel [C]
AH 18	28.c_Toes [C]

4.7.03. Ear Points on Antihelix Zones

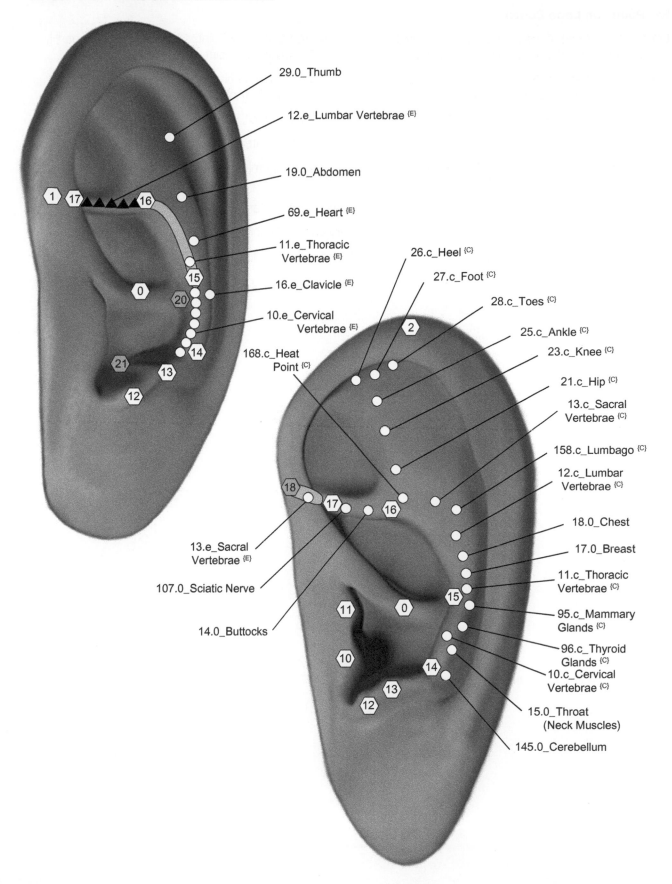

29.0_Thumb

12.e_Lumbar Vertebrae [E]

19.0_Abdomen

69.e_Heart [E]

11.e_Thoracic Vertebrae [E]

16.e_Clavicle [E]

10.e_Cervical Vertebrae [E]

26.c_Heel [C]

27.c_Foot [C]

28.c_Toes [C]

25.c_Ankle [C]

23.c_Knee [C]

21.c_Hip [C]

13.c_Sacral Vertebrae [C]

158.c_Lumbago [C]

12.c_Lumbar Vertebrae [C]

18.0_Chest

17.0_Breast

11.c_Thoracic Vertebrae [C]

95.c_Mammary Glands [C]

96.c_Thyroid Glands [C]

10.c_Cervical Vertebrae [C]

15.0_Throat (Neck Muscles)

145.0_Cerebellum

168.c_Heat Point [C]

13.e_Sacral Vertebrae [E]

107.0_Sciatic Nerve

14.0_Buttocks

FIGURE 4.11 The somatotopic organs that are represented in antihelix zones are shown from different perspectives of 3-D ear images.

Ear Points on Lobe Zones

LO 1   9.0_Master Cerebral Point, 151.e_Pre-Frontal Cortex, 164.0_Anxiety Point, 186.e_Master Omega [E], 47.c^2_Dental Analgesia 2, 118.e_Optic Nerve, 201.e_Prostaglandin Point [E]

LO 2   57.e_External Nose [E], 127.c^1_Dental Analgesia 1, 119.e_Olfactory Nerve, 139.e_Limbic System, 141.e_Amygdala, 150.e_Frontal Cortex, 182.e_Irritability Point [E] (Anti-Aggressivity Point)

LO 3   8.0_Master Sensorial Point, 4.0_Eye, 149.e_Parietal Cortex, 75.c^4_Tonsil 4, 180.c^6_Helix Point 6

LO 4   41.e_Frontal Sinus, 49.c_Tongue [C], 48.c^1_Palate 1, 48.c^2_Palate 2

LO 5   52.0_Face (Cheeks), 54.0_Lips, 58.c_Inner Ear [C], 132.e_Trigeminal Nucleus, 180.c^5_Helix Point 5, 197.c_Sneezing Point [C]

LO 6   42.0_Vertex of Head, 49.e_Tongue [E], 135.e_Striatum (Basal Ganglia), 148.e_Temporal Cortex

LO 7   51.0_Chin, 116.e_Trigeminal Nerve, 106.e_Salivary Glands [E], 212.e_Vomiting Reflex [E]

LO 8   44.0_Lower Jaw (Mandible), 45.0_Upper Jaw (Maxilla), 43.0_TMJ, 46.0_Teeth, 128.e_Pons, 140.e_Hippocampus, 190.e_Anti-Depressant Point [E]

4.7.04. Ear Points in Lobe Zones

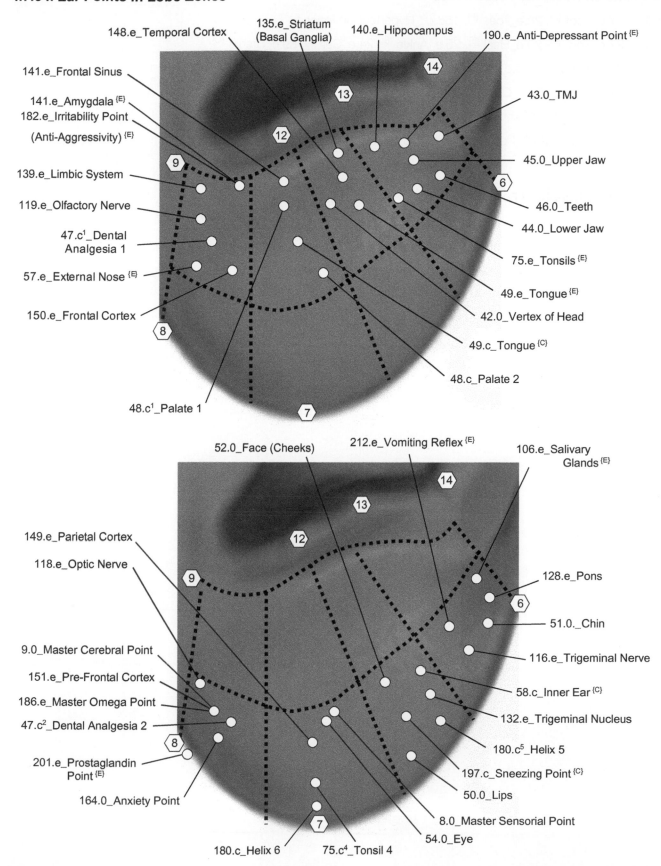

148.e_Temporal Cortex

135.e_Striatum (Basal Ganglia)

140.e_Hippocampus

190.e_Anti-Depressant Point [E]

141.e_Frontal Sinus

141.e_Amygdala [E]

182.e_Irritability Point (Anti-Aggressivity) [E]

139.e_Limbic System

119.e_Olfactory Nerve

47.c¹_Dental Analgesia 1

57.e_External Nose [E]

150.e_Frontal Cortex

48.c¹_Palate 1

43.0_TMJ

45.0_Upper Jaw

46.0_Teeth

44.0_Lower Jaw

75.e_Tonsils [E]

49.e_Tongue [E]

42.0_Vertex of Head

49.c_Tongue [C]

48.c_Palate 2

52.0_Face (Cheeks)

212.e_Vomiting Reflex [E]

106.e_Salivary Glands [E]

149.e_Parietal Cortex

118.e_Optic Nerve

9.0_Master Cerebral Point

151.e_Pre-Frontal Cortex

186.e_Master Omega Point

47.c²_Dental Analgesia 2

201.e_Prostaglandin Point [E]

164.0_Anxiety Point

128.e_Pons

51.0._Chin

116.e_Trigeminal Nerve

58.c_Inner Ear [C]

132.e_Trigeminal Nucleus

180.c⁵_Helix 5

197.c_Sneezing Point [C]

50.0_Lips

8.0_Master Sensorial Point

54.0_Eye

180.c_Helix 6

75.c⁴_Tonsil 4

FIGURE 4.12 The somatotopic organs that are represented in lobe zones are shown from different perspectives of 3-D ear images.

Ear Points on Triangular Fossa Zones

TF 6   27.e_Foot [E], 28.e_Toes [E], 156.c^1_Hypertension Point 1

TF 5   27.e_Foot [E], 26.e_Heel [E], 25.e_Ankle [E], 24.e_Calf [E], 89.c_Uterus [C]

TF 4   23.e_Knee [E], 153.c_Antihistamine Point [C], 155.c^1_Hepatitis 1

TF 3   22.0_Thigh, 154.c_Constipation [C]

TF 2   1.0_Shen Men (Spirit Gate)

TF 1   21.e_Hip [E], 20.0_Pelvis (Groin, Pubic Bone)

Ear Points on Scaphoid Fossa Zones

SF 6   30.0_Fingers

SF 5   29.0_Thumb, 31.0_Hand, 32.0_Wrist, 53.c_Dermatitis [C] (Urticaria), 78.c^1_Appendicitis 1, 195.e^1_Insomnia 1

SF 4   34.0_Elbow, 33.0_Forearm

SF 3   35.0_Upper Arm, 78.c^2_Appendicitis 2

SF 2   36.0_Shoulder

SF 1   37.0_Shoulder Joint, 16.c_Clavicle [C], 78.c^3_Appendicitis 3, 195.e^2_Insomnia 2

4.7.05. Ear Points in Triangular Fossa Zones

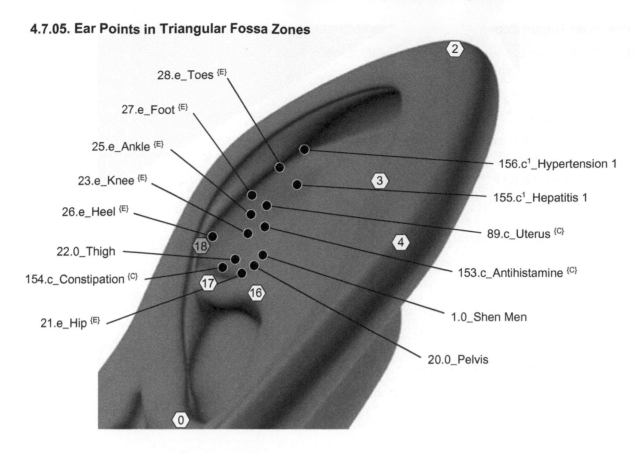

28.e_Toes $^{\{E\}}$

27.e_Foot $^{\{E\}}$

25.e_Ankle $^{\{E\}}$

23.e_Knee $^{\{E\}}$

26.e_Heel $^{\{E\}}$

22.0_Thigh

154.c_Constipation $^{\{C\}}$

21.e_Hip $^{\{E\}}$

156.c^1_Hypertension 1

155.c^1_Hepatitis 1

89.c_Uterus $^{\{C\}}$

153.c_Antihistamine $^{\{C\}}$

1.0_Shen Men

20.0_Pelvis

4.7.06. Ear Points in Scaphoid Fossa Zones

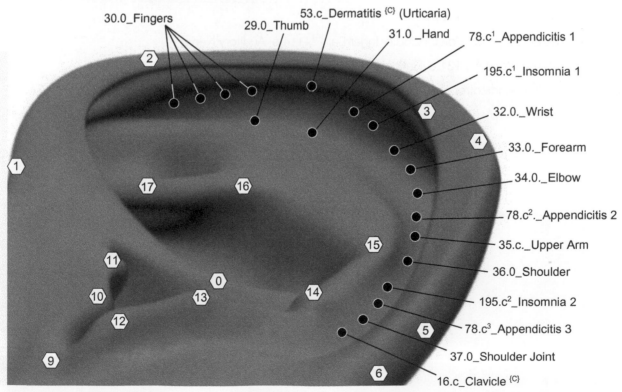

30.0_Fingers

29.0_Thumb

53.c_Dermatitis $^{\{C\}}$ (Urticaria)

31.0 _Hand

78.c^1_Appendicitis 1

195.c^1_Insomnia 1

32.0._Wrist

33.0._Forearm

34.0._Elbow

78.c^2._Appendicitis 2

35.c._Upper Arm

36.0_Shoulder

195.c^2_Insomnia 2

78.c^3_Appendicitis 3

37.0_Shoulder Joint

16.c_Clavicle $^{\{C\}}$

[FIGURE 4.13 The somatotopic organs that are represented in triangular fossa zones and scaphoid fossa zones are shown from different perspectives of 3-D ear images.

Ear Points on Tragus Zones

TG 5   59.c_External Ear [C], 69.c^2_Heart [C2], 193.e_Vitality Point [E], 209.e_Frustration Point [E], 210.e_Interferon Point [E]

TG 4   162.c_Thirst Point [C], 146.e_Corpus Callosum

TG 3   161.c_Appetite Control Point [C], 92.c_Adrenal Glands [C], 57.c_External Nose [C], 146.e_Corpus Callosum

TG 2   7.e_Tranquilizer Point, 156.c^2_Hypertension Point 2, 191.e_Mania Point [E], 192.e_Nicotine Point [E], 146.e_Corpus Callosum

TG 1   89.e_Pineal Gland [E] (Epiphysis), 55.c^1_Eye Disorder 1 (Mu 1)

Ear Points on Antitragus Zones

AT 3   38.0_Occiput, 147.e_Occipital Cortex

AT 2   39.0_Temples, 152.c_Asthma Point [C], 178.0_Apex of Antitragus

AT 1   40.0_Forehead, 55.c^2_Eye Disorder 2 (Mu 2)

Ear Points on Intertragic Notch Zones

IT 1   143.e_Cingulate Gyrus, 55.c^1_Eye Disorder 1, 157.c_Hypotension Point [C]

IT 2   5.0_Master Endocrine Point (Internal Secretion), 102.e_Thyrotrophins (TSH)

Ear Points on Subtragus Zones

ST 4   73.c_Pharynx [C], 74.c_Larynx [C]

ST 3   6.e_Master Oscillation Point [E], 58.e_Inner Ear [E], 114.e_Auditory Nerve

ST 2   56.c_Internal Nose [C], 131.e_Reticular Formation

ST 1   104.e_Adrenocorticotrophin (ACTH)

4.7.07. Ear Points in Tragus Zones and 4.7.08. Antitragus Zones

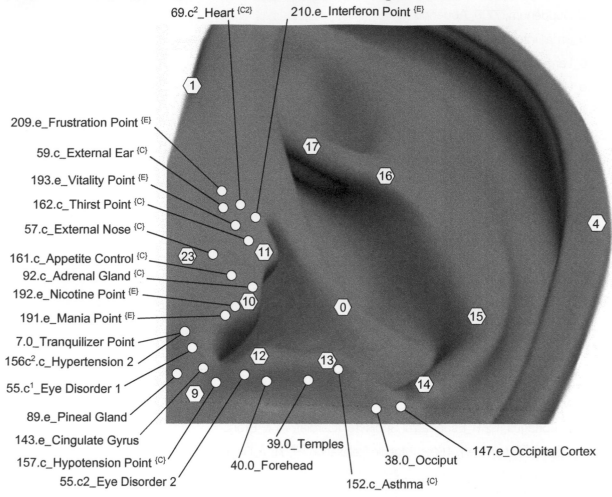

69.c²_Heart {C2}

210.e_Interferon Point {E}

209.e_Frustration Point {E}

59.c_External Ear {C}

193.e_Vitality Point {E}

162.c_Thirst Point {C}

57.c_External Nose {C}

161.c_Appetite Control {C}

92.c_Adrenal Gland {C}

192.e_Nicotine Point {E}

191.e_Mania Point {E}

7.0_Tranquilizer Point

156c².c_Hypertension 2

55.c¹_Eye Disorder 1

89.e_Pineal Gland

143.e_Cingulate Gyrus

157.c_Hypotension Point {C}

55.c2_Eye Disorder 2

39.0_Temples

40.0_Forehead

38.0_Occiput

152.c_Asthma {C}

147.e_Occipital Cortex

4.7.09. Ear Points in Subtragus Zones and 4.7.10. Intertragic Notch Zones

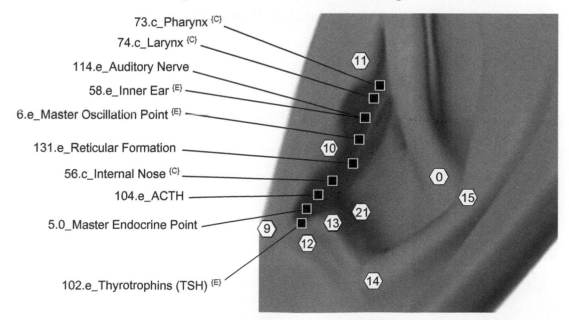

73.c_Pharynx {C}

74.c_Larynx {C}

114.e_Auditory Nerve

58.e_Inner Ear {E}

6.e_Master Oscillation Point {E}

131.e_Reticular Formation

56.c_Internal Nose {C}

104.e_ACTH

5.0_Master Endocrine Point

102.e_Thyrotrophins (TSH) {E}

⌈FIGURE 4.14 The somatotopic organs that are represented in tragus zones, antitragus zones, subtragus zones, and intertragic notch zones are shown from different perspectives of 3-D ear images.

Ear Points in Superior Concha Zones

SC 1   64.0_Duodenum, 77.0_Appendix

SC 2   65.0_Small Intestines, 187.e_Omega 1, 163.c_Alcoholic Point [C]

SC 3   66.0_Large Intestines

SC 4   87.e_Urethra [E], 88.c_Prostate [C], 67.e_Rectum [E], 174.c^2_Hemorrhoids 2, 111.e_Hypogastric Plexus [E]

SC 5   86.0_Bladder

SC 6   84.c_Kidney [C], 85.c_Ureter [C], 172.c_Ascites Point [C]

SC 7   83.0_Pancreas, 93.e_Cortisol Hormones

SC 8   82.0_Gall Bladder (*Right Ear*), 81.e_Spleen [E] (*Left Ear*)

Ear Points in Inferior Concha Zones

IC 1   99.e_Anterior Pituitary Gland [E], 100.e_Posterior Pituitary Gland [E], 105.e_Prolactin, 160.c_San Jiao [C] (Triple Warmer)

IC 2   70.c^2_Lung 2, 136.e_Anterior Hypothalamus

IC 3   72.0_Trachea, 73.e_Pharynx [E], 74.e_Larynx [E], 113.e_Vagus Nerve

IC 4   69.c^1_Heart [C1], 70.c^2_Lung 2, 166.c_Tuberculosis [C]

IC 5   70.c^1_Lung 1, 137.e_Posterior Hypothalamus

IC 6   60.0_Mouth, 55.c^3_Eye Disorder 3

IC 7   61.0_Esophagus, 62.0_Esophagial Sphincter (Cardia), 71.c_Bronchi

IC 8   81.c_Spleen [C] (*Left Ear*), 159.c_Muscle Relaxation [C], 76.e_Diaphragm [E]

Ear Points in Concha Ridge Zones

CR 1   63.0_Stomach

CR 2   79.0_Liver, 155.c^2_Hepatitis 2, 189.e_Wonderful Point [E] (Marvelous Point)

4.7.11. Ear Points in Superior Concha Zones

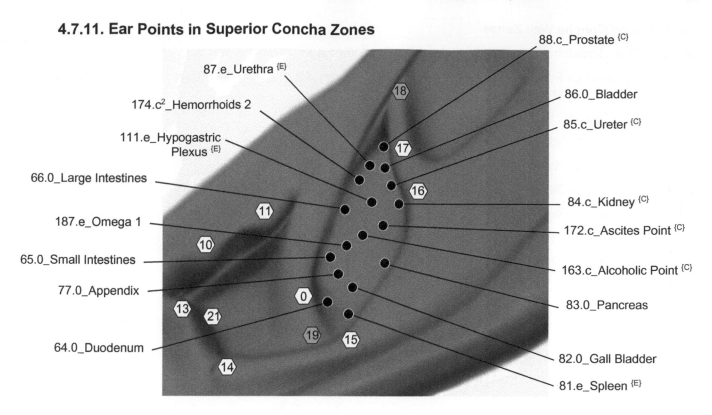

88.c_Prostate {C}

87.e_Urethra {E}

174.c²_Hemorrhoids 2

111.e_Hypogastric Plexus {E}

86.0_Bladder

85.c_Ureter {C}

66.0_Large Intestines

187.e_Omega 1

84.c_Kidney {C}

172.c_Ascites Point {C}

65.0_Small Intestines

163.c_Alcoholic Point {C}

77.0_Appendix

83.0_Pancreas

64.0_Duodenum

82.0_Gall Bladder

81.e_Spleen {E}

4.7.12. Ear Points in Inferior Concha Zones and 4.7.13. Concha Ridge Zones

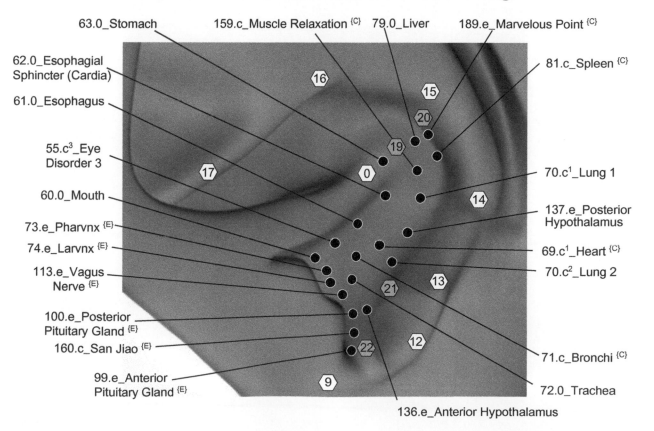

63.0_Stomach   159.c_Muscle Relaxation {C}   79.0_Liver   189.e_Marvelous Point {C}

62.0_Esophagial Sphincter (Cardia)

81.c_Spleen {C}

61.0_Esophagus

55.c³_Eye Disorder 3

60.0_Mouth

70.c¹_Lung 1

73.e_Pharvnx {E}

137.e_Posterior Hypothalamus

74.e_Larvnx {E}

69.c¹_Heart {C}

113.e_Vagus Nerve {E}

70.c²_Lung 2

100.e_Posterior Pituitary Gland {E}

160.c_San Jiao {E}

71.c_Bronchi {C}

99.e_Anterior Pituitary Gland {E}

72.0_Trachea

136.e_Anterior Hypothalamus

FIGURE 4.15 The somatotopic organs that are represented in superior concha zones, inferior concha zones, and concha ridge zones are shown from different perspectives of 3-D ear images.

Ear Points on Concha Wall Zones

CW 1   101.e_Gonadotrophins (FSH, LH), 91.c_Ovaries [C]/Testes [C]

CW 2   4.0_Thalamus Point (Subcortex), 4.c_ Nervous Subcortex, 68.e_Circulatory System, 106.c_Salivary Glands [C], 165.c_Excitement Point [C], 225.c_Epilepsy Point [C]

CW 3   138.c_Brain [C], 99.c_Pituitary Gland [C], 196.e_Dizziness Point [E]

CW 4   97.e_Parathyroid Gland, 127.c_Brainstem [C]

CW 5   96.e_Thyroid Glands [E], 95.e_Mammary Glands [E]

CW 6   94.e_Thymus Gland [E]

CW 7   92.e_Adrenal Glands [E], 109.e_Thoracic Sympathetic Ganglia

CW 8   109.e_Thoracic Sympathetic Ganglia

CW 9   109.e_Lumbar Sympathetic Ganglia

4.7.14. Ear Points on Concha Wall Zones

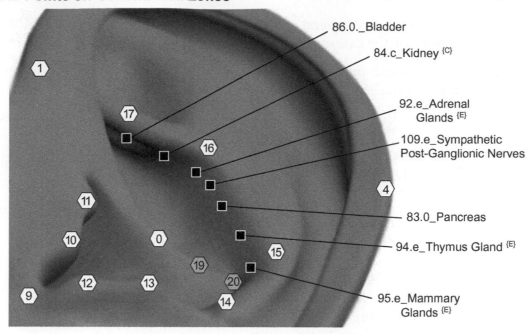

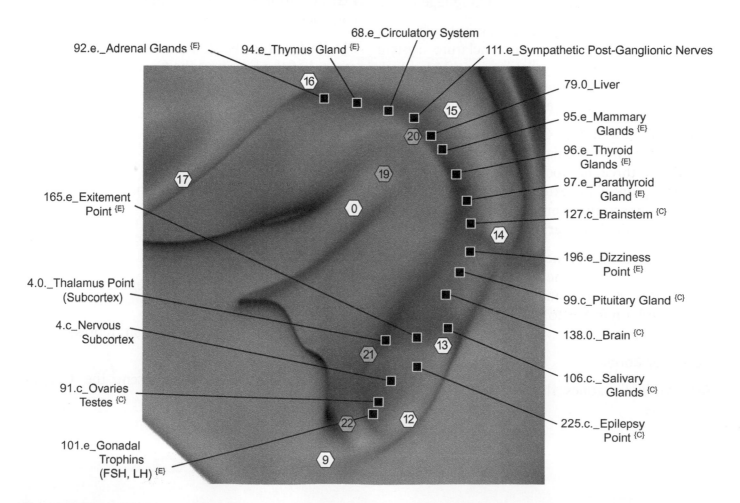

FIGURE 4.16 The somatotopic organs that are represented in concha wall zones are shown from different perspectives of 3-D ear images.

■ KEY TERMS FOR CHAPTER 4

AZ: Auricular zones use an alphanumeric code to designate specific regions of the external ear.

LM: Auricular landmarks are prominent structural features on the external ear that facilitate the distinction between one auricular area and another.

MA: Microsystem auricular is a term derived from the World Health Organization to designate the somatotopic microsystem on the external ear.

Nomina Anatomica: The internationally agreed upon text that was developed to create a standard terminology for human anatomy, first in 1895 and updated from an International Congress of Anatomists meeting in 1955. Most adopted phrases were derived from Latin, utilizing some words from the English language.

Romoli, Marco: The Italian doctor who has developed an auricular nomenclature system referred to as auricular sectograms (SA), which consist of a radial array of different pie-shaped regions of the external ear.

Wojak, Winfried: The German doctor who has developed an auricular nomenclature system based on three numbers—one Arabic number for the region of the external ear followed by two other numbers representing the x-axis and the y-axis of a rectilinear grid.

Zhou, Liqun: The Chinese doctor who has developed an auricular nomenclature system based on the WHO 1990 recommendations for using two letters and a number to designate each region of the external ear.

Auricular Zones

AH: Antihelix zones that represent the Spinal Vertebrae.

AT: Antitragus zones that represent the Head.

CR: Concha Ridge zones that represent the Stomach and the Liver.

CW: Concha Wall zones that represent the Endocrine Glands.

HX: Helix zones that represent the Anti-inflammatory treatments.

IC: Inferior Concha zones that represent the Thoracic Organs.

IT: Intertragic Notch zones that represent the Pituitary Gland.

LO: Ear Lobe zones that represent the Brain and the Face.

PC: Posterior Concha zones that represent motor control of internal organs.

PG: Posterior Lobe zones that represent motor control of Foot.

PL: Posterior Lobe zones that represent motor control of the Face and the Cortex.

PP: Posterior Lobe zones that represent motor control of the Upper Extremities.

PT: Posterior Lobe zones that represent motor control of the Lower Extremities.

SC: Superior Concha zones that represent the Abdominal Organs.

SF: Scaphoid Fossa zones that represent the Arm and Hand.

ST: Subtragus zones that represent the Inner Ear, Larynx, and Pharynx.

TF: Triangular Fossa zones that represent the Leg and Foot.

TG: Tragus zones that represent the Corpus Callosum and Adrenal Glands.

▪ CHAPTER 4 REVIEW QUESTIONS

1. Standardized, international, nomenclature terminology for all anatomical organs was first described in the text_____.
   a. *Nomina Anatomica*
   b. *Emperor's Classic of Internal Medicine*
   c. *Gray's Anatomy*
   d. *Materia Medica*

2. The World Health Organization Committee for Acupuncture Nomenclature determined that all body acupuncture and auricular acupuncture abbreviations should be indicated by_____.
   a. Arabic numeral values
   b. Roman numeral values
   c. one letter and a digital number
   d. two letters and a digital number

3. The microsystem auricular points for the Cervical and Thoracic Vertebrae are represented on_____ zones.
   a. Helix (HX)
   b. Antihelix (AH)
   c. Triangular Fossa (TF)
   d. Antitragus (AT)

4. The Scaphoid Fossa (SF) zones contain microsystem points that correspond to the_____.
   a. thoracic internal organs
   b. abdominal internal organs
   c. shoulder, arm, and hand
   d. upper and lower jaw

5. The abbreviation IT refers to the zones of the_____.
   a. Tragus
   b. Intertragic Notch
   c. Triangular Fossa
   d. Antitragus

6. The two-letter abbreviation for the zones of the Superior Concha is_____.
   a. LO
   b. CR
   c. IC
   d. SC

7. The Concha Ridge zones include auricular microsystem points for the_____.
   a. heart
   b. pancreas
   c. bladder
   d. stomach

8. The suffix ".c" or the superscript $^{\{C\}}$ refers to microsystem points indicated by_____.
   a. Cartesian coordinates
   b. Chinese ear acupuncture charts
   c. charts for the auricle designated by WHO
   d. Zones in the concha of the ear

9. Whereas the microsystem point for the Knee is represented on Antihelix (AH) zones in Chinese ear acupuncture charts, it is shown in_____ in European auricular acupuncture charts.
   a. Triangular Fossa (TF) zones
   b. Scaphoid Fossa (SF) zones
   c. Helix (HX) zones
   d. Antitragus (AT) zones

10. The master point found at Helix zone 1 (HX 1) is_____.
    a. Master Endocrine Point
    b. Master Cerebral Point
    c. Point Zero
    d. Shen Men Point

Answers

1 = a; 2 = d; 3 = b; 4 = c; 5 = b; 6 = d; 7 = d; 8 = b; 9 = a; 10 = c

Overview of Auricular Diagnosis Procedures

[5.0 | Overview of Auricular Diagnosis Procedures

CHAPTER 5 LEARNING OBJECTIVES

1. To delineate specific types of auricular diagnostic procedures.
2. To identify skin surface changes associated with auricular diagnosis.
3. To apply specific, tactile pressure to the auricle in order to evaluate degrees of tenderness of auricular acupoints.
4. To demonstrate clinical procedures for conducting electrical detection of auricular acupoints.
5. To compare the differences between Chinese pulse diagnosis and pulse diagnosis using the vascular autonomic signal (VAS).

5.1 Visual Observation of Skin Surface Changes on the Ear

Just as classical acupuncturists have observed distinct changes in the color and shape of the tongue and in the subtle qualities of the radial pulse, practitioners of ear acupuncture have emphasized the diagnostic value of visually examining the external ear (Kvirchishvili, 1974; Romoli and Vettoni, 1982; Huang, 1996). Although not as routinely found as other diagnostic indicators of reactive ear points, prominent physical attributes of the auricular skin surface have been associated with specific clinical conditions. This visual inspection of the auricle should be conducted before the ear surface is cleaned with alcohol or manipulated for other auricular procedures.

Dark Colored Spots

Shiny red, purple, or brown spots are observed at distinct regions on the auricular surface that typically indicate acute inflammations in the body. A spot that is bright red tends to indicate an acute reaction that is painful, whereas dark red is seen with patients who have a long history of disease. Dark gray or dark brown can indicate tissue de-differentiation or tumors that could be found in the correspondent organ. These colored spots are not to be confused with ordinary freckles that do not necessarily indicate a diagnostic condition. If pressure is applied to these colored regions of the auricle, that spot is usually painful to touch. The absence of these spots does not indicate the absence of any medical problem, but the occurrence of colored regions on the ear does suggest the high probability of some type of pathology in the correspondent part of the body. These colored spots only gradually go away when the health of the related body area improves. In some clinical cases of kidney stones, the appearance of a red spot over the auricular Kidney point was observed to move from its original position to a nearby auricular region closer to the auricular Bladder point, corresponding to the movement of the kidney stone in the body toward the urinary bladder in the body.

One of the most prominent examples that I have ever observed which demonstrated the discoloration of a specific part of the auricle was found on the external ear of an acupuncture colleague. Dr. Ralph Alan Dale has published numerous journal articles on the topic of microsystems. Dr. Dale had been wearing a gold ring on the fourth digit of his left hand at a time when he developed a serious illness, which temporarily caused swelling in his hands. He was unable to remove the gold ring for many weeks. When he finally did succeed in removing the ring, there remained a dark area of skin around the finger digit where the ring had been. Dr. Dale subsequently noticed that a small dark spot had appeared on the scaphoid fossa of his left external ear, at the exact auricular position that corresponds to the fingers. Because the skin condition never recovered, both the dark ring of skin on his finger and the small dark spot on his external ear remained for the remainder of Dr. Dale's life.

White, Flaky Skin

White flakes, crusty scales, peeling skin, shedding, and dandruff-like areas of desquamation on the auricle usually indicate a chronic condition in the body. Whiteness surrounded by redness in the auricular heart region typically indicates rheumatic heart disease. A close inspection of the ear of different patients may reveal a dryness on localized regions of the skin. If the auricle of that individual is cleaned, the white flaky regions tend to reappear within several days unless the correspondent condition is successfully treated. If a treatment is effective for healing that condition, the flaky regions on the ear do not reappear. This skin surface observation closely corresponds to the continued presence of a disorder, and when the physical disorder is alleviated, the white flakiness on the auricular surface disappears.

Although I have seen white, flaky skin on the auricles of many patients, one individual in particular always remains prominent in my mind. Upon my first meeting of this middle-aged man, I noticed that the inferior concha of his auricle was completely covered with powdery white skin, looking somewhat like very thick dandruff. At my suggestion, this man consulted with his medical doctor the next week, and the week after that he was scheduled for open heart surgery. The degree of flaky skin on the heart area of his auricle corresponded to a very severe coronary condition.

Physical Textures and Skin Protrusions

Specific areas of the auricular skin surface can exhibit spot-like protrusions, slight depressions, rough regions of thickened skin, or blister-like papules protruding above the skin surface. These papules are small, circumscribed, solid elevations of the auricular skin that could be normal in appearance or colored as red, white, or white papules surrounded by redness. Sometimes there is a dark gray protrusion.

One patient who was consulting with me about low back pain happened to have an open scar on the skin next to his external ear. This region on the helix root of the auricle is identified as the External Genitals in Chinese ear acupuncture charts. The patient reported that the scar had been there for several months and had not healed, despite the application of antibiotics for several weeks. I administered electrical stimulation around the edges of this scar on his ear, in addition to the treatment of ear points related to his back pain problems. Upon seeing this man a week later, not only did he report a reduction in back pain but also the scar on his ear had started to heal. At this point, the patient informed me, for the first time, that he had also been suffering from pain in his genital region. However, since his first auriculotherapy treatment, that genital pain had gone away. There was a direct correspondence between the presence of the skin disruption on the genital point of his ear and pain in his acutal genitals, and as the problem in the body improved following auriculotherapy treatment, the reactive point on his external ear started to go away.

Earlobe Crease

Diagonal folds in the skin over the ear lobe have been correlated with certain types of health disorders (Figures 5.1 and 5.2). Lichstein *et al.* (1974) and Mehta and Homby (1974) both published studies in the *New England Journal of Medicine* that correlated diagonal ear lobe creases with coronary problems. Their double blind clinical studies showed that the presence of a crease running diagonally from the intertragic notch to the bottom of the lobe was more predictive of the occurrence of a coronary problem than knowing either the patient's blood pressure level or serum cholesterol level. A psychologist colleague of mine had a very prominent ear lobe crease; he was also overweight and he had a family history of heart disease. After he took more disciplined care of his health, losing weight and switching to a more nutritious diet, the coronary ear lobe crease became less distinctive. However,

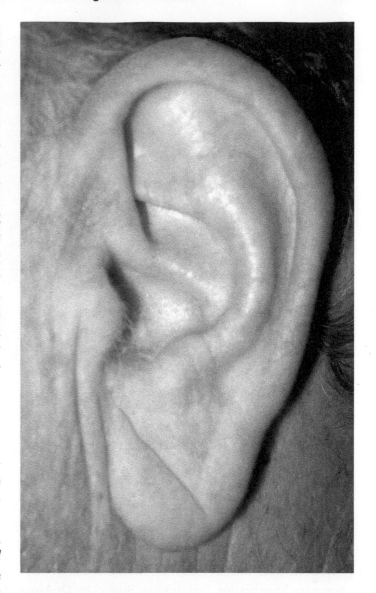

FIGURE 5.1 Photograph of an example of a diagonal ear lobe crease that has been related to coronary problems.

a few years later, he became less disciplined about his diet and exercise, which led to a large increase in weight and an increase in his blood pressure. The ear lobe crease became more prominent again and he suffered increased cardiovascular complications. There was a direct correspondence between the depth of the crease on his ear lobe and the severity of his health problem.

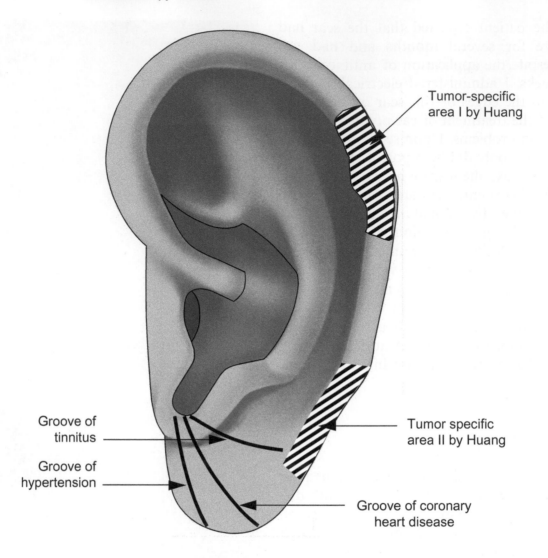

Tumor-specific
area I by Huang

Groove of
tinnitus

Groove of
hypertension

Tumor specific
area II by Huang

Groove of coronary
heart disease

FIGURE 5.2 Image of external ear that indicates diagonal ear lobe creases that have been related to hypertension, coronary heart disease, and tinnitus. Studies by Dr. Liqun Huang have been associated with regions of the helix that are associated with tumors.

5.2 Tactile Palpation of Auricular Tenderness

The most readily available technique for determining the reactivity of auricular reflex points is to apply localized pressure to specific areas of the auricle (Figure 5.3). Patients are often very surprised that palpation of one area of the external ear is so much more painful than identical pressure applied to a nearby auricular region. Even more amazing is how that specific area of the ear has been previously recognized on ear reflex point charts as indicative of pathological problems that the patient knows he or she is experiencing.

General Reactivity to Touch

Check broad regions of the external ear by using long stroking movements with your fingers and by applying generalized, pinching pressure to particular regions of the auricle. Determine areas of increased ear sensitivity of the patient to applied palpation with the thumb on the front of the ear and the index finger on the posterior side of the auricle. At the practitioner's preference, these positions may be reversed and the thumb placed at the back of the auricle and the index finger in front. Ask the patient if he or she notices whether one region is more tender than another while the palpation is taking place. Monitoring

(A)

(B)

(C)

(D)

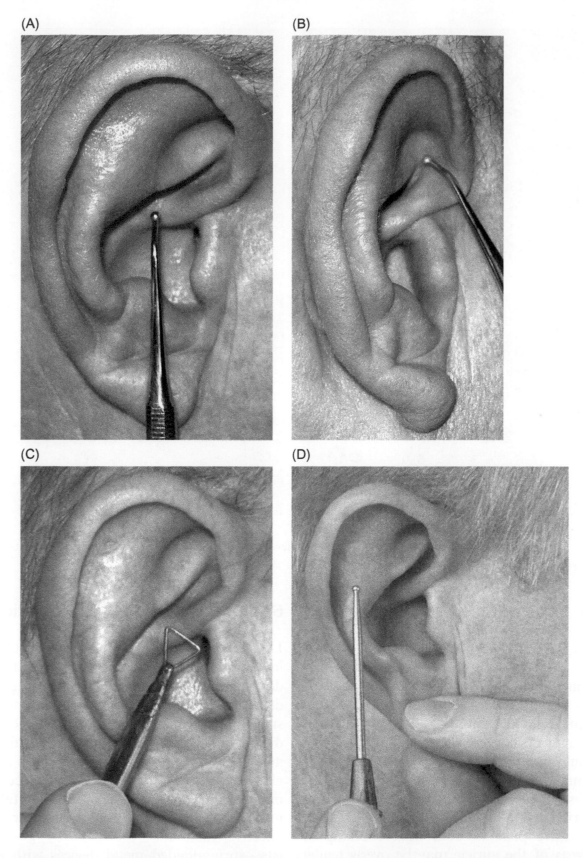

FIGURE 5.3 Photographs of palpation tools used for auricular diagnosis. Metal probe devices can be used to apply pressure to Point Zero (A) or the Sympathetic Autonomic point (B). A triangular stylus can be utilized on a sharp crevice at Point Zero (A), whereas a spring-loaded probe that maintains constant pressure can be used to detect reactive ear points on the antihelix (D).

(A)

(B)

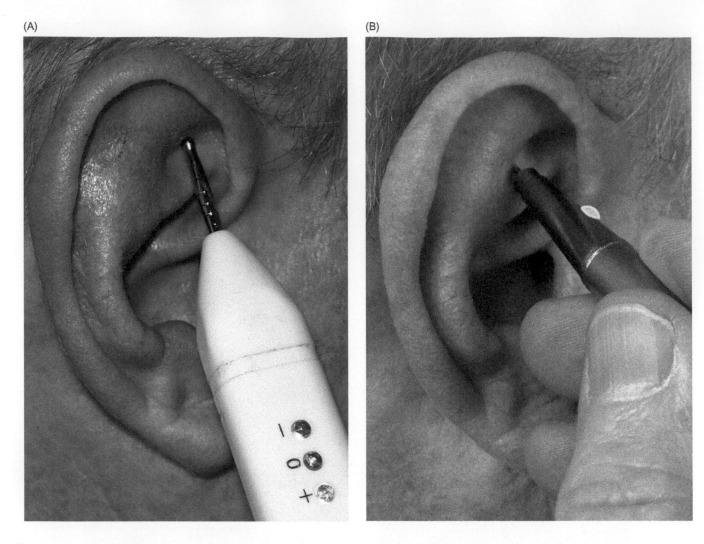

FIGURE 5.4 Different electrical point finders have been developed in China (A) and in the West (B) to determine the electrodermal skin conductance level of reactive ear points.

the individual's facial grimaces in response to tactile pressure is an excellent indicator that one has detected an appropriate diagnostic ear point.

Gently pinch the two sides of the auricle at different areas. It is important to develop tactile awareness of the different contours of the cartilaginous antihelix and the curving ridges around the helix. One should pull down on the fleshy ear lobe and feel throughout the depths of the concha. Note areas of skin surface that may be rough, bumpy, scaly, waxy, dry, oily, cold, or warm. For especially sensitive patients, even light touching of broad areas of the auricle may be overly tender for them, and one should proceed more softly with touching these individuals. For less sensitive patients, one can apply more selective palpation by a fingernail or the tips of one's fingers.

Specific Tenderness to Palpation

Localized tender areas on the external ear are investigated by utilizing a long metal probe designed with a small metal ball at the tip. The detecting probe should have a round, blunt, smooth metal tip ball, approximately 1.5 mm in diameter. Several pictures of such metal probes are shown in Figure 5.4. These probes are available at many acupuncture supply companies or at stores that sell medical or dental equipment. Some art supply stores also offer similarly effective tools that are used by graphic artists—spring-loaded metal devices with a small, spherical tip. Firmly stretch out the auricle with one hand as the tactile probe is held against the external ear with the other hand. Slowly glide the probe over the ear surface, stopping on small regions of skin that the patient informs you are sensitive to the lightly applied pressure. Direct pressure is applied to an auricular region that is suspected of representing a correspondent part of the body where the patient has indicated he or she has pathology.

If several points on the ear are found to be tender, selectively examine each point to determine which one is the most painful of the group. The degree of tenderness usually relates to the severity of the condition. The more sensitive the ear point, the more serious the associated body disorder. Heightened tenderness typically appears within 12 hours after a health problem occurs. The tenderness becomes more sensitive if the condition worsens, but it disappears within 7 days after the problem is alleviated. There is a distinct clinical skill in learning the level of pressure that is needed to discriminate the most appropriate ear point. The practitioner searches for the area of the ear that exhibits the highest intensity of tenderness without overly stressing the patient with unnecessarily severe discomfort.

Rating Responses to Tactile Pressure

The practitioner should request verbal ratings by the patient to indicate the degree of sensitivity that is felt at each point on the auricle when pressure is applied. Like the ashi points in body acupuncture, one rating procedure is to have the patient either say "There" or "That's it" when he or she feels that a specific region is especially tender. Alternatively, one can use a range of numerical or verbal responses to indicate the degree of tenderness. A value of "1" or "Slight" could indicate low-level tenderness, "2" or "Moderate" could indicate middle-level tenderness, "3" or "Strong" could indicate high-level tenderness, and "4" or "Very Strong" could indicate extremely high-level tenderness. Other practitioners use a 10-point rating scale.

Spontaneous facial grimace reactions or behavioral flinches in response to applied pressure should also be noted. A noticeable wince by the patient when you palpate a specific point

on the ear may not be comfortable for the patient, but it is one of the best predictors that you have detected an active reflex point that is appropriate for treatment. Nogier referred to the contraction of facial muscles in response to auricular palpation as the "sign of the grimace," the most reliable indication that one has a "real" ear reflex point. The Chinese have developed a grading system in which the degree of facial grimaces and verbal expressions is rated as follows: – for no pain, + for flinching or saying "ouch," ++ for frowning, +++ for wincing, and ++++ for dodging away or saying that "the pain is unbearable." The "+" symbols for the degree of facial grimaces can be replaced by the numerical values 1–4.

5.3 Electrical Detection of Ear Reflex Points

Of all the methods for conducting auricular diagnosis, examination of the auricle with an electrical point finder is the most reliable and least aversive (Figure 5.5). Even small changes in electrodermal skin resistance can be determined by electrical detection procedures. For many practitioners, the main consideration is either the cost of a quality point finder or the extra time it takes to first determine the most reactive ear points. Although both of these objections are understandable considerations, the increase in accuracy of discovering the most appropriate ear point for diagnosis and treatment of that client is worth the expense, time, and effort. One can learn to use even inexpensive but less sophisticated equipment in an effective manner.

Cleaning Skin Surface

To examine the ear with an electrical point finder, one must first clean the ear with alcohol to remove unwanted sources of interference to electrical detection. High electrical resistance impairs the electrical point finder's ability to discriminate active ear reflex points from normal regions of the auricle. Sources of such unwanted skin resistance could include earwax, oily surfaces,

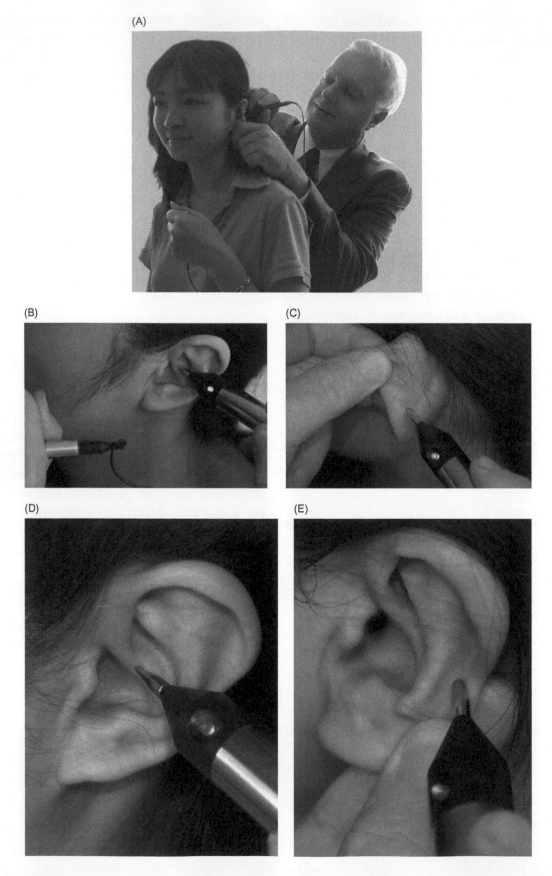

FIGURE 5.5 A photograph of an electrical diagnostic probe is shown with Dr. Oleson examining a female client. The practitioner holds the tip of the probe on the skin of the auricle while the client holds a reference electrode in her hand. A light on the probe comes on when an electrically conductive point is detected.

crusty skin, accumulated dust, facial makeup, or hair spray ingredients. Although it is possible to obtain electrodermal findings even when these substances are not removed, the auricular detection results are not as specific nor as reliable. One must allow several minutes after cleaning the ear with alcohol to let the skin surface dry.

Electrical Point Finders

A practitioner should utilize an electrical point finder specifically designed for the ear by both its size and its electrical amperage. Some probes designed for the body are inappropriate for the ear because the tips of the probes are too big or the instruments use too high of an electrical detecting voltage. Note that in order for an electrical detecting probe to function, a small level of electrical current is passed from the detecting probe into the skin of the auricle and then passes through the patient's body back to the reference probe and then back to the electronic equipment. Ear acupoints are smaller, closer to the surface, and have generally lower electrodermal skin resistance than body acupoints. Consequently, the tip of the detecting probe should be smaller for ear point finders than for body point finders. The point finder probe may be fixed in position, but it is preferred that the probe should be a spring-loaded rod, providing uniform pressure over different auricular surfaces. Even more selective than monopolar probes with one electrode probe touching the auricular skin surface are concentric, bipolar probes with two probes placed on the ear. A central detecting rod is surrounded by an outer barrel, allowing for differential amplification of the voltage difference between the two adjacent electrodes. This procedure allows for maximum discrimination of the difference in electrodermal skin resistance between the reactive ear point and adjacent skin areas, allowing for more precise detection of the lowest regions of electrodermal skin resistance. In each case, the auricular probe is applied to the ear by the practitioner while another lead is held in the patient's hand, providing a complete electrical circuit.

Electrodermal Measurements

The practitioner monitors decreased skin resistance, or inversely stated, increased skin conductance, as the electrodermal probe glides over the skin held by one hand. The practitioner's other hand is needed to stabilize the auricle and stretch out the ear for easier access to hidden areas. Electrodermal activity has also been designated as the galvanic skin response (GSR), a monitor of the degree of electrical current that flows through the skin from the detecting probe to the handheld neutral probe. Electricity must always flow between two points; thus, for some point finders that do not utilize a handheld probe, it is imperative that the practitioner touch the skin of the patient at the ear. Usually a light or a sound from the electrical point finder indicates a change in skin conductance. Depending on the equipment's design, a change in the electrodermal measurements leads to a change in auditory or visual signals that indicate the occurrence of reactive auricular points.

Electrical Threshold Settings

For some equipment, one must first set a threshold for a particular patient before assessing other ear points. To set the threshold, place the electrodermal probe on the Shen Men point or Point Zero on the auricle. Next, increase the detection sensitivity on the equipment until the sound, lights, or visual meter indicate that there is high electrical conductance, or low electrical resistance. Then, slightly reduce the sensitivity so that the Shen Men point or Point Zero is barely detected. It should be possible to find these two master points in most individuals who are examined. These two master points are usually reactive because they indicate the effects of everyday stress in a person's life. The Shen Men point and Point Zero may not be the most electrically conductive points on a person's ear, but they are the two ear points most consistently identified across different individuals.

Electrode Probe Procedures

Slowly glide the ear probe across all regions of the auricle to determine localized areas of increased skin conductance (decreased skin resistance). If one moves the probe too quickly, one can easily miss a reactive ear point. If one applies too much pressure with the probe, one can create false ear points that are just due to the increased electrical contact with the skin. Hold the auricular probe perpendicular to the stretched surface of the ear and then gently glide the probe over the ear, using firm but not overly strong pressure. Do not lift and poke with the probe because you may miss an active ear point. The therapist's other hand is used to support the back of the patient's ear. It is important to follow the contours of the auricle as one glides the probe over the auricle, checking both hidden and posterior surfaces as well as the anterior surface of the auricle. The back of the ear is often less electrically sensitive than the front of the auricle, but the posterior side of the ear is often more tender to applied pressure than is the front side of the ear. To more readily find an ear point on the posterior surface, first detect the appropriate point on the front side of the auricle, and then put a finger on that spot and bend the ear over. It is then easier to search the back of the ear for the identical region on the posterior surface once the ear point on the front of the auricle has been identified.

5.4 Nogier Vascular Autonomic Signal

The auricular cardiac reflex was first described by Paul Nogier in his 1972 text, *Treatise of Auriculotherapy*, and was only later renamed the Nogier vascular autonomic signal (N-VAS). Although this N-VAS pulse is often referred to as just VAS, "VAS" usually refers to the "visual analogue scale," a widely used assessment measure of pain intensity. For the N-VAS pulse, the practitioner first touches a specific part of the external ear and then monitors the radial pulse with the thumb to determine if there is either a decrease or an increase in pulse amplitude. The pulse may seem to diminish and collapse, or it may seem to

become sharper and more vibrant. The modification of the pulse can occur anywhere from the second pulse beat up to the tenth pulse beat following stimulation of the external ear. This change in the N-VAS can last for two to four pulse beats. The stimulus could be tactile pressure to the skin, but it also could be activated by holding a magnet over the ear surface, by pulsed laser stimulation, by placing a colored plastic filter over the auricle, or by using a slide that contains a specific chemical substance. The art of this auricular medicine technique is in learning to feel the subjective subtleties of the radial pulse.

Classical pulse diagnosis as it is practiced in Oriental medicine uses the practitioner's three middle fingers lightly placed on the radial artery at the wrist. The Nogier pulse technique requires placement of only the thumb over the radial artery. N-VAS is related to a change in pulse amplitude or pulse volume that occurs in response to stimulation of the auricle. In contrast, Oriental medical practitioners feel for steady-state qualities of the pulse, such as whether it is wiry, choppy, slippery, or tight. Mastery of either pulse technique requires many practice sessions with someone already skilled in this procedure (Figures 5.6 and 5.7).

Dr. John Ackerman (1999) proposed that N-VAS exists as a specific autonomic biophysical response system that constitutes one of the principal coordinating and integrating systems of the body. At the same time, N-VAS is viewed as a pathway by which the central nervous system receives information and modulates sympathetic outflow for precise modulation of the blood vascular system. N-VAS is thought to occur in every artery of the body and is expressed through changes in smooth muscle tone and blood influx. This vascular system is controlled by endothelium-derived factors, mainly by the vasodilator substance nitric oxide (NO). The chemical NO acts directly on vascular smooth muscle cells of the circulatory system to regulate vascular tone. The release of NO is modulated by wall shear stress, frequency of pulsatile flow, and amplitude of pulsatile flow.

From the standpoint of information theory, the autonomic controlled blood vascular supply could be represented as an analog system,

(A)   (B)   (C)

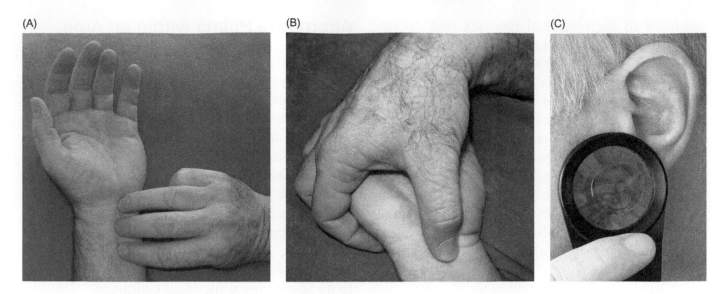

[**FIGURE 5.6** In Oriental medicine, pulse diagnosis is determined by placing three fingers over the radial artery at the wrist in order to detect specific qualities of the steady pulse (A). Practitioners of auricular medicine in Europe hold the wrist with only the thumb placed on the radial artery (B), which is referred to as the Nogier vascular autonomic signal. The practitioner feels for changes in the amplitude or the waveform of the pulse in reaction to the stimulation of the auricle by a light filter (C) or by laser light stimulators.

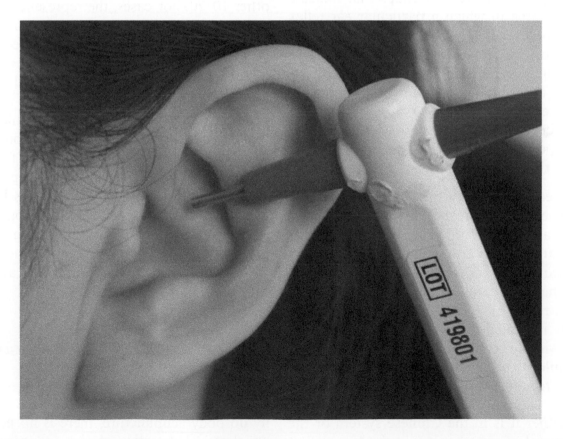

[**FIGURE 5.7** This photograph shows a magnetic probe with positive versus negative polarity placed over the external ear. A practitioner of auricular medicine feels for changes in the Nogier vascular autonomic signal in response to this magnetic probe.

contrary to the electrical neurons that operate as a digital system consisting of on or off neural impulses. As an analog system, the vascular system is regulated by the strength of flow, wavelength variations in its strength, and direction of flow. The adaptive capability of the vascular system results from mechanical stimuli such as wall shear stress and transmural pressure that is modulated by NO release and vascular muscle tone. It is now known that changes in vascular tone are reflected by signal strength-related parameters of the pulsatile blood flow curve, such as the area under the curve, the amplitude, and the flux.

5.5 Clinical Pearls for Auricular Diagnosis

Ear as Final Guide

The auricular charts depicting different organs of the body are somatotopic maps that indicate the general area in which a particular ear reflex point can be found. However, it is the measured reactivity of specific sites on the auricle that serves as the best determinant of the exact location of an appropriate ear point. By monitoring the heightened tenderness to applied pressure and the increased electrical conductance at a specific locus, one is able to select the most relevant ear points that represent body pathology.

Different ear charts indicate a territory of the auricle where the correct point may be found, but there are several possible spots within that region that one could choose. Only the most reactive ear points represent the actual location of the somatotopic site. If there is no reactive ear point in a region of the auricle, there is no body pathology indicated for treatment. If there is no pathology in the correspondent area of the body, there should be no tenderness or electrical activity at the related microsystem point on the ear. When choosing between different ear points to treat, whether it is in the Chinese system or the European system, whether it is in the Nogier first phase or second phase, this fundamental principle—that the ear itself is the final guide—should always be followed.

Alternative Points within an Area

The actual auricular point consists of a small site within a general area of the auricle indicated by the somatotopic auricular map. The ear reflex point representing a particular part of the body can be found in one of several possible locations within this area. In some individuals, the ear point will be found in one auricular location, whereas in other persons, it will be found in a nearby but different auricular location. The location of a point may change from one day to the next; thus, it is essential that one check for the ear point that exhibits the highest degree of reactivity at the time someone is examined.

Ipsilateral Ear Reactivity

In 80–90% of individuals, reactive ear reflex points are found on the same ear as the side of the body where there is pain or pathology. In the other 10–20% of cases, the representation is contralateral; thus, the most active ear point is found on the opposite side of the body. Because most clinical problems have a bilateral representation, it is common to treat both the right and the left ear on a patient. If the practitioner treats just one ear of a patient, it is usually best to stimulate the ear that is ipsilateral to the side of the body with the greatest degree of discomfort. Those few persons who exhibit contralateral auricular representation of a body problem are referred to as lateralizers or oscillators, and they need special consideration. Many clinical conditions, such as drug addictions, mental health disorders, or hypertension, are systemic in nature; thus, both the right and the left ear should be stimulated.

Electrodermal Detection versus Tenderness Palpation

For most acupuncture practitioners who primarily do body acupuncture, there is no need to use an electrical detection device in order to identify the most appropriate acupuncture point to treat. However, for auricular diagnosis, electrical ear point finders are an essential addition to the identification of ear points by tenderness palpation. The ear is a small, curving surface of circular contours, and the use of electrical detection devices may be difficult and confusing. Because most electronic devices designed for this purpose use monopolar probes with direct current, the longer one holds the detecting probe over the surface of the ear, the more electrical current will pass into the skin and essentially create a false ear point. The threshold setting used on many electronic detecting devices may be highly variable simply because the equipment is low on battery power. Even with constant-pressure probes, maintaining a consistent placement of the auricular probe against the patient's external ear is not always easy, leading to unreliable readings. There is a definite skill required to use these ear probes, and there needs to be supervised practice in order for one to master holding the ear probe while simultaneously holding the patient's ear in a firm and steady manner in order to obtain reliable results.

5.6 Assessment of Laterality Disorders

Persons who have difficulties with neural communication between the left and the right sides of the brain are referred to as having problems with laterality, also referred to as "oscillation" in the European school of auriculotherapy. This crossed-laterality condition is sometimes identified as "switched" or "crossed-wired" in American chiropractic schools. It is as if the two cerebral hemispheres are competing for control of the body rather than working in a complementary manner. Laterality problems are typically found in the 10–20% of the population that exhibits higher electrically conductivity at ear reflex points on the contralateral ear than on the ipsilateral ear. Usually these patients show high electrical conductance at the Master Oscillation point, but not everyone who has an active Master Oscillation point is an oscillator. Oscillation can also be due to severe stress or dental foci. The Master Oscillation point in patients with laterality disorders needs to be corrected with acupressure, needling, or electrication stimulation before

that patient can receive satisfactory medical treatment or acupuncture treatment.

It is believed that many functional disorders are due to dysfunctions in the interhemispheric connections through the corpus callosum, the anterior commissure, and the reticular formation of the brain. There is inappropriate interference of one side of the brain with the other side of the brain. Global relationships that should be processed by the right cerebral hemisphere are ineffectively analyzed by the left cerebral cortex. Verbal information that should be processed by the left cerebral hemisphere is inappropriately processed by the right cerebral cortex. Such individuals frequently exhibit dyslexia, learning disabilities, and problems with orientation in space, and they are susceptible to immune system disorders. When they were in elementary school, persons with laterality problems reported that they often had problems with poor concentration; they also suffered from stuttering, made many spelling mistakes, demanded a lot of attention, and felt "different" from others. As adolescents, these individuals reported that they experienced frequent anxiety, hyperactivity, gastrointestinal dysfunctions, and misgauged distances, or that they tripped over things. One way people may recognize that they are an oscillator is that they have overly sensitive or rather unusual reactions to prescription medications not observed in the average person. Dysfunctions of laterality and oscillation are found more often in left-handed or in ambidextrous persons. The proportion of dyslexia and other learning disorders is significantly higher in left-handers than in right-handers. Laterality problems are rarely noticeable before the age of 2 years, but cerebral organization begins to be definitively lateralized by 7 years, the "age of reason." It is during this age period that disorders of laterality may first appear.

Physical Tests for the Presence of Laterality Disorders

1. *Hand writing*: Have a person write something. Which hand did the person use, the right hand or the left hand? Many

individuals were trained to write with their right hand when they were children, even though they were naturally left-handed. For this reason, some of the following tests may be a more authentic appraisal of their actual laterality preference.

2. *Hand clap*: Have a person clap his or her hands as if the person were giving polite applause at a social function, with one hand on top of the other hand. Which hand is on top?

3. *Hand clasp*: Have a person clasp his or her hands, with the fingers interlocked. Which thumb is on top?

4. *Arm fold*: Have a person fold his or her arms, with one arm on top of the other. Which arm is on top? The arm that leads to the hand that touches the crease at the opposite elbow is considered the arm that is on top.

5. *Foot kick*: Have a person pretend to kick a football. Which foot does the person kick with, the right foot or the left foot?

6. *Eye gaze*: Have a person open both eyes and then line up the raised thumb of his or her outstretched hand toward a small point on the opposite wall. Alternatively, have the person make a circular hole by touching his or her middle finger to his or her thumb, and then the individual should look at the spot on the wall through the hole. In either case, next have the person close first one eye, open both eyes again, and then close the other eye. Which eye closure caused the greatest degree of movement from the point on the opposite wall? If there is a greater shift in the position of the spot with the right eye closed, then the person is right eye dominant; if the spot shifts more with closing the left eye, the individual is left eye dominant. One could alternatively have someone notice which eye he or she would leave open and which the person would close if he or she were to imagine shooting a target with a rifle. In the example of the rifle, the eye used for aiming the rifle would be the dominant eye.

7. *Laterality scoring system*: If a person scores 4 or more on the left side, that individual is likely to have a laterality dysfunction. The person might also have problems with spatial orientation, dyslexia, learning difficulties, attentional deficits, allergies, immune system disorders, and unusual medication reactions. Laterality does not necessarily produce a medical problem, because many individuals learn to compensate for this imbalance over the course of their lifetime. At the same time, they may have certain vulnerabilities that conventional medicine does not allow for. The dosage and incidence of side effects of Western medications are based on the average response by a large group of people. Such mean values do not take into account the idiosyncratic reactions of unusual individuals. Persons with laterality dysfunctions must be very careful about the treatments that they are given because of their high level of sensitivity.

5.7 Obstructions from Toxic Scars and Dental Foci

In addition to idiosyncratic problems attributable to laterality disorders, other factors may also interfere with subsequent pathologies that have a long-standing nature. The failure to completely heal from one condition may act as a source of disequilibrium that blocks the alleviation of newer health problems. Two such sources of obstruction are (1) toxic scars from old wounds or previous surgeries and (2) damaged tissue from invasive dental procedures. Toxic scars could occur on the skin surface or in deeper structures, creating a region of cellular disorganization that emits abnormal electrical charges. This pathological tissue generates a disharmonious resonance that is a source of chronic stress and interferes with general homeostatic balance. Abnormal sensations, such as itching, numbness, pain, or soreness, often occur in the region of toxic scars.

In addition to checking the region of the external ear that corresponds to a body area that was previously injured, one should examine the skin disorder region of the helix tail. Dental procedures, such as removing decayed teeth or drilling a root canal, are beneficial for dental care, but they may also leave a dental focus that interferes with general health maintenance. Dental foci may follow dental surgery, be related to bacterial foci under a filling, or result from an abscess or gum disease. There may also be pathogenic responses to mercury. The patients are often unaware that they have such a disorder because the consequence of these previous scars may not necessarily be experienced at a conscious level. These pathological regions may be electrically detected at the auricular area that corresponds to the site of the toxic scar or dental focus. They may also be discovered by monitoring the Nogier vascular autonomic signal response to stimulation of the affected region of the body. Only when this toxic scar region is successfully treated can other health care procedures be effective.

Sometimes one's own personal experience is the most impressive source of confirmation for accepting a new concept in health care. When I was an adolescent, I dislocated my right shoulder during a skateboarding accident. At approximately the same time in my teenage life, I also had my wisdom teeth removed by an oral surgeon. Several days after the dental surgery, my left lower jaw became swollen and inflamed, but it seemed to finally heal. As I became an adult, the chronic stress of everyday life was manifested as discomforting shoulder aches, but I never experienced jaw pain. Repeated acupuncture sessions, chiropractic adjustments, and massage treatments all produced temporary relief of the right shoulder pain, but there was no stable resolution of this condition. In 2000, I was given an auricular medicine diagnosis by Dr. Beate Strittmatter. She identified a toxic scar at the location of the wisdom tooth at the left lower jaw as well as an active shoulder point on the ear. The insertion of a needle at a point on the left ear Lower Jaw point was included with stimulation of the Shoulder point on the right auricle. This treatment of the dental obstruction as well as the correspondent shoulder ear point led to an immediate correction of the shoulder problem that has not returned since.

5.8 Scientific Evaluations of Auricular Diagnosis

Auricular diagnosis is primarily used for the detection of reactive points on the ear that need to be treated, rather than as a principal means of achieving the correct medical diagnosis of a patient. Nonetheless, findings from auricular diagnosis can reveal a clinical problem missed by other medical examination procedures or verify a problem only suspected from other diagnostic tests. Physical auricular reactions may appear before the body symptoms appear or leave a permanent reactive mark of pathology in the corresponding body organ. The auricular points change with the various stages of an illness or injury, including the initial occurrence, continued development, and ultimate resolution. Reactive auricular points reflect the ongoing information about a disease, not only the health condition occurring in the present. It can indicate the state of an illness or injury in the past or in the near future. Positive auricular points may have a different appearance in different stages of a disease and indicate when a pathology is completely healed.

At the 1995 International Symposium on Auricular Medicine in Beijing, China, several scientific studies indicated that auricular diagnosis has been used to detect malignant tumors, coronary heart disease, and pulmonary tuberculosis. One study found that 36 of 79 cases of colon cancer showed dark red capillaries in the superior concha, 54 of 78 cases of lung cancer revealed brown pinpoint depressions scattered in patches in the inferior concha, and 16 of 31 cases of uterine cancer showed spotted depressions in the internal genitals area of the concha wall. No such changes in the color or the morphology of corresponding ear points were found in normal control subjects. Another investigation showed that 116 of 1263 hospitalized patients had reactive liver points on the ear. Further examination of these 116 patients revealed 80 cases of hepatitis. Still another study found that of 84 cases diagnosed by ultrasound to exhibit gall bladder disease, 81% showed a dark red region in the gall bladder area of the auricle. In 93% of cases of chronic gastritis, the stomach and duodenum auricular regions appeared white, shiny, and bulgy. In contrast, these two points appeared deep red when there was an acute gastric disorder. The results of using pressure or electronic detection were essentially the same as visual observation.

Dr. Michel Marignan (1999) of Marseilles, France, reported on his investigations with digital thermography of the ear at the 1999 International Consensus Conference on Acupuncture, Auriculotherapy, and Auricular Medicine (ICCAAAM). Skin temperature radiations from the auricular surface that were measured with the help of an infrared camera were used with liquid nitrogen and a computer especially adapted for this procedure. The temperature variations of radiation across the human ear changed in response to stimulation of various areas of the ear pavilion. Marignan suggested that reactive auricular points are due to microscopic thermal regulation. The evidence of correspondence between anatomical localization and the auricular thermal reaction provided a possible scientific basis for auriculotherapy.

At the same 1999 ICCAAAM conference, Edward Dvorkin of Israel presented his work on reactive auricular points on skin samples obtained from humans undergoing surgery. By monitoring the Nogier vascular autonomic signal and by electrical detection of reactive ear points before the surgery, the skin samples from the external ear were identified as "active" or nonreactive. Small pieces of skin were taken from auricular regions that corresponded to the Thalamus point, the Allergy point, the Anti-Depression point, and the Aggressivity point. A neutral part of the auricular skin of each patient was also taken for comparison purposes. Electron microscopy examination of ultrathin sections of all the studied zones revealed the following findings: (1) thick nerve bundles with myelinated as well as nonmyelinated nerve fibers, (2) solitary thin bundles of nonmyelinated nerve fibers, (3) mast cells related to blood vessels and nerves, (4) numerous veins without innervation, and (5) solitary arteries without innervation. However, no specific ultrastructure or morphological substratum was found in this study for "active" ear reflex points compared to the neutral ear points. The distinctive characteristics of active auricular points must thus be based on physiological activity rather than physical structural differences. The earlier research by Marignan suggests that peripheral sympathetic

nerve control of blood vessels supplying the auricle can better account for active auricular points.

My own research on auricular diagnostic electrodermal activity began in the 1970s at the UCLA Pain Management Center. Oleson et al. (1980b) was the first double blind assessment to scientifically validate the somatotopic pattern of auricular reflex points. Some of the findings from this research were presented in Chapter 1 of this text. Forty patients with specific musculoskeletal pain problems were first evaluated by a doctor or nurse to determine the exact body location of their physical pain. A second medical doctor, who had extensive training in auricular acupuncture procedures, then examined each patient's ear. This second doctor had no prior knowledge of the subject's previously established medical diagnosis and was not allowed to verbally interact with the patient. There was a positive correspondence between auricular points identified as reactive and the parts of the body where there was musculoskeletal pain. "Reactive" was defined as auricular points that were tender to palpation and exhibited at least 50 microamps of conductivity. Nonreactive ear points corresponded to parts of the body from which there was no reported pain. The statistically significant, overall correct detection rate was 75.2%. When the pain was located on only one side of the body, electrical conductivity was significantly greater at the somatotopic ear point on the ipsilateral ear than at the corresponding area of the contralateral ear.

Another double blind assessment of auricular diagnosis did not occur until a decade later. Ear reflex points related to heart disorders were examined by Saku et al. (1993) in Japan. Reactive electropermeable points on the ear were defined as auricular skin areas that had conductance of electrical current greater than 50 microamps, indicating relatively low skin resistance. There was a significantly higher frequency of reactive ear points at the Chinese Heart points in the inferior concha (84%) and on the tragus (59%) for patients with myocardial infarctions and angina pain than for a control group of healthy subjects (11%). There was no difference between the coronary heart disease group and the control group regarding the electrical reactivity of auricular points that did not represent the heart. The frequency of electropermeable auricular points for the Kidney (5%), Stomach (6%), Liver (10%), Elbow (11%), or Eye (3%) was the same for coronary patients as for individuals without coronary problems, highlighting the specificity of this phenomenon.

Observations that acupuncture points exhibited lower levels of skin resistance than surrounding skin surface areas were first reported in the 1950s by Nakatani in Japan and by Niboyet in France. In the 1970s, Matsumoto showed that 80% of acupuncture points could be detected as low resistance points. The electrical resistance of acupuncture points was found to range from 100 to 900 kilohms, whereas the electrical resistance of non-acupuncture points ranged from 1100 to 11,700 kilohms. Reichmanis et al. (1975, 1976) further showed that meridian acupuncture points exhibit even lower electrical resistance when there is pathology in the organ they represent. For instance, electrodermal resistance on the Lung meridian is lower when one has a respiratory disorder, whereas skin resistance on the Liver meridian is lower when one has a liver disorder. Those acupuncture points that were ipsilateral to the site of body discomfort exhibited a lower electrical resistance than the corresponding meridian point on the contralateral side of the body. This work corroborated earlier findings (Bergsmann and Hart, 1973).

Subsequent research on the differential electrodermal activity of acupoints has continued to verify these earlier studies. Xianglong et al. (1992) of China examined 68 healthy adults for computerized plotting of low skin resistance points (LSRPs). A silver electrode was continuously moved over a whole area of body surface, while a reference electrode was fastened to the hand. Starting from the distal ends of the four limbs, investigators moved the electrode along the known meridians. The resistance of low skin impedance points (LSIPs) was approximately 50 kilohms, whereas the impedance at non-LSIPs was typically 500 kilohms. A total of 83.3% of LSIPs were located within 3 mm of a channel. In only a few cases could individual LSIPs be found in nonchannel areas. The topography of LSRPs in rats was examined by Chiou et al. (1998).

Specific LSRP loci were found to be distributed symmetrically and bilaterally over the shaved skin of the animal's ventral, dorsal, and lateral surface. The arrangement of these points corresponded to the acupuncture meridians found in humans. The LSRPs were hypothesized to represent zones of autonomic concentration, with the higher electrical conductivity due to higher neural and vascular elements beneath the points. The LSRPs gradually disappeared within 30 minutes after the animal's death.

Skin and muscle tissue samples were obtained by Chan et al. (1998) from four anesthetized dogs. Acupuncture points, defined by regions of low skin resistance, were compared to control points, which exhibited higher electrodermal resistance. The points were marked for later histological examination. Concentration of natural chemical substance P was significantly higher at skin acupuncture points (3.33 ng/g) than at control skin points (2.63 ng/g) that did not exhibit low skin resistance. Elevation of substance P concentration was also significantly higher in skin tissue samples (3.33 ng/g) than in the deeper, muscle tissue samples (1.81 ng/g). Substance P is known to be a spinal neurotransmitter found in nociceptive, afferent C-fibers (Kashiba and Ueda, 1991). This chemical plays an active role in pain transmission, stimulates contractility of autonomic smooth muscle, induces subcutaneous liberation of histamine, causes peripheral vasodilation, and leads to hypersensitivity of sensory neurons. Substance P seems to activate a somato-autonomic reflex that could account for the clinical observations of specific acupuncture points that are both electrically active and tender to palpation.

Experimentally induced changes in auricular reflex points in rats were examined by Kawakaita et al. (1991). The submucosal tissue of the stomach of anesthetized rats was exposed, and then acetic acid or saline was injected into the stomach tissue. Skin impedance of the auricular skin was measured by constant voltage, square wave pulses. A silver metal ball, the search electrode, was moved over the surface of the rat's ear and a needle was inserted into subcutaneous tissue to serve as the reference electrode. Injection of acetic acid led to the gradual development of lowered skin resistance points on central regions of the rats' ears, auricular areas that correspond to the gastrointestinal region of human ears. In normal rats and in experimental rats before the surgical operation, low impedance points were rarely detected on the auricular skin. After experimentally induced peritonitis, there was a significant increase in low impedance points (0–100 kilohms) and moderate impedance points (100–500 kilohms) but a decrease in high impedance points (>500 kilohms). Histological investigation could not prove the existence of sweat glands in the rat auricular skin. The authors suggested that the low impedance points are in fact related to sympathetic control of blood vessels.

Failure to find confirmation for the Nogier auricular somatotopic map was reported by Andersson et al. (2007). They recruited 25 patients from a chronic pain clinic in Sweden for double blind evaluation of auricular diagnosis, which had not been examined in a systematic scientific study since Oleson et al. (1980b). Patients were asked where they experienced musculoskeletal pain in 11 different areas of the body that hypothetically correspond to 11 somatotopic regions of the antihelix, scaphoid fossa, and triangular fossa. The experimental protocol was similar to that used by Oleson et al. (1980b), with the participant asked to not talk to the auricular examiner who was blind to the patient's condition and the patient's body was covered with a sheet except for the head. The auricular examiner used a spring-loaded stylus by Sedatelec to search for tender ear points. The patients reported their tenderness score on a "0" to "4" verbal rating scale, and wincing reactions by patients were also noted. Statistical analysis was applied to kappa values with regard to the agreement between patient pain reports of areas where they experienced musculoskeletal pain and the reports of tenderness to pressure applied to specific areas of the auricle. Whereas there was concurrence of 76% agreement between those patients who reported neck and shoulder pain and who also reported tenderness in the areas of the external ear that correspond to the neck and shoulder, there was not agreement between persons with no neck and shoulder pain and

who also stated lower ratings of tenderness over the areas of the auricle associated with the neck and shoulder. Only 51.1% of the patients who reported musculoskeletal pain in different areas of the body also reported tenderness in the corresponding regions of the auricle and reported no tenderness in auricular areas that corresponded to body regions with no reported pain. These values did not reach statistical significance. There are distinct differences between the study conducted by Andersson et al. and that conducted by Oleson et al. In our 1980 study, we utilized electrodermal detection by a highly skilled clinician to obtain the auricular diagnosis. We found that electrical detection values were far superior to tenderness palpation for specific identification of an accurate auricular diagnosis. One conclusion from the Andersson study would thus be that in order to obtain reliable findings for auricular diagnosis, it is very important to include an electrical point finder in the examination process. Most practitioners of body acupuncture do not need an electrical point finder to find body acupoints and thus are not highly skilled in the manual dexterity and electronic sophistication that is required to conduct an evaluation of the curving contours of the external ear. Extensive practice with a well-designed electrical detection probe is imperative for those practitioners who seek to be more proficient in auricular diagnosis.

■ KEY TERMS FOR CHAPTER 5

Auricular Tenderness: Response to tactile palpation of external ear to determine reactive ear acupoints that can correspond to pathological regions in the physical body.

Dental Foci: Toxic reactions in the physical body that are due to impaired healing following a dental procedure. Unless successfully treated, obstructions due to dental foci will impair the clinical results achievable with auriculotherapy or body acupuncture.

Earlobe Creases: Wrinkles on the lobe of the external ear that correspond to the occurrence of coronary disorders.

Electrical Detection: Use of electronic equipment to determine the degree of electrical activity of ear reflex points.

Electrical Threshold: The electrical setting at which one can detect a reactive acupuncture point on the auricle or on body acupuncture meridians.

Electrode Probe: A metal rod connected to an electronic device that allows the electrical detection of acupuncture points.

Electrodermal Measurements: The use of electronic equipment to assess the passage of electrical current through the skin.

Electrodermal Skin Conductance: The passage of electrical current through the skin. Reactive acupoints have *high* skin conductance.

Electrodermal Skin Resistance: The opposition to the passage of electrical current through the skin. Reactive acupoints have *low* skin resistance.

Ipsilateral Ear Reactivity: Most individuals show reactive ear reflex points that are found on the same ear as the side of body where there is pain or pathology. Although the ipsilateral ear is usually higher in reactivity, the corresponding contralateral ear is also active.

Laterality Disorders: Physical health disorders related to imbalances in the functional activity of the right and the left sides of the brain. Such disorders include ADHD, dyslexia, and immune system disorders.

Oscillation: The condition whereby dysfunctional interactions between the left side and the right side of the brain impair the effectiveness of other treatments.

Reactive Point: Auricular regions that are identified as areas of high sensitivity to pressure applied to the external ear and areas of high electrodermal conductivity.

Skin Surface Observations: Assessment of reactive points on the external ear based on skin surface changes in the color or texture of the skin surface.

Substance P: A natural chemical in subdermal tissue that has been found in higher concentrations below areas of low electrodermal skin resistance related to acupuncture points than at other areas of skin.

Toxic Scars: Obstructions to healing due to interference from some traumatized region of the body that never fully healed after an accident, injury, or illness.

Vascular Autonomic Signal (VAS): Delayed changes in the radial pulse amplitude or pulse wave form in response to stimulation of some area of the auricle or the body.

■ CHAPTER 5 REVIEW QUESTIONS

1. Observable changes on the auricular skin surface that tend to indicate a chronic health condition are typically characterized by_____.
   a. dark purple spots
   b. shiny red spots
   c. brown freckles
   d. white, flaky skin

2. A deep, diagonal crease on a patient's earlobe has been clinically associated with_____ disorders.
   a. coronary
   b. respiratory
   c. digestive
   d. urinary

3. Behavioral assessment of facial grimaces has been used to rate diagnostic responses to_____ applied to the auricle.
   a. visual inspection
   b. tactile pressure
   c. pulse amplitude
   d. electrodermal detection

4. An active auricular point exhibits *decreased*_____ at a specific region of the ear surface.
   a. biochemical changes
   b. tenderness to pressure
   c. electrodermal skin resistance
   d. electrodermal skin conductance

5. The Point Zero and Shen Men points on the auricle are often used to set electrical_____ by which to compare the electrical detection of other ear points.

   a. current intensities
   b. resistance interference
   c. pulse amplitude
   d. threshold levels

6. In contrast to pulse diagnosis in Oriental medicine, the pulse reaction to stimulation of the external ear in European auricular medicine is called the_____.

   a. vascular autonomic signal
   b. cardiac auricular reaction
   c. phase shift pulse
   d. auricular coronary reflex

7. The concept that_____ refers to the detection of active ear reflex points is more clinically effective than to simply determine the selection of ear points to treat based on standardized ear charts.

   a. the somatotopic guide
   b. the correspondent ear points
   c. the ear is the final guide
   d. the auricular activation principle

8. Difficulties in the neural communication between the right and left sides of the brain can often lead to_____.

   a. cerebral dominance activation
   b. laterality disorders
   c. ipsilateral focus
   d. identity dysfunction

9. The impact of previous dental surgeries on the treatment of other medical conditions is attributable to the detrimental effect of_____.

   a. invasive deterioration
   b. physical obstruction
   c. global disorganization
   d. toxic scars

10. The specific region of the body that is related to an active somatotopic ear point is labeled the_____ body area.

    a. correspondent
    b. representative
    c. identified
    d. organic

Answers

1 = d; 2 = a; 3 = b; 4 = c; 5 = d; 6 = a; 7 = c; 8 = b; 9 = d; 10 = a

Overview of Auriculotherapy Treatment Procedures

CONTENTS

6.0 Overview of Auriculotherapy Treatment Procedures

CHAPTER 6 LEARNING OBJECTIVES

1. To demonstrate awareness of different types of acupressure techniques used for auriculotherapy.

2. To apply the insertion of acupuncture needles into selective acupoints on the external ear.

3. To differentiate electrical stimulation procedures involved in auricular electroacupuncture and transcutaneous auricular stimulation.

4. To apply ear acubeads and semipermanent ear needles for continued auriculotherapy stimulation.

5. To evaluate precautions and hindrances associated with auriculotherapy.

6.1 Auricular Acupressure

General Tactile Massage: Stroke broad regions of the external ear by using one's thumb to rub against the front of the auricle, while the tip of the index finger, or the length of the distal segment of the finger, is held against the posterior side of the ear for support. These finger positions can be reversed at the discretion of the

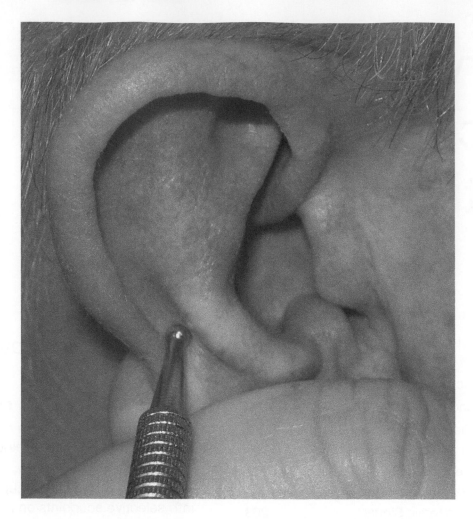

FIGURE 6.1 Ear acupressure massage can be activated with a metal stylus applied to specific points on the auricle while using the opposite hand of the practitioner to provide back pressure.

practitioner, with the index finger on the front of the auricle and the thumb on the posterior side of the ear. First, stroke down the tragus with the thumb, and then spread the strokes across the ear lobe to induce a general calming effect. Next, stroke the external ear from the beginning of the helix root at landmark zero, then rise up and around the curving helix, ending at the base of the helix tail. Proceed by stroking across the antihelix tail, beginning at the base, then working up the antihelix, in each case massaging across the inner ridge of the antihelix, and massage outward toward the scaphoid fossa and helix rim. End with gentle strokes throughout the superior concha, concha ridge, and inferior concha. If patients are taught to do this procedure on themselves, it is suggested that their index finger be placed upon the front of the external ear and their thumb be placed on the back of the auricle.

Specific Tactile Massage: Apply a metal stylus to the most reactive ear points that were discovered during auricular diagnosis. Such a metal probe should have a small metal ball at the tip that is approximately 1.5 mm in diameter. An example of such a probe is shown in Figure 6.1. One could also use the eraser end of a pencil or the blunt end of an acupuncture needle, but those approaches do not provide as specific or comfortable a surface for tactile massage. Hold the skin of the external ear taught with the opposite hand. Micromassage of any ear point may sometimes lead to an initial increase in pain at that area of the ear. As the localized auricular massage is continued, the pain will gradually diminish and disappear. The direction of massage that is adopted should be oriented such that it is the least uncomfortable for the individual to tolerate and the easiest for the practitioner to apply. For neck, back, and shoulder tension, place firm but gentle pressure on the antihelix tail, antihelix body, inferior crus, and scaphoid fossa. For headaches, specific pressure is applied to the antitragus and antihelix tail. Visceral dysfunctions are treated with the stylus probe pressed against specific regions of the concha.

Auriculopressure Techniques: Massage each tender ear point for 1 or 2 minutes, repeating the process once or twice daily. Apply massage with a circling, rotating motion, first noticing which direction produces the least uncomfortable effect. A long stroking massage along the outer helix rim or the antihelix ridge reduces muscle tension and sympathomimetic excess excitation, such as when a patient is anxious. Descending, longitudinal strokes tend to tonify muscles and excite sympathetic activity, whereas ascending, longitudinal strokes tend to relax muscles and enhance parasympathetic tone. A radial, centrifugal massage away from landmark zero and outward across the concha enhances parasympathetic sedation and visceral relaxation. Massaging the tragus downward and outward, from superior to inferior, can augment cellular reactions and interhemispheric communication, whereas massaging the tragus upward and inward, from inferior to superior, tends to slow down metabolism and calm interhemispheric cerebral communication.

6.2 Ear Acupuncture Needling Techniques

Cleaning Ear: After conducting any visual inspection necessary for auricular diagnosis, clean the ear with alcohol for sterilization and for removing earwax, skin oils, sweat, grease, makeup, or hair spray. Besides its antiseptic value, alcohol removes oily substances from the skin surface of the ear and improves the ability to detect auricular points with electrical point finders. One must allow several minutes after the external ear surface has dried before proceeding further with the treatment.

Prepare Needles: Unpackage at least five sterilized, 0.5-inch (15-mm) needles to be inserted ipsilaterally or bilaterally. Shorter needles are preferred because longer needles tend to fall out too easily. Thin or thick needles, with diameter sizes of #30 gauge (0.30 mm), #32 gauge (0.25 mm) or #34 gauge (0.22 mm), are preferred for the ear; thinner needles tend to bend on insertion, whereas thicker needles tend to induce excessive discomfort. Stainless-steel needles are appropriate for most clinical purposes, although better results are sometimes obtained by using gold needles on one ear and silver needles on the opposite ear. Knowledge of the Nogier vascular autonomic signal (N-VAS) is often necessary to determine whether gold or silver needles are more appropriate for which ear. For auricular acupuncture, it is not necessary to use guide tubes to surround and strengthen the needle. One needs one hand to insert the needle and the other hand to hold the ear steady, thus preventing the ability to hold a plastic tube.

Determine Treatment Plan: Examine the specific treatment plans listed in Chapter 9 to select the auricular points that are most appropriate for the condition being treated. Typically, treat the correspondent anatomic points, master points, and supportive ear points listed for that condition. You should not treat all of the ear points listed—only those points that have high tenderness and high electrical conductance. Utilize auricular diagnosis findings to use the ear reactivity as the final guide for determining point selection.

Select Order of Ear Points: Detect two to six points on each ear with an electrical point finder, selecting only the most reactive points. The point finder should be spring-loaded and will leave a brief indentation at the ear point when stronger pressure is applied when a reactive ear point is detected. The indentation mark left on the ear surface after pressure from a diagnostic probe precisely localizes the region of the auricle where the needle should be inserted. The order in which auricular points are needled depends more on

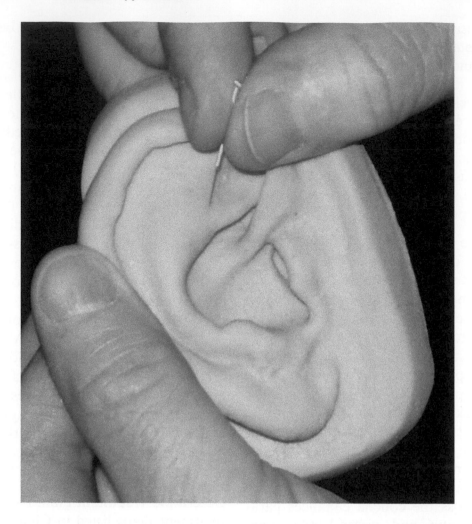

[**FIGURE 6.2** Practicing needle insertion techniques can be facilitated with the use a rubber ear model. A half-inch needle should be inserted with a quick jab followed by a spinning action to secure the needle placement.

the practical convenience of their location than on the priority of their importance for treating a specific condition. Needles are first inserted into ear points that are located in more central or hidden regions of the auricle because needles in more peripheral areas of the ear would get in the way of using more central ear points. Although needles on the front of the auricle may be first detected by auricular diagnosis, it is important to needle the acupoints on the posterior side of those same points before inserting needles onto the anterior side. Bending the ear to allow access to the posterior side of the auricle would be prevented if the needles to be used on the front of the ear were already in place.

Needle Insertion Procedures: First, stretch out the auricle with one hand while using the other hand to hold the needle over the appropriate ear point. Avoid doing one-handed ear acupuncture, only using the hand holding the needle. Insert the needle with a quick jab and a twist to a depth of 1 or 2mm. The needle should just barely penetrate the skin, but it is acceptable if it touches the cartilage. The needle should be inserted deep enough so that it holds firmly but not so deep that it pierces through to the other side. The practitioner should also be careful not to let the needle stick the practitioner's hand that is used to stabilize the patient's ear. Beginning students often find it helpful to practice needle insertion techniques with a rubber ear, as shown in Figure 6.2.

It is usually more comfortable for the patient if the practitioner inserts the needle on the patient's exhalation breath, after first taking a deep inhalation breath. The patient may gasp or

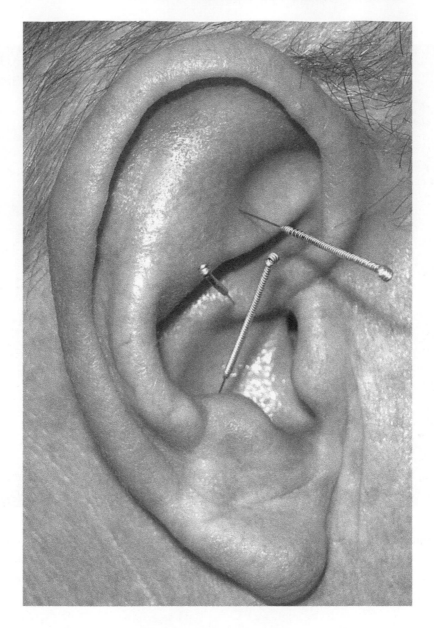

[**FIGURE 6.3** This photograph shows half-inch needles inserted into the auricular acupoints Shen Men, Point Zero, and Thalamus point.

flinch when a needle is inserted into a particularly sensitive region, but sometimes there is no discomfort. Although the needle may produce intense discomfort on first insertion, this aversive effect is short-lived and the pain quickly subsides. The intensity of pain at an auricular point is usually a sign that the point is most appropriate for treatment of that patient's condition. Figure 6.3 shows the insertion of acupuncture needles into the ear acupoints Shen Men, Point Zero, and Thalamus point. As presented in Figure 6.4A, needles used in acupuncture have a specific shape and are contained in a

sterilized packet that must first be opened; hair clips are often necessary to keep strands of hair off of the ear. Figure 6.4B shows the location of five needles inserted into the external ear according to the National Acupuncture Detoxification Association (NADA) addiction protocol.

Guide tubes that are often used to insert needles into body acupuncture points are not necessary for auriculotherapy. The plastic hollow tubes that allow an acupuncturist to simply tap the needle deep into the skin of the body are needed in auricular acupuncture because of the shallow depth of ear points. It is much better

(A)

(B)

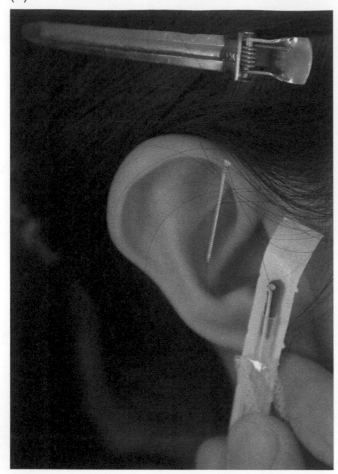
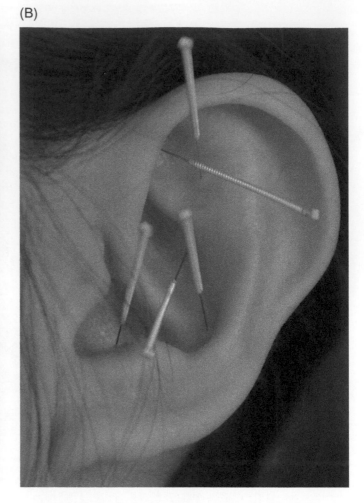

FIGURE 6.4 This photograph of the type of acupuncture needles used in auriculotherapy (A) shows one needle inserted into the auricle and another needle held still in the sterilized package from which it came. Shown in the opposite ear are needles inserted into the five ear points used in the NADA protocol for drug detoxification (B): Shen Men, Sympathetic point, Kidney point, Liver point, and Lung point.

to visually hold the needle precisely over an ear point that has been previously identified by a skin surface indentation mark. The hand that would hold the guide tube is needed to be free to hold the ear stable. With the other hand, insert all the needles you plan to use at one time and leave them in place. You may periodically twirl the needles to maintain their firm connection in the skin, which also serves to further stimulate activation of that auricular point by the repeated twirling.

Bleeding may occur when a needle is withdrawn from the ear, but gentle pressure with a cotton ball can be applied to that ear point to stop the bleeding within a few seconds.

Treatment Duration: Leave all the inserted needles in place for 10–30 minutes, and then remove them and place the used needles in an approved sharp's container. Some needles fall out before the session is over, which tends to indicate that the particular ear points where these needles were inserted received sufficient stimulation.

Number of Sessions: Treat one to three times a week for 2–10 weeks, and then gradually space out the treatment sessions. A given condition may require as few as 2 sessions and as many as 12 sessions, depending on the chronicity and severity of the problem and on the energy level of the patient. If after 3 sessions there is no improvement in the condition, either utilize a different set of ear points or try another form of therapy.

6.3 Auricular Electroacupuncture Stimulation

Ear Needling Techniques: For electroacupuncture, use the needling techniques described in the previous section to detect the appropriate ear points and to insert needles into the skin.

Tape Needles Securely: In order to hold the inserted needles securely in place, tape the needles across the ear with medical adhesive tape. Without this tape, needles will tend to pull out the external ear when you attach the stimulating electrodes; the electrodes need to be held in place with protective tape. Fasten the electrode leads securely in place, either to the patient's clothes or to office equipment.

Attach Electrode Leads: Use microgator clip electrode leads from an electronic stimulator to connect to the inserted needles (Figure 6.5). Because these moveable clips may pull out the inserted needles when attached, one must make sure that the needles are first securely taped in place. It is also wise to fasten the electrode wires to a secure anchor so that these wires will not drag on the needles and pull them out by accident.

Determine Electrode Pairs: One always needs to stimulate between two needles because electricity flows from a positive pole to a negative pole. It does not usually matter which pole of the stimulator is attached to which ear point, but if the patient reports any increase in pain, one can try switching the electrode leads to the opposite polarity.

Set Frequency Parameters: Preset the electrical frequency rate to either a slow 2 or 10 Hz frequency or to a parameter known as dense–disperse, in which 2 Hz frequencies are alternated with 100 Hz frequencies (Figure 6.6). Lower frequencies (10 Hz or less) most affect enkephalins, endorphins, and visceral and somatic disorders, whereas higher frequencies (100 Hz or higher) affect dynorphins and neurological dysfunctions.

Adjust Current Intensity: Gradually raise the electrical current intensity to a perceptible level and then reduce it to a subpain threshold. The electrical stimulation intensity should not be overly uncomfortable.

Number of Sessions: As with auricular acupuncture without electrical stimulation, leave the needles in place and maintain the stimulation current for 10–30 min. Treat the patient one to three times a week for 2–10 weeks. Although more cumbersome to apply than needle insertion alone, electroacupuncture is typically more powerful and more successful in relieving pain and alleviating the problems of addiction.

6.4 Transcutaneous Auricular Stimulation

Transcutaneous Stimulation Overview: In this treatment method, the practitioner detects and stimulates each ear point with the same electrical probe (Figure 6.7). The auricular point is sequentially detected and then immediately treated with microcurrent stimulation before moving on to the next ear point. It is a form of transcutaneous electrical nerve stimulation (TENS) or neurostimulation and can be medically billed as such. Before beginning auriculotherapy, it is best to have the patient repeat those movements, or maintain those postures, that most aggravate his or her painful condition. It is also useful for the practitioner to put physical pressure on those body areas that are painful, which further intensifies the patient's experience of the problem. One can thus establish a behavioral baseline from which there can be seen a change in experience as a result of the auriculotherapy treatment. Because the same movements, postures, or applied pressures are repeated prior to and following the treatment, the patient can experience the immediate benefit of the treatment. This practice tends to eliminate doubts about the auriculotherapy procedure that often occur when only subjective impressions of improvement are elicited. Patients often demonstrate facial grimaces, limited range

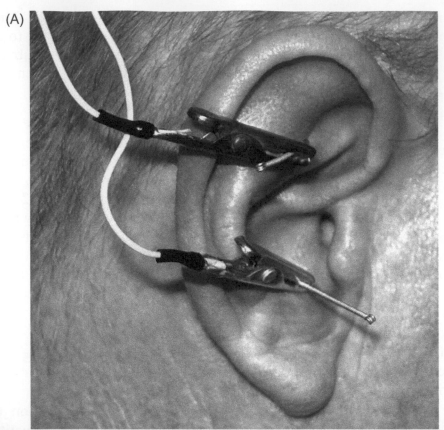

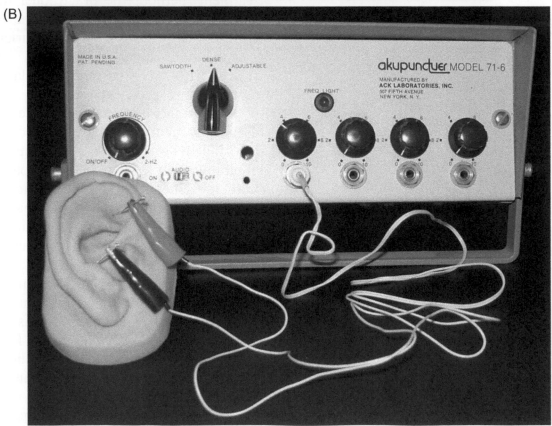

⟦FIGURE 6.5 Photographs of an ear with alligator clip electrodes connected to needles inserted into the Shen Men and Lung points (A). Electroacupuncture stimulation equipment is shown with electrode wires leading to a rubber ear model (B).

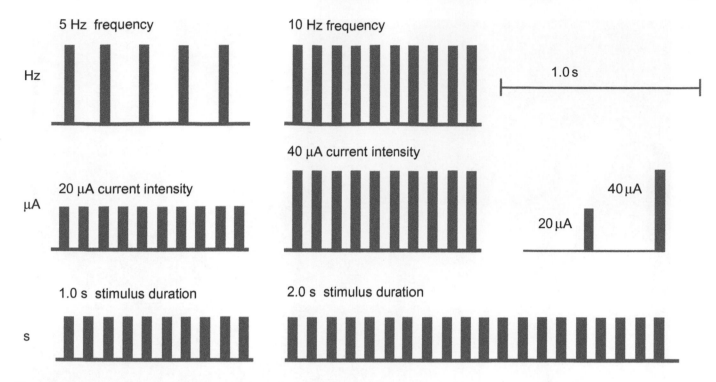

[**FIGURE 6.6** The parameters that distinguish different aspects of electrical stimulation include differences in frequency, the number of pulses per second, and intensity, the amplitude of each pulse.

of movements, or verbal response to pressure when the area of pain or pathology in the body is activated. Using diagnostic assessments of the body, both before and after stimulation of an ear point, is much more convincing to patients than subjective verbal assessments.

Cleaning Ear: Clean the external ear with alcohol to eliminate skin oil and surface flakiness. Having a clean auricular surface is very important for determining the accuracy of reactive ear points that will be treated with transcutaneous electrical stimulation.

Determine Treatment Plan: As with other auricular procedures, consult the specific treatment plans listed later in this book to select the auricular points that seem most appropriate for the condition being treated. First, treat local anatomic points corresponding to specific body symptoms. If there is more than one local point, only treat the most tender and most electrically conductive local points. Next, treat master points and then stimulate supportive ear points.

Set Stimulation Frequency: On some electronic equipment, specific dials on the instrument allow you to change the frequency of stimulation that will be applied. Preset the frequency rate of stimulation, measured in cycles per second or Hertz (Hz). Paul Nogier identified the specific zones of the ear that are most optimal for stimulation by the type of body tissue to be treated. Whereas Asian electronic equipment is often supplied with only one frequency, usually 2 or 10 Hz, American and European electronic equipment is often supplied with a range of frequency rates from which to choose. The specific frequencies developed by Dr. Nogier are as follows: 2.5 Hz for the subtragus; 5 Hz for the concha; 10 Hz for the antihelix, antitragus, and helix arch; 20 Hz for the tragus and intertragic notch; 40 Hz for the helix tail; 80 Hz for the peripheral ear lobe; and 160 Hz for the medial ear lobe. The type of organ tissue being treated is also a factor, with 5 Hz used for visceral disorders, 10 Hz for musculoskeletal disorders, 40 Hz for neuralgias, 80 Hz for subcortical dysfunctions, and 160 Hz for cerebral dysfunctions. For instance, if one were treating a spinal cord disorder by treating an active point found in the concha, one would stimulate that point with 40 Hz rather than 5 Hz.

(A)

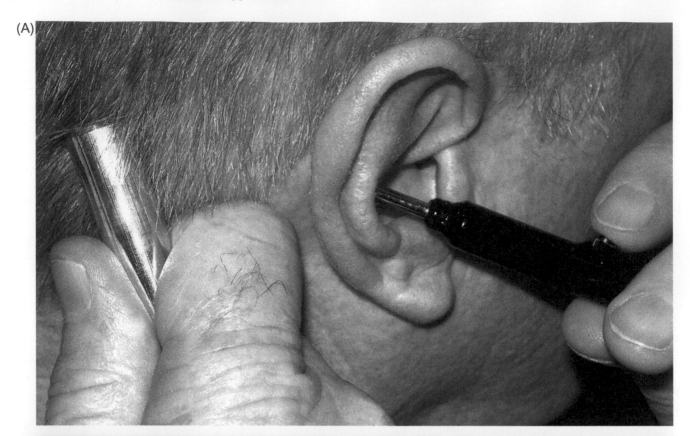

(B)

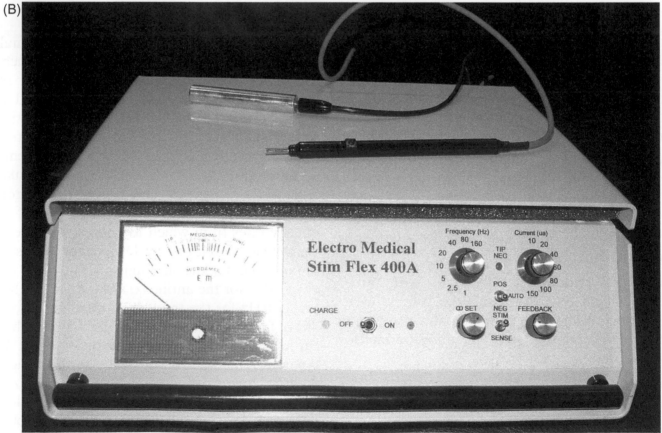

⌈FIGURE 6.7 Transcutaneous electrical stimulation of the skin surface of an auricular acupoint (A) is referenced to an electrode held in the patient's hand. The Stim Flex 400A electrical stimulation equipment (B) shows that the frequency of stimulation can range from 1 Hz (cycles per second) to 160 Hz, and the current intensity is usually set between 10 and 80 microamps.

If one has electronic equipment that does not provide these very specific frequencies, many different frequencies of stimulations can have clinical benefit.

Adjust Stimulation Intensity: Prepare to set the intensity of auricular stimulation by the patient's pain tolerance, usually ranging from 10 to 80 microamps, most typically at 40 microamps. The current intensity is lowered if the patient complains of pain from even weak auricular stimulation. If even the lowest intensity is experienced as painful, then only auricular acupressure should be used at that ear point. A major problem with electrical stimulators that are designed for treating the body as well as the ear is that the skin surface on the body has a much higher electrical resistance than does the ear. Consequently, electrical current levels that are sufficient to activate body acupoints are too intense for stimulating auricular points. Practitioners should be clear to not confuse stimulation frequency with stimulation intensity. Frequency refers to the number of pulses of current in a period of time, whereas intensity refers to the amplitude or strength of the electric current. Only increased electrical intensity is related to perceived pain, whereas different frequencies are perceived slight sensations related to the different patterns of pulses.

Set Threshold Intensity Level: Some instruments require the practitioner to first set a threshold level by raising the sensitivity of the unit so that one can electrically detect the Shen Men point or Point Zero. Most reactive correspondent points are typically more electrically conductive than Shen Men or Point Zero, but these two master points are more consistently active in a majority of clients. Sometimes by first stimulating one of these two master points, other auricular points become more identifiable for detection. This process is called "lighting up the ear."

Apply Auricular Probe: Apply the auricular detecting and stimulating probe to the external ear, stretching the skin tightly to reveal different surfaces of the ear. The practitioner's other hand supports the back of the ear so that both it and the probe are steady. Gently glide the auricular probe over the ear, holding the probe perpendicular to the ear surface. Do *not* pick up the probe and jab at different areas of the ear. The patient usually holds a common lead in one of his or her hands in order to complete a full electrical circuit. Electric current flows from the stimulating equipment to the electrode leads to the ear probe to the patient's auricle through the patient's body to the patient's hand to the metal common lead to the return electrode wires and back to the electronic equipment. Figure 6.8 shows the different angles at which the ear probe should be held against the ear when finding the master points on the auricle. If there is some problem with stimulation, be sure that all parts of the circuit are complete. There could be a break in electrode wires or the patient may fail to continue holding the reference lead.

Initiate Direct Current Detection Mode: Diagnosis of reactive ear points is achieved with low-level direct current (DC). The microcurrent levels used for detection are usually only 2 microamps in strength. The detecting cycle is usually indicated by a change in a continuous tone or by a light that flashes when a reactive point is detected. Because of the gradually accumulating electrical current, the continued application of the detecting probe upon the auricular skin surface may lead to the development of an active auricular point that was not previously active. Continued DC current applied to the ear surface can create a false ear point.

Activate Alternating Current Stimulation Mode: Reactive ear points discovered during auricular diagnosis are stimulated with alternating current (AC) during the treatment mode. The practitioner presses a button on the auricular probe to turn the stimulation on or off. The probe must be touching the surface of the auricle while it is held in place at a reactive ear point. After the practitioner has detected and stimulated one ear point, he or she then proceeds to the next reactive ear point. The microcurrent levels used for treatment are only 10–80 microamps in strength. The stimulation frequency is usually indicated by rapidly pulsating tones or flickering lights, which are unlike the gradually changing sounds and lights observed during the detection mode.

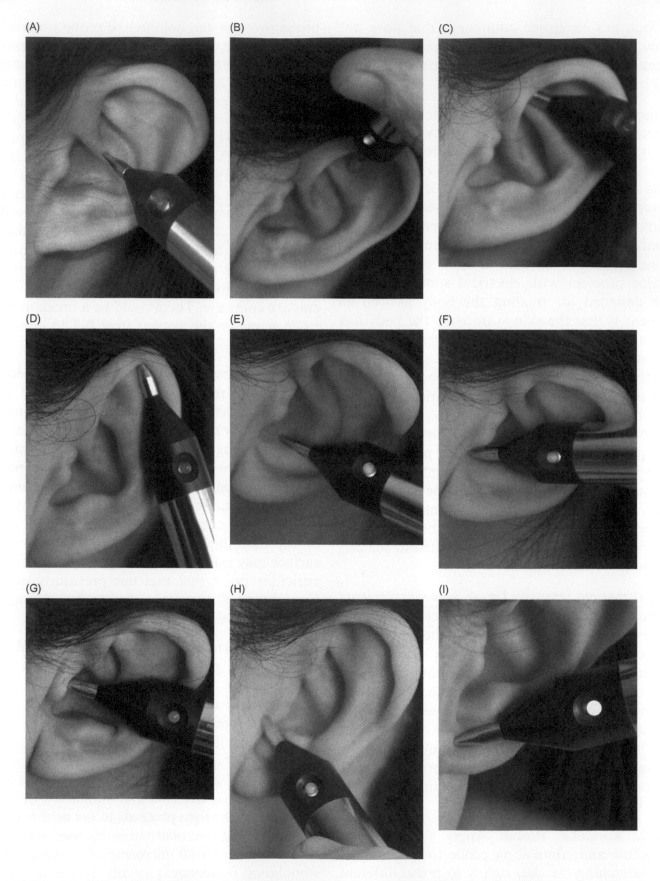

FIGURE 6.8 This series of photographs shows an electrical point finder applied to the auricular master points identified as Point Zero (A), Shen Men (B), Sympathetic point (C), Allergy point (D), Thalamus point (E), Master Endocrine point (F), Master Oscillation point (G), Tranquilizer Point Zero (H), and Master Cerebral point (I).

Determine Stimulation Duration: Treat each ear point for 8–30 seconds, sometimes treating for as long as 2 minutes for chronic conditions or for drug addictions. Longer stimulation is used for chronic ailments of long-standing duration or for very severe symptoms. One tends to treat anatomic points for more than 20 seconds, whereas master points may only require 10 seconds of stimulation. Stimulation of 10 ear points for 20 seconds each would require a treatment duration of less than 10 minutes.

Limit Number of Ear Points: Treat 5–15 points per auricle, using as few ear acupoints as possible. Usually treat the external ear that is ipsilateral to the correspondent body area where there is pathology. Treat the opposite ear as well if there is time to do so.

Bilateral versus Unilateral Stimulation: When finished treating all of the points on the ipsilateral ear, one should usually then stimulate points on the opposite ear because most health problems are bilaterally represented. Even when the problem is localized to one side of the body, it is often useful to treat the master points on both ears.

Assess Perception of Patient: Determination of the ear points that are detected is partially dependent on the degree of tenderness experienced by that particular patient. Ratings of tenderness can be determined by verbal descriptors of pain or patients can be asked to use numbers ranging from 0 to 4, which represent increasing levels of discomfort. Continue to ask patients to monitor their bodily discomfort during stimulation of their ear. If their symptoms start to diminish, or if they notice sensations of warmth in the affected area of the body, the auricular stimulation of an ear point should be maintained. If no symptom changes are noticed within 30 seconds, stimulate another ear point.

Number of Sessions: Two to ten auriculotherapy sessions are usually required to completely relieve a condition, but significant improvement can be noticed within the first two sessions. By monitoring perceived pain level in a body region, and by determining the range of movement of musculoskeletal areas, one can more easily determine the progress of the auriculotherapy treatments. These behavioral assessments should be conducted before and after an auriculotherapy session. For internal organs and neuroendocrine disorders, there is often no specific symptom to notice; thus, one must wait to observe a change in the patient's condition. Even for musculoskeletal problems, there may not be a marked relief of pain until several hours later; thus, the patient should continue to monitor his or her symptoms for 24 hours after a session.

Laser Stimulation: The procedures described for transcutaneous electrical stimulation can also be used for transcutaneous laser stimulation. Both transcutaneous laser stimulation and transcutaneous electrical stimulation are noninvasive procedures, and they seem to yield similar clinical results. However, the U.S. Food and Drug Administration has only recently approved the use of laser stimulation for auriculotherapy in the United States; thus, there are few clinical findings to substantiate the treatment outcome effects following laser stimulation. A principal benefit that has been clinically reported for the use of laser stimulators on the external ear is that the stimulation with lasers is often less uncomfortable for the patient than either needle insertion or transcutaneous electrical stimulation. One would follow the previously presented steps with a laser stimulator just as one would do with an electrical stimulator.

Medical Billing Procedures: To bill for auriculotherapy as TENS, one can assign the CPT Code 64550 for peripheral nerve neurostimulation or the CPT Code 97032 for electrical stimulation with constant practitioner attendance. One could also use the CPT Code 97781 for acupuncture with electrical stimulation for auricular electroacupuncture stimulation.

Stimulation Equipment: Various American, European, and Asian manufacturers produce electronic equipment designed for auricular stimulation, ranging in price from $80 to $8,000 (US). Included in the units available in the United States are the Acuscope, the Stim Flex 400, the Hibiki 7, the Neuroprobe, and the Pointer Plus. Contact information for these manufacturers is found at the back of this book.

Bipolar versus Monopolar Probes: Many of the auricular diagnostic and auriculotherapy treatment probes that are available today use monopolar probes, whereas some use bipolar probes. A monopolar probe places only one electrode stylus against the auricular skin surface, with the reference probe usually held in the patient's hand. A bipolar probe places two electrode probes against the auricular skin surface, with the reference probe held in the patient's hand serving as a neutral region for comparing the electrical findings between the two probes placed against the ear. The bipolar probes placed against the external ear are usually set up in a concentric design, with an inner stylus located within an outer barrel. For detection, the bipolar probe uses differential amplification of the electrical resistance between each auricular probe and the handheld reference probe. For treatment, the bipolar probe limits stimulation to localized regions of the auricle, whereas monopolar probes lead to diffuse activation of broad regions of the external ear. Paul Nogier (1972) noted that bipolar detection of ear reflex ear points not only led to the discovery of low electrical resistance points but also allowed for the identification of high skin resistance ear points. These high resistance points can be as significant in the selection of ear acupoints to be used for successful treatment of a health condition as low electrical resistance points.

6.5 Auricular Medicine and the Nogier Vascular Autonomic Signal

European doctors who monitor N-VAS to determine which ear points to stimulate refer to this clinical procedure as auricular medicine rather than auriculotherapy. The somatotopic cartography of the auricle is verified by a change in radial pulse amplitude following tactile pressure at specific points on the auricle. The N-VAS can also be activated by the positive or negative poles of a magnet. Different sides of a two-prong polarized probe are used to elicit the change in pulse qualities that indicate the reactivity of specific areas of the ear. Needles are then inserted into

the identified ear points, or sometimes they are treated with laser stimulation. Because the focus of this book is the description of auriculotherapy procedures, rather than auricular medicine, further explanation of this technique would require another text.

6.6 Seven Frequency Zones Associated with Auricular Medicine

Dr. Nogier identified seven specific regions of the body that resonated with seven basic frequency zones (Figure 6.9). The specific frequency associated with each body region was determined by holding different colored transparency slides over the auricle and noting whether the different colors could balance disturbances in the N-VAS response. Alternatively, Nogier would stimulate the ear or the body with different frequencies of a flashing white strobe light. The body regions were differentiated with letters "A" through "G." Each letter also indicated certain types of health conditions that were related to the type of tissue of that organ region. The color and number of a Kodak–Wratten filter that relates to each frequency zone of the body is presented in the second and third columns of Table 6.1. Individual colors have different frequencies of oscillating photons of light. The primary frequencies of light are visible in a rainbow or when sunlight shines through a crystal prism. The lowest frequency of red light progresses to the higher frequencies of orange light, yellow light, green light, blue light, and violet-colored light. Nogier determined that the effects of progressively shorter wavelengths of different colored light filters on body tissue could also be found with progressively higher frequencies of flashing light, faster frequencies of electrical pulses, or higher frequencies of laser stimulation.

The electrical frequencies for each zone of the body are presented in the fourth column of Table 6.1, and the exact body resonance rates are presented in the fifth column. Each rate is twice the rate of the frequency below it. The concha and visceral disorders are stimulated at 5 Hz, the

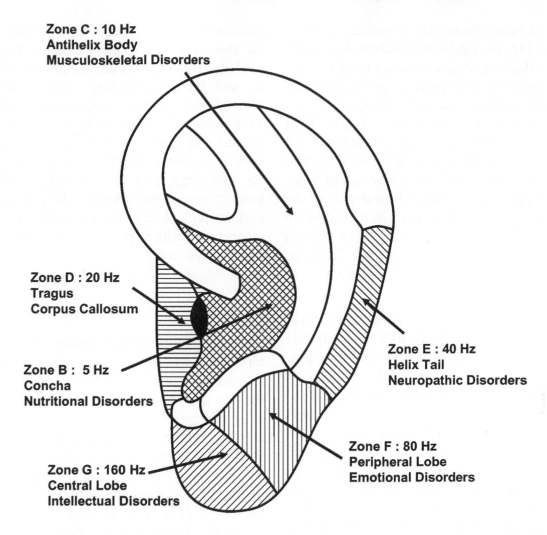

Zone C : 10 Hz
Antihelix Body
Musculoskeletal Disorders

Zone D : 20 Hz
Tragus
Corpus Callosum

Zone B : 5 Hz
Concha
Nutritional Disorders

Zone E : 40 Hz
Helix Tail
Neuropathic Disorders

Zone G : 160 Hz
Central Lobe
Intellectual Disorders

Zone F : 80 Hz
Peripheral Lobe
Emotional Disorders

[**FIGURE 6.9** Seven frequency zones on the auricle are shown for subtragus zone A at 2.5 Hz, concha zone B at 5 Hz, antihelix zone C at 10 Hz, tragus zone D at 20 Hz, helix tail zone E at 40 Hz, peripheral ear lobe zone F at 80 Hz, and central ear lobe zone G at 160 Hz.

TABLE 6.1	Colored Filters, Electrical Frequencies, and Laser Stimulation Frequencies.					
Zone	Color	Wratten Filter	Electrical Frequency (Hz)	Exact Rate (Hz)	Laser Frequency (Hz)	Auricular Areas
A	Orange	#22	2.5	2.28	292	Subtragus
B	Red	#25	5.0	4.56	584	Concha
C	Yellow	#4	10.0	9.12	1,168	Antihelix, Antitragus
D	Orange	#23	20.0	18.25	2,336	Tragus
E	Green	#44	40.0	36.50	4,672	Helix Tail
F	Blue	#98	80.0	73.00	9,334	Peripheral Ear Lobe
G	Purple	#30	160.0	146.00	18,688[a]	Medial Ear Lobe

[a]In clinical practice, the harmonic resonance frequency of 146 Hz is used for laser stimulation because such a rapid frequency rate of 18 kHz tends to overheat the laser equipment.

antihelix and musculoskeletal disorders are stimulated at 10 Hz, on up to the highest frequency of 160 Hz, which is used to correct cerebral and learning disorders. The corresponding frequencies for laser stimulation are presented in the sixth column, with the last column reserved for the areas of auricular anatomy related to each frequency zone. Some practitioners of auricular medicine have suggested that these seven resonant frequencies are related to the energies of the seven primary chakras of Ayurvedic medicine. In some energetic systems, each chakra is associated with the different colors of the rainbow, from red to orange to yellow to green to blue to violet to white light.

Zone A: Cellular Vitality: This zone runs up the midline of the physical body like the acupuncture channels of the conception vessel and governing vessel in Oriental medicine and like the nadi points of Ayurvedic medicine. The auricular area for this 2.5 Hz zone is the subtragus. Zone A affects primitive reticular energy and the primordial forces that affect cellular organization. This frequency often occurs at the site of scars and tissue disturbance and relates to the embryonic organization of cellular tissue. It is used to treat cellular hyperactivity, cellular proliferation, inflammatory processes, neoplastic cancers, tumors, or tissue de-differentiation.

Zone B: Nutritional Metabolism: This zone affects internal organs and 5 Hz is the optimal frequency for stimulating points in this zone, located in the concha of the auricle. Zone B affects vagal nerve projections to visceral organs. The 5 Hz frequency is utilized to treat nutritional disorders, digestive assimilation disorders, tissue malnutrition, neurovegetative dysfunctions, organic allergies, constitutional dysfunctions, and parasympathetic imbalance. When treating endodermal visceral organ points, the 5 Hz frequency moves with the territory related to that phase. Consequently, 5 Hz is used for internal organ tissue whether in the Territory 2 concha in Phase I, in the Territory 3 ear lobe regions in Phase II, or in the Territory 1 antihelix regions in Phase III.

Zone C: Kinetic Movements: This zone affects proprioception, kinetic movements, and the musculoskeletal body. The resonant frequency for this zone is 10 Hz, which is the frequency used to treat auricular points on the antihelix and the surrounding areas of the auricle, such as the scaphoid fossa and triangular fossa. This zone affects myofascial pain, sympathetic nervous system arousal, somatization disorders, cutaneous allergies, motor spasms, muscle pathology, and any disorder aggravated by kinetic movement. When stimulating mesodermal, musculoskeletal points related to the Nogier second and third phases, the 10 Hz frequency rate moves with the territory related to that phase. A rate of 10 Hz is used throughout the Territory II concha in Phase II and throughout the Territory III tragus and ear lobe in Phase III.

Zone D: Global Coordination: This 20 Hz zone represents the corpus callosum and anterior commissure, which coordinates associations between the two sides of the brain. It is represented on the external tragus of the auricle that lies immediately above the subtragal zone A. It corresponds to crossed-laterality dysfunctions—problems of cerebral symmetry versus divergence that lead to lack of coordination between the two sides of the body. This zone D frequency affects asymmetrically bilateral pain problems and strictly midline pain problems. In a right-handed person, the right tragus corresponds to the anterior side of the body conception vessel and the left tragus corresponds to the posterior body governing vessel (Figure 6.10). In each case, the body is represented upside down, with the upper body toward the inferior tragus and the lower body toward the superior tragus. For a left-handed person, who is often an oscillator, the opposite is the case. In a left-hander, the left tragus corresponds to the anterior side of the body and the right tragus corresponds to the posterior side of the body.

Zone E: Neurological Interactions: This zone represents the spinal cord and peripheral nerves, and it corresponds to the helix tail of the auricle. The 40 Hz frequency is used for spinal disorders, skin disorders, dermatitis, skin scars, neuropathies, neuralgias, and herpes zoster.

Zone F: Emotional Reactions: This 80 Hz zone represents the brainstem, thalamus, limbic system, and striatum and is represented on the

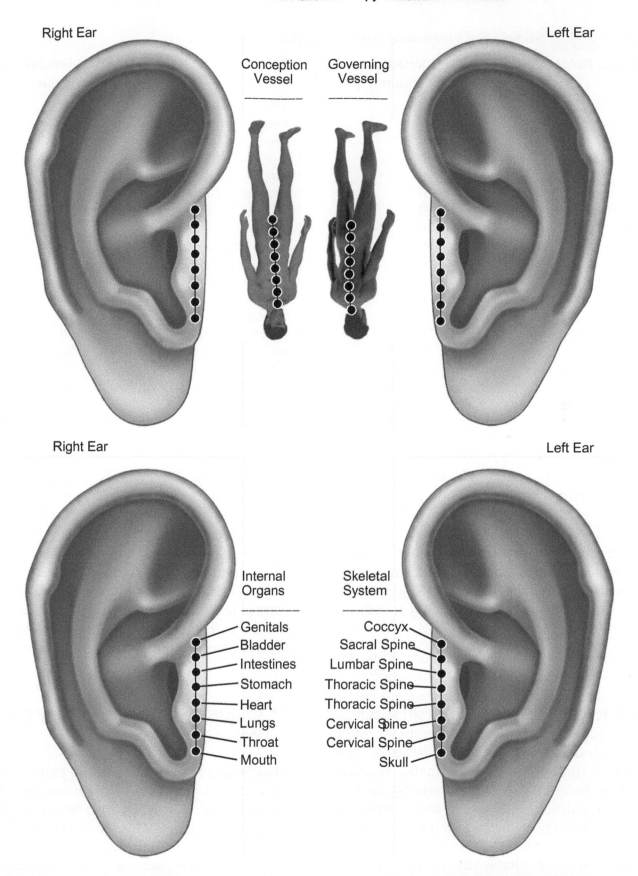

Right Ear

Conception Vessel

Governing Vessel

Left Ear

Right Ear

Left Ear

Internal Organs

Genitals
Bladder
Intestines
Stomach
Heart
Lungs
Throat
Mouth

Skeletal System

Coccyx
Sacral Spine
Lumbar Spine
Thoracic Spine
Thoracic Spine
Cervical Spine
Cervical Spine
Skull

〔FIGURE 6.10 The Conception Vessel meridian is represented on the tragus region of the right ear, whereas the Governing Vessel meridian is represented on the tragus region of the left ear. Somatotopic representation of an inverted body is shown for internal organs on the right tragus, whereas the skull and spinal vertebrae are shown on the tragus of the left ear.

TABLE 6.2 Stimulation Frequencies for Specific Auricular Points.

Auricular Point	Stimulation Frequency (Hz)	Auricular Point	Stimulation Frequency (Hz)
Master Oscillation point	2.5	Gastrointestinal Organs	5
Point Zero	10	Lung and Respiratory Organs	5
Shen Men	10	Abdominal Organs	5
Autonomic Sympathetic point	10	Urogenital Organs	10
Allergy point	10	Heart Muscle Activity	10
Endocrine point	20	Musculoskeletal Spine	10
Tranquilizer point	20	Musculoskeletal Limbs	10
Thalamus point	80	Musculoskeletal Head	10
Master Sensorial point	160	Sensory Organs	10
Master Cerebral point	160	Endocrine Glands	20
Muscle Relaxation point	5	Peripheral Nerves	40
Wind Stream	10	Spinal Cord	40
San Jiao (Triple Warmer)	20	Brainstem	80
Appetite Control point	20	Thalamus and Hypothalamus	80
Vitality point	20	Limbic System and Striatum	80
Anti-Depressant point	80	Corpus Callosum	20
Aggressivity point	80	Cerebral Cortex	160
Psychosomatic point	160		

peripheral lobe of the auricle. It corresponds to problems related to unconscious postures, conditioned reflexes, tics, muscular spasms, stammering, headaches, facial pain, overly sensitive sensations, clinical depression, and emotional disturbances. When treating ectodermal neuroendocrine points related to the Nogier second and third phase, the 80 Hz frequency moves with territory related to that phase.

Zone G: Intellectual Organization: This zone represents psychological functions affected by the frontal cortex that are represented on the medial lobe of the auricle. The 160 Hz stimulation frequency is utilized for pyramidal, motor neuron dysfunctions, memory disorders, intellectual dysfunctions, psychosomatic reactions, obsessive nervousness, chronic worry, malfunctioning conditioned reflexes, and deep-seated psychopathology. When treating ectodermal cerebral cortex points related to the Nogier second and third phase, the 160 Hz frequency moves with territory related to that phase. The placement of colored filters or the selection of electrical or laser stimulation frequencies is based on the type of disorder and the region of the

ear that corresponds to each zone (Table 6.2). The progressive rise in resonance frequencies going from zone A to zone G reflects the increasing evolutionary complexity of organic tissue organization. As one ascends from basic cellular metabolism to visceral organs to musculoskeletal tissue to peripheral nerves to subcortical brain structures to the hierarchal structure of the cerebral cortex, the frequencies that relate to each successive zone become increasingly faster.

6.7 Semipermanent Auricular Pellet Procedures

Ear Acubeads: Small stainless-steel balls or small seeds soaked in an herbal solution can be placed on a specific ear point and then held there by a small adhesive patch (Figure 6.11). Ear acubeads are also called ear seeds, acupoint pellets, ion spheres, semen vaccaria grains, otoacupoint beads, or magrain pellets. The small adhesive strips used to hold the seeds are best handled with forceps or tweezers to place them in difficult to reach areas of the ear (Figure 6.12). In Chinese

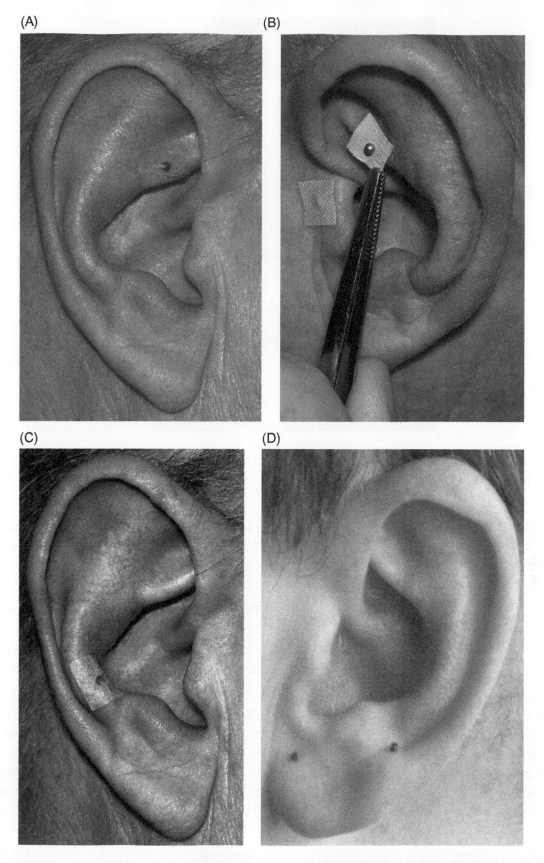

FIGURE 6.11 Different types of ear pellets are shown with Band-Aid tapes that hold the pellets in place. Pellets can include vaccaria seeds taped onto the low back region (A) or the neck region (C) of the auricle. A magnetized gold metal ball is held with forceps before it is applied to the auricle (B). Semipermanent needles can be inserted for prolonged stimulation of points on the ear lobe (D).

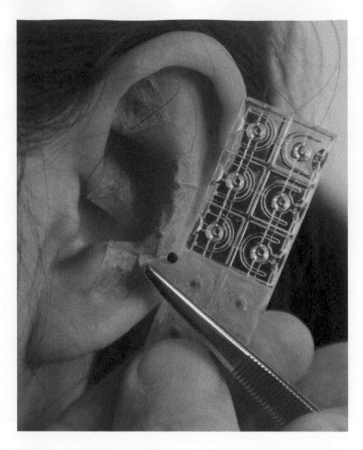

[FIGURE 6.12 This photograph shows several ear seeds that are taped onto the external ear and also shows tweezers removing an individual ear seed from the plastic holder from which it came.

ear acupuncture, the ripe seeds from the vaccaria plant have become a popular replacement for ear needles. The ear seeds are often used as the sole method of auricular stimulation. The seeds can be as effective as needles, are less painful, and have less chance of leading to infections. Even after needle insertion treatments, ear acubeads are left in place at reactive ear points in order to sustain the benefits of auricular acupuncture. They should not be left on the auricle for longer than 1 week. Spontaneous sweating on the ear surface and daily bathing may make it difficult for ear pellets to stay attached. Although patients are often encouraged to periodically press on the acubeads during the week, this added procedure runs the risk of knocking the acubead out of the correct place for optimal treatment effects.

Ear Magnets: These magnets appear similar to the acupoint pellets, but they consist of small magnets held onto the auricular surface with a Band-Aid-like adhesive. Double blind, controlled trials by acupuncturist Lorna Suen in Hong Kong showed that gold acubeads that were magnetized were significantly more effective than nonmagnetized acubeads placed over identical ear points.

Press Needles and Ear Tacks: These are small, semipermanent needles or indwelling, thin tacks that are inserted into the ear to be left in place for several days (Figure 6.13). These types of needles provide stronger stimulation than the ear pellets.

Staple-Puncture: A surgical staple gun is used to apply staple needles into the skin at specific ear points. This procedure has been most commonly used for the treatment of weight loss by a staple inserted into the stomach and esophagus points. However, prominent concerns about potential infections have discouraged the long-term use of staples.

Aquapuncture: Novocain, saline, vitamins, or an herb solution are subcutaneously injected into a specific region of the ear. The subdermal pressure as well as the ingredients of the injected solution provide prolonged stimulation of an ear point.

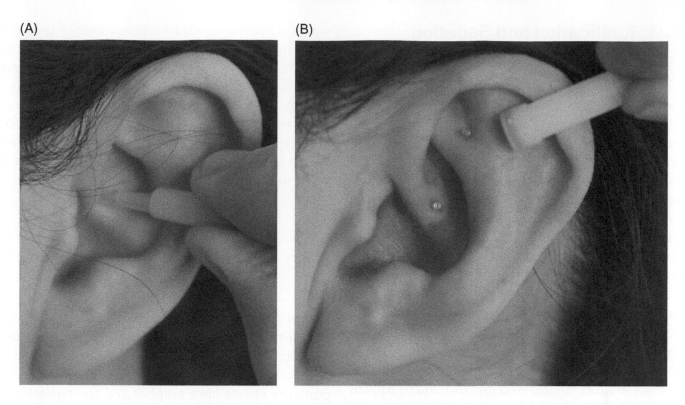

(A)　(B)

[**FIGURE 6.13** This photograph shows an ASP needle being inserted into Point Zero (A) and the magnetic end of the ASP needle held over the Shen Men point (B) to further stimulate that ear point.

6.8 Selection of Auricular Acupoints for Treatment

Correspondent Ear Points: Select ear points according to the corresponding area on the body that exhibits pain or pathology.

Reactive Ear Points: Select ear points that exhibit selective reactivity, as indicated by abnormal color or shape, tenderness, or increased electrodermal response. The repeated refrain is to "let the ear be the final guide."

VAS Diagnosis: Select points that exhibit reactivity based on changes in N-VAS.

TCM Diagnosis: Select ear points according to differentiations of zang–fu syndromes related to Traditional Chinese Medicine (TCM) theory and the flow of qi in acupuncture channels.

Physiological Conditions: Select ear points according to modern physiological understanding of the neurobiological mechanisms underlying a medical disorder.

Reports from Clinical Findings: Select ear points according to their function based on clinical writings and scientific studies.

Symptomatic Observations: Select ear points according to the presenting clinical symptoms, requiring a general medical diagnosis of the patient to differentiate superficial complaints from underlying pathology.

Practitioner's Previous Experiences: Select ear points based on personal clinical experience. Some auricular loci are found to elicit therapeutic effects for a certain disease that seem to have nothing to do with either conventional Western medicine or TCM.

6.9 Tonification and Sedation Procedures in Auricular Acupuncture

Tonification of Master Points: The Chinese refer to tonification as the activation or augmentation of areas with weak energy. Use a brief, 6- to 10-second duration train of electrical pulses for activating weak functions. One often tonifies master points and functional points with this brief stimulation. In auricular acupuncture needling, tonify by inserting gold needles into the ear ipsilateral to the problem, turning the needles in a clockwise rotation. Gold activates the sympathetic nervous system; thus, tonification procedures are utilized to treat parasympathetic disorders, hyporeactions, and energetic vacuums. One tends to treat the dominant side of the body when there is doubt. A pain that is aggravated by rest and requires mobilization to diminish symptoms indicates the need for a gold needle.

Sedation of Overactive Correspondent Points: The Chinese refer to sedation as the dispersion of excessive energy to diminish its overactivity. Use a 12- to 30-second duration train of electrical pulses, negative electrical polarity to diminish overactive organs or excessive reactions due to stress or tension. One should rarely transcutaneously stimulate an ear point for more than 2 minutes. One typically sedates local points representing a specific area of the body by treating them with more prolonged stimulation. In auricular acupuncture, one may sedate by inserting silver needles into the reactive ear point, turning the needle in a counterclockwise rotation. Silver is said to activate the parasympathetic nervous system. Most reactive points on the ear require sedative procedures because they represent muscle tension, sympathetic arousal, stressful reactions, and excessive energy use. For some individuals, one may also need to treat the ear contralateral to the area of the body where there is a problem, the nondominant side. Any patient complaint that is aggravated by movement or exercise will often indicate the need for a silver needle. One can stimulate a point with a strong stimulus over a short period of time or a weak stimulus over a prolonged period of time.

6.10 Relationship of TCM Yin Organs to Ear Acupoints

The principal organs utilized to balance the acupuncture channels in TCM can also be activated by stimulation of the corresponding auricular points. Recent revisions of the Chinese ear acupuncture charts have emphasized the representation of the lung, heart, liver, spleen, and kidney points on the posterior surface of the auricle as well as in the concha of the anterolateral surface. The location of these Yin organs is presented in Figure 6.14.

Lung Ear Point: Affects respiratory disorders, drug detoxification, substance abuse, skin diseases, and problems with hair or nails.

Heart Ear Point: Produces mental calming, relieves nervousness, and improves memory impairment.

Liver Ear Point: Affects blood, muscles, tendons, inflammations, sprains, and eye diseases.

Spleen Ear Point: Affects digestion, reduces muscle tensions, and facilitates physical relaxation.

Kidney Ear Point: Affects urinary disorders, bone fractures, back pain, and hearing disorders.

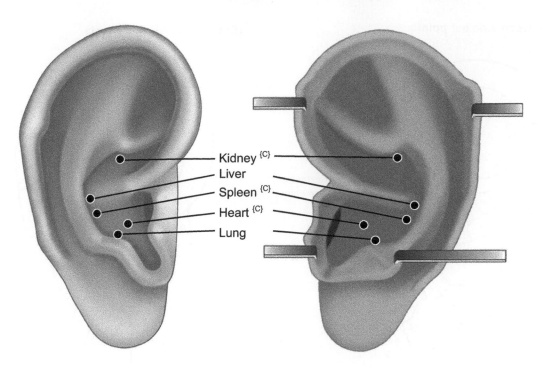

Kidney {C}
Liver
Spleen {C}
Heart {C}
Lung

⟦FIGURE 6.14 The five ear points that represent primary Yin organs on the auricle.

6.11 Geometric Ear Points at 30° Angles

Nogier and his colleagues discovered that after treating correspondent ear points indicated by somatotopic maps, it was also possible to discern a series of reactive auricular points that occurred along an imaginary straight line. These lines were referred to as geometric because they occurred at 30° angles to each other. The practitioner would first configure an imaginary line that extended from point zero to the correspondent point and outward to the peripheral helix that intersected with that line. Stimulation of any reactive ear points along this line was found to augment the treatment effects seen with auriculotherapy. In addition to treating the helix point,

30° angles extending from this helix location were used to create additional imaginary lines that were also stimulated. These configurations are depicted in Figures 6.15 and 6.16. According to Bahr (1977), the application of these 30° angles may account for the Chinese ear acupuncture points used for appendix disorders found in the scaphoid fossa and tonsil points found on the helix. There is also a 30° angle between the Chinese hypertension point in the triangular fossa, a second hypertension point on the tragus, and the European marvelous point, which is also used to treat high blood pressure. The technical complexity of this geometric procedure, however, limits its usefulness to those clinical cases that do not respond to more straightforward applications of auriculotherapy.

(A) **Geometric ear points**

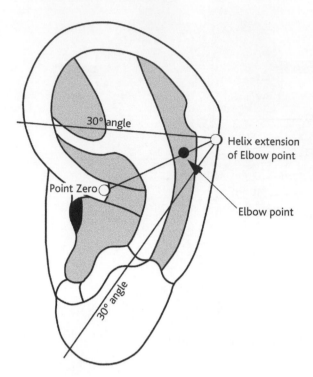

(B) **Chinese helix ear points**

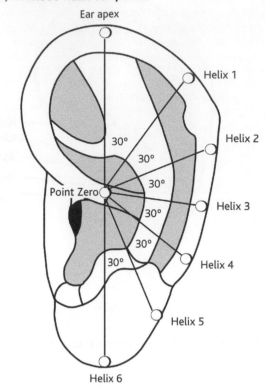

(C) **Chinese Appendix ear points**

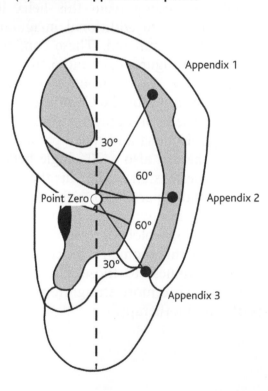

(D) **Chinese Tonsil ear points**

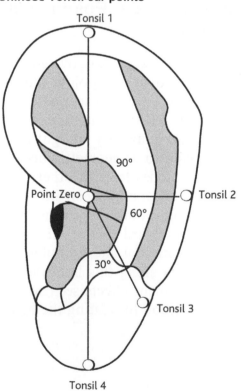

FIGURE 6.15 Geometric ear points can occur at 30° angles from a radial line that extends from Point Zero to the helix (A). Chinese ear acupuncture points are also found at 30° angles located on the helix (B), found in the scaphoid fossa for appendix disorders (C), and found on the helix for tonsillitis disorders (D).

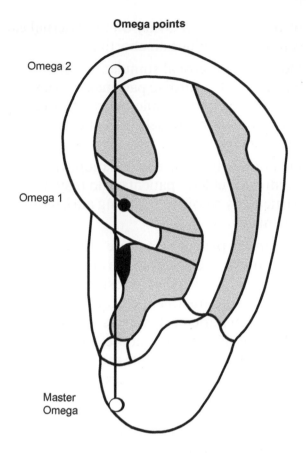

Omega points

Omega 2

Omega 1

Master
Omega

[**FIGURE 6.16** Omega points in European auricular medicine are found along a vertical line that connects Master Omega at the Master Cerebral point on the ear lobe, Omega 1 at the Intestines point in the superior concha, and Omega 2 near the Allergy point on the helix arch.

6.12 Inverse Relationships of the External Ear to the Physical Body

When treating the muscles attached to the spinal vertebrae and the peripheral limbs, it has been found in both auriculotherapy and manipulative therapies that it is possible to treat opposing regions of the musculoskeletal body. By this technique, one can stimulate reactive points on the cervical spine to relieve a condition in the lumbosacral spine or one can treat the foot to affect pain relief in the shoulder. These specific relationships are presented in Table 6.3. For example, one would search for a reactive point on the part of the auricle that represents the sixth cervical vertebrae to affect the fifth lumbar vertebrae, and one would treat the first lumbar vertebrae to affect the third thoracic vertebrae. One could treat the region of the auricle representing the right wrist in order to alleviate a dysfunction in the left ankle or treat the ear point representing the left hip to relieve tension in the right shoulder. The occurrence of these reciprocal relationships may explain the observation of some reactive ear points at auricular areas not related to the correspondent body organ.

TABLE 6.3	Opposing Relationships between Inverse and Contrary Body Regions.		
Upper Spine Region	**Inverse Region of Lower Spine**	**Right Side of Body**	**Contrary Side of Opposing Body**
Cervical Spine 1	Sacral Spine 5	Right hand	Left foot
Cervical Spine 2	Sacral Spine 4	Right wrist	Left ankle
Cervical Spine 3	Sacral Spine 3	Right elbow	Left knee
Cervical Spine 4	Sacral Spine 2	Right shoulder	Left hip
Cervical Spine 5	Sacral Spine 1	Right hip	Left shoulder
Cervical Spine 6	Lumbar Spine 5	Right knee	Left elbow
Cervical Spine 7	Lumbar Spine 4	Right ankle	Left wrist
Thoracic Spine 1	Lumbar Spine 3	Right foot	Left hand
Thoracic Spine 2	Lumbar Spine 2		
Thoracic Spine 3	Lumbar Spine 1		
Thoracic Spine 4	Thoracic Spine 12		
Thoracic Spine 5	Thoracic Spine 11		
Thoracic Spine 6	Thoracic Spine 10		
Thoracic Spine 7	Thoracic Spine 9		
Thoracic Spine 8	Thoracic Spine 8		

6.13 Precautions Associated with Auriculotherapy

- The most common adverse side effect from auriculotherapy is that the ear may become red and tender to touch after the treatment. Inform the patient that this redness and tenderness are only temporary.

- Although it is very uncommon for patients to report adverse reactions to the auriculotherapy treatment, this is a possibility. In this case, the practitioner should closely monitor the patient for several days after the treatment.

- Administer antibiotics to patients if the ear becomes infected. Any bleeding after the insertion of an acupuncture needle into the ear is usually very brief and rarely leads to an infection. However, staple-puncture techniques, in which a surgical staple tack is left in place for several days, can possibly lead to infection.

- Some patients may become sleepy or dizzy after a treatment and they may need to lie down for a while. This sedation effect has been attributable to the release of endorphins and is considered more beneficial than unwanted.

- Allow nervous, anxious, weak, or hypertensive patients some time for a rest after the treatment. It is helpful to offer patients warm tea while they recover.

- Avoid treating patients when they are excessively weak, anemic, tired, fasting, hypoglycemic, or have just eaten a heavy meal. The treatment will not be as effective.

- Do not treat any pain needed to diagnose an underlying problem until that underlying condition has been fully evaluated.

- Do not relieve any pain needed by patients to limit them from engaging in inappropriate physical activity that could aggravate their condition.

- Be cautious when treating pregnant women. This precaution is mostly required for malpractice reasons, rather than any known clinical evidence regarding possible harmful effects of auriculotherapy on a fetus or pregnant woman. Nonetheless, Chinese studies have suggested that strong stimulation of the Uterus and Ovary on the external ear can possibly induce an abortion.

- Do not use electrical stimulation on patients with a cardiac pacemaker, even though the electrical microcurrents used in auriculotherapy are delivered at extremely small intensity levels.

- Do not use aggressive stimulation with children or elderly patients who may be particularly sensitive to strong auriculotherapy treatments.

- Inform the patient to not use alcohol or recreational drugs before the auriculotherapy treatment because these substances may interfere with treatment efficacy. At the same time, when auriculotherapy is used for the treatment of substance abuse, auriculotherapy can be effective even while the patient is still using recreational substances.

6.14 Hindrances to Treatment Success

If a patient's disorder persists after auriculotherapy treatment of the correspondent ear points, there may be a therapeutic blockage due to a toxic scar or dental focus. The practitioner should inquire of the patient's medical history and previous accidents or surgeries. Sometimes a hindrance to treatment is due to an allergy, which is an excess of energy. Other times, there is an obstacle to the transmission of the cellular information because of a region of energy deficiency. The loss of energy may be attributable to the aftereffects of an accident or surgery that caused a toxic scar and a short-circuit in the energy of that person. A different type of toxic scar is a dental focus related to continued inflammation from a prior dental procedure. Silver amalgam in tooth fillings or chronic infection of the gingiva can also produce a dental focus.

Allow that some medical problems presented by a patient cannot be effectively treated by auriculotherapy because they are due to either (1) a structural imbalance that needs to be corrected by some physical therapy procedure or (2) psychological dysfunctions that need to be addressed by some type of psychotherapeutic intervention. Dr. Nogier often combined auriculotherapy with osteopathic manipulations in order to provide structural integration to the neuromuscular changes that could be achieved with auriculotherapy. When the obstacle is due to an unresolved emotional state, stimulation of Point Zero can bring balance to the psychosomatic resistance.

Although psychosomatic disorders are often dismissed by physicians and patients alike, there is ample evidence that psychological factors have a profound impact on many physical conditions. Until emotional issues related to anxiety, depression, loneliness, resentment, and shame are satisfactorily resolved, a patient's unconscious motivations may defeat the most skillful of clinicians. Even when patients strongly vocalize that they want to be relieved of their physical suffering, those same individuals are not consciously aware of their own thoughts, attitudes, and behaviors that have the opposite effect. Gentle but firm confrontation regarding the possibility that such psychological barriers exist is often necessary before proceeding further with any medical treatment. Many practitioners are not comfortable addressing such issues with resistant patients, but such confrontations are often very necessary for the eventual improvement of a person's health problems.

6.15 Clinical Pearls for Auriculotherapy Treatments

- Treat as few ear points as possible.
- Only treat ear points that are tender to palpation or are electrically conductive.
- Treat a maximum of three problems at a time, treating the primary problem first.
- Treat ipsilateral ear reflex points for unilateral problems, and treat both ears for bilateral conditions. If the patient exhibits a laterality or oscillation disorder, the Master Oscillation point should be treated first, and then correspondent points on both auricles should be stimulated.

- Treat the front of the external ear for relieving the sensations of pain, and then treat the back of the ear for relieving muscle spasms that produce muscle tension and limit range of motion.
- Hold the external ear taught with one hand while using the other hand to hold a detecting probe to the ear or a treatment probe or acupuncture needle.
- After treating the anatomic points that correspond to the area of the bodily symptom, treat the master points. Lastly, treat supportive functional points.
- The most commonly used master points are Point Zero, Shen Men, Autonomic Sympathetic point, Thalamus point, Endocrine point, and Master Cerebral point.
- Anatomic points that are often used to alleviate other disorders include ear points for the Occiput, the Chinese Kidney, the Heart, the Lung, the Liver, and the Stomach.
- The most commonly used Chinese functional points are Muscle Relaxation point, Appetite Control point, Brain (Central Rim), Windstream (Lesser Occipital Nerve), and San Jiao (Triple Warmer).
- The most frequently utilized European functional points are Antidepressant point, Anti-Aggressivity point, Vitality point, and Psychosomatic point.
- Treat Nogier Phase II and Phase III points if successful results are not obtained with Phase I points or with Chinese ear points. Phase II points are indicated for chronic deficient conditions, whereas Phase III ear points are indicated for chronic excess conditions.
- Evaluate the patient for the presence of physical hindrances or psychological obstacles that could interfere with the treatment. One might also notice if treating reactive points on the ear related to geometric, inverse, or contrary relationships improves the clinical effectiveness of the auriculotherapy treatment.
- Auriculotherapy works very well with other treatment modalities. It is quite common to combine ear acupuncture and body acupuncture in the same treatment session.

- Chinese herbs, moxibustion, homeopathic substances, and acupressure massage can be effectively integrated with auriculotherapy as well as body acupuncture.

- Postural adjustments with osteopathic or chiropractic manipulations serve to facilitate the reduction of muscle spasms attained with auricular stimulation.

- Biofeedback, hypnosis, meditation, and yoga all serve to augment the general relaxation effect seen with auriculotherapy.

- Patients with psychosomatic disturbances would probably benefit from psychotherapeutic interventions if they could accept the perspective that unconscious, emotional conflicts could be a contributing factor to their physical health problem.

- Any procedure used as standard medical practice for the condition being treated can be further enhanced by the use of auriculotherapy.

■ KEY TERMS FOR CHAPTER 6

Alternating Current (AC): The bidirectional flow of electrical charge from one polarity to a different polarity, going back and forth, repeatedly changing its direction or strength, usually at a certain frequency or range of frequencies. In North America, the frequency of alternation of the direction of flow used by power stations is 60 Hz, or 60 cycles per second, whereas in other areas of the world it is 50 Hz. The standard amplitude of 60 Hz current is usually 120 volts, whereas the amplitude of 50 Hz current is usually 220 volts. The microcurrent levels used in auriculotherapy are typically less than 100 microamps.

Auricular Acupressure: Application of pressure from one's fingers or a metal stylus onto reflex points on the external ear.

Auricular Electroacupuncture (AES): Electrical stimulation through pairs of acupuncture needles inserted into the skin surface of the external ear.

Auricular Medicine: Utilization of the Nogier vascular autonomic signal (N-VAS) to determine the most reactive ear points to be used for auricular acupuncture stimulation.

Bilateral Versus Unilateral Stimulation: Stimulation of ear acupoints on one side of the body (unilateral) versus stimulation of ear acupoints on both sides of the body (bilateral).

Bipolar Versus Unipolar Probes: Metal probes for the stimulation of ear acupoints that include one probe on the auricular surface and one probe in the hand (unipolar probes) versus two probes on the auricular surface and one probe in the hand (bipolar probes).

Detection Mode: Diagnosis of reactive ear points is achieved with low intensities of direct current.

Direct Current (DC): The unidirectional flow of electrical charge from one pole of an electrical source to a different location, in only one direction. Because there is no alternating flow of current, there is no frequency for DC current, but there are different amplitudes of current intensity.

Ear Acubeads: Small stainless-steel balls or small seeds soaked in an herbal solution can be placed on a specific ear point and held there by an adhesive Band-Aid.

Ear Acupuncture Needling: The insertion of acupuncture needles into the skin surface of the external ear.

Ear Magnets: These acupoint pellets consist of small magnets held onto the auricular surface with a Band-Aid-like adhesive.

Ear Pellets: Small stainless-steel balls or small seeds soaked in an herbal solution can be placed on a specific ear point and held there by an adhesive Band-Aid.

Frequency Zones: Seven different regions of the external ear have been associated with the following specific stimulation frequencies: 2.5, 5, 10, 20, 40, 80, and 160 Hz.

Geometric Ear Points: Determination of a series of reactive auricular points that are found along straight lines which typically occur at 30° angles to each other.

Laser Stimulation: The application of coherent laser light for noninvasive stimulation of auricular acupoints.

Press Needles: These are small, semipermanent needles or indwelling, thin tacks that are inserted into the ear to be left in place for several days.

Sedation: The Chinese principle of the dispersion of excessive energy to diminish overactivity at an acupuncture point.

Staple Puncture: A surgical staple gun is used to apply staple needles into the skin at specific ear points.

Stimulation Duration: The length of time that electrical stimulation is applied to an ear point.

Stimulation Equipment: Electronic equipment specifically designed for auricular stimulation.

Stimulation Frequency: Frequency rate of electrical or laser stimulation that is measured in cycles per second or Hertz (Hz).

Stimulation Intensity: The amplitude of electrical stimulation pulses measured in microamps.

Stimulation Mode: Reactive ear points discovered during auricular diagnosis are treated with microcurrent levels of AC.

Threshold Level: A level of current intensity that is set to establish an optimal level of detecting current to compare the electrical reactivity of one ear acupoint to another.

Tonification: The Chinese principle of augmentation of acupoints with weak energy.

Transcutaneous Auricular Stimulation (TAS): Electrical stimulation through metal probes applied to the surface of the skin over the external ear, with no penetration of the skin by acupuncture needles.

■ CHAPTER 6 REVIEW QUESTIONS

1. Compared to acupuncture needles inserted into body acupuncture points, the insertion of needles into ear acupoints typically involves needles that are_____.
   a. several inches long and wide in diameter
   b. less than 1 inch long and narrow in diameter
   c. enclosed by guide tubes that surround the needle
   d. require a different type of metal

2. The order of placement of needles into the external ear usually requires that needles be inserted into the anterior auricular surface_____.
   a. after electrical stimulation through those needles
   b. before electrical detection of those ear points
   c. after insertion of needles onto the posterior auricle
   d. before insertion of needles onto the posterior auricle

3. Auricular electroacupuncture requires that electrode leads from an electrical stimulation device be_____.
   a. attached to two different needles inserted into the auricle
   b. connected to one ear acupoint and one body acupoint
   c. activated by unilateral current
   d. activated by bilateral current

4. The current intensity level used for auricular electrical stimulation should be optimally set at_____.
   a. the highest levels possible
   b. the lowest levels possible
   c. higher levels than are used for body acupuncture stimulation
   d. the highest levels that accommodate patient tolerance

5. The electrical stimulation frequency that has been shown to be optimal for the activation of ear acupoints related to musculoskeletal movement disorders is_____.

   a. 5 Hz
   b. 10 Hz
   c. 20 Hz
   d. 100 Hz

6. The type of electrical current that is more likely to be used for auriculotherapy treatment rather than auricular diagnosis is_____.

   a. direct current
   b. continuous current
   c. disrupted current
   d. alternating current

7. Bilateral auricular stimulation refers to the activation of ear acupoints_____.

   a. on the right side of the head
   b. on the left side of the head
   c. on the same side of the head
   d. on both sides of the head

8. Transcutaneous auricular stimulation refers to the stimulation of ear acupoints by electrodes_____.

   a. attached to needles inserted into the auricle
   b. applied to the skin surface on the auricle
   c. connected to small pellets on the ear
   d. activated by laser light

9. According to TCM theory, the ear point that is most appropriate for the treatment of substance abuse is the _____.

   a. Kidney point
   b. Liver point
   c. Lung point
   d. Stomach point

10. The most frequent caution that would lead to limitations in the application of auricular electrical stimulation is the presence of_____ in the patient.

   a. pregnancy
   b. cancer
   c. a coronary disorder
   d. a respiratory disorder

Answers

1 = b; 2 = c; 3 = a; 4 = d; 5 = b; 6 = d; 7 = d; 8 = b; 9 = c; 10 = a

Somatotopic Representations on the External Ear

[7.0 | Somatotopic Representations on the External Ear

CHAPTER 7 LEARNING OBJECTIVES

1. To identify the location and function of Master points on the auricle.

2. To identify the location and function of Musculoskeletal points on the auricle.

3. To identify the location and function of Internal Organ points on the auricle.

4. To identify the location and function of Neuroendocrine points on the auricle.

5. To identify the location and function of Functional points on the auricle.

6. To identify the differences in location for Nogier Phase I, Phase II, and Phase III acupoints on the auricle.

More than 25 books specifically devoted to auricular acupuncture have been consulted to determine the anatomical location and somatotopic function of specific regions of the ear. The first English language texts of the Chinese system of ear acupuncture included the works of Helena Huang (1974), Nahemkis and Smith (1975), and Mario Wexu (1975). Textbooks describing the Chinese ear acupuncture maps have been written in several other European languages, including Dutch (Van Gelder, 1985), French (Grobglas and Levy, 1986), German (König and Wancura, 1993), and Italian (Romoli, 2009). More recent textbooks that have focused on Chinese approaches to auricular diagnosis and ear acupuncture treatment were written by Li-Chun Huang (1996), an international expert on auricular acupuncture who served as Director of the Auricular Acupuncture Department at the Beijing University of Chinese Medicine before coming to the United States.

The European perspective of the somatotopic representations upon the external ear was initiated by the pioneering work of Paul Nogier. Originally published in French in the 1950s, Nogier's discoveries were subsequently published in English, including the *Treatise of*

Auriculotherapy in 1972, *From Auriculotherapy to Auriculomedicine* in 1983, *Points Réflexes Auriculaires* in 1987, and *Compléments des Points Réflexes Auriculaires* in 1989. Subsequent books that have further described the European approach to auriculotherapy include works by Bahr (1977), Bourdiol (1982), Kropej (1984), Strittmatter (1998, 2001), and Rubach (2001).

A synthesis of information from all of these texts was used to determine the location and function of the auricular points that are described in the present text. Although the variations in locations delineated in the Chinese and the European auricular maps are often perceived as confusing to beginning students, there is actually more congruence than disparity between the two auriculotherapy systems. When there are distinct differences between the two auricular systems, the acupoints associated with a specific body organ are usually located nearby, on an adjacent region of the external ear. For instance, whereas the Hip, Knee, and Foot are found on the antihelix superior crus in the Chinese ear charts, the somatotopic representations of these same lower extremity limbs are found in the nearby triangular fossa in the European cartography. The Chinese ear charts show that the Kidney organ is represented in the superior concha of the external ear, whereas the European texts depict the Kidney on the undersurface of the internal helix that lies beneath the helix root, near the superior concha.

After conducting auricular diagnosis on hundreds of patients for more than 35 years, it has become my clinical perspective that both auricular systems are accurate. For some patients, the reactive ear points conform to the localization presented by the Chinese ear charts, whereas for other clients, the most conductive and tender ear points better fit the European auricular charts. I tend to prefer the European ear charts for the treatment of musculoskeletal pain and neurological disorders, whereas the Chinese ear charts seem to more accurately represent the location of internal, visceral organs. Oriental medicine is principally focused on the constitutional factors associated with the internal organs for which each meridian channel is named, whereas

European practitioners of auriculotherapy tend to place greater emphasis on the neurophysiological control of the musculoskeletal system and the nervous system. The Nogier system of three different phases related to three different territories on the auricle may at first seem overly complex and confusing, but the clinical applicability of these phases becomes easier with continued practice. Understanding all these systems provides the most optimal background for successful clinical application of auriculotherapy.

The number for an auricular point in this text is designated by a decimal and the letter ".c" when it is an ear acupoint in the Chinese system of auriculotherapy, whereas it is designated by ".e" when it is an ear acupoint in the European system of auriculotherapy. The corresponding name for that auricular point is followed by the superscript letter "[C]" or the letter "[E]" and is surrounded by the grammatical signs "{ }."

{C} = Auricular acupuncture point in Chinese system

{E} = Auricular acupuncture point in European system

When referring to an auricular acupuncture point, the name of an organ is capitalized, whereas when referring to the actual organ in the physical body, the name is left lowercase. Different anatomical regions of the external ear, such as antihelix tail and inferior concha, are left lowercase. The following sentence illustrates this format.

The Elbow point in the scaphoid fossa represents both the muscles and the tendons that connect to the elbow joint, representing forearm problems due to muscle spasms or to tendonitis.

Each auricular point presented in this text is thus identified with a number, with that point's principal name, with alternative names for that point, and with the auricular zone (AZ) where it is found. If auricular zone locations are shown with a "/" symbol, the ear point occurs at the junction of two adjacent zones.

The location of each ear point is also described with regard to a specific region of auricular anatomy and the nearest auricular landmark (LM). The physiological function of the correspondent organ and the health disorders affected by a particular ear point are presented after the identification of the location of that ear point.

It should be continually kept in mind that the name of an ear acupoint after a region of the body or some internal organ does not represent that anatomical structure when it is functioning appropriately. Rather, an ear acupoint only appears when there is some pathology or dysfunction in the correspondent organ.

7.1 Master Points on the External Ear

The master points are so identified because they are typically active in most patients and they are useful for the treatment of a variety of health disorders. The practitioner should first stimulate the appropriate anatomic point that corresponds to the location of pathology or dysfunction, and then the clinician should stimulate the master points that are specifically indicated for that medical condition. These master points are also called "Tune-Up" points.

No.	Auricular Microsystem Point *(Alternative Name)*	[Auricular Zone]

0.0   Point Zero *(Ear Center, Point of Support, Solar Plexus, Navel)*   [HX 1/CR 1]

Location: Found in a notch on the helix root at LM_0, where the vertically ascending helix root rises from the more horizontal concha ridge.

Function: This master point is the geometrical and physiological center of the whole auricle. It brings the whole body toward homeostasis, producing a balance of energy, a balance of hormones, and a balance of brain activity. It supports the actions of other auricular points and returns the body to the idealized state that was originally present in the womb.

On the auricular somatotopic map, Point Zero is located where the umbilical cord would rise from the abdomen of the inverted fetus pattern found on the ear. It has consequently been utilized to treat disorders related to birth trauma and diseases affecting newborn infants. As the Solar Plexus point, Point Zero serves as the "autonomic brain" that controls visceral organs through the activity of peripheral nerve ganglia. Point Zero is frequently combined with the Shen Men point for treatment of most health disorders.

1.0   Shen Men *(Spirit Gate, Divine Gate)*   [TF 2]

Location: Found superior and central to the tip of the triangular fossa, between the junction of the superior crus and the inferior crus of the antihelix. It is located slightly inward and slightly upward from the tip of the triangular fossa.

Function: The purpose of Shen Men is to tranquilize the mind and to facilitate a state of harmony, serenity, and a deeper connection to one's essential spirit. This master point alleviates stress, pain, tension, anxiety, depression, insomnia, restlessness, and excessive sensitivity. The Chinese also believe that Shen Men affects excitation and inhibition of the cerebral cortex, which is similar in function to Nogier's Phase II Thalamus point that is found in this same area of the ear.

Shen Men is utilized in almost all treatment plans, including auricular acupuncture analgesia for surgery. It was one of the first points emphasized for the application of ear acupuncture for the detoxification from addictive drugs and for the treatment of alcoholism and substance abuse. It is also used to reduce coughs, fever, inflammatory diseases, epilepsy, and high blood pressure. When it is difficult to find electrically active ear points, stimulation of either Shen Men or Point Zero heightens the reactivity of other auricular points, thus making them easier to detect.

No.   Auricular Microsystem Point *(Alternative Name)*   [Auricular Zone]

2.0   Sympathetic Autonomic Point   [IH 4/AH 7]

Location: Found at LM_19, the junction of the internal helix and the adjacent section of the inferior crus of the antihelix. The Sympathetic point is covered by the brim of the helix root above it, thus making it difficult to view directly from the external surface of the ear. The tip of an ear pointer probe should be directed along a horizontal plane parallel to the inferior crus below, aimed toward the medial side of the ear next to the head.

Function: This master point balances the complementary divisions of the autonomic nervous system, reducing excess excitement of sympathetic nervous system overactivation and facilitating the calming effects of parasympathetic sedation. The Sympathetic point is the primary ear point for diagnosing visceral pain and for enhancing general sedation. It improves blood circulation by facilitating vasodilatation, thus improving either hypertension or hypotension. This point is reactive when someone suffers from an irregular heart rate, rapid heartbeats, angina pain, Raynaud's disease, visceral pain from dysfunctional internal organs, spasms in smooth visceral muscles, or neurovegetative disequilibrium. It is used for the treatment of kidney stones, gallstones, asthma, gastric ulcers, abdominal distension, and other dysfunctions of the autonomic nervous system.

3.c   Allergy Point 1 *(Apex of Auricle, Ear Apex)*   [HX 7/HX 8]

Location: Found on the external side of the ear apex, at LM_2.

Function: An anti-pyretic point to reduce general inflammation reactions related to allergies, rheumatoid arthritis, and asthmatic breathing difficulties. It alleviates fever, heat, swelling, blood pressure, inflammation, delirium, and pathogenic wind. This point has analgesic, anti-pyretic, and anti-inflammatory properties. The apex of the ear is often used for bloodletting by the prick of a needle at the very top of the ear to balance excess qi. It is used for the elimination of toxic substances and the excretion of metabolic wastes, and it can be used for anaphylactic shock.

3.e   Allergy Point 2   [IH 7/IH 8]

Location: Found on the internal side of the ear apex, below LM_2.

4.0   Thalamus Point *(Subcortex)*   [CW 2/IC 4]

Location: Found at the base of the concha wall on the vertical section which lies behind the antitragus. One follows a vertical ridge on the concha wall that descends from the apex of the antitragus at LM_13 down to the concha floor at LM_21.

For Paul Nogier, the whole concha wall behind the antitragus represents the many different nuclei of the thalamus of the brain. The ear point immediately located at LM_21 is referred to in French as the Point du Thalamus, the primary thalamus point that regulates sensory information going to the cerebral cortex, regulates general arousal activated by the reticular formation, and is the highest neurological level of the gate control system for pain.

In the Nogier phase system, the Phase I Thalamus is found on the front surface of the antitragus, the Phase II Thalamus is located in the triangular fossa region near the Shen Men point, and the Phase III Thalamus is located behind the antitragus, where Nogier's Point du Thalamus was previously identified at LM_21.

Function: This master point represents the whole diencephalon of the brain, including the thalamus and the hypothalamus. It affects the relay of sensory information to the cerebral cortex and modulates hypothalamic regulation of autonomic nerves and endocrine glands. The Thalamus is like a preamplifier for signals sent to the cerebral cortex, organizing the neural message and eliminating meaningless background noise. The Thalamus balances overexcitation of cortical neurons by the inhibition of those cortical neurons.

The Thalamus is the highest level of the supraspinal gate control system. It is used for alleviating most pain disorders, both acute and chronic. It is used in the treatment of neurasthenia, anxiety, depression, schizophrenia, overexcitement, sweating, swelling, shock, hypertension, coronary disorders, cardiac arrhythmias, Raynaud's disease, gastritis, nausea, vomiting, diarrhea, constipation, liver disorders, and gall bladder dysfunctions.

No.   Auricular Microsystem Point *(Alternative Name)*   [Auricular Zone]

5.0   Master Endocrine Point *(Internal Secretion, Pituitary Gland)*   [IT 2]

Location: Found on the wall of the intertragic notch, between LM_9 and LM_22.

Function: This master point brings Endocrine hormones to their appropriate homeostatic balance, either raising or lowering glandular secretions. The pituitary gland receives neurophysiological messages from the brain above it and then releases tropic hormones that affect specific endocrine glands in the body. The pituitary is the master gland controlling all other endocrine glands. It improves many of the symptoms associated with hyperthyroidism, hypothyroidism, diabetes mellitus, irregular menstruation, sexual dysfunction, hypersensitivity, rheumatism, and urogenital disorders. It also has anti-allergic, anti-rheumatic, and anti-inflammatory effects. In TCM theory, the Endocrine point reduces dampness and relieves swelling and edema.

6.e   Master Oscillation Point *(Laterality Point)*   [ST 3]

Location: Found on the underside of the subtragus, underneath the inferior tragus protrusion at LM_10.

Function: This master point balances laterality disorders related to dysfunctional interactions between the left and the right cerebral hemispheres. It anatomically represents the corpus callosum and the anterior commissure which joins the two sides of the brain. This point is often active in individuals who are left-handed or mixed dominant in handedness.

Whereas 80% of individuals show ipsilateral representation of body organs, 20% of patients exhibit contralateral representation of body organs. These latter individuals are viewed as "oscillators" in the European school of auriculotherapy. This same dysfunction is labeled "switched" in some chiropractic schools. Stimulation of this auricular point in oscillators is often necessary before any other treatment can be effective.

7.0   Tranquilizer Point *(Valium Analogue Point, Hypertensive Point)*   [TG 2]

Location: Found on the inferior tragus as it joins the face, this ear point lies halfway between LM_9 at the intertragic notch and LM_10 on the lower protrusion of the tragus, occurring on the stiff ridge of the cartilage rather than the soft tissue of the adjacent jaw.

Function: This master point produces a general sedation effect, facilitates overall relaxation, relieves generalized anxiety, reduces high blood pressure, and calms the effects of chronic stress.

8.0   Master Sensorial Point *(Eye Point)*   [LO 4]

Location: Found in the middle of the ear lobe, vertically inferior to LM_13 at the antitragus peak and vertically superior to LM_7 at the bottom of the ear lobe.

Function: This master point modulates the perception of sensory signals sent to the cerebral cortex, including tactile sensations in the parietal lobe, auditory sensations in the temporal lobe, and visual sensations in the occipital lobe. It is used to reduce any unpleasant or excessive sensation, such as tactile paresthesia, ringing in the ears, or blurred vision. It can also alleviate irritability due to strange smells, intense sounds, or extreme sensitivity to touch. This ear point is often reactive when a chronic pain problem is experienced more as a sensory phenomenon than a psychological phenomenon.

9.0   Master Cerebral Point *(Master Omega, Nervousness, Worry Point)*   [LO 1]

Location: Found where the medial ear lobe meets the face. It lies vertically inferior to the intertragic notch, below LM_9 and above LM_8, where the ear lobe attaches to the jaw.

Function: This master point represents the prefrontal lobe of the brain, the part of the cerebral cortex that perceives higher order thinking and initiates conscious action. The prefrontal lobe is often referred to as the "executive brain" because it is essential for making voluntary decisions that a person chooses to engage in specific actions. Stimulation of this auricular point tends to diminish nervousness, anxiety, fear, worry, dream-disturbed sleep, poor memory, obsessive–compulsive disorders, and psychosomatic disorders. This master point is often reactive when negative, self-critical, pessimistic thinking accompanies chronic pain problems.

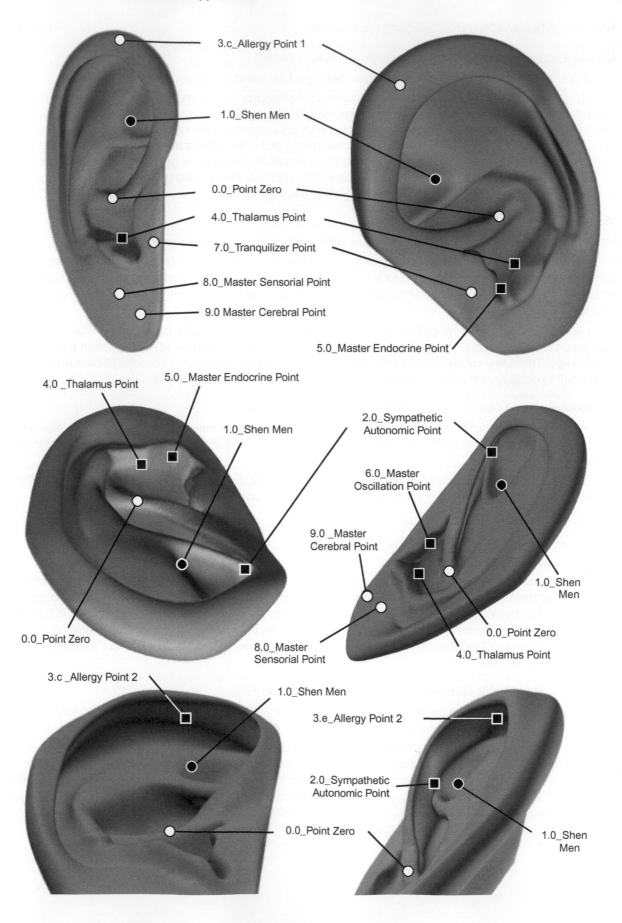

FIGURE 7.1 Master points found on a 3-D image of the external ear.

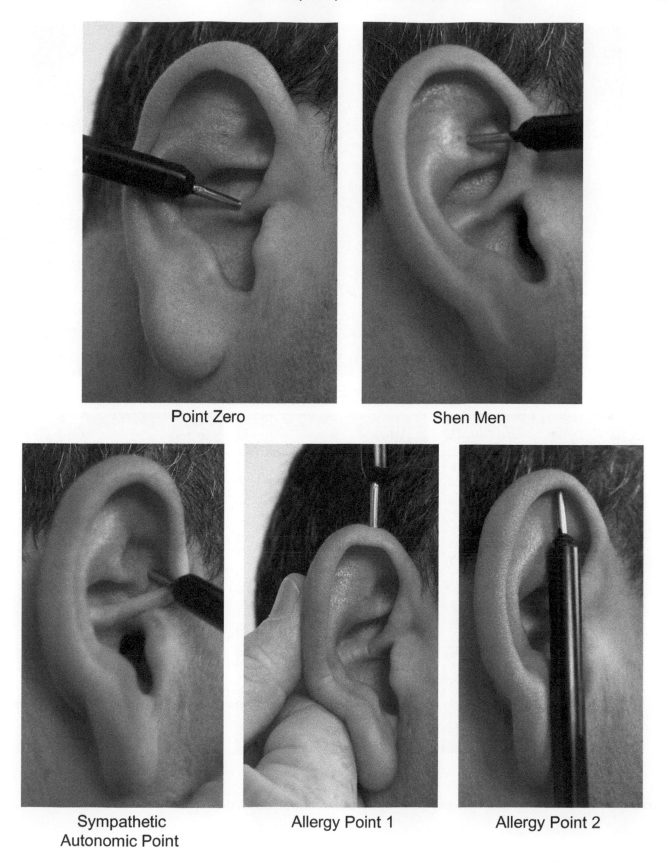

Point Zero

Shen Men

Sympathetic
Autonomic Point

Allergy Point 1

Allergy Point 2

FIGURE 7.2 Photographs of detecting probes placed at master points on the auricle.

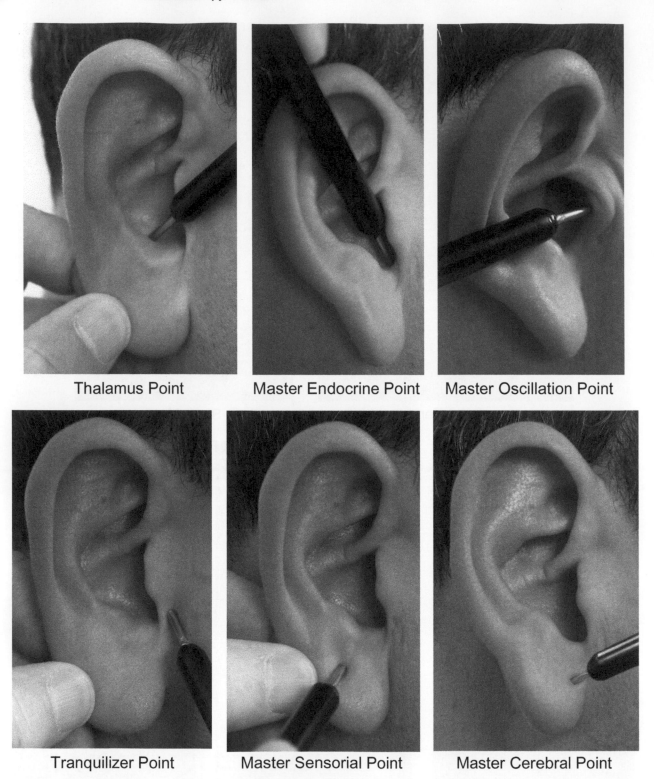

Thalamus Point   Master Endocrine Point   Master Oscillation Point

Tranquilizer Point   Master Sensorial Point   Master Cerebral Point

FIGURE 7.3 Photographs of detecting probes placed at master points on the auricle.

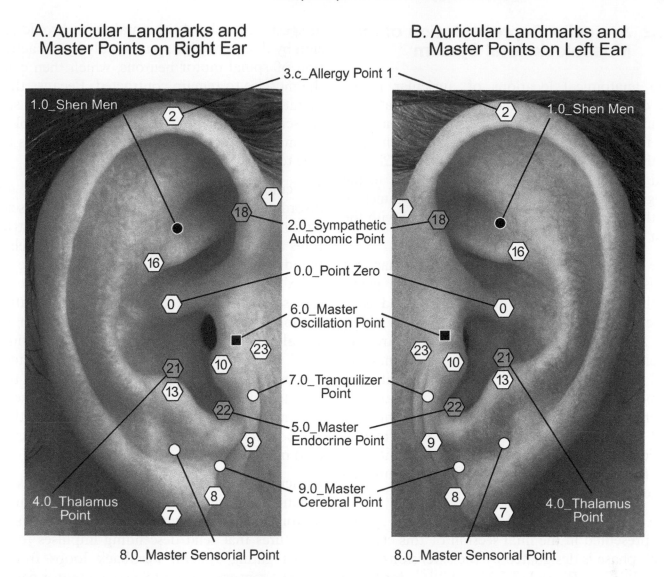

A. Auricular Landmarks and
Master Points on Right Ear

B. Auricular Landmarks and
Master Points on Left Ear

3.c_Allergy Point 1

1.0_Shen Men

1.0_Shen Men

2.0_Sympathetic
Autonomic Point

0.0_Point Zero

6.0_Master
Oscillation Point

7.0_Tranquilizer
Point

5.0_Master
Endocrine Point

9.0_Master
Cerebral Point

4.0_Thalamus
Point

4.0_Thalamus
Point

8.0_Master Sensorial Point

8.0_Master Sensorial Point

FIGURE 7.4 Photographs of master points found near auricular landmarks.

7.2 Auricular Representation of the Musculoskeletal System

The anatomical locations of auricular points are described verbally and are also indicated by their zone location. If there are several auricular regions that represent a correspondent part of the body, such as differences between Chinese and European ear points, or differences in the Nogier phase location of a point, the function of that ear point may only be presented with the first citation of that point.

The nomenclature system described in Chapter 4 is used with each auricular microsystem point. Each anatomical area of the body and each functional condition is designated by a different Arabic number. Chinese ear points are represented by the extension ".c" after the number and the superscript "$^{\{C\}}$" after the capitalized name of that point. European ear points are represented by the extension ".e" after the number and the superscript "$^{\{E\}}$" after the name of that auricular point. The numbers of ear points that are the same in both systems are represented by the extension ".0".

The three phases of the Nogier phase system are presented in the final section of this chapter. Each phase is designated by the extensions ".F1" and "$^{\{F1\}}$" for Phase I, ".F2" and "$^{\{F2\}}$" for Phase II, and ".F3" and "$^{\{F3\}}$"for Phase III. The musculoskeletal ear points are found in Territory 1 in Phase I, Territory 2 in Phase II, and Territory 3 in Phase III.

Most pain problems are due to myofascial pain created by chronic re-stimulation of sensory neuron feedback from a muscle in spasm. Sensory feedback from excessive tension in the muscles reactivates spinal interneurons that re-stimulate motor neuron excitation, which thus leads to a further increase in muscle contraction. Spinal reflex pathways may cause the muscles to stay in spasm. Muscles do not maintain chronic tension by themselves but, rather, only by the activation of spinal motor neurons, which then cause the muscles to remain contracted. Because these maintained muscle spasms are regulated by subconscious spinal reflexes, conscious control by the motor cortex and the premotor cortex is not able to stop the pain spasms.

Musculoskeletal auricular points represent any disorder associated with movement, muscles, tendons, ligaments, and the skeletal bone structures of the corresponding body area, as well as blood vessel circulation to that area. These ear reflex points for the musculoskeletal body represent somatic nervous system reflexes that affect pathological maintenance of reflex arcs in the spinal cord. These reflexes may be overstimulated by somatosensory neurons or repeatedly re-stimulated by proprioceptive muscles, thus maintaining dysfunctional, postural movements. Autonomic sympathetic reflexes affected by these ear points impair vascular supply to the associated body region.

Auricular acupuncture stimulation seems to function through unconscious, extrapyramidal motor reflex pathways and limbic system structures that send descending impulses to the spinal gating system. Feedback loops from a somatic sensory neuron to a spinal motor neuron keep a muscle in contraction. Auriculotherapy can disrupt these pathological feedback loops and can also facilitate autonomic regulation of blood circulation to a particular muscle region. Patients receiving auriculotherapy often report a sense of warmth in the body area that corresponds to the ear point being treated—a phenomenon related to increased vasodilatation in that body region.

Clinical problems treated by ear reflex points include relief of motor problems in the corresponding body area. Such problems include

A. Three Auricular Territories

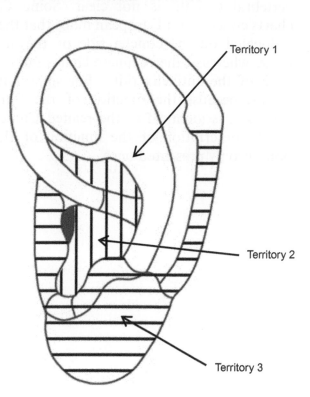

B. Musculoskeletal Somatotopic Ear

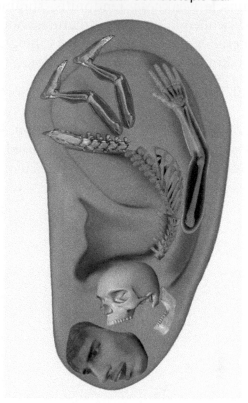

C. Visceral Organs Somatotopic Ear

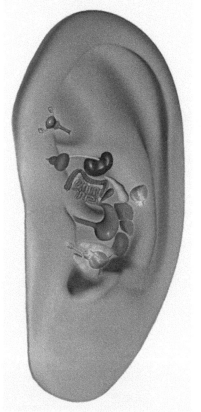

D. Nervous System Somatotopic Ear

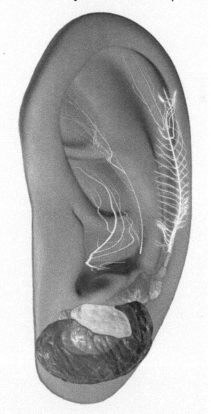

FIGURE 7.5 Somatotopic representations on three territories on the external ear.

muscle tension, muscle strain, muscle tremors, muscle weakness, tendonitis, sprained ligaments, swollen joints, bone fractures, bone spurs, peripheral neuralgias, arthritis, shingles, sunburns, skin irritations, and skin lesions.

For all ear reflex points, the anterior surface of the ear is used to treat the sensory neuron aspects of nociceptive pain sensation, whereas the posterior surface of the ear is used to treat the motor neuron aspects of muscular spasm.

The consensus for the Chinese location of the vertebral column is not clear. Some Chinese charts concur with European maps that the spine is located on the concha side of the antihelix ridge, whereas other Chinese charts put it at the peak of the antihelix ridge. For some auricular points, because the function of the European ear point is identical to the related Chinese ear points, description of the function of that ear point is only presented once.

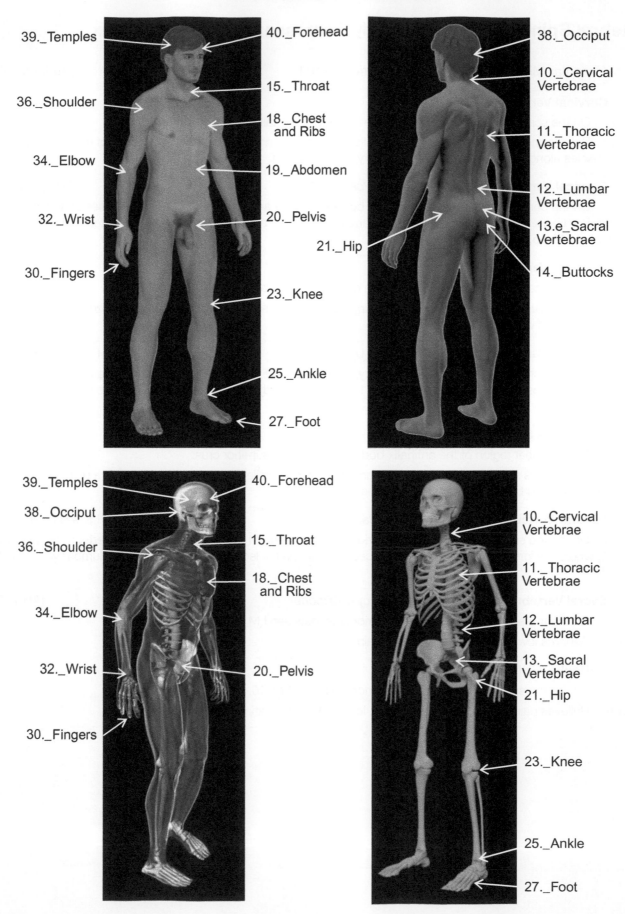

39._Temples
40._Forehead
38._Occiput
10._Cervical Vertebrae
15._Throat
11._Thoracic Vertebrae
36._Shoulder
18._Chest and Ribs
34._Elbow
19._Abdomen
12._Lumbar Vertebrae
32._Wrist
20._Pelvis
13.e_Sacral Vertebrae
21._Hip
30._Fingers
14._Buttocks
23._Knee
25._Ankle
27._Foot

39._Temples
40._Forehead
38._Occiput
10._Cervical Vertebrae
36._Shoulder
15._Throat
11._Thoracic Vertebrae
18._Chest and Ribs
34._Elbow
12._Lumbar Vertebrae
32._Wrist
20._Pelvis
13._Sacral Vertebrae
21._Hip
30._Fingers
23._Knee
25._Ankle
27._Foot

[**FIGURE 7.6** Identification of terms for major anatomical structures of the musculoskeletal body.

Vertebral Spine and Anterior Body Represented on the Antihelix

No.	Auricular Microsystem Point *(Alternative Name)*	[Auricular Zone]

10.c   Cervical Vertebrae {C}   [AH 8]

Location: On the scaphoid fossa side of the ridge of the antihelix tail.

Function: Relieves neck strain, neck pain, torticollis, headaches, and TMJ. Improves the range of motion related to tight muscles along the neck, increasing flexibility and circulation.

10.e   Cervical Vertebrae {E} *(Cervical Spine, Posterior Neck)*   [AH 1, AH2, PG 2]

Location: On the concha side of the antihelix tail, between LM_14 and LM_15. The C1 vertebra lies central to the antitragal–antihelix groove and runs along the narrow ridge of the antihelix tail up to the C7 vertebra at the antihelix midpoint at LM_15.

11.c   Thoracic Vertebrae {C}   [AH 9, AH 10]

Location: On the scaphoid fossa side of the ridge of the antihelix body.

Function: Relieves upper back pain, low back pain, shoulder pain, arthritis, shoulder tension, frozen shoulder, elbow dysfunctions, and wrist pain.

11.e   Thoracic Vertebrae {E} *(Thoracic Spine, Upper Back)*   [AH 3, AH 4, PG 3, PG 4]

Location: On the concha side of the antihelix body, between LM_15 and LM_16. The T1 vertebra lies above the concha ridge, across from LM_0, whereas the T12 vertebra lies adjacent to the beginning of the inferior crus at LM_16.

12.c   Lumbar Vertebrae {C} *(Lower Back)*   [AH 11]

Location: On the upper region of the antihelix body, but below the superior crus.

Function: Represents sacroiliac muscles and ligaments, this point relieves low back pain, sciatica pain, and peripheral neuralgia. It relieves back strain and disc degeneration.

12.e   Lumbar Vertebrae {E} *(Lumbar Spine, Sacroiliac)*   [AH 5, AH 6, PG 5, PG 6]

Location: On the top surface of the antihelix inferior crus, between LM_16 and LM_17. The L1 vertebra occurs at LM_16, where the inferior crus begins, and proceeds along the flat ledge of the inferior crus to lumbar vertebra L5 at LM_17.

13.e   Sacral Vertebrae {E} *(Sacral Spine, Coccyx, Tailbone)*   [AH 7, PG 7]

Location: On the top surface of the antihelix inferior crus, between LM_17 and LM_18.

Function: Relieves low back pain and sciatica pain.

14.0   Buttocks *(Gluteus Maximus Muscles)*   [AH 5, PG 5]

Location: On the top surface of the antihelix inferior crus, near LM_16.

Function: Relieves pain in the buttocks muscles, low back pain, sciatica pain, and hip pain.

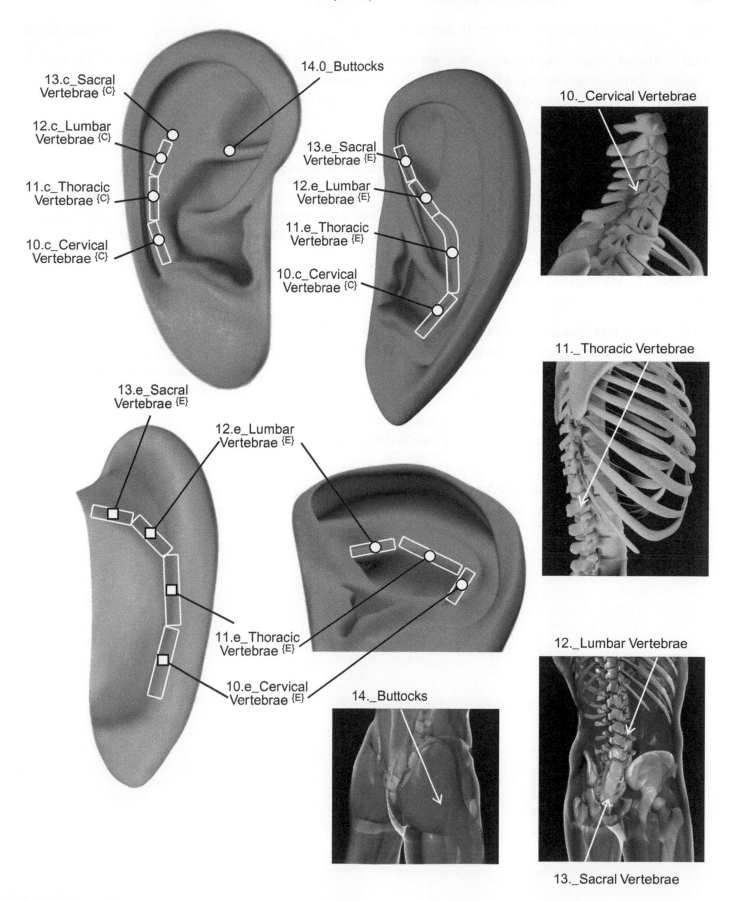

FIGURE 7.7 Musculoskeletal spinal vertebrae represented on the auricle.

No.   Auricular Microsystem Point *(Alternative Name)*   [Auricular Zone]

15.0   Throat *(Anterior Neck Muscles, Scalene Muscles)*   [AH 8, AH 9, PP 1, PP 3]

Location: On the scaphoid fossa side of the antihelix tail, between LM_14 and LM_15.

Function: Relieves neck tension, sore throats, torticollis, TMJ, and hyperthyroidism.

16.c   Clavicle {C} *(Collarbone)*   [SF 1]

Location: In the inferior scaphoid fossa groove peripheral to the Throat point.

Function: Relieves clavicle fractures, shoulder pain, arthritic shoulder, and rheumatism.

16.e   Clavicle {E} *(Scapula, Shoulder Blade)*   [AH 9, PP 3]

Location: On the more superior region of the scaphoid fossa, where it lies peripheral to the cervical and chest points. It lies on the peripheral side of the antihelix at the junction of the antihelix body and the antihelix tail at LM_15.

17.0   Breast *(Mammary Glands)*   [AH 10]

Location: On the scaphoid fossa side of the antihelix body, superior to LM_15.

Function: Relieves perimenstrual symptoms, breast tenderness, and breast cancer.

18.0   Chest and Ribs *(Pectoral Muscles, Thorax, Ribcage, Sternum)*   [AH 10, PP 3]

Location: On the antihelix body, superior to LM_15 and near the breast point.

Function: Relieves chest pain, chest heaviness, intercostal pain, angina pectoris, coughs, asthma, and hiccups.

19.0   Abdomen *(Abdominal Muscles)*   [AH 11, AH 12, PP 5]

Location: On the superior side of the antihelix body, below the superior crus.

Function: Relieves abdominal pain, low back pain, and hernias.

20.0   Pelvis *(Pelvic Girdle, Pelvic Cavity, Pubic Bone, Groin)*   [TF 1, PG 8]

Location: At the tip of the triangular fossa, above LM_16 and below the Shen Men point.

Function: Relieves groin pain, pelvic strain, pain during pregnancy, low back pain, hernias, and digestive disorders.

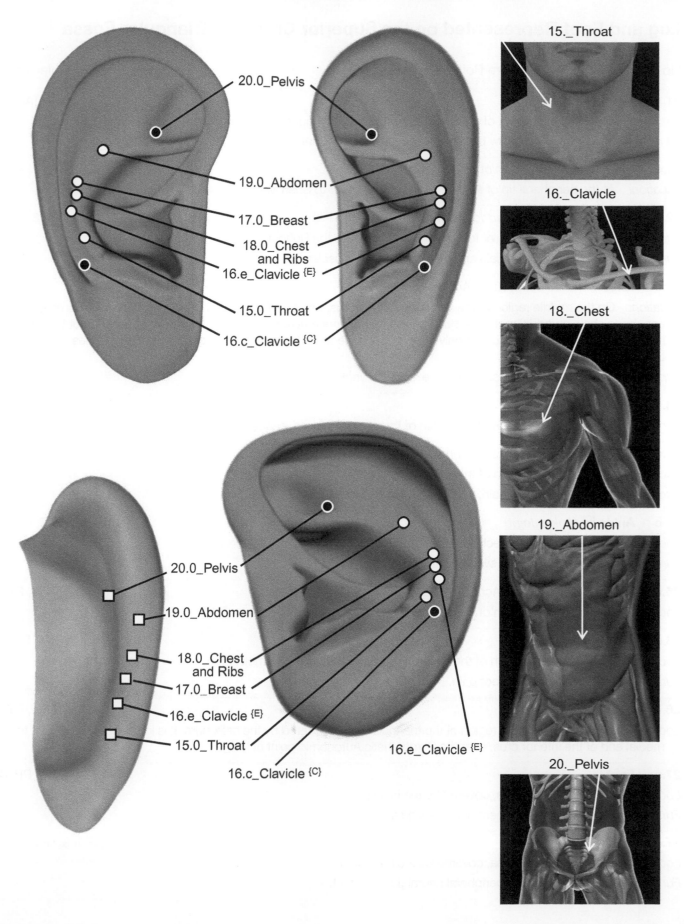

20.0_Pelvis

19.0_Abdomen

17.0_Breast

18.0_Chest
and Ribs

16.e_Clavicle {E}

15.0_Throat

16.c_Clavicle {C}

15._Throat

16._Clavicle

18._Chest

19._Abdomen

20._Pelvis

20.0_Pelvis

19.0_Abdomen

18.0_Chest
and Ribs

17.0_Breast

16.e_Clavicle {E}

15.0_Throat

16.c_Clavicle {C}

16.e_Clavicle {E}

FIGURE 7.8 Anterior torso represented on the auricle.

Leg and Foot Represented on the Superior Crus and Triangular Fossa

No.	Auricular Microsystem Point (Alternative Name)	[Auricular Zone]

21.c   Hip {C} (Hip Joint)   [AH 13]
Location: On the lower aspect of the antihelix superior crus, peripheral to Shen Men.
Function: Relieves hip pain, low back pain, and inflamed hip joint.

21.e   Hip {E} (Coxofemoral Joint)   [TF 1, PT 1]
Location: At the peripheral tip of the triangular fossa, inferior to Shen Men.

22.0   Thigh (Upper Leg, Quadriceps Muscles, Femur)   [TF 3, PT 1]
Location: In the inferior triangular fossa, immediately above the Buttocks point.
Function: Relieves upper leg pain and pulled hamstring muscles.

23.c   Knee {C} (Knee Joint, Knee Articulation)   [AH 15]
Location: On the middle region of the antihelix superior crus, peripheral to the triangular fossa Knee {E}. Some Chinese
    ear charts show an additional Knee point on the more peripheral region of the antihelix superior crus, but that point
    has not been found to be as commonly observed in patients as the primary Chinese Knee point that lies superior to
    the Chinese Hip point.
Function: Relieves knee pain, strained knee, and dysfunctions related to knee injuries.

23.e   Knee {E} (Patella, Knee Joint)   [TF 3/TF 4, PT 2]
Location: At the middle section of the depth of the triangular fossa, central to Shen Men.

24.e   Calf {E} (Lower Leg, Gastrocnemius Muscle, Tibia and Fibula Bones)   [TF 5, PT 3]
Location: On the central region of the triangular fossa.
Function: Relieves lower leg pain, muscle cramps of the calf muscle.

25.c   Ankle {C} (Ankle Joint)   [AH 17, PP 12]
Location: On the superior aspect of the antihelix superior crus, below the helix brim.
Function: Relieves ankle pain, swollen ankles.

25.e   Ankle {E} (Ankle Joint, Achilles Tendon)   [TF 5/TF 6, PT 3]
Location: On the central region of the triangular fossa, below the helix brim.

26.c   Heel {C}   [AH 17, PP 12]
Location: On the highest region of the antihelix superior crus, under the helix brim.
Function: Relieves heel pain, foot pain.

26.e   Heel {E} (Tarsus)   [TF 5, PT 3]
Location: On the most central region of the triangular fossa, covered by the helix brim. It is immediately adjacent to the
    medial end of the inferior crus, near the Sympathetic Autonomic point at LM_18.

27.c   Foot {C}   [AH 17, AH 18, PP 12]
Location: On the superior crus, covered by the helix brim.
Function: Relieves foot pain, peripheral neuralgia in the feet.

27.e   Foot {E} (Metatarsals)   [TF 5 & TF 6, PT 3]
Location: In the triangular fossa, covered by the helix brim.
Function: Relieves foot pain, peripheral neuralgia in the feet.

No.	Auricular Microsystem Point *(Alternative Name)*	[Auricular Zone]

28.c   Toes {C}   [AH 18, PP 12]

Location: On the superior crus, covered by the helix brim. The Toes are more peripheral toward the outside of the ear than the ear points for the Heel.

Function: Relieves pain in toes, strained toe, inflamed toe, frostbite, peripheral neuralgia.

28.e   Toes {E}   [TF 6, PT 3]

Location: In the triangular fossa, covered by the helix brim. The large Toe is the highest point on the triangular fossa, close to the top of the superior crus of the antihelix. The small Toe is located closer to the Heel point.

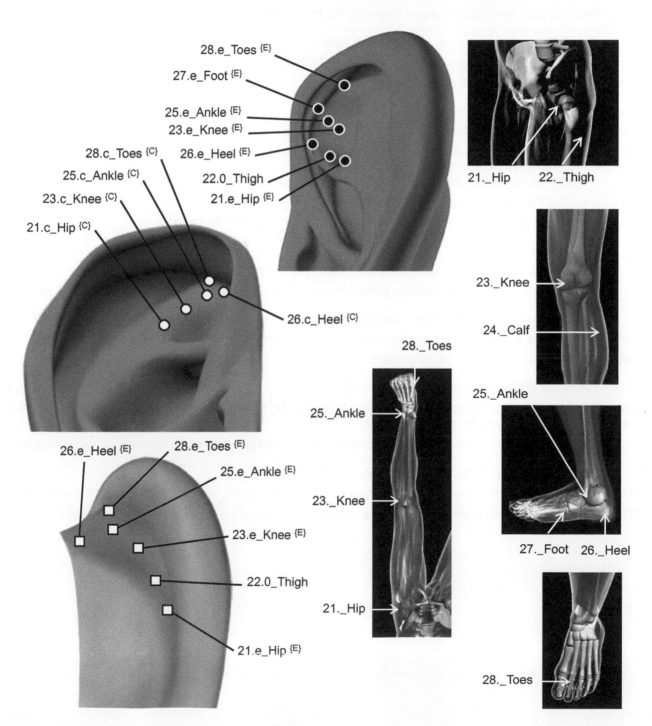

FIGURE 7.9 Lower extremities of hip, knee, and foot represented on the auricle.

Arm and Hand Represented on the Scaphoid Fossa

No.	Auricular Microsystem Point (Alternative Name)	[Auricular Zone]

29.0 **Thumb**   [AH 14 & AH 16, PP 9]
Location: Found on the antihelix superior crus, alongside the scaphoid fossa.
Function: Relieves pain of sprained thumb, sore thumbs, burns to thumb.

30.0 **Fingers** *(Digits, Phalanges)*   [SF 6, PP 10]
Location: Found on the uppermost scaphoid fossa, covered by the helix brim.
Function: Relieves pain, swelling, peripheral neuralgia, frostbite, and arthritis in fingers.

31.0 **Hand** *(Palm, Carpal bones, Metacarpal bones)*   [SF 5 & AH 14, PP 9]
Location: Found on the upper scaphoid fossa, central to LM_3 and Darwin's Tubercle.
Function: Relieves pain and swelling in the hand.

32.0 **Wrist** *(Wrist Joint)*   [SF 5, PP 7]
Location: Found in the scaphoid fossa, central to LM_4 of Darwin's Tubercle.
Function: Relieves carpal tunnel syndrome and alleviates pain, strain, sprain, arthritis, and swelling in the wrist joint.

33.0 **Forearm** *(Ulna Bone, Radius Bone, Brachioradialis Muscle)* [SF 4, PP 7]
Location: Found in the superior scaphoid fossa, inferior to the Wrist point.
Function: Relieves tennis elbow and alleviates tendonitis, pain, and strain in the forearm.

34.0 **Elbow** *(Elbow Joint)*   [SF 3, PP 5]
Location: Found in the scaphoid fossa, directly peripheral to the antihelix body.
Function: Relieves tennis elbow and alleviates tendonitis, pain, strain, soreness, and swelling in the elbow joint.

35.0 **Upper Arm** *(Biceps and Triceps Muscles, Humerus Bone)*   [SF 3, PP 5]
Location: Found in the scaphoid fossa, superior to the Shoulder point.
Function: Relieves pain and spasms in upper arm.

36.0 **Shoulder** *(Pectoral Girdle, Deltoid Muscles)*   [SF 2, PP 3]
Location: Found in the scaphoid fossa, peripheral to LM_0 and LM_15, where the antihelix region representing the neck meets the auricular area for the upper back.
Function: Relieves frozen shoulder and alleviates pain, tenderness, swelling, and arthritis in the shoulder muscles.

37.0 **Shoulder Joint** *(Master Shoulder, Scapula, Trapezius Muscles)* [SF 1, PP 1]
Location: Found in the inferior scaphoid fossa, inferior to the Shoulder point, central to LM_5, near the ear lobe.
Function: Relieves pain, tenderness, strain, arthritis, and swelling in the shoulder joint as well as the trapezius muscles.

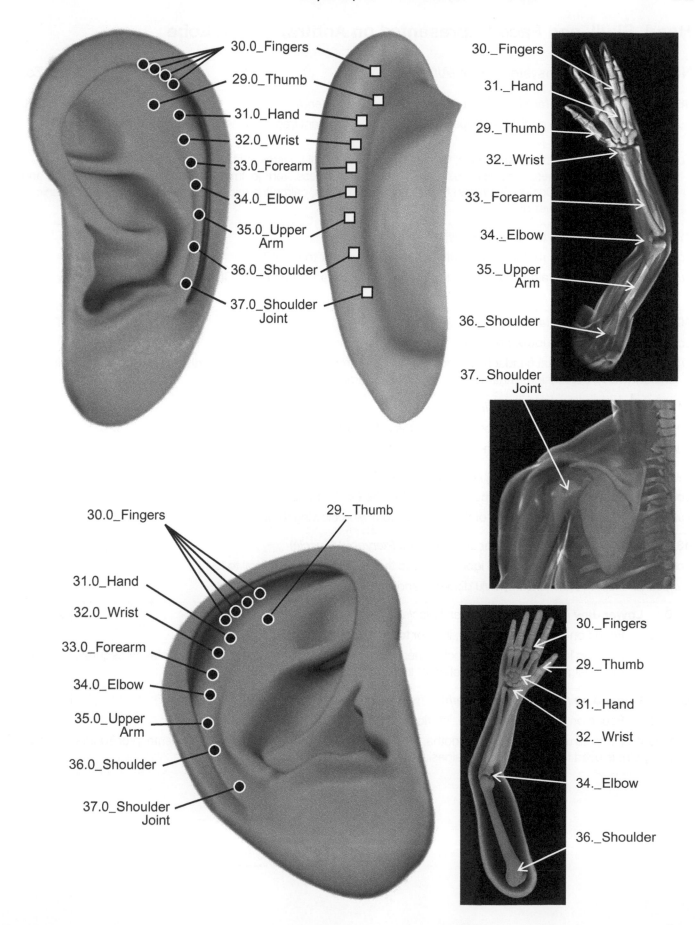

30.0_Fingers
29.0_Thumb
31.0_Hand
32.0_Wrist
33.0_Forearm
34.0_Elbow
35.0_Upper Arm
36.0_Shoulder
37.0_Shoulder Joint

30._Fingers
29._Thumb
31._Hand
32._Wrist
33._Forearm
34._Elbow
35._Upper Arm
36._Shoulder
37._Shoulder Joint

30.0_Fingers
29._Thumb
31.0_Hand
32.0_Wrist
33.0_Forearm
34.0_Elbow
35.0_Upper Arm
36.0_Shoulder
37.0_Shoulder Joint

30._Fingers
29._Thumb
31._Hand
32._Wrist
34._Elbow
36._Shoulder

FIGURE 7.10 Upper extremities of shoulder, knee, wrist, and hand represented on the auricle.

Head, Skull, and Face Represented on Antitragus and Lobe

No.	Auricular Microsystem Point (*Alternative Name*)	[Auricular Zone]

38.0   Occiput (*Occipital Skull, Occipitalis Muscle, Atlas of Head*)   [AT 3, PL 4]

Location: Found on the peripheral, superior antitragus, near the antitragal–antihelix groove, between LM_13 and LM_14.

Function: Relieves occipital headaches, tension headaches, facial spasms, stiff neck, epileptic convulsions, brain seizures, shock, dizziness, sea sickness, car sickness, air sickness, vertigo, impaired vision, insomnia, coughs, and asthma. In TCM, the Occiput is utilized for all nervous disorders, calms the mind, clears heat, dispels pathogenic wind, and nourishes liver qi.

39.0   Temple (*Temporal–Parietal Skull*)   [AT 2, PG 1]

Location: Found on the middle section of the antitragus, inferior to LM_13.

Function: Relieves migraine headaches, temporal headaches, and tinnitus. In TCM, this point affects the body acupoint Tai Yang and dispels harmful wind.

40.0   Forehead (*Frontal Skull*)   [AT 1, PL 2]

Location: Found on the lower antitragus, near LM_12 and the intertragic notch.

Function: Relieves frontal headaches, sinusitis, dizziness, impaired vision, insomnia, distractibility, neurasthenia, anxiety, worry, depression, lethargy, and disturbing dreams.

41.0   Frontal Sinus (*Maxillary Sinus*)   [LO 1]

Location: Found on the central lobe, inferior to the antitragus point for the Forehead.

Function: Relieves frontal headaches, sinusitis, and rhinitis.

42.0   Vertex (*Top of Head, Apex of Head, Crown of Head*)   [LO 6]

Location: Found on peripheral, superior lobe, below the Occiput point.

Function: Relieves pain at the top of the head, as from wind blowing through one's hair.

43.0   TMJ (*Temporal–Mandibular Joint, Lateral Pterygoid Muscle*)   [LO 8, PL 4/PL 6]

Location: Found on the peripheral lobe, inferior to the scaphoid fossa, central to LM_6.

Function: Relieves jaw tension, TMJ disorder, and bruxism.

44.0   Lower Jaw (*Mandible, Masseter Muscle, Lower Teeth*)   [L0 8, PL 6]

Location: Found on the peripheral lobe, inferior to the TMJ point.

Function: Relieves lower jaw tension, toothaches, TMJ, bruxism, anxiety, and pain from dental procedures. Used in acupuncture analgesia for tooth extraction of lower teeth.

45.0   Upper Jaw (*Maxilla, Upper Teeth*)   [L0 8, PL 4]

Location: Found on the peripheral lobe, inferior and central to the Lower Jaw point.

Function: Relieves upper jaw tension, toothaches, TMJ, bruxism, anxiety, and pain from dental procedures. The Upper Jaw point is used for acupuncture analgesia for tooth extraction of upper teeth.

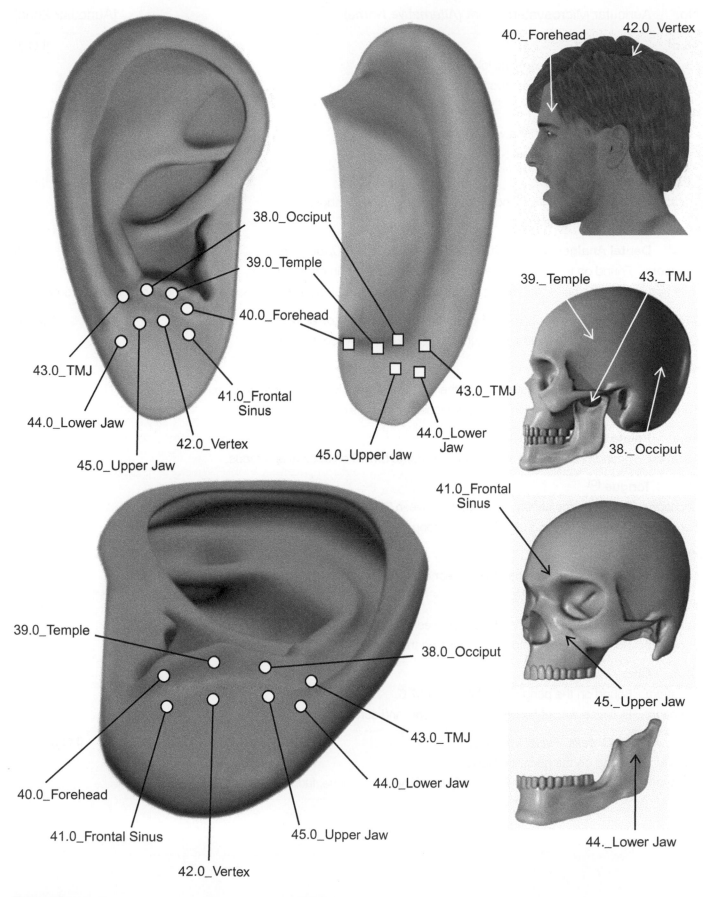

40._Forehead

42.0_Vertex

38.0_Occiput

39.0_Temple

40.0_Forehead

43.0_TMJ

44.0_Lower Jaw

41.0_Frontal Sinus

42.0_Vertex

45.0_Upper Jaw

43.0_TMJ

44.0_Lower Jaw

45.0_Upper Jaw

39._Temple

43._TMJ

39._Temple

38._Occiput

41.0_Frontal Sinus

38.0_Occiput

43.0_TMJ

44.0_Lower Jaw

45._Upper Jaw

45.0_Upper Jaw

40.0_Forehead

41.0_Frontal Sinus

42.0_Vertex

44._Lower Jaw

FIGURE 7.11 Head and jaw represented on the auricle.

No.	Auricular Microsystem Point *(Alternative Name)*	[Auricular Zone]

46.c¹ Toothache 1   [LO 8]

Location: Found on the peripheral lobe.

Function: Relieves toothaches, tooth decay.

46.c² Toothache 2   [CW 3]

Location: Found on the concha wall behind the antitragus.

Function: Relieves toothaches.

46.c³ Toothache 3   [IC 5]

Location: Found on the inferior concha, below the antitragus ridge.

Function: Relieves toothaches.

47.c¹ Dental Analgesia 1 *(Tooth Extraction Anesthesia 1, Upper Teeth)*   [LO 2]

Location: Found on the central lobe, inferior to LM_9 and the intertragic notch.

Function: Used for pain relief during dental procedures, gum disease, tooth decay, and periodontal inflammations.

47.c² Dental Analgesia 2 *(Tooth Extraction Anesthesia 2, Lower Teeth)*   [LO 1]

Location: Found on the central Lobe, inferior to the Dental Analgesia 1 point.

48.c¹ Palate 1 *(Lower Palate)*   [LO 4/AT 1]

Location: Found on the upper, center of the lobe, inferior to LM 12 on the antitragus.

Function: Relieves sores, ulcers, and infections in the gums of the mouth.

48.c² Palate 2 *(Upper Palate)*   [LO 4/LO 5]

Location: Found on the center of the lobe, inferior to LM 13 on apex of antitragus.

49.c Tongue {C}   [LO 4]

Location: Found on the center of the lobe, between Palate 1 and Palate 2.

Function: Relieves pain and bleeding of the tongue.

49.e Tongue {E}   [LO 5, PL 5, PL 6]

Location: Found on the peripheral lobe, near ear reflex points for the Upper Jaw.

50.0 Lips   [LO 5, PL 5]

Location: Found on the peripheral lobe, between LM_6 and LM_7.

Function: Relieves chapped lips, cold sores on the lips.

51.0 **Chin**   [LO 7]

Location: Found on the peripheral lobe, near LM_6.

Function: Relieves pain of broken chin, skin sores and scrapes on the chin.

52.0 Face *(Cheeks, Facial Muscles)*   [LO 5, PL 5]

Location: Found on the peripheral lobe.

Function: Relieves facial spasms, tics, trigeminal neuralgia, acne, facial paralysis.

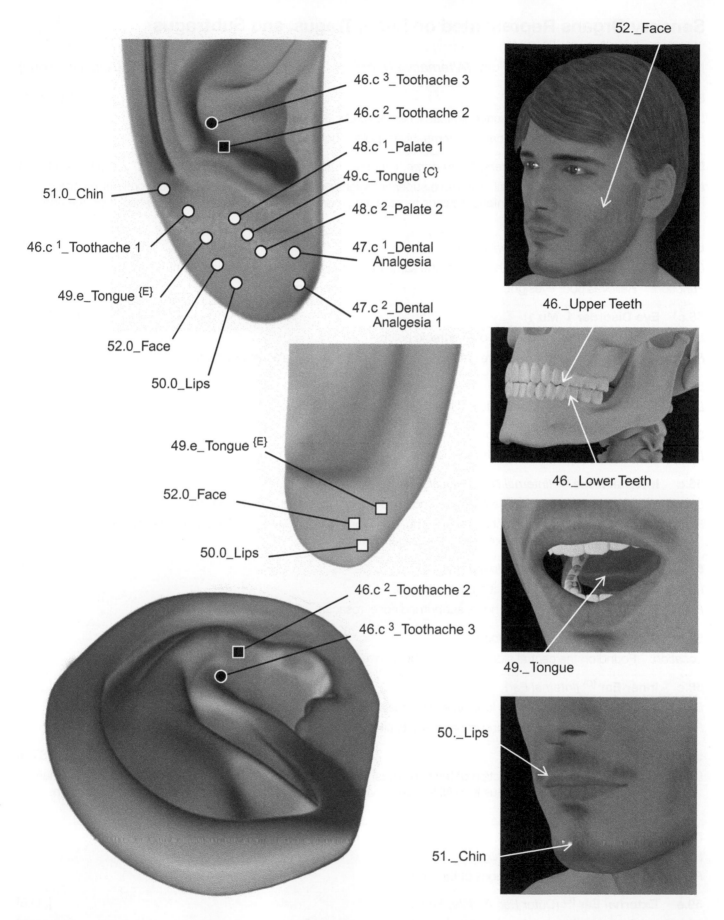

52._Face

46.c ³_Toothache 3

46.c ²_Toothache 2

48.c ¹_Palate 1

49.c_Tongue {C}

48.c ²_Palate 2

47.c ¹_Dental Analgesia

47.c ²_Dental Analgesia 1

51.0_Chin

46.c ¹_Toothache 1

49.e_Tongue {E}

52.0_Face

50.0_Lips

46._Upper Teeth

49.e_Tongue {E}

52.0_Face

50.0_Lips

46._Lower Teeth

46.c ²_Toothache 2

46.c ³_Toothache 3

49._Tongue

50._Lips

51._Chin

[FIGURE 7.12 Dental and facial features represented on the auricle.

Sensory Organs Represented on Lobe, Tragus, and Subtragus

No.	Auricular Microsystem Point (Alternative Name)	[Auricular Zone]

53.c   Dermatitis {C} (Urticaria)   [SF 5/IH 11]

Location: Found on the superior scaphoid fossa, central to LM_3, near the Hand point.

Function: Relieves dermatitis, urticaria, eczema, hives, poison oak.

53.e   Dermatitis {E} (Skin Disorders, Dermatome, Urticaria, Eczema)   [HX 12–HX 15]

Location: Found along the helix tail, with more superior regions of helix tail representing lumbosacral dermatomes over the lower extremities and more inferior regions representing thoracic dermatomes overlying the body and the upper extremities.

54.0   Eye (Retina, Master Sensorial Point)   [LO 4]

Location: Found at the center of the lobe, at the same location as the Master Sensorial point.

Function: Relieves poor eyesight, blurred vision, eye irritation, glaucoma, stye.

55.c^1 Eye Disorder 1 (Mu 1)   [IT 1/TG 1]

Location: Found on the central side of intertragic notch.

Function: Relieves blurred vision, eye irritation, glaucoma, retinitis, myopia, astigmatism.

55.c^2 Eye Disorder 2 (Mu 2)   [IT 1/AT 1]

Location: Found on the peripheral side of the intertragic notch.

55.c^3 Eye Disorder 3 (New Eye Point)   [IC 6]

Location: Found in the inferior concha, immediately below the helix root.

56.c   Internal Nose {C} (Internal Nose, Nasal Cavity)   [ST 2]

Location: Found on the middle of subtragus, underneath the tragus protrusion at LM_10.

Function: Relieves running nose, chronic sneezing, common colds, flu, sinusitis, rhinitis, nasal bleeding, profuse nasal discharge, nasal obstruction, allergies, and pathogenic wind.

57.c   External Nose {C} (Outer Nose)   [TG 3]

Location: Found on the middle section of the tragus.

Function: Relieves pain of broken nose, sunburned nose, rosacea.

57.e   External Nose {E} (Outer Nose)   [LO 1]

Location: Found on the central side of the ear lobe, between LM_8 and LM_9.

58.c   Inner Ear {C} (Internal Ear)   [LO 5]

Location: Found on the peripheral lobe, inferior to the Lower Jaw point.

Function: Relieves deafness, hearing impairment, tinnitus, dizziness, vertigo.

58.e   Inner Ear {E} (Cochlea)   [ST 3]

Location: Found on the middle section of the subtragus, near the Chinese Internal Nose. One procedure for alleviating sensorineural deafness and tinnitus is to fill the ear canal with saline and then electrically treat the inner ear with pulsed electrical stimulation.

59.c   External Ear {C} (Outer Ear, Auricle, Pinna)   [TG 5]

Location: Found on the superior tragus.

Function: Relieves pain and infections of the external ear.

59.e   External Ear {E} (Outer Ear, Auricle, Pinna)   [LO 5]

Location: Found on the peripheral ear lobe, near the Chinese Inner Ear.

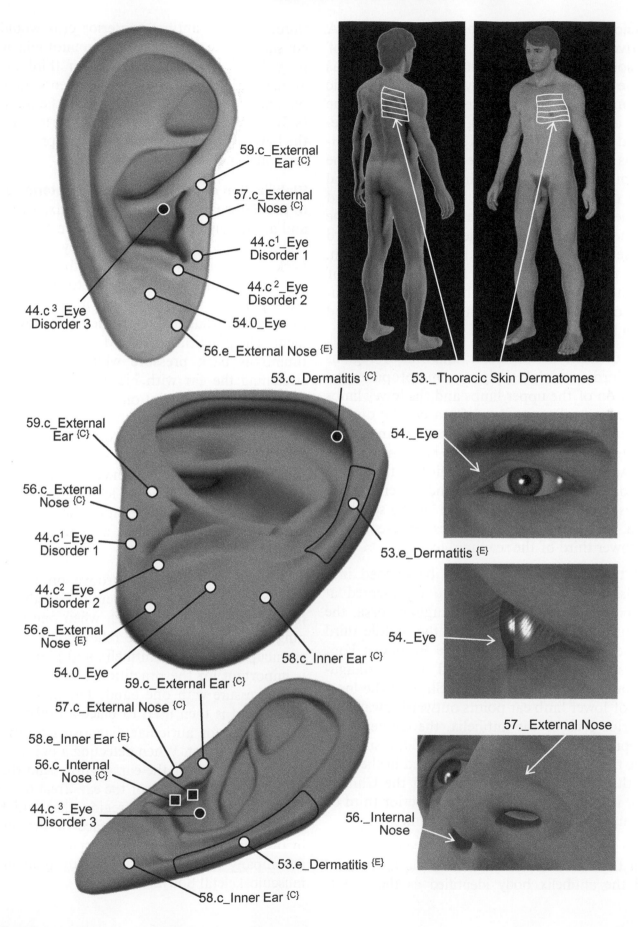

59.c_External Ear {C}

57.c_External Nose {C}

44.c¹_Eye Disorder 1

44.c²_Eye Disorder 2

44.c³_Eye Disorder 3

54.0_Eye

56.e_External Nose {E}

53.c_Dermatitis {C}

53._Thoracic Skin Dermatomes

59.c_External Ear {C}

56.c_External Nose {C}

44.c¹_Eye Disorder 1

44.c²_Eye Disorder 2

56.e_External Nose {E}

54.0_Eye

59.c_External Ear {C}

57.c_External Nose {C}

58.e_Inner Ear {E}

56.c_Internal Nose {C}

44.c³_Eye Disorder 3

53.e_Dermatitis {E}

58.c_Inner Ear {C}

58.c_Inner Ear {C}

54._Eye

53.e_Dermatitis {E}

54._Eye

57._External Nose

56._Internal Nose

FIGURE 7.13 Sensory organs represented on the auricle.

Division of Anatomical Regions by Thirds: A relatively simple procedure for identification of the somatotopic representation of certain areas of the musculoskeletal body is to divide specific anatomical regions into thirds. For example, the skull and muscles overlying the skull are represented on the antitragus. The "L-shaped" antitragus can be divided into equal thirds, with the Occiput represented on the upper, peripheral third of the antitragus, the Temples represented on the middle third of the antitragus, and the Forehead represented on the lower, central third of the antitragus, next to the intertragic notch. Both the Chinese and the European system of auriculotherapy concur with regard to the location of the Occiput, Temples, and Forehead along these equal regions of the antitragus.

This division of auricular anatomical regions into thirds can also apply to somatotopic representation of the upper limbs and the lower limbs of the body. The scaphoid fossa can be divided into equal thirds that run vertically from the ear lobe to the top of the helix. The hand and fingers are represented on the upper third of the scaphoid fossa; the forearm, elbow, and upper arm are represented on the middle third of the scaphoid fossa; and the whole shoulder is represented on the lower third of the scaphoid fossa.

The triangular fossa can also be divided into thirds, with the European Hip represented at the peripheral third of the triangular fossa, the European Knee represented in the middle third of the triangular fossa, and the European Foot represented in the central third of the triangular fossa, below the helix rim. Shifting the location of lower limb ear points outward toward the superior crus of the antihelix, the Chinese Hip is represented at the lower third of the superior crus, the Chinese Knee is represented in the middle third of the superior crus, and the Chinese Foot is represented in the most superior third of the superior crus, below the helix rim.

If the antitragus of the auricle is divided into thirds, with the antihelix tail considered the lower third and the antihelix body identified as the middle third, then the antihelix inferior crus would be considered the upper third. Somatotopic mapping thus indicates that the upper third of the antihelix inferior crus region represents the lumbosacral spine, the middle third of the antihelix body represents the thoracic spinal vertebrae, and the lower third of the antihelix tail represents the cervical spinal vertebrae.

Stabilization of the Anterior and Posterior Sides of the External Ear: Because the helix, antihelix, and antitragus are curving ridges on the peripheral aspect of the external ear, they tend to flap back and forth when scanning the ear for an ear reflex point. It is necessary to provide firm back pressure when detecting an ear acupoint for auricular diagnosis or auriculotherapy treatment. The practitioner should use his or her own thumb as back pressure while simultaneously stretching the ear with his or her index finger. When detecting a point on the posterior surface of the ear, slightly bend the ear over, revealing the back of the ear more prominently. Typically treat the exact same posterior auricular region that had been detected on the anterior surface of the auricle. This procedure for treating both the back of the ear and the front of the ear provides relief of muscle spasms that may accompany the sensory aspects of pain.

The scaphoid fossa is a groove on the most peripheral part of the external ear that also tends to flap back and forth when one is scanning the ear for an active reflex point. As with ear acupoints on the antihelix and antitragus, it is important for the practitioner to provide firm back pressure with one hand. The practitioner's other hand is then used to place a probe on the external ear for auricular diagnosis or auriculotherapy treatment. When detecting a point on the posterior surface of the ear, slightly bend the ear over, revealing the back of the ear. Treat the exact same posterior auricular region that had been detected on the anterior surface of the auricle in order to relieve the muscle spasms that may accompany the sensory aspects of pain in the musculoskeletal body.

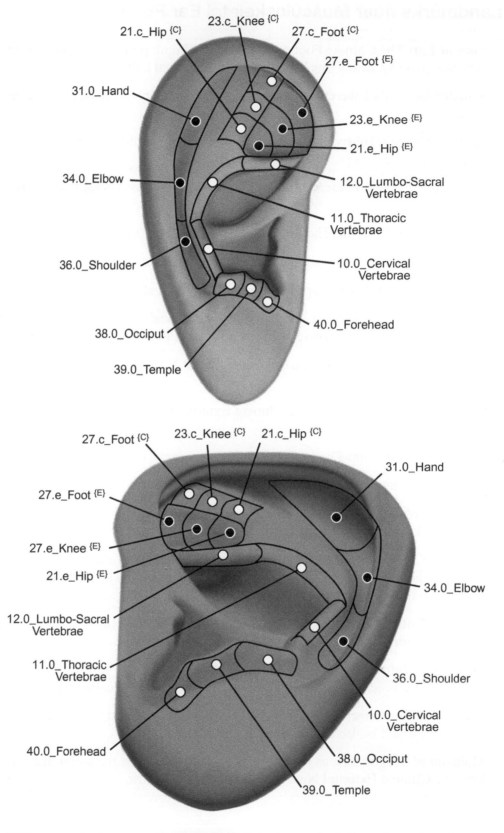

FIGURE 7.14 Different auricular areas are divided by thirds. The cervical, thoracic, and lumbosacral vertebrae are represented on three divisions of the antihelix. The hip, knee, and foot are represented on three divisions of the superior crus in the Chinese system and on three divisions of the triangular fossa in the European system. The shoulder, elbow, and hand are represented on three divisions of the scaphoid fossa, whereas the forehead, temple, and occiput are represented on three divisions of the antitragus.

Auricular Landmarks near Musculoskeletal Ear Points

LM_2	**Apex of Ear:** The Chinese Foot points and the Thumb point are located on the antihelix superior crus just below this landmark on the internal helix.
LM_3	**Superior Darwin's Tubercle:** The Hand point in the scaphoid fossa is found central to this landmark.
LM_4	**Inferior Darwin's Tubercle:** The Wrist point in the scaphoid fossa is found central to this landmark.
LM_5	**Helix Curve:** The Shoulder Joint point in the scaphoid fossa is located central to this landmark.
LM_6	**Lobular–Helix Junction:** The Lower Jaw and TMJ points are located central to LM_6.
LM_7	**Bottom of Lobe:** The Lips and Face are located superior to LM_7.
LM_8	**Lobular Insertion:** The European External Nose is located superior to LM_8.
LM_9	**Intertragic Notch:** The Mu 1 Eye Disease point is located just central to this landmark, whereas the Mu 2 Eye Disease point is located just peripheral to it.
LM_10	**Inferior Tragus Protrusion:** The Chinese External Nose is located halfway between LM_10 and LM_11 at LM_23.
LM_11	**Superior Tragus Protrusion:** The Chinese External Ear is located just superior to this landmark.
LM_12	**Antitragus Protrusion:** The Forehead on the antitragus is located near this landmark.
LM_13	**Apex of Antitragus:** The Temples on the antitragus are found inferior to this landmark.
LM_14	**Base of Antihelix:** The upper Cervical Vertebrae are located central to this landmark, the upper Neck Muscles just peripheral to it.
LM_15	**Antihelix Curve:** The division between the upper Thoracic Vertebrae and the lower Cervical Vertebrae is located at this landmark. The Shoulder point is located just peripheral to LM_15, in the scaphoid fossa.
LM_16	**Antihelix Notch:** The upper Lumbar Vertebrae are located central to this landmark, whereas the Elbow point is located peripherally in the scaphoid fossa.
LM_17	**Midpoint of Inferior Crus:** The division of the Upper Sacral Vertebrae from the lower Lumbar Vertebrae is located at this landmark, which is also called the Sciatica point.
LM_18	**Central Inferior Crus:** The most inferior Sacral Vertebrae and Coccyx are located at this landmark, which is also called the Sympathetic point.
LM_23	**Midpoint of Tragus:** Just as the cartilage of the tragus joins the softer fleshy tissue of the face, the Chinese External Nose is found at this landmark.

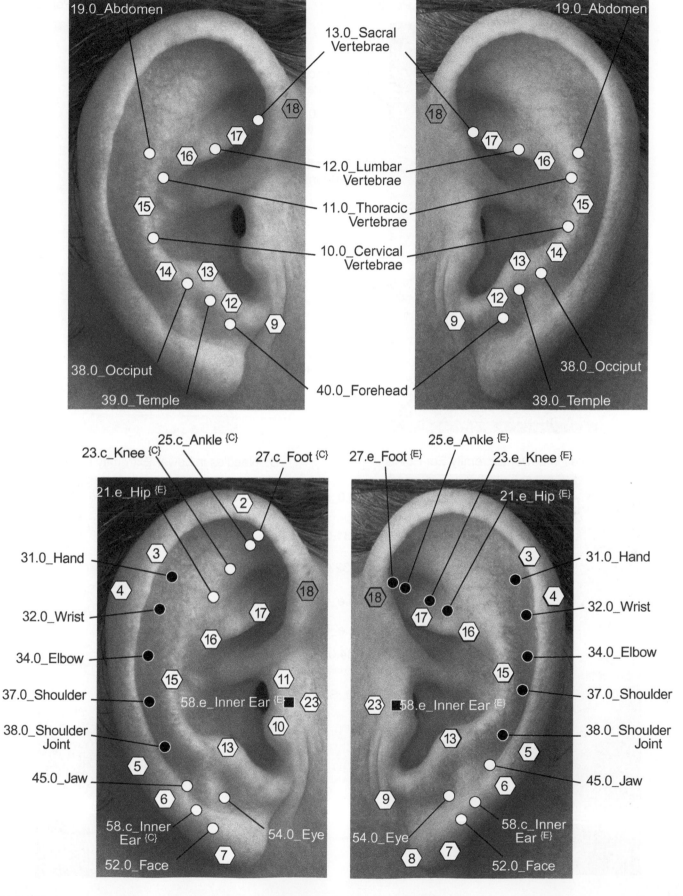

FIGURE 7.15 Photographs of auricular landmarks near musculoskeletal ear points.

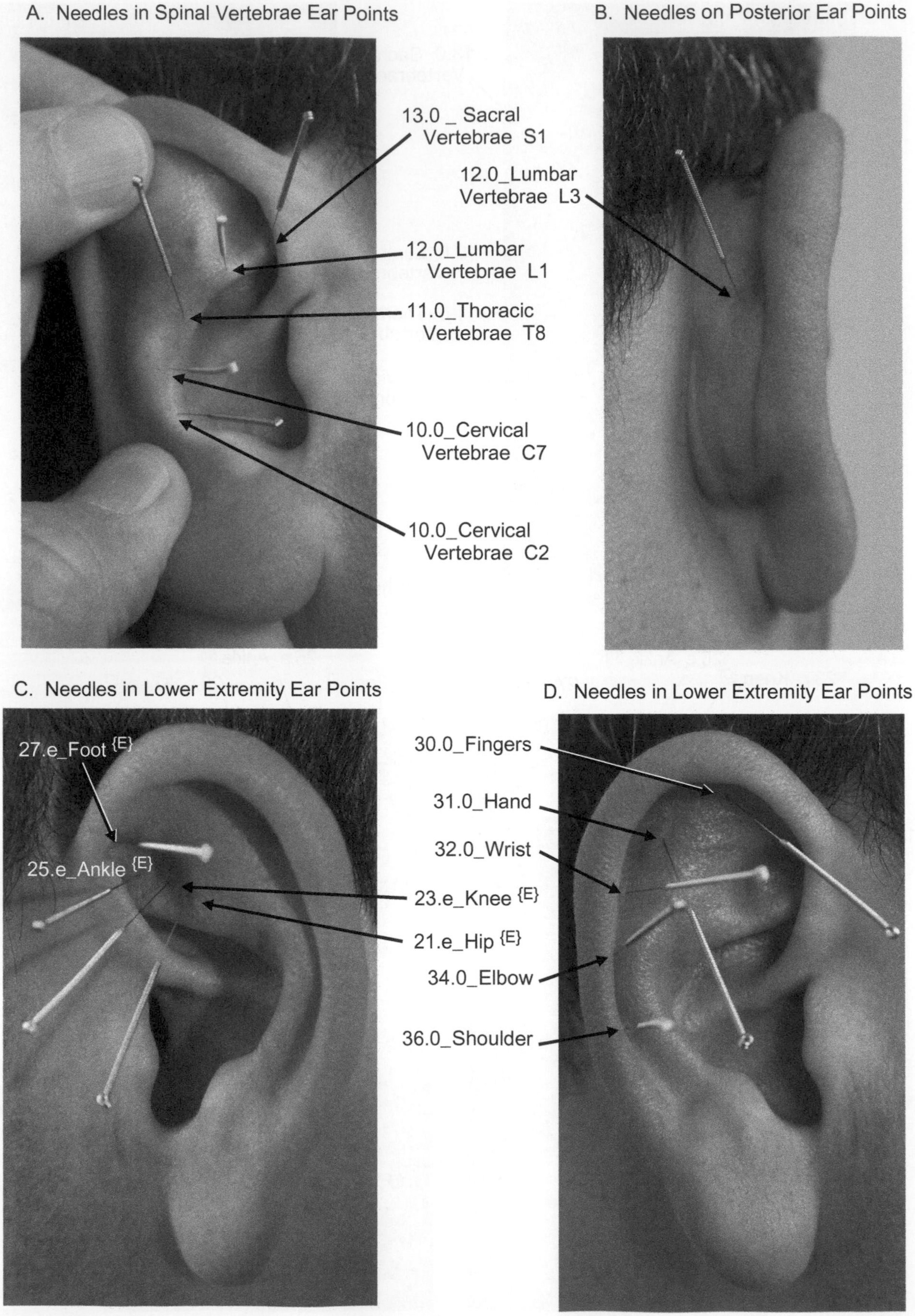

A. Needles in Spinal Vertebrae Ear Points

13.0 _ Sacral Vertebrae S1

12.0_Lumbar Vertebrae L3

12.0_Lumbar Vertebrae L1

11.0_Thoracic Vertebrae T8

10.0_Cervical Vertebrae C7

10.0_Cervical Vertebrae C2

B. Needles on Posterior Ear Points

12.0_Lumbar Vertebrae L3

C. Needles in Lower Extremity Ear Points

27.e_Foot {E}

25.e_Ankle {E}

D. Needles in Lower Extremity Ear Points

30.0_Fingers

31.0_Hand

32.0_Wrist

23.e_Knee {E}

21.e_Hip {E}

34.0_Elbow

36.0_Shoulder

FIGURE 7.16 Photographs of acupuncture needles inserted into musculoskeletal points.

7.3 Auricular Representation of Internal Visceral Organs

The arrangement of the location of internal organs on the auricle is based on the same anatomical organization as the organs are found in the internal body, only upside down. The auricular points represent physiological disturbances affecting an organ, not the actual anatomical tissue of that organ.

Digestive System: The gastrointestinal system, or alimentary canal, converts food that has been chewed into smaller fragments, allowing basic nutrients to be absorbed into the body to serve as the source of metabolic energy and to form the basic building blocks for muscles, bones, and cellular tissue.

Mouth: This soft tissue lining of the oral cavity or buccal cavity includes the gums, palate, tongue, and salivary glands, where food is masticated, tasted, and mixed with digestive fluids for better digestion. Pathological conditions that are represented on the Mouth auricular point include mouth sores, gum disease, and taste hunger cravings.

Esophagus: The gullet is a long tube that delivers food from the mouth to the stomach. Pathological conditions that are represented on the Esophagus auricular point include heartburn and indigestion.

Esophageal Sphincter: This smooth muscle valve closes off gastric juices from rising up out of the stomach. Pathological conditions that are represented on the Esophagus auricular point include heartburn, indigestions, and gastroesophageal reflux disorder (GERD).

Stomach: This hollow organ is a temporary storage tank for food. Through mechanical churning and mixture with gastric acid chemicals, food received from the mouth is further broken down into a mushy chime substance. Pathological conditions that are represented on the Stomach auricular point include nausea, vomiting, gastritis, and appetite control.

Small Intestines: This very long tube winds back on itself many times, allowing for the gradual absorption of food nutrients into the body. It begins at the duodenum that is connected to the stomach and ends at the ileum connected to the large intestines. Pathological conditions that are represented on the Small Intestines auricular point include malnutrition, digestive disorders, and intestinal distress.

Large Intestines: This final tube progresses from the ascending colon to the transverse colon to the descending colon, ending in the rectum. The colon withdraws water from indigestible food or releases excess fluid. Pathological conditions that are represented on the Large Intestines auricular point include colitis, constipation, and diarrhea.

Rectum: This sphincter valve holds back feces in the intestines before defecation occurs. It can be related to rectal sores, inflamed rectum, diarrhea, or constipation.

Circulatory System: This hydraulic system begins with the cardiac muscle in the thoracic chest cavity, which sends oxygen-rich blood through the arteries to deliver it to all parts of the body and receives oxygen-deficient blood from the veins. The lymphatic vessels collect excess fluid, metabolic wastes, and immune system breakdown products so that they can be eliminated from the body.

Heart: This primary cardiac muscle pumps blood to all parts of the body. Pathological conditions that are represented on the Heart auricular point include cardiac arrhythmias, hypertension, angina, panic attacks, and anxiety.

Blood Vessels: A long system of arteries branch out from the heart to the rest of the body, becoming progressively smaller as they turn into arterioles and finally into capillaries that distribute blood cells and fluids to local tissue, which then is collected into veins and returned to the heart. Blood vessels are found throughout the body; thus, they are somatotopically found throughout all regions of the external ear. Pathological conditions that are represented on the Circulatory Blood Vessels auricular points include poor circulation, cold feet, hypertension, and Raynaud's disorder.

Respiratory System: The tubular organs of this system allow the exchange of air and carbon dioxide, absorbing oxygen with each inhalation and releasing CO_2 upon exhalation.

Pharynx: This opening to the lungs includes the mouth lining, pharynx, larynx, and trachea. Pathological conditions that are represented on the Throat auricular point include sore throats, laryngitis, and difficulty swallowing.

Lungs: This primary organ for exchange of air gases includes the branching bronchial tubes and many thin alveoli sacs that facilitate the exchange of gases. Pathological conditions that are represented on the Lung auricular point include asthma, bronchitis, coughs, respiratory allergies, and smoking cessation.

Diaphragm: This smooth muscle membrane below the thoracic cavity allows inhalation to occur and separates the thorax from the abdomen. Pathological conditions that are represented on the Diaphragm auricular point include hiccups.

Abdominal Organs: Organs in the abdomen that function with other visceral systems.

Liver: This accessory digestive organ lies next to the stomach. The liver converts blood glucose into glycogen, incorporates amino acids into proteins, releases enzymes to metabolize toxic substances in the blood, and produces bile. The bile is released into the small intestines, where it facilitates digestion of fats. Pathological conditions that are represented on the Liver auricular point include hepatitis.

Gall Bladder: This muscular sac stores bile created by the liver. Pathological conditions that are represented on the Gall Bladder auricular point include gallstones.

Spleen: This lymphatic organ next to the stomach filters the blood and removes defective blood cells and bacteria. It is a site for producing additional immune cells. Pathological conditions that are represented on the Spleen auricular point include HIV disease, cancer, and immune system impairments.

Pancreas: This accessory endocrine–exocrine gland produces digestive enzymes, the hormone insulin to facilitate energy inside cells, and the hormone glucagon to raise blood sugar levels. Pathological conditions that are represented on the Pancreas auricular point include diabetes mellitus.

Appendix: This pouch attached to the large intestine contains lymphatic tissue. Pathological conditions that are represented at this ear point include appendicitis.

Urogenital Organs: Abdominal and pelvic organs of the urinary system and reproductive systems.

Kidney: This primary urinary organ filters toxic substances from the blood and releases them into the urine. It may retain or release body fluids and mineral salts. Pathological conditions that are represented on the Kidney auricular point include kidney stones and kidney infections.

Ureter: Two tubes that lead from each kidney to the bladder. Pathological conditions that are represented on the Ureter auricular point include urinary infections.

Bladder: The urinary bladder receives urine from the ureter and kidney and holds it for later release. Pathological conditions that are represented on the Bladder auricular point include bladder infections and an inflamed bladder.

Urethra: The final tube that connects the bladder and gonads to the outside world. Pathological conditions that are represented on the Urethra auricular point include urethritis and painful urination.

Prostate: The accessory reproductive organ in males that contributes milky substances to the semen. Pathological conditions that are represented on the Prostate auricular point include prostatitis and prostate cancer.

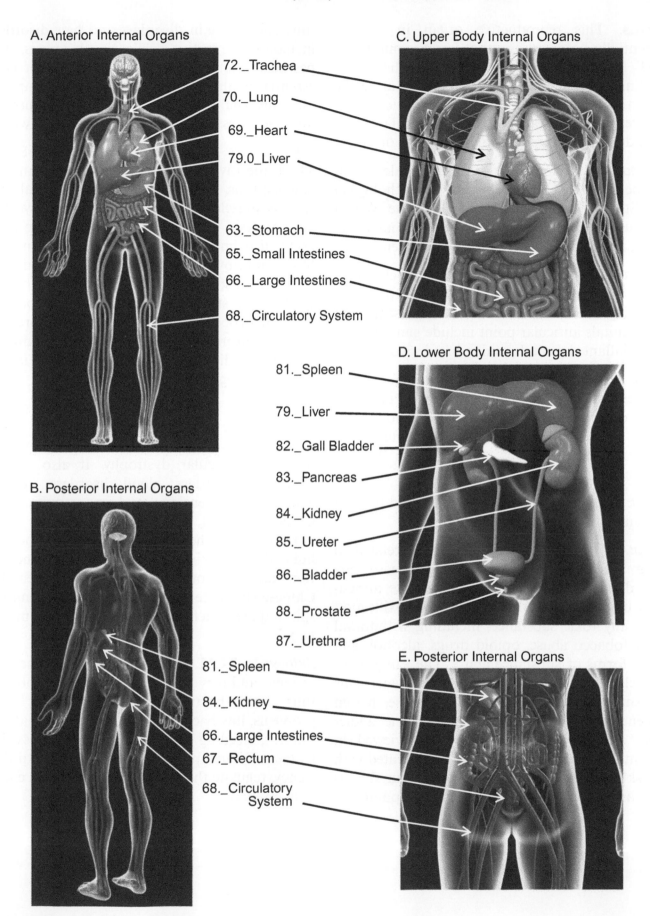

A. Anterior Internal Organs

72._Trachea
70._Lung
69._Heart
79.0_Liver
63._Stomach
65._Small Intestines
66._Large Intestines
68._Circulatory System

B. Posterior Internal Organs

81._Spleen
84._Kidney
66._Large Intestines
67._Rectum
68._Circulatory System

C. Upper Body Internal Organs

D. Lower Body Internal Organs

81._Spleen
79._Liver
82._Gall Bladder
83._Pancreas
84._Kidney
85._Ureter
86._Bladder
88._Prostate
87._Urethra

E. Posterior Internal Organs

FIGURE 7.17 Identification of terms for internal organs of the body.

Uterus: This reproductive organ in females potentially holds an egg that has become fertilized. If fertilization does not occur, the vascular lining of the uterus is discharged during the menstrual period. Pathological conditions that are represented on the Uterus auricular point include infertility and perimenstrual syndrome.

Vagina: This reproductive organ in females serves as the antechamber to the uterus. Pathological conditions that are represented on the Vagina auricular point include vaginitis, vaginal infections, and reduced sexual desire in women.

Genitals: The penis in the male and the clitoris in the female are used during sexual performance. Pathological conditions that are represented on the Genitals auricular point include genital infections, inflamed genitals, and reduced sexual desire.

TCM Five Element Functions: Traditional Chinese Medicine has designated energetic functions of specific organs that are not necessarily related to the physiological function of these internal organs as understood in Western conventional medicine.

Heart: The Heart auricular point is used to calm the mind and enhance one's spirit.

Lung: In TCM, the Lung points are related to drug detoxification because they release carbon dioxide with each exhalation. The auricular Lung point can thus facilitate detoxification from any toxic substance, including withdrawal from tobacco abuse, opioid drugs, alcohol, and other forms of substance abuse. The Lung point is included in auriculotherapy treatment plans for smoking withdrawal, alcohol abuse, heroin dependence, opiate withdrawal, cocaine addiction, and amphetamine abuse. As viewed in Oriental medicine, lung qi is also associated with the skin because we breathe through our skin as well as our lungs. Treating the Lung point can thus alleviate skin disorders and hair disorders, including dermatitis, urticaria, psoriasis, herpes zoster, and shingles. The Lung point is an essential analgesic point used for auricular acupuncture analgesia. Finally, this point is used to disperse excess lung qi and dispel invasive wind.

Liver: Insert Liver text from page 268: "In TCM, the Liver affects tendons, sinews, and ligaments; thus, this ear point is used to heal joint sprains, muscles strains, muscle spasms, myasthenia paralysis, and soft tissue injuries. The Liver point also improves blood circulation, enriches blood, improves eyesight, and relieves fainting, digestive disorders, convulsions, and paralysis due to a stroke. The auricular Liver point is used for hypochondriac pain, dizziness, premenstrual syndrome, and hypertension. According to Oriental medicine, the Liver nourishes Yin and restrains Yang by purging Liver Fire.

Spleen: "In TCM, the Spleen nourishes muscles; thus, the Spleen ear point is used to relieve muscle tension, muscle spasms, muscular atrophy, and muscular dystrophy. It also relieves lymphatic disorders, blood disorders, anemia, abdominal distension, and menstruation. In Chinese thought, the Spleen governs the transportation and the transformation of food and fluid, thus affecting digestive disorders, indigestion, gastritis, stomach ulcers, and diarrhea. The Chinese stimulate the Spleen point to strengthen spleen qi, stomach qi, and to regulate the middle jiao."

Kidney: In TCM, the Kidney affects bone conditions, auditory function, and hair problems; thus, it can be used for bone fractures, tooth problems, low back pain, ear disorders, deafness, tinnitus, bleeding gums, hair loss, and stress. The Chinese Kidney point can tonify kidney qi deficiency, regulate the passage of fluids , and enrich vital essence.

Digestive System Found in the Concha Region around Helix Root

No.	Auricular Microsystem Point (Alternative Name)	[Auricular Zone]

60.0 Mouth *(Fauces, Soft Palate)* [IC 6]

Location: Found on the inferior concha, next to the ear canal and below the helix root.

Function: Representing the soft tissue lining of the inner mouth, gums, and tongue, this ear point relieves eating disorders, mouth ulcers, cold sores, and glossitis.

61.0 Esophagus [IC 7]

Location: Found on the inferior concha, peripheral to the Mouth point.

Function: Representing the long tube that connects the mouth to the stomach, this ear point relieves indigestion, acid reflux, difficulty swallowing, epigastric obstructions, hiccups, and sore throats.

62.0 Esophageal Sphincter *(Cardia, Cardiac Orifice)* [IC 7]

Location: Found on the inferior concha, below LM_0, and below the central concha ridge.

Function: Representing the opening between the esophagus and the stomach, this ear point relieves indigestion, acid reflux, stomach heartburn, hiatal hernias, nausea, vomiting, difficulty swallowing, and GERD.

63.0 Stomach [CR 1, PC 2]

Location: Found on the medial concha ridge, just peripheral to LM_0. Control of the smooth muscle activity of the Stomach is also affected by stimulating the posterior concha region behind the concha ridge.

Function: Relieves eating disorders, overeating, poor appetite, diarrhea, indigestion, nausea, vomiting, stomach ulcers, gastritis, and stomach cancer. It also alleviates toothaches, headaches, and stress. It is the most commonly used auricular point for appetite control and weight reduction. However, treating this ear point only diminishes the physiological craving for food when one is on a diet plan. It does not override one's will. If there is not a conscientious effort to reduce food intake and increase physical exercise, the Stomach point on the ear is insufficient to reduce obesity. In TCM, this point reduces stomach fire excess.

64.0 Duodenum [SC 1, PC 3]

Location: Found on the superior concha, above the concha ridge Stomach point.

Function: Representing the opening from the stomach to the small intestines, this ear point relieves duodenal ulcers, duodenal cancers, diarrhea, and eating disorders.

65.0 Small Intestines *(Jejunum, Ileum)* [SC 2, PC 3]

Location: Found on the medial superior concha, near the helix root.

Function: Representing the long, winding tubes that absorb digested food, this ear point relieves diarrhea, indigestion, malnutrition, and abdominal distention.

| No. | Auricular Microsystem Point *(Alternative Name)* | [Auricular Zone] |

66.0   Large Intestines *(Colon)*   [SC 3 & SC 4, PC 4]

Location: Found on the central, narrow portion of the most medial, superior concha.

Function: Representing the ascending, descending, and transverse colons that move digested food refuse released toward the rectum after the nutritional aspects of food have been absorbed by the small intestines, this ear point relieves diarrhea, constipation, colitis, hemorrhoids, enteritis, and loose bowels.

67.c   Rectum {C} *(Lower Segment of Rectum)*   [HX 3]

Location: Found on the external surface of the helix root, above the Large Intestines point in the superior concha below.

Function: Representing the final portion of the rectum, this ear point relieves diarrhea, constipation, rectal sores, hemorrhoids, hernias, colitis, fecal incontinence, and dysentery.

67.e   Rectum {E} *(Anus, Hemorrhoid Point)*   [IH 2/SC 4, PC 4]

Location: Found on the innermost aspect of superior concha, where the internal helix and the inferior crus meet.

Auricular Microsystem Reflex Points and Yang Meridians: All yang meridians connect directly to the ear and vice versa. Stimulation of the Stomach, Small Intestines, and Large Intestines points on the external ear can alleviate qi stagnation, qi deficiency, or overactivity of qi respectively associated with the stomach, small intestine, and large intestine meridian channels.

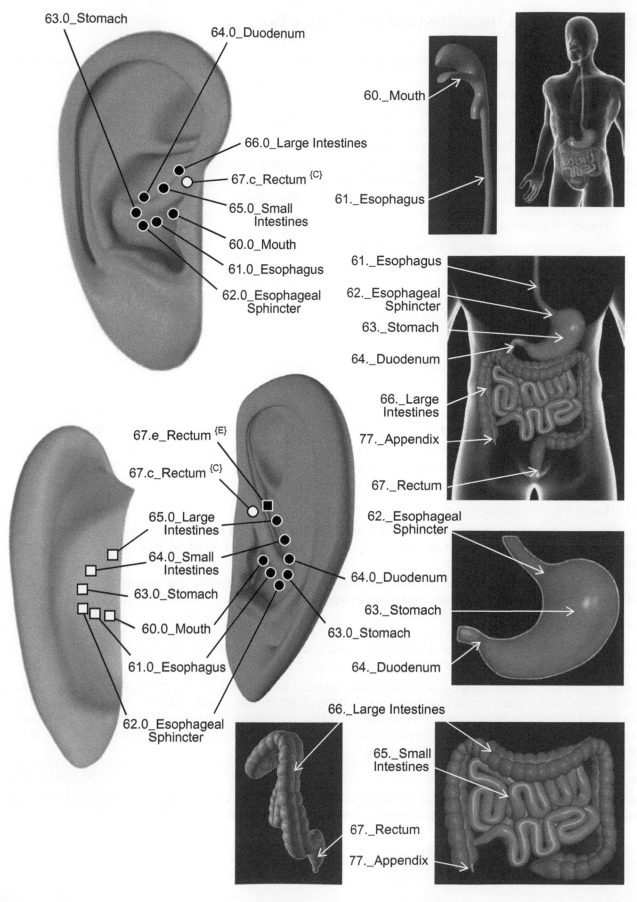

63.0_Stomach

64.0_Duodenum

66.0_Large Intestines

67.c_Rectum {C}

65.0_Small Intestines

60.0_Mouth

61.0_Esophagus

62.0_Esophageal Sphincter

60._Mouth

61._Esophagus

67.e_Rectum {E}

67.c_Rectum {C}

65.0_Large Intestines

64.0_Small Intestines

63.0_Stomach

60.0_Mouth

61.0_Esophagus

62.0_Esophageal Sphincter

64.0_Duodenum

63.0_Stomach

61._Esophagus

62._Esophageal Sphincter

63._Stomach

64._Duodenum

66._Large Intestines

77._Appendix

67._Rectum

62._Esophageal Sphincter

63._Stomach

64._Duodenum

66._Large Intestines

65._Small Intestines

67._Rectum

77._Appendix

FIGURE 7.18 Gastrointestinal organs represented on the auricle.

Thoracic Organs Represented on Inferior Concha

No.	Auricular Microsystem Point *(Alternative Name)*	[Auricular Zone]

68.e   Circulatory System *(Cardiovascular Blood Vessels)*   [CW 2–CW 9]

Location: The primary blood vessels are found all along the concha wall below the antihelix and the antitragus ridge. The arteries and veins are widely distributed throughout the body, found in every area of the auricle where the somatotopic image of the body area is represented.

Function: This auricular region represents the peripheral arteries and veins and the sympathetic nerves that control vasoconstriction and vasodilation. This set of auricular points relieves coronary disorders, heart attacks, hypertension, circulatory problems, cold hands, cold feet, arthrosclerosis, and anemia.

69.c^1 Heart $^{\{C1\}}$ *(Coronary Point)*   [IC 4, PC 2]

Location: Found in the deepest, most central area of the inferior concha.

Function: This ear point Relieves heart palpitations, tachycardia, arrhythmias, chest pain, angina, hypertension, hypotension, post-heart attack dysfunctions, and poor blood circulation. In TCM, the heart functions to tranquilize the mind it can thus be used to relieve anxiety, insomnia, neurasthenia, poor memory, perspiration, and night sweats and to regulate blood and reduce heart fire excess.

69.c^2 Heart $^{\{C2\}}$ *(Cardiac Point)*   [TG 5]

Location: Found on the superior tragus, near LM_11.

69.e   Heart $^{\{E\}}$ [AH 3, PG 4]

Location: This mesodermal coronary organ is found on the middle range of the antihelix body. The motor control of cardiac muscle is represented on the posterior groove, immediately behind the Heart point on the antihelix body.

Function: The European Heart point on the antihelix body is used to relieve physiological disorders such as heart palpitations, tachycardia, arrhythmias, chest pain, angina, hypertension, hypotension, post-heart attack dysfunctions, and poor blood circulation.

70.c^1 Lung 1 *(Contralateral Lung)*   [IC 4/IC 5]

Location: Found on the peripheral region of the inferior concha, below the concha ridge. Nogier contended that the lungs were located throughout the inferior concha. The Chinese limit the Lung 1 point to that region of the inferior concha peripheral to the Heart point.

Function: Relieves respiratory disorders such as asthma, bronchitis, pneumonia, emphysema, coughs, tuberculosis, sore throats, edema, chest stuffiness, and night sweats.

70.c^2 Lung 2 *(Ipsilateral Lung)*   [IC 4/IC 2]

Location: Found on the lower region of the inferior concha, inferior to the Chinese Heart point. In Nogier's work, he states that the whole inferior concha represents the lungs.

Function: Like the Chinese Lung 1 point, this second ear point for the lungs relieves problems related to all respiratory disorders, addiction disorders, and skin disorders. Although some texts state that the Chinese Lung 1 point is more often used for respiratory disorders and the Chinese Lung 2 point is more often used for addiction disorders, both Lung points seem to be equally effective for either type of health problem. The more critical variable is to determine which Lung point is more electrically conductive.

70.e   Lungs $^{\{E\}}$ [IC 2, IC 4, IC 5, IC 7]

Location: This endodermal organ is found throughout the inferior concha of Territory 2. The Nogier representation of the lung in the inferior concha incorporates the Chinese ear points for Lung 1, Lung 2, and Bronchi.

No.	Auricular Microsystem Point *(Alternative Name)*	[Auricular Zone]

71.c   Bronchi   [IC 7]

Location: Found on the upper region of the inferior concha, near the Esophagus point.

Function: This ear point is considered a third Chinese Lung point. It is used to relieve bronchitis, bronchial asthma, pneumonia, and coughs and helps dispel excess phlegm.

72.0   Trachea *(Windpipe)*   [IC 3]

Location: Found on the central region of the inferior concha, near the ear canal.

Function: Relieves sore throats, hoarse voice, laryngitis, common cold, and coughs with profuse sputum. It also dispels phlegm.

73.c   Pharynx {C} *(Throat Lining)*   [ST 4]

Location: Found on subtragus, underneath LM_10 and LM_11, above the ear canal.

Function: Relieves sore throats, hoarse voice, pharyngitis, tonsillitis, asthma, and bronchitis.

73.e   Pharynx {E} *(Throat Lining, Epiglottis)*   [IC 3]

Location: Found on edge of inferior concha that is next to the ear canal.

74.c   Larynx {C} *(Voice Box)*   [ST 4]

Location: Found on the underside of the subtragus, immediately above the ear canal.

Function: Relieves laryngitis, sore throats, and problems with vocalization.

74.e   Larynx {E} *(Voice Box)*   [IC 3]

Location: The voice box is found on the inferior concha, near the ear canal.

| No. | Auricular Microsystem Point *(Alternative Name)* | [Auricular Zone] |

75.c¹   Tonsil 1   [HX 9]

Location: Found on top of superior helix, peripheral to LM_2.

Function: Relieves tonsillitis, sore throats, laryngitis, pharyngitis, and acute inflammations. The whole helix tail is used in Chinese auricular treatment plans for alleviating inflammatory conditions, allergies, and immune system disorders.

75.c²   Tonsil 2   [HX 14]

Location: Found on the middle section of the helix tail, peripheral to LM_15.

75.c³   Tonsil 3   [HX 15]

Location: Found on the curve of the helix tail, where it joins the lobe at LM_6.

75.c⁴   Tonsil 4   [LO 3]

Location: Found on the bottom of the lobe, near LM_7.

75.e   Tonsil {E}   [SF 1]

Location: Found at the base of scaphoid fossa, near LM_6.

76.c   Diaphragm {C}   [HX 2]

Location: Found on the helix root, diagonally above LM_0.

Function: Relieves hiccups, diaphragmatic spasms, and visceral bleeding.

76.e   Diaphragm {E}   [IC 8/CR 2]

Location: Found on the peripheral inferior concha and the concha ridge.

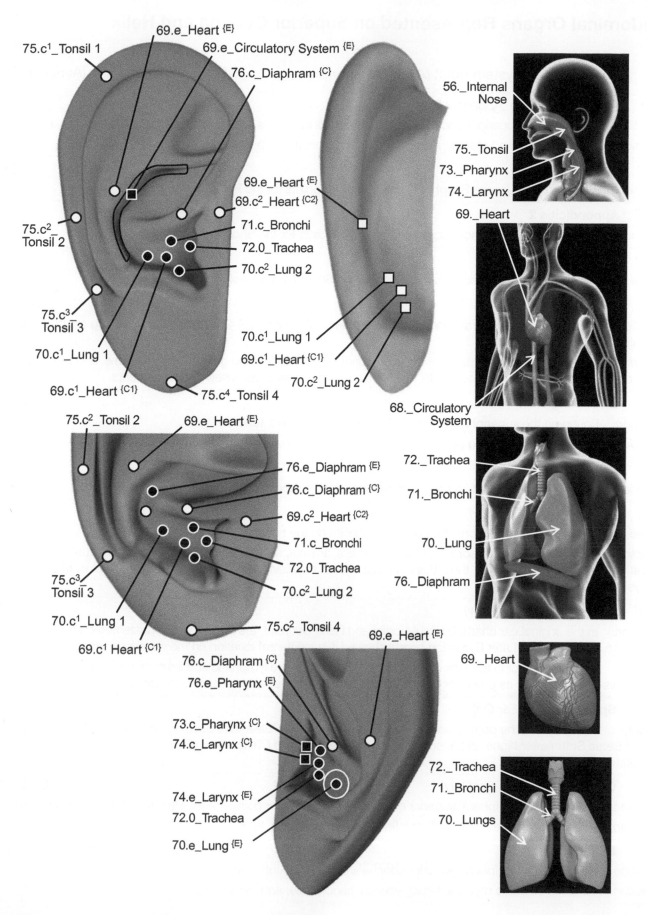

FIGURE 7.19 Thoracic organs represented on the auricle.

Abdominal Organs Represented on Superior Concha and Helix

No.	Auricular Microsystem Point *(Alternative Name)*	[Auricular Zone]

77.0   Appendix *(Primary Appendix Point)* [SC 1/SC 2]

Location: Found on the superior concha, between the Small Intestines and Large Intestines points on the auricle.

Function: Relieves acute and chronic appendicitis, toxic scars from appendectomy.

78.c¹   Appendicitis 1 [SF 6]

Location: Found on the superior Scaphoid Fossa, near ear points for the Fingers.

78.c²   Appendicitis 2 [SF 3]

Location: Found on the middle scaphoid fossa, near ear points for the Shoulder.

78.c³   Appendicitis 3 [SF 1]

Location: Found on the inferior scaphoid fossa, near the Shoulder Joint point.

79.0   Liver [CR 2, PP 6]

Location: Found on the peripheral concha ridge, between LM_19 and LM_20, sometimes occurring on the concha wall next to the concha ridge.

Function: Relieves hepatitis, cirrhosis of the liver, jaundice, alcoholism, and gall bladder problems, and regulates blood disorders, hypertension, and anemia. In TCM, the Liver affects tendons, sinews, and ligaments.

80.c¹   Liver Yang 1 [HX 10]

Location: Found on the superior helix, at LM_3, superior to Darwin's Tubercle.

Function: In TCM, the Liver Yang points calm the liver and suppress yang excess and hyperactivity.

80.c²   Liver Yang 2 [HX 11]

Location: Found on the helix tail, at LM_4, inferior to Darwin's Tubercle.

81.c   Spleen {C} *(Left Ear Only)* [IC 8, PC 3]

Location: Found on inferior concha, below the Liver point on the concha ridge.

Function: Relieves lymphatic disorders, blood disorders, anemia, abdominal distension, and menstruation. In TCM, the Spleen nourishes muscles; thus, this ear point is used to relieve muscle tension, muscle spasms, and muscular dystrophy.

81.e¹   Spleen {E1} *(Left Ear Only)* [SC 8]

Location: In the original ear charts by Paul Nogier and René Bourdiol, the Spleen was represented on the superior concha above LM_20. Later European charts showed it in a different location on the superior concha.

Function: Western medicine focuses on the role of the spleen in the lymphatic and immune systems; thus, Europeans use this point solely for its physiological rather than its energetic effects according to Oriental medicine.

81.e²   Spleen {E2} *(Left Ear Only)* [SC 6]

Location: In contrast to the original ear charts by Paul Nogier, the Spleen has been represented by Raphael Nogier and Beate Strittmatter higher in the superior concha, between the Chinese ear point for the Kidney and the Small Intestines point.

82.0   Gall Bladder *(Right Ear Only)* [SC 8, PC 3]

Location: Found on the peripheral superior concha, between the ear points for the Pancreas and the Duodenum.

Function: Relieves gallstones, gall bladder inflammations, deafness, tinnitus, and migraines.

83.0   Pancreas [SC 7 & CW 7, PC 4]

Location: Found on the peripheral superior concha and the adjacent concha wall.

Function: Relieves diabetes mellitus, hypoglycemia, pancreatitis, and dyspepsia.

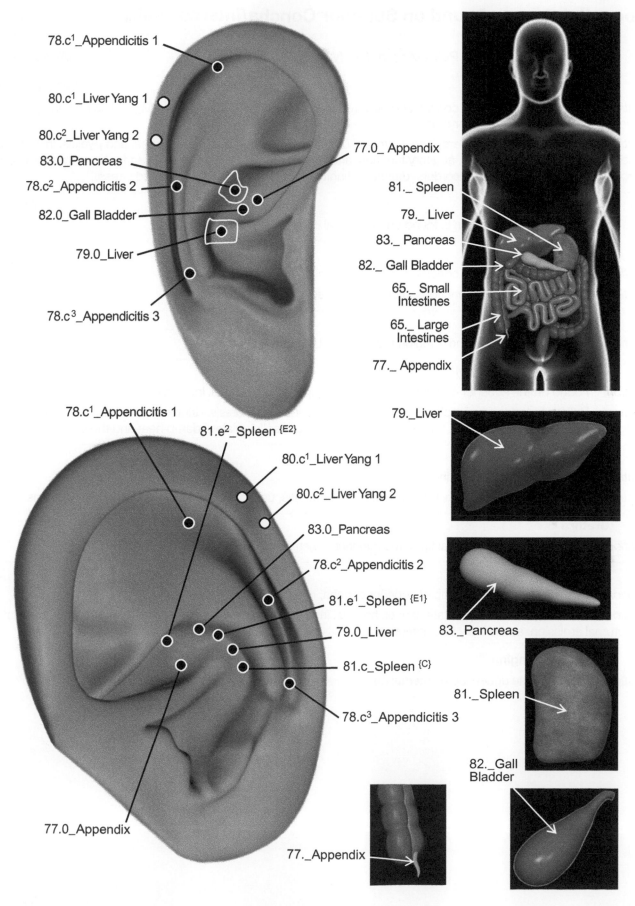

[**FIGURE 7.20** Abdominal organs represented on the auricle.

Urogenital Organs Found on Superior Concha/Internal Helix

No.	Auricular Microsystem Point (Alternative Name)	[Auricular Zone]

84.c   Kidney {C}   [SC 6/CW 8. PL 4]

Location: Found on the superior concha and nearby concha wall, immediately below LM_16. It is hidden by the overhanging ledge of the inferior crus.

Function: Relieves kidney disorders, kidney stones, urination problems, nephritis, diarrhea, and pyelitis. In TCM, the Kidney affects bone conditions, auditory function, and hair problems; thus, it can be used for bone fractures, tooth problems, low back pain, ear disorders, deafness, tinnitus, bleeding gums, hair loss, and stress.

84.e   Kidney {E}   [IH 4 & IH 5]

Location: This mesodermal organ is found on the medial internal helix of Territory 1.

85.c   Ureter {C}   [SC 6]

Location: Found on the superior concha, between the Chinese Kidney and Bladder points.

Function: Relieves bladder dysfunctions, urinary tract infections, and kidney stones.

85.e   Ureter {E}   [IH 4]

Location: Found on the internal helix region that overlies LM_18.

86.0   Bladder (*Urinary Bladder*)   [SC 5]

Location: Found on the superior concha, below LM_17, superior to the Small Intestines.

Function: Relieves bladder dysfunctions, cystitis, frequent urination, enuresis, dripping or retention of urine, bedwetting, pyelitis, and sciatica, migraines. In TCM, the bladder "regulates" damp heat and the Lower Jiao.

87.c   Urethra {C}   [HX 3]

Location: Found on the helix root, inferior to LM_1.

Function: Relieves painful urination, urethral infections, urethritis, urinary incontinence, and bladder problems.

87.e   Urethra {E}   [SC 4]

Location: Found on the most medial tip of the superior concha.

88.c   Prostate {C}   [SC 4]

Location: Found on the innermost tip of superior concha, near the European Urethra point.

Function: Relieves prostatitis, prostate cancer, hernias, impotency problems, painful urination, premature ejaculation, nocturnal emission, and urinary tract infection.

88.e   Prostate {E}/Vagina {E}   [IH 2]

Location: Found on the underside of internal helix.

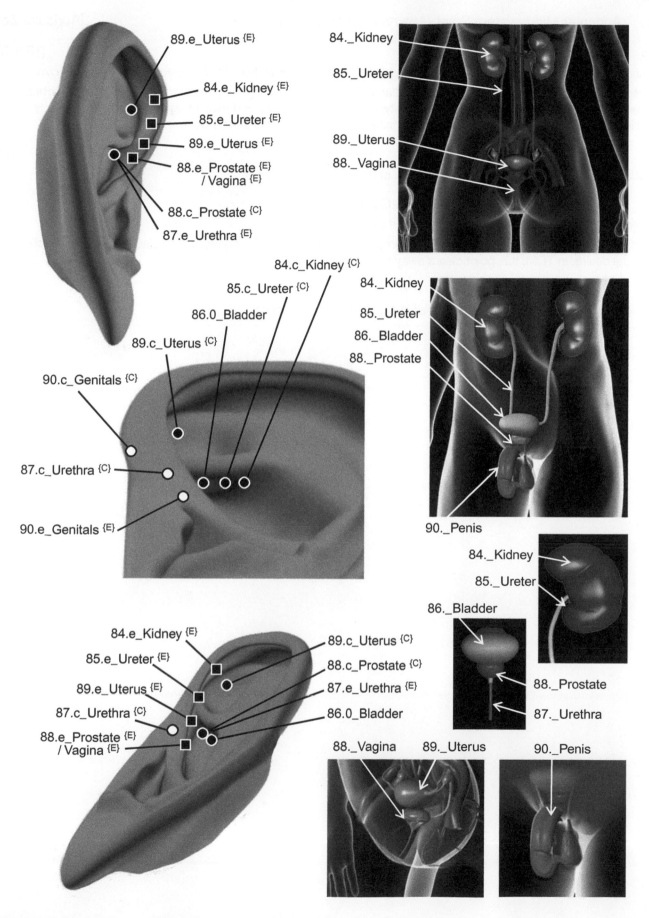

89.e_Uterus {E}

84.e_Kidney {E}

85.e_Ureter {E}

89.e_Uterus {E}

88.e_Prostate {E} / Vagina {E}

88.c_Prostate {C}

87.e_Urethra {E}

84._Kidney

85._Ureter

89._Uterus

88._Vagina

84.c_Kidney {C}

85.c_Ureter {C}

86.0_Bladder

89.c_Uterus {C}

90.c_Genitals {C}

87.c_Urethra {C}

90.e_Genitals {E}

84._Kidney

85._Ureter

86._Bladder

88._Prostate

90._Penis

84._Kidney

85._Ureter

86._Bladder

88._Prostate

87._Urethra

84.e_Kidney {E}

85.e_Ureter {E}

89.e_Uterus {E}

87.c_Urethra {C}

88.e_Prostate {E} / Vagina {E}

89.c_Uterus {C}

88.c_Prostate {C}

87.e_Urethra {E}

86.0_Bladder

88._Vagina   89._Uterus

90._Penis

FIGURE 7.21 Urogenital organs represented on the auricle.

No.   Auricular Microsystem Point *(Alternative Name)*   [Auricular Zone]

89.c   Uterus {C}   [TF 5/TF 6]

Location: Found on the central aspects of the triangular fossa, across from the European Kidney point above it.

Function: Relieves premenstrual problems, inflammations of uteral lining, irregular menstruation, dysmenorrhea, uterine bleeding, sexual dysfunctions, infertility, pregnancy problems, and miscarriages and can induce early childbirth deliveries. In TCM, this point replenishes Kidney qi and nourishes essence.

89.e   Uterus {E} *(Fallopian Tubes)*   [IH 3]

Location: This point is found on the underside of the internal helix root.

90.c   Genitals {C} *(Penis or Clitoris, External Genitals)*   [HX 4]

Location: Found on the helix region that leaves the face, at LM_1.

Function: Relieves scrotal rashes, groin pain, impotency, low back pain, and premature ejaculation, and it facilitates sexual desire. In TCM, this point clears away heat and dampness.

90.e   Genitals {E} *(Penis or Clitoris, External Genitals, Bosch Point)*   [HX 1]

Location: Found on the helix root area that is adjacent to the superior tragus.

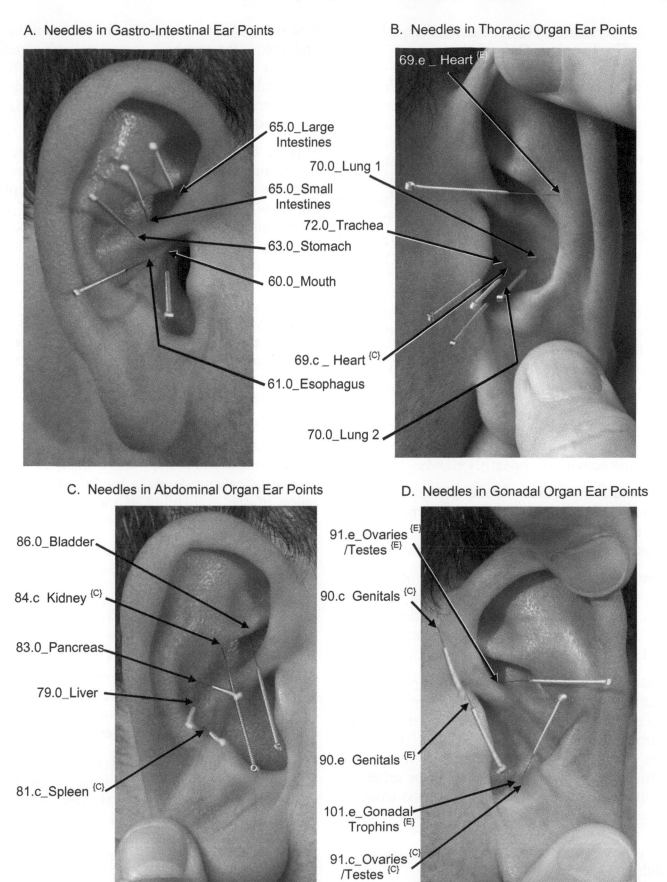

A. Needles in Gastro-Intestinal Ear Points

65.0_Large Intestines

65.0_Small Intestines

63.0_Stomach

60.0_Mouth

61.0_Esophagus

B. Needles in Thoracic Organ Ear Points

69.e _ Heart {E}

70.0_Lung 1

72.0_Trachea

69.c _ Heart {C}

70.0_Lung 2

C. Needles in Abdominal Organ Ear Points

86.0_Bladder

84.c Kidney {C}

83.0_Pancreas

79.0_Liver

81.c_Spleen {C}

D. Needles in Gonadal Organ Ear Points

91.e_Ovaries /Testes {E}

90.c Genitals {C}

90.e Genitals {E}

101.e_Gonadal Trophins {E}

91.c_Ovaries /Testes {C}

FIGURE 7.22 Photographs of acupuncture needles inserted into internal organ points.

7.4 Auricular Representation of Endocrine Glands

The endocrine glands are referred to as the internal secretion system because chemical hormones manufactured and released by these glands are secreted directly into the circulatory system. In the blood vessels, they are carried to all other parts of the body and exert some selective effect on specific target cells. Chemical substances released by the hypothalamus at the base of the brain are sent to cells in the pituitary gland beneath the hypothalamus. The pituitary gland subsequently releases tropic hormones that have selective action on target glands along the midline of the body. The target glands are directed to release their own hormones, depending on the level of tropic hormone received from the pituitary gland. Sensors in the hypothalamus monitor the blood levels of each target hormone circulating in the blood and determine whether the hypothalamus directs the pituitary to release more or less tropic hormones to activate or suppress the activity of the target glands.

Hypothalamic–Pituitary Axis (HPA): This term refers to the central role of the hypothalamus that controls the anterior pituitary to release hormones that control the target endocrine glands.

Anterior Pituitary: This anterior part of the pituitary gland contains only chemical secretory cells, which can release adrenocorticotrophins (ACTH), thyrotrophins (TSH), gonadotrophins (FSH, LH), endorphins, or growth hormone.

Posterior Pituitary: This posterior part of the pituitary gland contains special neurons that descend from the hypothalamus and secrete anti-diuretic hormone or oxytocin into the blood. The anti-diuretic hormone ADH directs the kidneys to reabsorb more water from urine and return that water to the general bloodstream to increase overall fluid level. Oxytocin induces uterine contractions during childbirth and has been associated with empathetic bonding in adults.

Pineal Gland: This gland lies above the midbrain and below the cerebral cortex, releasing melatonin at night to facilitate sleep, and it affects the regulation of day–night circadian rhythms. Deficiencies in melatonin are sometimes related to depression as well as sleep disorders.

Thyroid Gland: This gland lies at the base of the throat and releases thyroxin hormone in response to the release of pituitary thyrotrophin hormone. Thyroxin accelerates the rate of cellular metabolism throughout the body, affecting virtually every cell of the body by stimulating enzymes concerned with glucose oxidation. Iron deficiency reduces the ability of the thyroid gland to produce thyroxin, thus leading to goiter. Hyperthyroid activity can lead to Grave's disease, an autoimmune system disorder that causes elevated metabolic rate and nervousness, whereas hypothyroidism produces symptoms of lethargy and depression.

Parathyroid Gland: This gland lies at the base of the throat next to the thyroid gland and releases parathormone into the blood when it senses decreasing calcium levels in the blood. By facilitation of the availability of calcium, parathormone affects nervous system excitability.

Mammary Gland: This gland in the breasts affects milk production in nursing women.

Thymus Gland: This gland lies behind the sternum in the chest and affects the differentiation of basal white blood cells made in the bone marrow into active immune cells. The specific differentiated immune cells can become T-helper cells, T-suppressor cells, or T-killer cells. Impaired Thymus gland activity is related to AIDS/HIV, cancer, and autoimmune problems.

Pancreas Gland: This gland lies next to the stomach and releases the hormone insulin to facilitate the transport of glucose from the bloodstream into individual cells, where it can become available as energy. The pancreas releases the hormone glucagon to promote higher blood glucose levels.

Adrenal Gland: This gland lies at the top of the abdomen, on top "ad" of each "renal" kidney. It is divided into the inner adrenal medulla, which releases the hormone adrenalin in response to activation by sympathetic nerves, and the adrenal cortex, which releases cortisol and other stress-related hormones in response to the pituitary adrenocorticotrophin hormone ACTH.

Gonads: These sex glands lie at the base of the body.

Ovaries: The sex gland in women lies in the pelvic cavity, sequentially releasing estrogen and progesterone in response to the pituitary gonadotrophin

hormones FSH and LH. Estrogen facilitates ovulation and enhances female sex drive, whereas progesterone facilitates implantation of a fertilized egg in the uterus and maternal behavior.

Testes: The sex gland in men releases the hormone testosterone, which increases sex drive, energy level, and aggressiveness. Overly high levels of testosterone, referred to as hypergonadism, lead to precocious sexual development, excessive growth, extreme irritability, and manic behaviors. Low levels of testosterone, referred to as hypogonadism, can lead to low sex drive, lack of energy, and emotional depression.

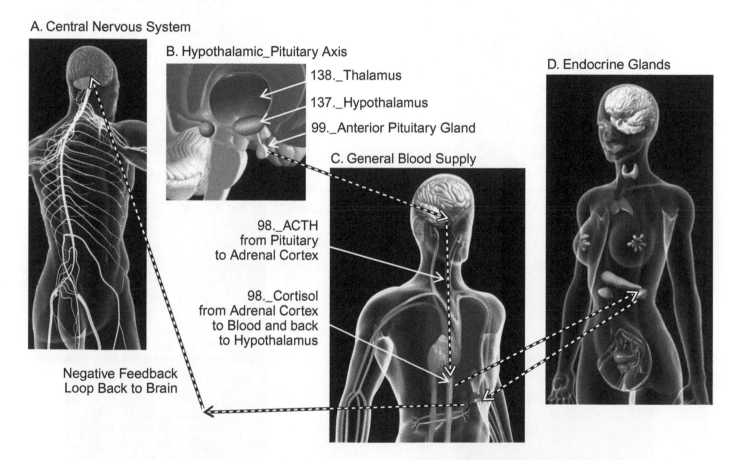

A. Central Nervous System

B. Hypothalamic_Pituitary Axis

138._Thalamus

137._Hypothalamus

99._Anterior Pituitary Gland

C. General Blood Supply

D. Endocrine Glands

98._ACTH from Pituitary to Adrenal Cortex

98._Cortisol from Adrenal Cortex to Blood and back to Hypothalamus

Negative Feedback Loop Back to Brain

FIGURE 7.23 The hypothalamic–pituitary pathway is shown in the brain, endocrine glands, and circulatory system.

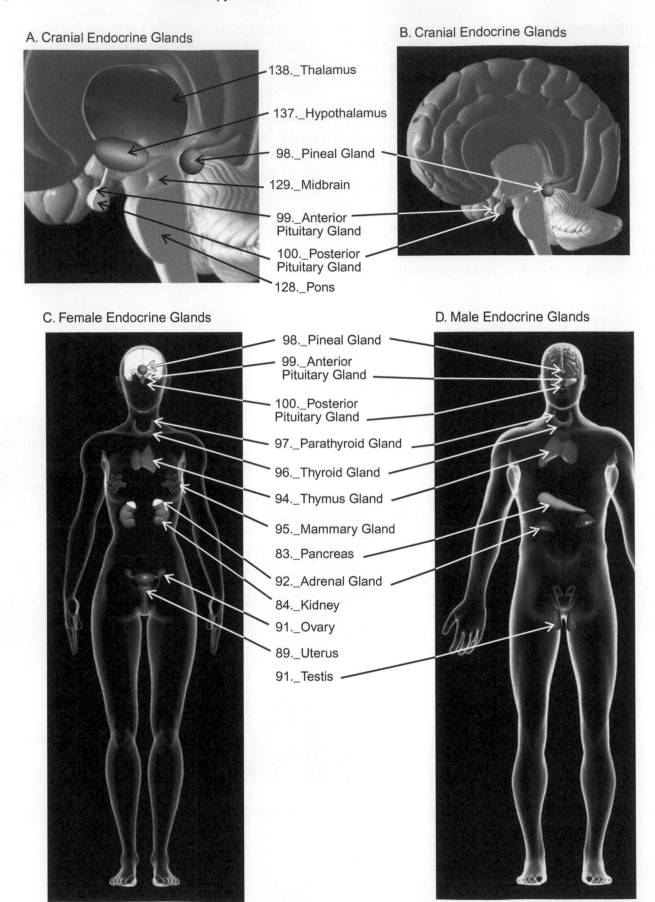

A. Cranial Endocrine Glands

138._Thalamus
137._Hypothalamus
98._Pineal Gland
129._Midbrain
99._Anterior Pituitary Gland
100._Posterior Pituitary Gland
128._Pons

B. Cranial Endocrine Glands

C. Female Endocrine Glands

D. Male Endocrine Glands

98._Pineal Gland
99._Anterior Pituitary Gland
100._Posterior Pituitary Gland
97._Parathyroid Gland
96._Thyroid Gland
94._Thymus Gland
95._Mammary Gland
83._Pancreas
92._Adrenal Gland
84._Kidney
91._Ovary
89._Uterus
91._Testis

FIGURE 7.24 Identification of terms for endocrine glands in the body.

Peripheral Endocrine Glands Represented along the Concha Wall

No.	Auricular Microsystem Point (Alternative Name)	[Auricular Zone]

91.c   Ovaries {C}/Testes {C} (Gonads, Internal Genitals, Sex Glands)   [CW 1]

Location: Found on the concha wall near the intertragic notch. Located toward the bottom of the auricle, this Chinese point is inconsistent with other points that reflect an inverted fetus orientation because the gonads are found toward the base of the body, not the head. In contrast, this point is consistent with the Nogier location for the pituitary gonadal hormones FSH and LH. These two pituitary hormones would be appropriately found on the inferior part of the external ear that represents the head, where the actual pituitary gland is located.

Function: Relieves sexual dysfunctions, testitis, ovaritis, impotency, and frigidity.

91.e   Ovaries {E}/Testes {E} (Gonads, Internal Genitals, Sex Glands)   [IH 1]

Location: This European location for the gonads which lies under the internal helix root more logically corresponds to the inverted fetus model of the external ear because this helix root region of the ear represents other urogenital organs that are found in the lower body, not the head.

92.c   Adrenal Glands {C} (Suprarenal Gland, ACTH)   [TG 2/TG 3]

Location: Found on the prominent knob of the inferior tragus protrusion at LM_10. Because this lower tragal and intertragic notch region of the auricle generally represents tropic hormones released by the pituitary gland, the Chinese Adrenal Gland may actually correspond to the pituitary hormone ACTH that regulates the adrenal cortex. Nogier reported that several points on the auricle represent the release of the adrenal hormone Cortisol; one of those locations occurs at the same region of the tragus as the Chinese location for the Adrenal Glands.

Function: Affects adrenocortical hormones that assist one in dealing with stress. Relieves stress-related disorders, fevers, inflammatory disorders, infections, hypersensitivity, rheumatism, allergies, coughs, asthma, skin disorders, hypertension, hypotensive shock, profuse menstruation, and blood circulation problems. It is used for disturbances of adrenocortical functions, such as Addison's disease and Cushing's syndrome.

92.e   Adrenal Glands {E}   [CW 7]

Location: Found on the concha wall, below LM_16, near the Chinese Kidney point. The actual adrenal glands in the body sit on top "ad" of each "renal" kidney.

93.e   Cortisol   [SC 6]

Location: This hormone is found on the superior concha, below the Chinese Kidney.

Function: This corticosteroid hormone from the adrenal cortex gland is utilized to modulate the effects of stress and reduce inflammations, but prolonged release of cortisol tends to suppress the immune system.

94.e   Thymus Gland   [CW 6]

Location: This endodermal endocrine gland is found on the peripheral concha wall near the Pancreas point.

Function: The thymus gland affects the development of T cells of the immune system. This ear point is used to treat the common cold, flues, allergies, cancer, HIV, AIDS, and autoimmune disorders. This point has anti-inflammatory, anti-rheumatic, and anti-allergic effects by stimulating the immune system.

No.	Auricular Microsystem Point (Alternative Name)	[Auricular Zone]

95.c   Mammary Glands {C}   [AH 10]

Location: Found on each side of the antihelix body, just superior to the antihelix tail.

Function: This point is used to treat problems with milk secretion, breast development, or breast cancer.

95.e   Mammary Glands {E}   [CW 5]

Location: Found on the concha wall above the concha ridge, central to Chinese Mammary points.

96.c   Thyroid Glands {C}   [AH 8]

Location: Found on the antihelix tail, alongside the scaphoid fossa.

Function: Thyroxin that is released by the Thyroid Gland affects overall metabolic rate and general arousal. Relieves hyperthyroidism, hypothyroidism, goiter, and sore throats.

96.e   Thyroid Glands {E}   [CW 5]

Location: This endocrine gland is found on the concha wall, above the junction of the concha ridge and the inferior concha at LM_20.

97.e   Parathyroid Glands   [CW 4]

Location: Found on the concha wall, inferior to the European Thyroid point.

Function: The parathyroid gland affects calcium metabolism. This point relieves muscle cramps, muscle spasms, weak bones, and frequent fractures.

Cranial Endocrine Glands Represented at Intertragic Notch

No.	Auricular Microsystem Point (Alternative Name)	[Auricular Zone]

98.e   Pineal Gland (Epiphysis, Point E)   [TG 1]

Location: Found on the most inferior aspects of the tragus, at LM_9.

Function: The pineal gland releases melatonin hormone to affect circadian rhythm and day–night cycles. This ear point is used to relieve jet lag, irregular sleep patterns, insomnia, and depression.

99.c   Pituitary Gland {C}   [CW 3]

Location: Found on the edge of the junction of the concha wall and the apex of the antitragus, between LM_13 and LM_14.

Function: The Pituitary is the master endocrine gland, releasing pituitary hormones to control the release of hormones from all other endocrine glands. This ear point relieves hypersensitivity, allergies, rheumatism, skin diseases, reproductive disorders, menstrual distress, diseases of blood vessels, and digestive disorders.

99.e   Anterior Pituitary {E} (Adenohypophysis, Internal Secretion, Master Gland)   [IC 1]

Location: Found on the most inferior part of inferior concha, below the intertragic notch.

Function: The Anterior Pituitary is considered the master endocrine gland, releasing pituitary hormones to regulate the release of hormones from all other endocrine glands. This ear point relieves hypersensitivity, allergies, rheumatism, skin diseases, reproductive disorders, menstrual distress, diseases of blood vessels, and digestive disorders.

100.e   Posterior Pituitary {E} (Neurohypophysis)   [IC 3]

Location: Found on the inferior concha near inferior side of the ear canal.

Function: The Posterior Pituitary contains neurons from the hypothalamus, which then releases hormones into the general bloodstream that affect the kidneys. The posterior pituitary releases anti-diuretic hormone that affects thirst, water retention, and salt metabolism.

| No. | Auricular Microsystem Point *(Alternative Name)* | [Auricular Zone] |

101.e   Gonadotrophin Hormones *(FSH, LH, Genital Control Point)*   [CW 1]

Location: Found on concha wall near intertragic notch. It is the same ear point as the Chinese Ovaries and Testes point on the concha wall.

Function: Gonadal pituitary hormones FSH and LH regulate the release of sex hormones by the ovaries or testes. This point relieves sexual dysfunctions, low sex drive, infertility, irregular menstruation, premenstrual syndrome, testitis, ovaritis, fatigue, and depression.

102.e   Thyrotrophin Hormones *(TSH, Thyroid-Stimulating Hormone)*   [IT 2]

Location: Found on the concha wall of the intertragic notch, midway between LM_9 and LM_22.

Function: Thyroidal pituitary hormone TSH regulates the release of thyroxin hormone by the thyroid gland. This ear point reduces metabolic rate, hyperthyroidism, hypothyroidism, hyperactivity, and Grave's disease.

103.e   Parathyrotrophin Hormones *(PSH, Parathyroid-Stimulating Hormone)*   [IT 2]

Location: Found on the most central part of wall of intertragic notch, below LM_9.

Function: The parathyroid pituitary hormone PSH regulates parathormone release by the parathyroid gland. This point facilitates calcium metabolism and reduces muscle tetanus.

104.e   Adrenocorticotrophin Hormones (ACTH) *(Adrenal Control Point)*   [ST 1]

Location: This pituitary gland hormone point is somatotopically found near the intertragic notch and inferior to the Chinese Adrenal point.

Function: This pituitary hormone is activated by the hypothalamus, and once it is released into the general bloodstream, it activates the adrenal cortex gland to release cortisol hormone as part of the body's response to stress. Levels of ACTH and cortisol are regulated by negative feedback by the hypothalamic–pituitary–adrenal axis.

105.e   Prolactin *(LTH)*   [IC 1]

Location: Found on the inferior region of the inferior concha, peripheral to the ear canal.

Function: This pituitary hormone regulates the activity of the mammary glands, initiating lactation and milk secretion.

106.c   Salivary Glands [C] *(Parotid Gland)*   [CW 2]

Location: Found on the concha wall just behind the apex of antitragus, LM_13.

Function: The salivary glands are controlled by the parasympathetic nervous system in response to food. These salivary glands are actually exocrine glands rather than endocrine glands. This point relieves dry mouth, xerostomia, mumps, inflammations of the salivary gland, and skin diseases.

106.e   Salivary Glands [E] *(Parotid Gland)*   [LO 8]

Location: Found on the peripheral region of the lobe, at the base of the scaphoid fossa.

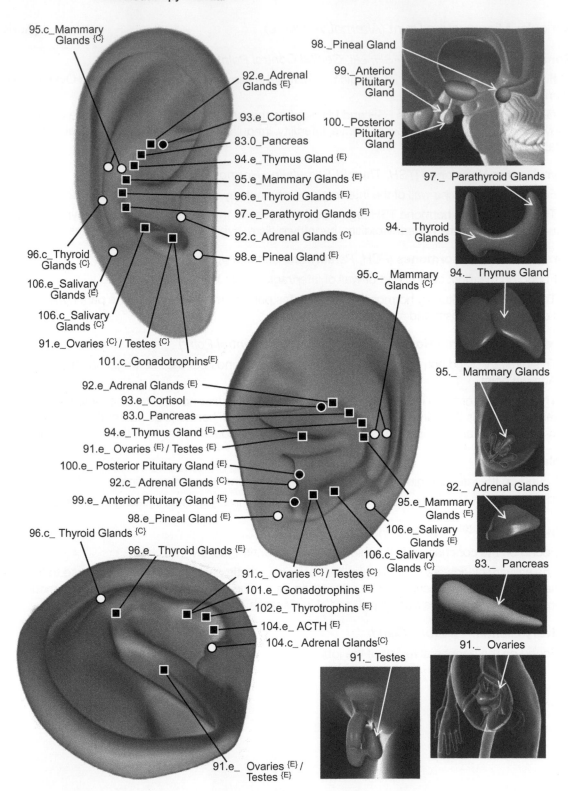

FIGURE 7.25 Endocrine glands represented on the auricle.

7.5 Auricular Representation of Nervous System

The nervous system is primarily represented on the helix and lobe, but it is found throughout all parts of the external ear as the nervous system connects to every part of the body.

Central Nervous System: The core of the nervous system consists of the brain and spinal cord, which respond to and regulate all other parts of the body.

Peripheral Nervous System: The peripheral nerves consist of sensory neurons that send messages to the spinal cord from the skin, muscles, and visceral organs or to motor neurons that travel from the spinal cord out to the muscles and organs of the body.

Somatic Nervous System: This division of the peripheral nervous system consists of sensory neurons that receive afferent messages from the skin and control motor neurons that control the activity of skeletal muscles. The somatic nerves are voluntarily controlled by the more conscious aspects of the pyramidal system of the motor cortex descending to alpha motor neurons that send out impulses to contract striate muscles. Subtle shifts in the manner of movement and in muscle tone are regulated by gamma motor neurons that are modulated by the less conscious, subcortical, extrapyramidal system. Sensory somatic neurons enter the dorsal root of the spinal cord and ascend the dorsal columns of the spinal white matter to synapse in the brainstem, the thalamus, and ultimately arrive at the somatosensory cortex on the post-central gyrus of the parietal lobe. It is the somatic nerves that sustain the pathological reflexes associated with the chronic muscle tension that leads to myofascial pain.

Autonomic Nervous System: This division of the peripheral nervous system consists of those nerves that connect the spinal cord to the visceral organs of the body. This system is regulated unconsciously by the subcortical hypothalamus in the brain. All autonomic nerves leaving the central nervous system have preganglionic nerves that travel from the spinal cord to a peripheral ganglion which synapses onto postganglionic nerves that travel from that ganglion to a visceral organ. Every internal organ sends sensory neurons to the spinal cord or brain, which then send the visceral message to the hypothalamus. Each visceral organ also receives descending motor messages from the hypothalamus.

Sympathetic Nervous System: This subdivision of the autonomic nervous system consists of those autonomic nerves that leave the spinal cord in the region of the thoracic and lumbar vertebrae and travel to a chain of ganglia alongside the spinal vertebrae. From this sympathetic chain, postganglionic nerves branch out to internal organs. Sympathetic nerves cause excitation and arousal of bodily energy in times of stress, strong emotion, or physical exercise. This system leads to an increase in heart rate, blood pressure, vasoconstriction, sweating, and pupillary dilation, accompanied by the release of the hormone adrenalin from the adrenal medulla gland. Sympathetic postganglionic nerves are adrenergic, utilizing the neurotransmitter norepinephrine.

Parasympathetic Nervous System: This subdivision of the autonomic nervous system consists of those autonomic nerves that leave the central nervous system from either the cranium or the sacral vertebrae. These preganglionic nerves travel out into the body and synapse on postganglionic nerves near a visceral organ. Parasympathetic nerves lead to sedation and conservation of bodily energy. They cause decreases in heart rate and blood pressure while producing increases in vasodilation, pupillary constriction, salivation, and digestion of food. Parasympathetic synapses are cholinergic, utilizing the neurotransmitter acetylcholine.

- **Sympathetic Preganglionic Nerves**: These autonomic nerves travel from the thoracic–lumbar spine to the sympathetic chain of ganglia outside the spinal vertebrae.

- **Sympathetic Postganglionic Nerves**: These autonomic nerves travel from the sympathetic chain of ganglia outside the spinal vertebrae to the actual visceral organ.

- **Splanchnic Nerves**: These peripheral, sympathetic nerves connect to lower visceral organs.

A. Anterior, Motor Nerves

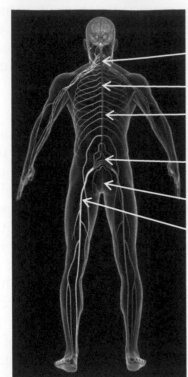

126._Cervical Spinal Cord

125._Thoracic Spinal Cord

112._Solar Plexus

124._Lumbo-Sacral
Spinal Cord

111._Hypogastric Plexus

107._Sciatic Nerve

B. Posterior, Sensory Nerves

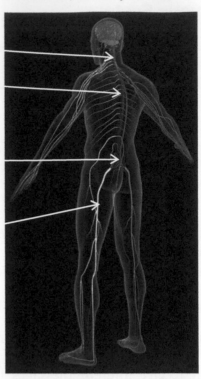

C. Brainstem Nuclei

146._Corpus Callosum

151._Pre-Frontal Cortex

128._Pons

116._Trigeminal Nerve

130._Midbrain
Tegmentum & PAG

133._Red Nucleus

134._Substantia
Nigra

145._Cerebellum

131._Reticular
Formation

126._Cervical
Spinal Cord

D. Peripheral Nerves

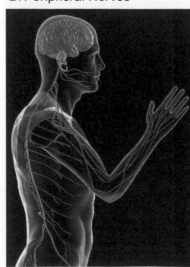

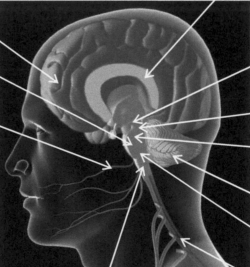

127._Brainstem Medulla Oblongata

FIGURE 7.26 Brainstem, spinal cord, and peripheral nerves in the head and body.

- **Vagus Nerve**: This primary parasympathetic nerve connects to most visceral organs.
- **Sciatic Nerve**: This somatic nerve travels from the lumbar spinal cord down to the leg.
- **Trigeminal Nerve**: This somatic nerve affects sensations of the face and partially controls facial movements.
- **Facial Nerve**: This somatic nerve controls major facial movements.
- **Oculomotor Nerve**: This somatic nerve controls eye movements.
- **Optic Nerve**: This cranial nerve responds to visual sensations from the eye.
- **Olfactory Nerve**: This cranial nerve responds to smell sensations from the nose.
- **Auditory Nerve**: This cranial nerve responds to hearing sensations from the ear and affects one's sense of physical balance and equilibrium.

Central Nervous System Regions of the Brain:
Cortical Brain Regions: This highest level of the brain determines the intellectual processes of thinking, learning, and memory. The cerebral cortex initiates voluntary movements and is consciously aware of sensations and feelings.

- **Prefrontal Cortex**: This most evolved region of the human cortex initiates conscious decisions. It is referred to as the "executive brain" because it is involved in all intentional actions regarding different choices that one takes.
- **Frontal Cortex**: This cortical region contains the pre-central gyrus motor cortex which initiates specific, voluntary movements by activating upper motor neurons in the pyramidal system that send direct neural impulses to lower motor neurons in the spinal cord.
- **Parietal Cortex**: This posterior region contains the somatosensory cortex on the post-central gyrus. This region consciously perceives the sensations of touch and the general awareness of spatial relationships.
- **Temporal Cortex**: This posterior and lateral cortical region contains the hearing centers of the brain. The left temporal lobe processes the verbal meaning of language and the rational logic of math, whereas the right temporal lobe processes the intonation and rhythm of sounds.

- **Occipital Cortex**: This most posterior cortical region processes conscious, visual perceptions. The left occipital lobe can consciously read words, whereas the right occipital lobe is superior at recognizing faces and emotional expressions.
- **Corpus Callosum**: This broad band of myelinated axon fibers connects the left cerebral hemisphere cortical lobes with their respective lobes on the right cerebral hemisphere.

Subcortical Brain Regions: These regions of the brain serve as an intermediary between the cerebral cortex above and the spinal cord below, operating outside of conscious awareness.

- **Cerebellum**: The second largest structure of the brain lies beneath the occipital lobe and above the pons. It is part of the extrapyramidal system control of semivoluntary movements and postural adjustments.
- **Thalamus**: This spherical nucleus relays sensory messages from lower brainstem regions up to a specific locus on the cerebral cortex. The thalamus also contains neurons that participate in the supraspinal gating of pain and modulate general arousal or sedation. The subconscious thalamus is considered the gateway to the conscious cerebral cortex.
- **Anterior Hypothalamus**: This nucleus lies below the thalamus, where it connects to the limbic system, the pituitary gland, and the parasympathetic nervous system. This nucleus produces general sedation.
- **Posterior Hypothalamus**: This nucleus connects to the limbic system and the pituitary gland. It activates the sympathetic nervous system, producing brain arousal and behavioral aggression.
- **Limbic System**: This collection of subcortical nuclei affects emotions and memory.
- **Cingulate Cortex**: This paleocortex limbic region lies immediately beneath the higher neocortex.
- **Hippocampus**: This semicircular limbic structure lies beneath the neocortex but outside the thalamus. It affects attention span,

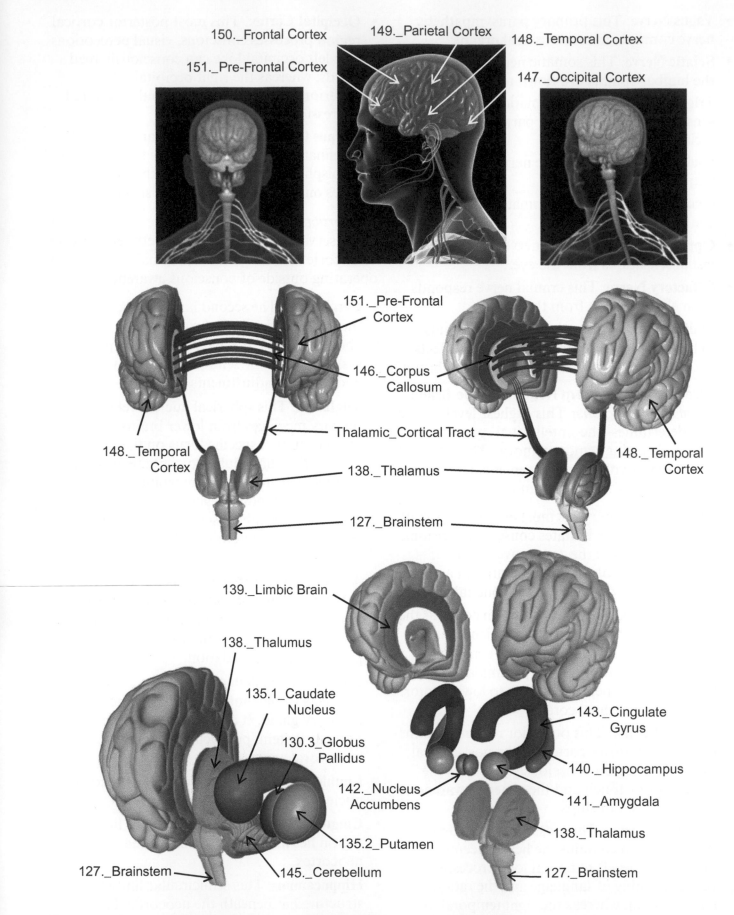

FIGURE 7.27 Cerebral cortex, limbic brain, and striatum structures in the head.

long-term memory storage, and emotional experiences.

- **Amygdala Nucleus**: This spherical limbic nucleus lies under the lateral temporal lobe and modulates increases or decreases in aggressiveness, irritability, and mania.

- **Septal Nucleus**: This medial limbic structure is involved in pleasure and reward.

- **Nucleus Accumbens**: This midline nucleus occurs next to the septal nucleus and is the primary dopaminergic control center for the reward pathways of the brain. It plays a significant role in the brain's response to all substances that are addictive in nature. Neurons in this nucleus are excited by alcohol, opium, cocaine, and methamphetamine. Stimulation of this nucleus produces strong pleasure cravings.

- **Striatum**: These basal ganglia nuclei lie along the limbic system, below the cerebral cortex and outside the thalamus. Specific basal ganglia nuclei include the goat horn-shaped caudate nucleus, the spherical putamen, and the spherical globus pallidus, all of which are part of the extrapyramidal system control of semivoluntary movements.

- **Brainstem**: This term refers to the medulla oblongata of the brainstem. It affects basic unconscious control of body metabolism, respiration, and heart rate.

- **Pons**: This brainstem area lies below the cerebellum and affects REM sleep and dreams.

- **Midbrain Tectum**: This roof of the midbrain contains the superior colliculus and the inferior colliculus, which respectively control visual and auditory reflexes.

- **Midbrain Tegmentum (Ventral Tegmental Area, Periaqueductal Gray)**: This part of the midbrain affects basic metabolism, the dopamine mesolimbic reward pathway, and the inhibition of pain by the periaqueductal gray.

- **Reticular Formation**: This region in the midbrain tegmentum activates general arousal. The nearby raphe nuclei affect the ability to fall asleep.

- **Red Nucleus and Substantia Nigra**: This region within the midbrain tegmentum affects the extrapyramidal system and the striatum, regulating semivoluntary movements. The substantia nigra sends dopaminergic neurons to the striatal nuclei.

Peripheral Nervous System Represented on the Ear

No.	Auricular Microsystem Point (*Alternative Name*)	[Auricular Zone]

107.0   Sciatic Nerve (*Sciatica Point*)   [AH 6]
Location: Found on a notch at the midpoint of antihelix inferior crus, at LM_17.
Function: Relieves sciatic neuralgia, lower limb paralysis, and post-polio syndrome.

108.e   Sympathetic Preganglionic Nerves   [HX 12–HX 14]
Location: Found along the length of the helix tail as it joins the scaphoid fossa.
Function: Relieves reflex sympathetic dystrophy, vasospasms, and neuralgias.

109.e   Sympathetic Postganglionic Chain (*Paravertebral Nerves*)   [CW 5–CW 9]
Location: Found along the length of the concha wall above the superior concha.
Function: Relieves back pain, reflex sympathetic dystrophy, neuralgias, vasospasms, and poor blood circulation.

110.e¹   Parasympathetic Cranial Nerves   [IC 1]
Location: Found in the inferior concha near the intertragic notch landmark LM_22.
Function: Relieves autonomic nervous disorders affecting the upper body and the head.

110.e²   Parasympathetic Sacral Nerves (*Pelvic Splanchnic Nerve*)   [IC 6]
Location: Found in the inferior concha, superior to the ear canal.
Function: Relieves visceral spasms, pelvic pain, and sexual desire.

111.e   Hypogastric Plexus (*Lumbosacral Splanchnic Nerves, Omega 1*)   [SC 4/SC 5]
Location: Found in the central region of the superior concha.
Function: This plexus distributes lumbar sympathetic nerves to the rectum, bladder, ureter, and genital organs. Relieves pelvic dysfunctions, ureter, irritable bladder, and constipation.

112.e   Solar Plexus (*Celiac Plexus, Splanchnic Nerves, Abdominal Brain*)   [HX 1]
Location: Found on the helix root, diagonally above Point Zero and LM_0.
Function: Relieves abdominal dysfunctions, gastrointestinal spasms, and pathology in the viscera of upper abdominal organs, such as the stomach, liver, spleen, pancreas, and adrenal glands.

113.e   Vagus Nerve (*Tenth Cranial Nerve, X n.*)   [IC 3]
Location: Found in the inferior concha, next to the ear canal, and throughout the concha.
Function: The vagus nerve affects parasympathetic nervous system control of most internal organs. This point relieves diarrhea, heart palpitations, and anxiety.

114.e   Auditory Nerve (*Eighth Cranial Nerve, VIII n., Cochleovestibular Nerve*)   [ST 3]
Location: Found on the underside of the subtragus.
Function: Affects hearing and vestibular disorders, deafness, tinnitus, and equilibrium imbalance.

115.e   Facial Nerve (*Seventh Cranial Nerve, VII n., Nucleus of Solitary Tract*)   [PL 6]
Location: Found on the peripheral region of the posterior ear lobe.
Function: Relieves facial muscle spasms, tics, and facial paralysis.

No.	Auricular Microsystem Point *(Alternative Name)*	[Auricular Zone]

116.e   **Trigeminal Nerve** *(Fifth Cranial Nerve, V n.)*   [LO 5, PL 5]

Location: Found along the peripheral edge of the ear lobe.

Function: Relieves trigeminal neuralgia and dental analgesia.

117.e   **Oculomotor Nerve** *(Third Cranial Nerve, III n.)*   [PL 3]

Location: Found along the peripheral edge of the ear lobe.

Function: Affects control of eye movements and relieves eye twitches.

118.e   **Optic Nerve** *(Second Cranial Nerve, II n.)*   [LO 1]

Location: Found on the central side of the ear lobe, inferior to the intertragic notch at LM_9.

Function: Relieves visual disorders and eyesight dysfunctions.

119.e   **Olfactory Nerve** *(First Cranial Nerve, I n.)*   [LO 2]

Location: Found on the central side of the ear lobe, inferior to the intertragic notch at LM_9.

Function: Relieves problems with smell sensations.

120.e   **Inferior Cervical Ganglia** *(Stellate Ganglion, Cervical-Thoracic Ganglia)*   [CW 5]

Location: Found on the junction of the inferior concha ridge and the concha wall.

Function: Affects thoracic sympathetic control, migraines, and whiplash.

121.e   **Middle Cervical Ganglia** *(Wonderful Point, Marvelous Point)*   [CR 2/CW 4]

Location: Found on the junction of the inferior concha and the concha wall.

Function: Balances excessive sympathetic arousal, reduces hypertension, affects blood vascular regulation, and relieves muscle tension, post-concussion syndrome, and reflex sympathetic dystrophy.

122.e   **Superior Cervical Ganglia**   [CW 4]

Location: Found on the junction of inferior concha and concha wall, below LM_14.

Function: Affects cranial sympathetic control, migraines, and facial pain.

123.c   **Minor Occipital Nerve** *(Lesser Occipital Nerve, Windstream)*   [IH 11/SF 5]

Location: Found on the junction of the internal helix with the superior scaphoid fossa.

Function: Alleviates migraine headaches, occipital headaches, blood vessel spasms, post-traumatic brain syndrome, arteriosclerosis, neuralgias, numbness, spondylopathy, neurasthenia, and anxiety. It is used in Chinese ear acupuncture like a master point to tranquilize the mind and clear zang–fu meridian channels.

Spinal Cord and Brainstem Represented on Helix Tail and Lobe

No.   Auricular Microsystem Point *(Alternative Name)*   [Auricular Zone]

124.e   Lumbosacral Spinal Cord   [HX 12, PP 8]

Location: Found on the superior helix tail, below Darwin's tubercle, at LM_4.

Function: The anterior, front side of the helix tail represents the sensory, dorsal horn cells of the lumbosacral spinal cord, whereas the posterior, back side of the helix tail represents motor, ventral horn cells of the lumbosacral spinal cord. This point relieves peripheral neuralgias in the region of the lower limbs, including shingles, post-herpetic neuralgia, sunburns, poison oak, and poison ivy. It is used very effectively with patients who have neuralgic side effects from medication treatment of AIDS or cancer or for diabetic patients with poor peripheral circulation to the feet.

125.e   Thoracic Spinal Cord   [HX 13, PP 6]

Location: Found on the helix tail, peripheral to LM_15.

Function: Anterior side of the helix tail affects sensory neurons of the thoracic spinal cord, whereas the posterior side affects motor neurons of the thoracic spinal cord. Relieves shingles, sunburns, and poison oak or poison ivy on the body or arms.

126.e   Cervical Spinal Cord   [HX 14, PP 4]

Location: Found on the inferior helix tail, above LM_5.

Function: Relieves sunburned neck, neuralgias, shingles, and poison oak on neck. The anterior, front side of the helix tail affects sensory cervical neurons, whereas the posterior, back side affects motor cervical neurons.

127.c   Brainstem [C] *(Medulla Oblongata)*   [CW 4]

Location: Found on the central side of concha wall, just below the base of antihelix, LM_14.

Function: Affects body temperature, respiration, cardiac regulation, shock, meningitis, brain trauma, and hypersensitivity to pain. This point tonifies the brain, invigorates the spirit, arrests epileptic convulsions, reduces overexcitement, abates fever, and calms pathogenic wind.

127.e   Medulla Oblongata [E] *(Brainstem)*   [LO 8, PP 2]

Location: Found on the inferior helix tail, between LM_5 and LM_6.

Function: Affects body temperature, respiration, and cardiac regulation.

128.e   Pons   [LO 7, PL 6]

Location: Found on the peripheral lobe.

Function: Affects sleep and arousal, paradoxical REM sleep, and emotionally reparative dreams, and it relieves insomnia, disturbing dreams, dizziness, and psychosomatic reactions.

129.e   Midbrain Tectum *(Super Colliculus, Inferior Colliculus)*   [LO 6]

Location: Found on the peripheral ear lobe.

Function: The midbrain tectum nuclei include the superior colliculus, which affects subcortical reflexes for visual stimuli, and the inferior colliculus, which affects subcortical reflexes for auditory stimuli.

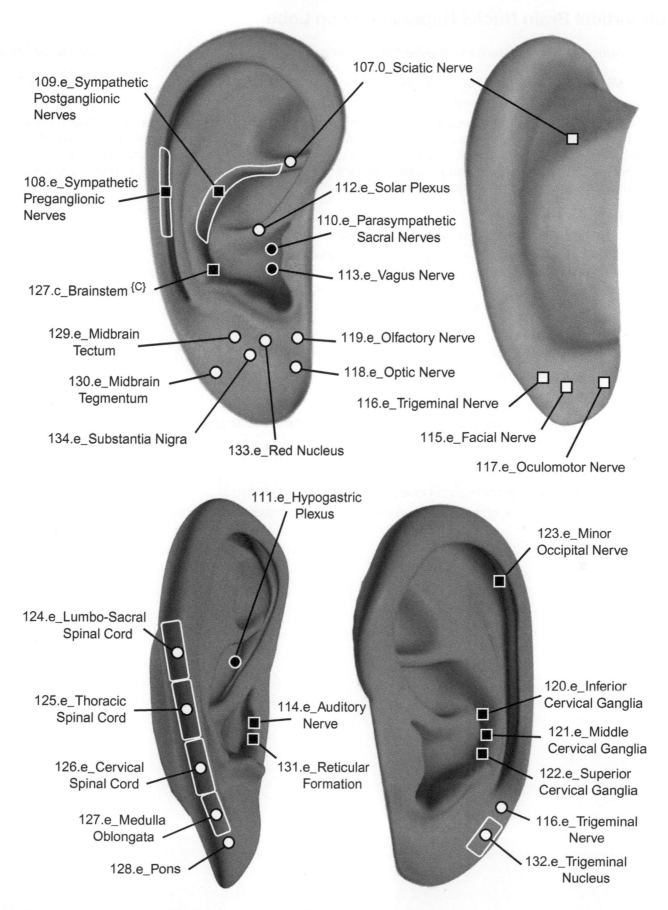

107.0_Sciatic Nerve

109.e_Sympathetic Postganglionic Nerves

108.e_Sympathetic Preganglionic Nerves

112.e_Solar Plexus

110.e_Parasympathetic Sacral Nerves

113.e_Vagus Nerve

127.c_Brainstem {C}

129.e_Midbrain Tectum

119.e_Olfactory Nerve

130.e_Midbrain Tegmentum

118.e_Optic Nerve

116.e_Trigeminal Nerve

134.e_Substantia Nigra

115.e_Facial Nerve

133.e_Red Nucleus

117.e_Oculomotor Nerve

111.e_Hypogastric Plexus

123.e_Minor Occipital Nerve

124.e_Lumbo-Sacral Spinal Cord

125.e_Thoracic Spinal Cord

114.e_Auditory Nerve

120.e_Inferior Cervical Ganglia

126.e_Cervical Spinal Cord

131.e_Reticular Formation

121.e_Middle Cervical Ganglia

122.e_Superior Cervical Ganglia

127.e_Medulla Oblongata

116.e_Trigeminal Nerve

128.e_Pons

132.e_Trigeminal Nucleus

[FIGURE 7.28 Brainstem, spinal cord, and peripheral nerves represented on the auricle.

Subcortical Brain Nuclei Represented on Lobe

No.	Auricular Microsystem Point (Alternative Name)	[Auricular Zone]

130.e Midbrain Tegmentum (*Ventral Tegmental Area, Periaqueductal Gray*)   [LO 5, PL 5]

Location: Found on the peripheral ear lobe.

Function: The midbrain tegmentum contains the red nucleus and substantia nigra nuclei that affect extrapyramidal control of semivoluntary muscles and motor integration of voluntary movements. Also located in this region of the midbrain is the periaqueductal gray, which is a primary area of the brainstem that releases endorphinergic and serotonergic neurotransmitters to reduce pain. This point also relieves parkinsonian tremors, torticollis, and writer's cramp, and it can be used in substance abuse problems.

131.e Reticular Formation   [ST 2, ST3]

Location: Found on the subtragus, opposite to the ear canal.

Function: The reticular activating system (RAS) of the brainstem activates arousal, attention, alertness, vigilance, and integration of nociceptive input, and it affects brain laterality. It reduces unstable reflex behaviors, oscillation disorders, insomnia, and problems with circadian rhythms, such as jet lag. The nearby Raphe nuclei, which contain serotonin, serve to facilitate sleep.

132.e Trigeminal Nucleus   [LO 7, PL 5]

Location: Found on the peripheral ear lobe.

Function: Relieves symptoms of trigeminal neuralgia, dental pain, and facial tremors.

133.e Red Nucleus   [LO 6, PL 6]

Location: Found on the superior region of ear lobe, below the peripheral antitragus.

Function: Regulates semivoluntary acts and relieves extrapyramidal muscle tremors.

134.e Substantia Nigra   [LO 6, PL 6]

Location: Found on the superior region of lobe, below the peripheral antitragus.

Function: Regulates semivoluntary acts and relieves extrapyramidal muscle spasms related to Parkinson's disease.

Subcortical Brain Nuclei Represented on Concha Wall and Lobe

No.	Auricular Microsystem Point (Alternative Name)	[Auricular Zone]

135.e   Striatum (Basal Ganglia, Extrapyramidal Motor System)   [LO 4, PL 4]

Location: Found on the superior region of the ear lobe, below the antitragus.

Function: Affects muscle tone, elaboration of automatic and semiautomatic movements, and inhibition of involuntary movements. Relieves parkinsonian disease, tremors, and spasms.

135.e[1]   Caudate Nucleus: This striatum nucleus is located below the cerebral cortex and outside the thalamus. It is shaped like a goat horn and regulates excessive ongoing motor activity.

135.e[2]   Putamen: This striatum nucleus facilitates coordinated, learned motor activity.

135.e[3]   Globus Pallidus: This striatum nucleus facilitates ongoing motor activity.

136.e   Anterior Hypothalamus   [IC 2]

Location: Found in the inferior concha region near the intertragic notch.

Function: Affects parasympathetic sedation and balances both hypertension and hypotension. Affects fertility disorders, sexual disorders, thermoregulation, and perspiration.

137.e   Posterior Hypothalamus   [IC 5]

Location: Found in the inferior concha, near the Thalamus point at LM_21.

Function: Facilitates sympathetic arousal and relieves hypertension and cardiac acceleration. Affects secretion of adrenalin, vigilance, and wakeful consciousness, and it decreases digestion.

138.c   Brain [C] (Thalamic Nuclei, Diencephalon, Central Rim)   [CW 3]

Location: On the upper edge of the concha wall, behind the occiput on the antitragus. Dr. Li Chun Huang (2005) of the Beijing University of Chinese Medicine has conducted extensive clinical research on ear acupuncture in China. She has suggested that there are actually three Subcortex points on the concha wall behind the antitragus. These three points form an equilateral triangle when viewed in association with each other. All three Subcortex points lie between the primary Thalamus point at LM_21 and the Endocrine point near LM_22. These subdivisions of the Subcortex have selective actions on the nervous system, with predominant effects for neural dysfunctions, for digestive system dysregulation, or for impaired blood circulation.

138.c[1]   Nervous Subcortex   [CW 2]

138.c[2]   Digestive Subcortex   [CW 1]

138.c[3]   Coronary Vascular Subcortex   [CW 1]

Function: Alleviates the deficiency of blood supply to the brain, cerebral concussion, restlessness, cerebellar ataxia, epilepsy, attention deficit disorder, hyperactivity, addictions, clinical depression, asthma, sleep disturbance, and low intellectual functioning. It also affects hypothalamic control of the pituitary gland and endocrine glands. Relieves glandular disturbances, irregular menstruation, sexual impotence, diabetes mellitus, and brain tumors.

138.e   Thalamic Nuclei [E] (Brain, Diencephalon)   [CW 1–CW 3]

Location: Found on the concha wall behind the antitragus ridge. For Paul Nogier, the whole concha wall behind the antitragus represents the many different nuclei of the thalamus of the brain, including pain, sensory, and limbic arousal functions.

No.   Auricular Microsystem Point *(Alternative Name)*   [Auricular Zone]

139.e   Limbic Brain *(Rhinencephalon, Reactional Brain, Visceral Brain)*   [LO 2]

Location: Found on the ear lobe below the intertragic notch at LM_9.

Function: Affects memory, amnesia, retention of lived-through emotional experiences, sexual arousal, aggressive impulses, and compulsive behaviors.

140.e   Hippocampus *(Memory Brain, Fornix)*   [LO 6/LO 8, PL 6]

Location: Found on the superior ear lobe immediately inferior to the length of the antitragus.

Function: This limbic nucleus affects memory, amnesia, and retention of lived-through emotional experiences.

141.e   Amygdala *(Emotional Brain, Anti-Aggressivity Point)*   [LO 2/AT 1]

Location: Found in the notch on the superior lobe as it joins the peripheral intertragic notch.

Function: This limbic nucleus affects anger, irritability, excessive aggressiveness, mania, sexual compulsions, and sexual dramas.

142.e   Nucleus Accumbens *(Septal Nucleus, Sexual Brain, Pleasure Center)*   [LO 2/IT 1]

Location: Found on the central ear lobe, just inferior to the intertragic notch and LM_12.

Function: This limbic nucleus affects pleasure, reinforcement, and instinctive responses and seems to be the primary contributing brain region to substance abuse and addiction.

143.e   Cingulate Gyrus *(Paleocortex, Emotional Reactivity)*   [IT 1]

Location: Found on the central intertragic notch, above LM_9.

Function: This limbic region of the brain alleviates chronic pain, reduces emotional suffering, and improves memory.

144.e   Olfactory Bulb *(Smell Brain)*   [LO 2]

Location: Found on the central ear lobe as it meets the face, between LM_8 and LM_9.

Function: Affects sense of smell.

145.e   Cerebellum   [AH 1/AT 3, PL 4]

Location: Found on the inferior antihelix tail and the posterior lobe.

Function: Affects motor coordination and postural tonus. Relieves intentional muscle tremors, spasms, semiautomatic movements, coordination of axial movements, postural tonus, perfection of intentional cortical movements, vertigo, vestibular equilibrium, and clinical depression.

Cerebral Cortex Represented on the Ear Lobe and Tragus

No.	Auricular Microsystem Point (Alternative Name)	[Auricular Zone]

146.e   Corpus Callosum   [TG 2–TG 4]

Location: Found along the whole length of the vertically ascending tragus.

Function: Affects brain laterality of the left and right cerebral hemispheres. The interactions between the two sides of the brain are represented on the tragus in an inverted pattern. The callosal radiations to the frontal cortex are projected onto the inferior tragus, near LM_9; the temporal–occipital cortex radiations are projected onto the middle of the tragus, between LM_10 and LM_11; and the parietal cortex radiations are projected onto the superior tragus. The tragus also represents the anterior Conception Vessel (Ren mai channel) and the posterior Governing Vessel (Du mai channel) in an inverted position, with the head down toward zone TG 1 and the base of the body up toward zone TG 5.

Cerebral Laterality: The right ear in a right-handed person represents the logical, linguistic, left cerebral cortex, and the left ear represents the rhythmic, artistic right cerebral hemisphere. These representations are reversed in some left-handed individuals and in patients with oscillation problems. An oscillator might have the left cerebral cortex projected onto the left ear and the right cerebral cortex represented on the right ear.

147.e   Occipital Cortex *(Occipital Lobe, Visual Cortex)*   [AT 3, LO 8]

Location: Found on the peripheral antitragus and the ear lobe below it.

Function: Affects visual neurological disorders and impaired visual perception.

148.e   Temporal Cortex *(Temporal Lobe, Auditory Cortex, Acoustic Line)*   [LO 6, LO 8]

Location: Found on the peripheral ear lobe.

Function: Affects auditory disorders and impaired tone discriminations.

149.e   Parietal Cortex *(Post-Central Gyrus, Parietal Lobe, Somatic Cortex)*   [LO 3, LO 5, LO 6]

Location: Found over the middle of the ear lobe.

Function: Affects tactile paresthesia, musculoskeletal pain, and stroke symptoms.

150.e   Frontal Cortex *(Pre-Central Gyrus, Frontal Lobe, Pyramidal System)*   [LO 3, PL 3]

Location: Found on the central ear lobe.

Function: Initiates motor action. Relieves motor paralysis and muscle tonus.

151.e   Prefrontal Cortex *(Executive Brain, Master Cerebral Point)*   [LO 1, PL 1]

Location: Found on the central ear lobe as it joins the face, between LM_8 andLM_9.

Function: Facilitates decision making and relieves poor concentration, obsessions, and worry.

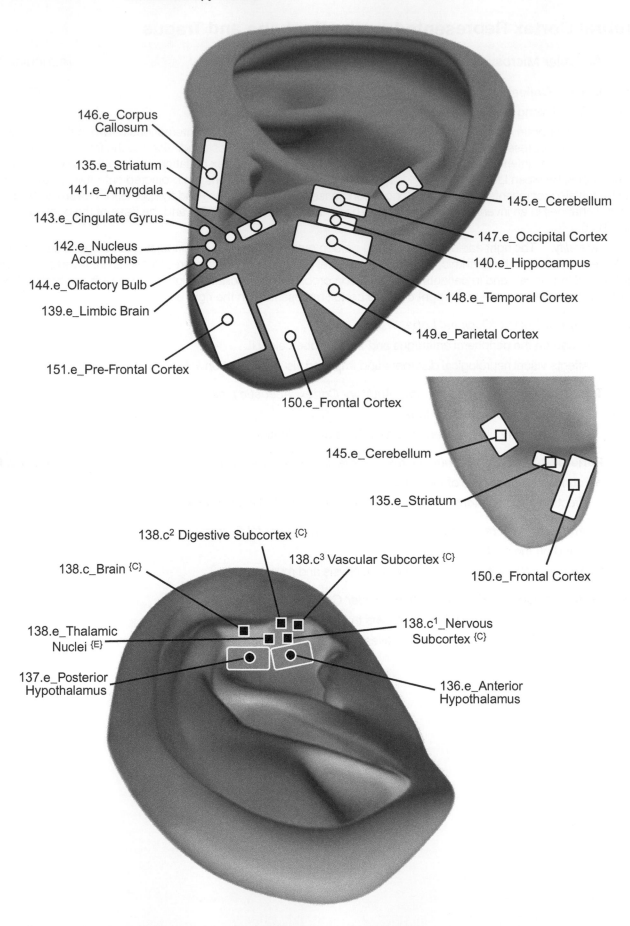

146.e_Corpus Callosum

135.e_Striatum

141.e_Amygdala

143.e_Cingulate Gyrus

142.e_Nucleus Accumbens

144.e_Olfactory Bulb

139.e_Limbic Brain

151.e_Pre-Frontal Cortex

150.e_Frontal Cortex

145.e_Cerebellum

147.e_Occipital Cortex

140.e_Hippocampus

148.e_Temporal Cortex

149.e_Parietal Cortex

145.e_Cerebellum

135.e_Striatum

150.e_Frontal Cortex

138.c² Digestive Subcortex {C}

138.c³ Vascular Subcortex {C}

138.c_Brain {C}

138.e_Thalamic Nuclei {E}

138.c¹_Nervous Subcortex {C}

137.e_Posterior Hypothalamus

136.e_Anterior Hypothalamus

[FIGURE 7.29 Cerebral cortex, limbic brain, and striatum represented on the auricle.

7.6 Auricular Representation of Functional Points

Chinese Functional Points Represented on the Ear

No.   Auricular Microsystem Point (Alternative Name)   [Auricular Zone]

152.c   Asthma Point {C} (Ping Chuan)   [AT 2]

Location: Found on the apex of the antitragus, at LM_13.

Function: Relieves symptoms of asthma, bronchitis, coughs, difficulty breathing, and itching.

153.c   Antihistamine Point {C}   [TF3/TF 4]

Location: Found in the middle of the triangular fossa, near the European Knee point.

Function: Relieves symptoms of colds, allergies, asthma, bronchitis, and coughs.

154.c   Constipation {C}   [TF 3]

Location: Found on the triangular fossa, superior to LM_17 on the antihelix inferior crus.

Function: Relieves constipation and indigestion.

155.c^1 Hepatitis 1   [TF 4]

Location: Found on the superior aspects of the triangular fossa as it curves upward toward the antihelix superior crus.

Function: Reduces liver dysfunctions and liver inflammations.

155.c^2 Hepatitis 2 (Hepatomeglia, Cirrhosis)   [CR 2]

Location: Found on the peripheral inferior concha, at the Liver point.

156.c^1 Hypertension 1 (Depressing Point, Lowering Pressure Point)   [TF 6]

Location: Found on the superior triangular fossa, near the European points for the toes.

Function: Reduces high blood pressure and induces relaxation.

156.c^2 Hypertension 2 (High Blood Pressure Point)   [TG 2]

Location: Found on the inferior tragus at the Tranquilizer point.

156.c^3 Hypertension 3 (Hypertensive Groove)   [PG 4 & PG 8]

Location: Found on the superior, posterior groove, behind the antihelix body.

157.c   Hypotension Point {C} (Raising Blood Pressure Point)   [IT 1]

Location: Found on intertragic notch, between Eye Disorders Mu 1 and Mu 2.

Function: Elevates abnormally low blood pressure.

158.c   Lumbago {C} (Lumbodynia, Coxalgia)   [AH 11 & AH12]

Location: Found on the middle of the antihelix body.

Function: Relieves the functional or psychosomatic aspects of low back pain.

159.c   Muscle Relaxation {C}   [IC 7/IC 8]

Location: Found on the peripheral inferior concha, near the Chinese Spleen and Liver points.

Function: This point is one of the most clinically effective points on the auricle for reducing muscle tension, with almost the status of a master point because it is used so often to reduce pain and stress.

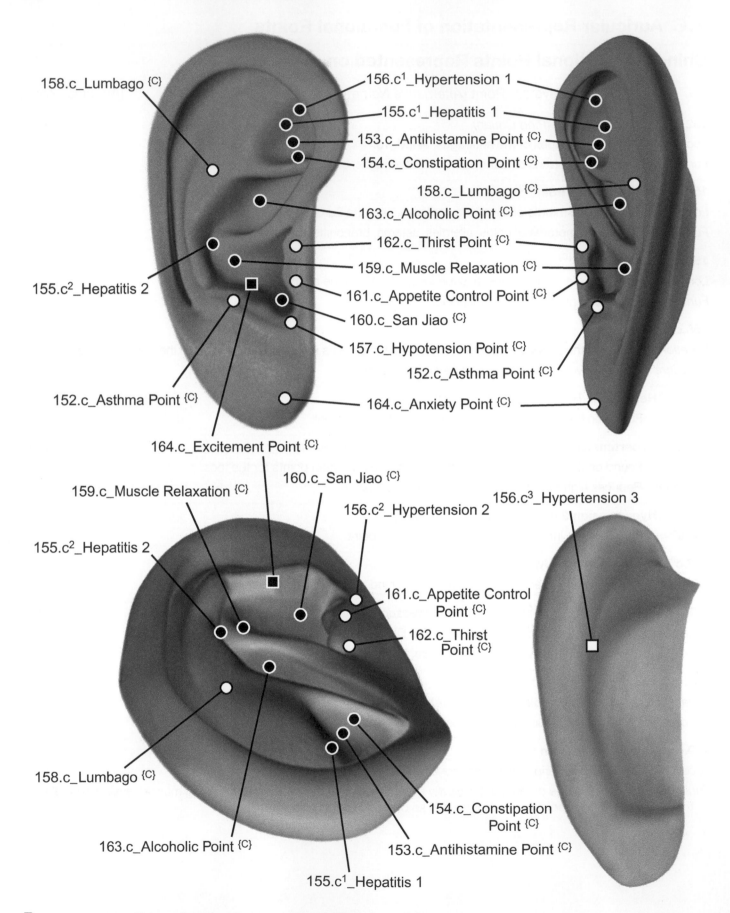

FIGURE 7.30 Chinese functional points represented on the auricle.

No. Auricular Microsystem Point *(Alternative Name)* [Auricular Zone]

160.c San Jiao *(Triple Warmer, Triple Heater, Triple Burner, Triple Energizer)* [IC 1]

Location: Found on the inferior concha, near the Pituitary Gland point, the gland that regulates anti-diuretic hormone that controls fluid levels released in urine.

Function: Affects diseases of the internal organs and the endocrine glands. Affects the circulatory system, respiratory system, and thermoregulation. It relieves indigestion, shortness of breath, anemia, hepatitis, abdominal distension, constipation, and edema. San jiao regulates water circulation and fluid distribution related to the Lower Jiao, Middle Jiao, and Upper Jiao.

161.c Appetite Control Point {C} *(Hunger Point, Weight Control)* [TG 3]

Location: Found on the middle of tragus, between LM_10 and LM_11.

Function: Diminishes appetite, nervous overeating, overweight disorders, hyperthyroidism, and hypertension. This ear point is combined with stimulation of the Stomach point for reduction of the food cravings that impair one's commitment to a diet plan and exercise program. However, it does not replace the need to use one's willpower to maintain commitment to a comprehensive weight reduction program.

162.c Thirst Point {C} [TG 4]

Location: Found on the tragus, just inferior to the superior tragus protrusion, LM_11.

Function: Diminishes excessive thirst related to diabetes insipidus and diabetes mellitus. In TCM, it nourishes yin and promotes the production of body fluids to reduce thirst.

163.c Alcoholic Point {C} *(Drunk Point)* [SC 2]

Location: Found on the superior concha, between the Small Intestines point and the Chinese Kidney point.

Function: Relieves hangovers and facilitates the treatment of alcohol abuse. Just as the Appetite Control point can only facilitate but not overrule the effects of one's willpower for weight reduction, so too does this Alcoholic point facilitate alcohol withdrawal but does not replace the need for one's conscious volition to sobriety. An alcoholic patient must commit himself or herself to a life of sobriety and some type of support group or empowerment group, such as a 12-step program.

164.0 Anxiety Point *(Nervousness, Neurasthenia, Worry Point)* [LO 1]

Location: Found on the central ear lobe, near LM_8 and the Master Cerebral point.

Function: Relieves anxiety, worry, neurosis, and neurasthenia.

165.c Excitement Point {C} [CW 2]

Location: Found on the concha wall below the apex of the antitragus at LM_13 and above the Thalamus point at LM_21.

Function: This point induces excitation of the cerebral cortex to relieve drowsiness, lethargy, depression, hypogonadism, sexual impairment, impotency, and obesity.

No.	Auricular Microsystem Point *(Alternative Name)*	[Auricular Zone]

166.c   Tuberculosis Point {C}   [IC 5]

Location: Found on the inferior concha, at center of the Lung region.

Function: Relieves tuberculosis, pneumonia, and breathing difficulties.

167.c   Bronchitis {C}   [IC 6/IC 7]

Location: Found on the inferior concha, at the Bronchi point, inward from the Lung region.

Function: Relieves bronchitis, pneumonia, and breathing difficulties.

168.c   Heat Point {C}   [AH 11]

Location: Found on the antihelix body, at the junction of the inferior and superior crus.

Function: Produces peripheral vasodilation, reducing vascular inflammation and sensation of being warm or feverish. It is used for acute strains, low back pain, Raynaud's disease, and phlebitis.

169.c   Cirrhosis {C}   [CR 2]

Location: Found on the peripheral concha ridge, within the Liver region.

Function: Relieves cirrhosis damage to the liver and hepatomeglia.

170.c   Pancreatitis {C}   [SC 7]

Location: Found on the peripheral superior concha, within the Pancreas region.

Function: Relieves inflammation and deficiencies of the pancreas, diabetes, and indigestion.

171.c   Nephritis {C}   [SF 1/HX 15]

Location: Found on the inferior helix tail as it meets the gutter of the scaphoid fossa, near LM_5.

Function: Reduces kidney inflammations.

172.c   Ascites Point {C}   [SC 6]

Location: Found on the superior concha, between the duodenum and Chinese Kidney points.

Function: Reduces excess abdominal fluid, cirrhosis, and flatulence.

173.c   Mutism Point {C} *(Dumb Point)*   [ST 3]

Location: Found on the underside of subtragus, superior to the Internal Nose point.

Function: Used to assist problems with speaking clearly or with stuttering.

174.c[1]   Hemorrhoids 1   [IH 6]

Location: Found on the underside of the internal helix, near the European Kidney point.

Function: Alleviates hemorrhoids.

174.c[2]   Hemorrhoids 2   [SC 4]

Location: Found on the central superior concha, near the Chinese Prostate point.

| No. | Auricular Microsystem Point *(Alternative Name)* | [Auricular Zone] |

175.c   Windstream {C} *(Lesser Occipital Nerve, Minor Occipital Nerve)*   [IH 11]

Location: Found on the peripheral internal helix as it joins the superior scaphoid fossa. It is found near the Chinese Dermatitis or Urticaria point.

Function: Alleviates allergies, bronchial asthma, allergic rhinitis, coughs, dermatitis, urticaria, and allergic constitutions. This point is utilized in Chinese ear acupuncture treatments to dispel the effects of pathogenic, "evil wind." It has antihistamine, anti-inflammatory, and anti-allergic effects.

176.c   Central Rim {C}   [CW 3]

Location: Found on the portion of the concha wall below the junction of the antihelix tail and the antitragus.

Function: Alleviates basic metabolic symptoms of stress, neurological problems, and addiction disorders. In TCM, it replenishes spleen qi and kidney qi, nourishes the brain, and tranquilizes the mind.

177.c   Apex of Tragus {C}   [TG 5]

Location: Found on the tragus superior protrusion, at LM_11.

Function: Reduces inflammation, fever, swelling, and arthritic pain. It has analgesic, anti-pyretic, and anti-inflammatory properties.

178.c   Apex of Antitragus {C}   [AT 2]

Location: Found on the antitragus superior protrusion, at LM_13.

Function: Reduces inflammation, fever, and swelling.

179.c   Apex of Auricle {C} *(Ear Apex, Allergy Point 1)*   [HX 7]

Location: Found on the external side of the apex of the ear, at LM_2.

Function: An anti-pyretic point to reduce general inflammation reactions related to allergies, rheumatoid arthritis, and asthmatic breathing difficulties. It alleviates fever, heat, swelling, blood pressure, inflammation, delirium, and pathogenic wind. This point has analgesic, anti-pyretic, and anti-inflammatory properties.

The apex of the auricle is often used for bloodletting by the prick of a needle at the very top of the ear to balance excess qi. It is used for the elimination of toxic substances, the excretion of metabolic wastes, and can be used for anaphylactic shock.

180.c[1]   Helix 1   [HX 11]

Location: Found on the peripheral helix, at Darwin's Tubercle, between LM_3 and LM_4.

Function: Antipyretic ear points reduce inflammation, fever, swelling, and blood pressure.

180.c[2]   Helix 2   [HX 13]

Location: Found on the helix tail, within the region of the lumbosacral spinal cord.

180.c[3]   Helix 3   [HX 14]

Location: Found on the helix tail, within the region of the cervical spinal cord.

180.c[4]   Helix 4   [HX 15]

Location: Found on the helix tail, where the helix meets the lobe at LM_6.

180.c[5]   Helix 5   [LO 7]

Location: Found on the peripheral ear lobe, midway between LM_6 and LM_7.

180.c[6]   Helix 6   [LO 3]

Location: Found on the bottom of the ear lobe, at LM_7, below the Chinese Tonsil 4 point.

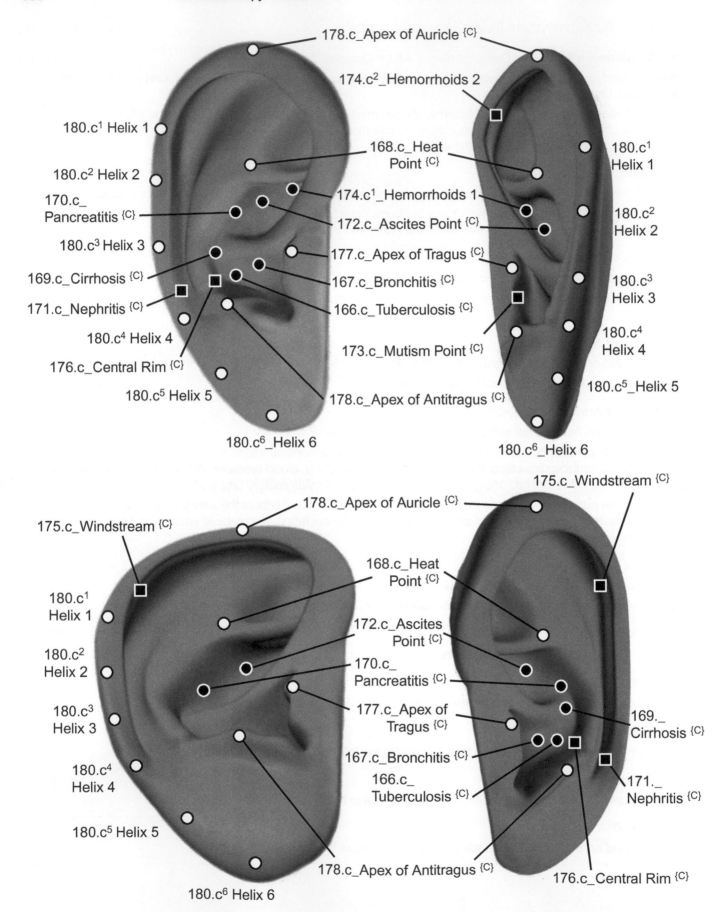

FIGURE 7.31 Chinese functional points represented on the auricle.

Chinese Functional Ear Points Most Commonly Used in Treatment Protocols:

Ear Point Number	Name	Zone Location
152.c	Asthma point [C]	[AT 2]
153.c	Antihistamine point [C]	[TF 4]
154.c	Constipation [C]	[TF 3]
156.c[1]	Hypertension 1	[TF 3]
156.c[2]	Hypertension 2	[TG 2]
156.c[3]	Hypertension 3	[PG 4 & PG 8]
158.c	Lumbago [C]	[AH 11 & AH 12]
159.c	Muscle Relaxation [C]	[IC 7/IC 8]
160.c	San Jiao (Triple Warmer)	[IC 1]
161.c	Appetite Control point [C]	[TG 3]
164.c	Anxiety point	[LO 1]
165.c	Excitement point [C]	[CW 2]
168.c	Heat point [C]	[AH 11]
175.c	Windstream [C]	[IH 11]

European Functional Points Represented on the Ear

No.	Auricular Microsystem Point (Alternative Name)	[Auricular Zone]

181.e   Auditory Line *(Language Area of Auditory Cortex on Temporal Lobe)*   [LO 6]

Location: Found as a horizontal line on the ear lobe, inferior to the antitragus.

Function: The auditory line represents the auditory cortex on the temporal lobe, with stimulation of high-frequency sounds more present on the central part of this line and representation of low-frequency sounds more present on the peripheral part of this line. It is used to relieve deafness, tinnitus, Meniere's disease, and other hearing disorders.

182.e   Irritability Point {E} *(Anti-Aggressivity Point)*   [LO 2/AT 1]

Location: Found in notch at the junction of the ear lobe to the medial side of the antitragus, central to LM_12.

Function: Reduces irritability, aggression, frustration, rage, mania, and drug withdrawal. This auricular region represents the limbic system nucleus called the amygdala, a brain area that can increase or decrease aggressive behaviors.

183.e   Psychosomatic Point {E} *(Psychotherapeutic Point, Point R, Bourdiol Point)*   [HX 4/HX 5]

Location: Found on the superior helix root as it joins the face at LM_1. It is located near the Chinese ear reflex point for the Genitals.

Function: Alleviates psychological disorders and can help psychotherapy patients remember long forgotten memories, repressed emotional experiences, and psychotic thinking. It also facilitates the mental processing of vivid, intense, disturbing dreams.

184.e   Sexual Desire {E} *(Bosch Point, Libido Point)*   [HX 1]

Location: Found on the helix root as it joins the superior edge of tragus, at the European ear point for the Genitals, the Penis and Clitoris.

Function: Increases libido, enhances sexual arousal.

185.e   Sexual Suppression {E} *(Jerome Point, Sexual Compulsive Disorders)*   [HX 15]

Location: Found on the scaphoid fossa as it joins the helix tail near LM_5.

Function: Lowers libido, calms sexuality, and alleviates insomnia.

186.e   Master Omega *(Master Cerebral Point, Anxiety, Worry, Angst)*   [LO 1]

Location: Found on the inferior ear lobe near the face, midway between LM_8 and LM_9. It is the same point as the Master Cerebral point and the Chinese Neurasthenia points. It is in the region of the ear reflex point for the prefrontal cortex. A vertical line can be drawn between this master Omega point and the functional points Omega 1 and Omega 2.

Function: Affects psychological stress, such as obsessive–compulsive disorders, fear, worry, ruminating thoughts, angst, psychosomatic disorders, and general analgesia.

187.e   Omega 1 *(Master Vegetative Point, Hypogastric Plexus)*   [SC 2]

Location: Found on the superior concha, central to the Small Intestines point.

Function: Affects vegetative stress, such as digestive disorders and visceral pain.

188.e   Omega 2 *(Master Inflammatory Point)*   [HX 6]

Location: Found on the superior helix, central to the Allergy 1 point at LM_2.

Function: Affects somatic stress, reducing rheumatoid arthritis and inflammations of the limbs.

189.e   Marvelous Point {E} *(Wonderful Point, Middle Cervical Plexus)*   [CR 2/CW 4]

Location: Found on the peripheral concha ridge, in the region of the Liver ear point.

Function: Balances excessive sympathetic arousal, reduces hypertension, affects blood vascular regulation, and relieves muscle tension.

No.	Auricular Microsystem Point *(Alternative Name)*	[Auricular Zone]

190.e   Anti-Depressant Point {E} *(Cheerfulness Point, Joy Point)*   [LO 8]
Location: Found on the peripheral ear lobe, central to the TMJ ear point.
Function: Relieves endogenous depression, reactive depression, and dysphoric mood.

191.e   Mania Point {E}   [TG 2]
Location: Found on the inferior tragus edge below LM_10, below the Adrenal Gland {C} ear point.
Function: Relieves hyperactive behavior, mania, and addictions.

192.e   Nicotine Point {E}   [TG 2]
Location: Found on the inferior tragus edge that lies over the concha at LM_10, between the Mania point and the Chinese Adrenal Gland {C} ear point.
Function: Reduces nicotine craving in persons withdrawing from smoking. This point becomes more prominent if the patient has not smoked for a while.

193.e   Vitality Point {E}   [TG 4]
Location: Found on the superior tragus, superior to LM_11, above the Thirst Point {C}.
Function: Affects immune system disorders, AIDS, cancer, and chronic fatigue.

194.e   Alertness Point {E}   [HX 12/HX 13]
Location: Found on the helix tail, below Darwin's Tubercle at LM_4.
Function: Induces arousal, activation, and alertness.

195.e[1]   Insomnia 1 *(Sleep Disorder 1)*   [SF 5]
Location: Found on the superior scaphoid fossa, near the Wrist ear point.
Function: Relieves insomnia, nervousness, and depression.

195.e[2]   Insomnia 2 *(Sleep Disorder 2)*   [SF 1]
Location: Found on the inferior scaphoid fossa, near the Shoulder Joint ear point.
Function: Relieves insomnia, sleep difficulties, nervous dreams, and inability to dream.

196.e   Dizziness Point {E} *(Vertigo)*   [CW 4]
Location: Found on the concha wall, below the first Cervical Vertebrae ear points.
Function: Relieves dizziness and vertigo.

197.e   Sneezing Point {E}   [LO 5]
Location: Found on the peripheral ear lobe.
Function: Reduces sneezing related to illness, symptoms of allergies.

198.e   Weather Point {E}   [HX 3]
Location: Found on the helix root, superior to the Chinese Rectum ear point.
Function: Alleviates any symptoms due to changes in weather.

199.e   Laterality Point {E}   [Jaw]
Location: Found on the sideburns area of the face, central to LM_23 on the tragus.
Function: Facilitates balance of left and right cerebral hemispheres, reduces oscillation.

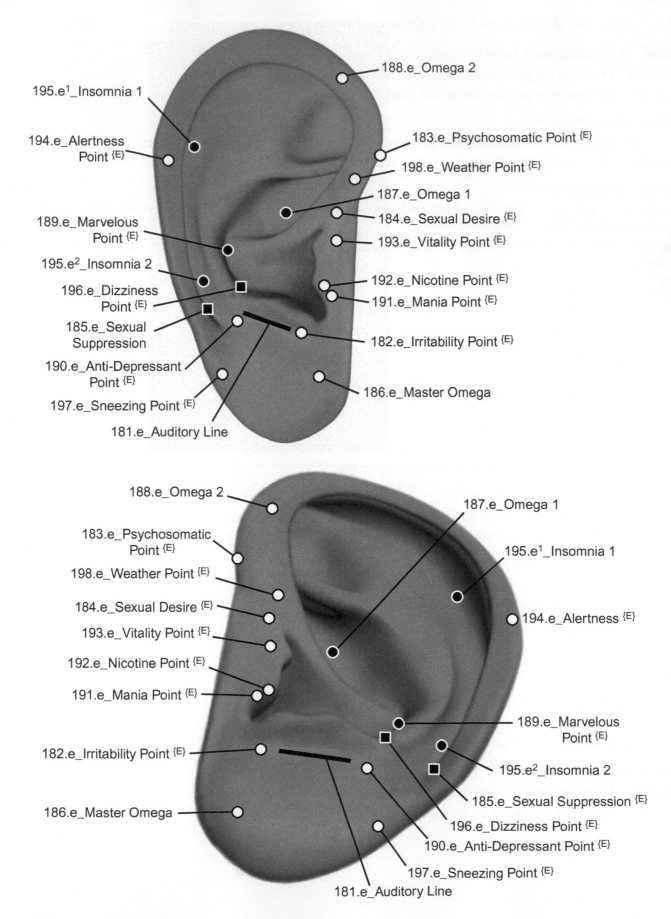

FIGURE 7.32 European functional points represented on the auricle.

No.	Auricular Microsystem Point (*Alternative Name*)	[Auricular Zone]

200.e **Darwin's Point** [E] (*Bodily Defense*) [HX 11]

Location: Found on the Darwin's tubercle on the helix, between LM_3 and LM_4.

Function: Relieves pain in the lower back and lower limbs related to neurological dysfunctions in the spinal cord.

201.e **Prostaglandin Point** [E] [LO 1/PL 1]

Location: On the posterior underside of the ear lobe where it joins the neck at LM_8.

Function: Reduces inflammatory pain, rheumatism, and hypotension.

202.e **Progesterone** [IH 6]

Location: Found on the region of the internal helix above the European Kidney ear point.

Function: Used to alleviate PMS symptoms.

203.e **Oxytocin** [CW 3]

Location: Found on the concha wall behind the antitragus.

Function: Used to enhance maternal bonding and empathetic connection to others.

204.e **Angiotensin Point** [E] (*Renin Point*) [IH 6]

Location: On underside of the internal helix, between the European Kidney ear point and the Progesterone ear point.

Function: Reduces hypertension.

205.e **Analgesia Point** [E] [SC 7]

Location: Found on the superior concha, near the Duodenum point.

Function: Used to facilitate pain relief for surgeries.

206.e **Hypnotic Point** [E] [HX 13]

Location: Found on the helix tail, horizontally across from LM_15.

Function: Used to tranquilize and sedate.

207.e **Barbiturate Point** [E] [SF 3]

Location: Found on the scaphoid fossa, near the Elbow point.

Function: Used to tranquilize and sedate, and alleviates insomnia.

208.e **Beta-1 Receptor** [SF 4/IH 12]

Location: Found on the peripheral internal helix above the Barbiturate ear point.

Function: Alleviates cardiovascular disorders and complications to anti-hypertensive medications.

209.e **Frustration Point** [E] [TG 5/HX 2]

Location: Found on the superior region of the tragus, below the helix root and adjacent to the face.

Function: Used to alleviate frustration, aggressive behaviors, and irritability.

210.e **Interferon Point** [E] [TG 5/HX 1]

Location: Found on the edge of the supratragus region where it meets the helix root, above LM_11 and closer to concha than the Frustration Point [E].

Function: Used to enhance immune defense, reduce fever, and produce anti-inflammatory responses.

211.e **Mercury Toxicity Point** [E] [SC 6]

Location: Found on the superior concha, near the Bladder point.

Function: Used to relieve the effects of metal toxicity reactions.

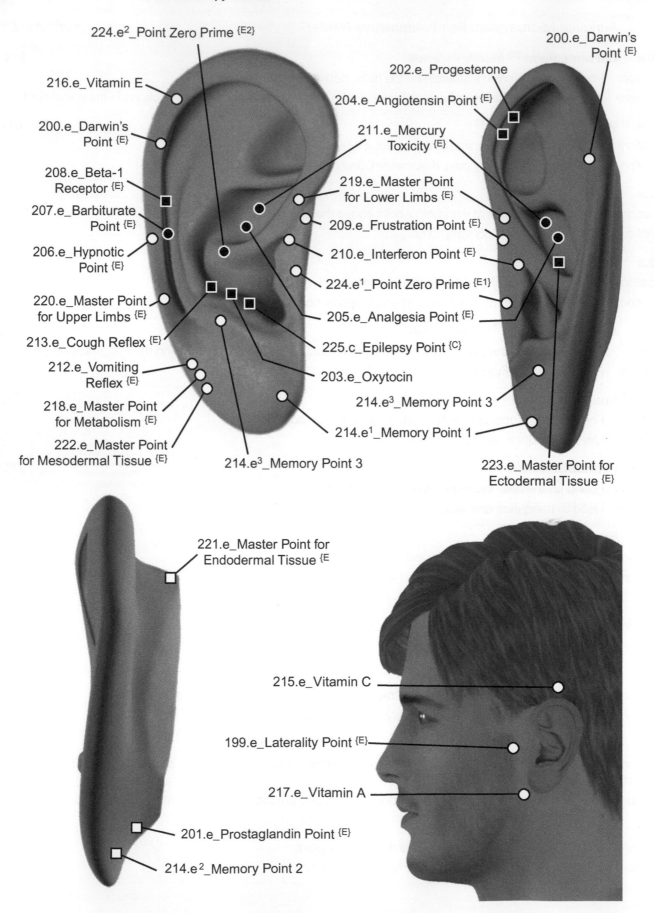

224.e²_Point Zero Prime {E2}

216.e_Vitamin E

200.e_Darwin's Point {E}

208.e_Beta-1 Receptor {E}

207.e_Barbiturate Point {E}

206.e_Hypnotic Point {E}

220.e_Master Point for Upper Limbs {E}

213.e_Cough Reflex {E}

212.e_Vomiting Reflex {E}

218.e_Master Point for Metabolism {E}

222.e_Master Point for Mesodermal Tissue {E}

214.e³_Memory Point 3

202.e_Progesterone

204.e_Angiotensin Point {E}

211.e_Mercury Toxicity {E}

219.e_Master Point for Lower Limbs {E}

209.e_Frustration Point {E}

210.e_Interferon Point {E}

224.e¹_Point Zero Prime {E1}

205.e_Analgesia Point {E}

225.c_Epilepsy Point {C}

203.e_Oxytocin

214.e³_Memory Point 3

214.e¹_Memory Point 1

200.e_Darwin's Point {E}

223.e_Master Point for Ectodermal Tissue {E}

221.e_Master Point for Endodermal Tissue {E

215.e_Vitamin C

199.e_Laterality Point {E}

217.e_Vitamin A

201.e_Prostaglandin Point {E}

214.e²_Memory Point 2

FIGURE 7.33 European functional points represented on the auricle.

No.	Auricular Microsystem Point *(Alternative Name)*	[Auricular Zone]

212.e   Vomiting Reflex {E}   [LO 7]

Location: Found on the peripheral ear lobe.

Function: Alleviates emesis, morning sickness, and dysfunctional pharyngeal reflexes.

213.e   Cough Reflex {E}   [CW 4]

Location: Found on the concha wall, near the Chinese Brainstem ear point.

Function: Alleviates uncontrolled cough reflexes.

214.e^1 Memory 1   [LO 1]

Location: Found on the central ear lobe, in the region of the Prefrontal Cortex ear point.

Function: Facilitates improvement in memory and attention.

214.e^2 Memory 2   [LO 6]

Location: Found on the superior ear lobe, in the region of the Hippocampus ear point.

Function: Facilitates improvement in memory and attention.

214.e^3 Memory 3   [PL 2]

Location: Found on the posterior ear lobe, in the region of the Prefrontal Cortex ear point.

Function: Facilitates improvement in memory and attention.

215.e   Vitamin C   [Head]

Location: Found on the head, superior to the apex of the ear at LM_2.

Function: Relieves stress and symptoms of colds or flu similar to vitamin C.

216.e   Vitamin E   [HX 9]

Location: Found on the helix arch, peripheral to Allergy 1 at LM_2.

Function: Used to amplify effects of taking vitamin E.

217.e   Vitamin A   [Neck]

Location: Found on the neck, inferior to the ear lobe at LM_8.

Function: Used to amplify the effects of taking vitamin A.

218.e   Master Point for Metabolism {E}   [LO 7]

Location: Found on the peripheral ear lobe.

Function: Affects treatment of any metabolic disorder.

219.e   Master Point for Lower Limbs {E}   [HX 2]

Location: Found on the helix root, above the European Genitals point.

Function: Relieves pain and swelling in the legs and feet.

220.e   Master Point for Upper Limbs {E}   [HX 15]

Location: Found on the helix tail, in the region of the European Medulla Oblongata.

Function: Relieves pain and swelling in the arms, hands, and fingers.

221.e   Master Point for Endodermal Tissue {E} *(Deep Tissue)*   [PG 7]

Location: Found on the posterior ear behind LM_1.

Function: Affects treatment of internal organ and endocrine disorders.

222.e   Master Point for Mesodermal Tissue {E} *(Middle Tissue)*   [LO 7]

Location: Found on the peripheral ear lobe below LM_6.

Function: Affects treatment of musculoskeletal disorders.

No.	Auricular Microsystem Point *(Alternative Name)*	[Auricular Zone]

223.e   Master Point for Ectodermal Tissue {E} *(Superficial Tissue)*   [IH 1]

Location: Found on the internal helix above LM_0.

Function: Affects treatment of ectodermal tissue of skin and nervous system.

224.e¹   Point Zero Prime 1   [TG 3]

Location: Found at LM_23 on the Tragus, halfway between LM_1 and LM_8.

Function: Balances dysfunctions throughout the body, including laterality disorders.

224.e²   Point Zero Prime 2   [CR 1/CR 2]

Location: Found on the concha ridge, at LM_19.

Function: Balances dysfunctions throughout the body.

225.c   Epilepsy Point {C}   [CW 2]

Location: Found on the concha wall below the apex of the antitragus at LM_13.

Function: Used to alleviate epileptic seizures.

European Functional Ear Points Most Commonly Used in Treatment Protocols:

Ear Point Number	Name	Zone Location
182.e	Irritability point {E}	[LO 2/IT 1]
183.e	Psychosomatic point {E}	[HX 4]
184.e	Sexual Desire {E}	[HX 1]
185.e	Sexual Suppression {E}	[HX 15]
190.e	Anti-Depressant point {E}	[LO 8]
192.e	Nicotine point {E}	[TG 2]
193.e	Vitality point {E}	[TG 4]
195.e¹	Insomnia 1	[SF 5]
195.e²	Insomnia 2	[SF 1]
196.e	Dizziness point {E}	[CW 3]
198.e	Weather point {E}	[HX 3]
201.e	Prostaglandin point {E}	[PL 1]

7.7 Auricular Representation of Nogier Phases I, II, and III

In subsequent revisions of the original somatotopic representation of the body on the external ear, Dr. Paul Nogier described three different somatotopic maps on the ear. He postulated that two additional auricular microsystems are distinct from the original inverted fetus pattern. Each anatomical region of the external ear can represent more than one microsystem point. Nogier has referred to these different representations as *phases*. The use of this term can be related to the phases of the moon or to phase shifts in the frequency of light as it passes through a crystal prism to create different colored beams of light. The vascular autonomic signal (VAS) that is utilized in auricular medicine responds to different colored light filters depending on the particular phase to which an ear point corresponds.

Phase I: The *inverted fetus* pattern is used to treat the majority of medical conditions and directly corresponds to the Chinese ear reflex points. Phase I represents the tissues and organs of the actual physical body. This phase is the primary source for correcting somatic tissue disorganization, which is the principal manifestation of most medical conditions. Phase I ear points tend to indicate yang excess reactions.

Phase II: The *upright man* pattern is used to treat more difficult, chronic conditions that have not responded successfully to treatment of the Phase I microsystem points. Phase II represents psychosomatic reactions and neurophysiological connections to bodily organs. This phase is useful for correcting central nervous system dysfunctions and mental confusion that contribute to the psychosomatic aspects of pain and pathology of chronic illnesses. Phase II points are often related to yin degenerative conditions.

Phase III: The *horizontal man* pattern is used the least frequently, but it can be very effective for relieving unusual conditions or idiosyncratic reactions. Phase III affects basic cellular energy. This phase can correct the energy disorganization that affects cellular tissue. It produces subtle changes in the electromagnetic energy fields that surround physical organs. Phase III points often indicate prolonged yang inflammatory conditions.

Phase IV: The *motor upside down man* pattern is represented on the posterior side of external ear and essentially mirrors the Phase I inverted fetus pattern on the anterolateral side of the auricle. The Phase IV points are used to treat muscle spasm aspects of a condition, whereas Phase I points reflect the sensory aspects of pain. To find a specific Phase IV point on the posterior side of the auricle, first place your finger on the corresponding point on the anterolateral, front side of the ear, and then bend the ear over and locate where the region you are pressing is most prominent on the back side of the ear.

A basic reason why Dr. Nogier developed the concept of the phases was his contention that each type of embryological tissue has a certain frequency or resonance. Different anatomical regions of the ear respond to phase shifts in the resonance of the corresponding part of the body. The location of the three territories is based on their differential innervation by the trigeminal nerve, with its mesodermal, somatic muscular actions in Phase I; the vagus nerve, with its endodermal, autonomic, visceral effects in Phase I; and the cervical plexus nerves, which exert ectodermal, nervous system activity in Phase I. The shifts in the embryological tissue represented in each territory as one proceeds from Phase I to Phase II to Phase III are presented in Table 7.1.

Nogier proposed his three phases partly as an attempt to account for some of the discrepancies between the French and the Chinese ear acupuncture charts. Three of the mesodermal internal organs represented on the ear—the heart, kidney, and spleen—are all examples of yin meridians that the Chinese say are indirectly connected to the ear acupuncture points. Taoism describes the flow of qi energy from various states of yang energy and yin energy. These two forces can be compared to the binary code used in computers as well as to the active versus resting states of a neuron. The Chinese have developed specific symbols wherein yang

TABLE 7.1	Phase Shifts on the External Ear.		
	Territory 1	**Territory 2**	**Territory 3**
Phase I	Mesodermal	Endodermal	Ectodermal
Phase II	Ectodermal	Mesodermal	Endodermal
Phase III	Endodermal	Ectodermal	Mesodermal

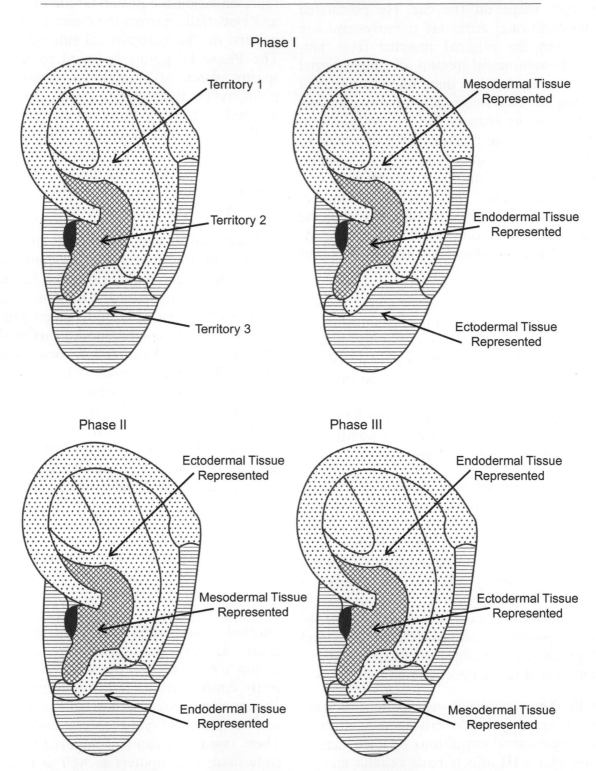

FIGURE 7.34 Nogier phases represented on the three territories of the external ear.

is represented by a solid line and yin is symbolized by a broken line. Specific combinations of three such lines form what is known as a trigram. Helms (1995) cited the work of the French acupuncturist Maurice Mussat in presenting eight such trigrams rotating around the yin–yang symbol of Taoism.

The yang trigrams are diametrically opposite to their corresponding yin trigram. Each trigram code reflects a specific interaction of three basic components of the universe: matter, movement, and energy. From a tripartite phase perspective, Phase I represents solid matter, Phase II represents the control of movement by the nervous system, and Phase III represents the echo reverberation of the energy of the spirit. Disturbance of the dynamic symmetry of composition of these three functional interactions can result in an imbalance of energy.

Dr. Richard Feely of Chicago has suggested that these three energy states in Chinese philosophy can be compared to Nogier's three microsystem phases. Sequential shifts in interactions from the initial yang reactions manifested in Phase I to the resonance reverberations of the yin reactions of Phases II to the energetic manifestations of Phase III.

Auricular Zones for Different Phases of Mesodermal Tissue

Vertebral Column: For both the Chinese system and the Nogier Phase I system, the vertebral column is found in Territory 1 on the antihelix tail and antihelix body. The Chinese state in their charts that the whole vertebral column is limited to just the body and tail of the antihelix, whereas Nogier has indicated that the Phase I Cervical Vertebrae are found on the antihelix tail, the Thoracic Vertebrae are found on the antihelix body, and the Lumbosacral Vertebrae extend onto the inferior crus of the antihelix. The Cervical Vertebrae in Phase I thus lie between LM_14 and LM_15, the Thoracic Vertebrae lie between LM_15 and LM_16, the Lumbar Vertebrae lie between LM_16 and LM_17, and the Sacral Vertebrae lie between

LM_17 and LM_18. The Chinese charts do show the Buttocks point and the Sciatica point on the inferior crus, but their charts do not include the Lower Vertebrae on this area.

In Nogier's Phase II, Cervical Vertebrae are found along the inferior side of the concha ridge of Territory 2, between LM_19 and LM_20. The Phase II Thoracic Vertebrae are found along the concha ridge of Territory 2, between LM_20 and LM_0. The Phase II Lumbosacral Vertebrae are found on the helix root, above LM_0. However, some of Nogier's texts showed the orientation of the Phase II Spinal Vertebrae in one pattern, but these same Phase II Spinal Vertebrae are shown in an opposite orientation in a different text, with the Cervical and Thoracic Vertebrae depicted on the helix root and the Lumbosacral Vertebrae depicted on the concha ridge.

In Oriental medicine, either representation of the Spinal Vertebrae would be found in the same area of the auricle as the internal organs Liver, Spleen, and Stomach. In Phase III, the Cervical, Thoracic, and Lumbosacral Vertebrae lie along the surface of the tragus in Territory 3, which previously had represented the Corpus Callosum in European texts and the Ren mai or Du mai meridians in Oriental medicine. However, as was indicated for the Phase II Spinal Vertebrae, different Nogier texts show the vertebral column oriented in one of two opposite orientations, and there is not yet a common consensus in the clinical community with regard to which pattern is most correct.

Upper and Lower Extremities: The Chinese placed the Hip, Knee, and Foot on the Territory 1 antihelix superior crus, whereas Nogier placed the Phase I lower extremity points in the triangular fossa, which is a nearby area of Territory 1. In both the Chinese system and Phase I of Nogier's system, the Shoulder, Elbow, and Hand are found in identical areas of the scaphoid fossa.

In Nogier's Phase II, the upper extremities shift to the inferior concha within Territory 2, whereas the lower extremities are found in the superior concha of Territory 2. The Phase II Hip is located near the Endocrine master point, the

Phase II Knee is located near the Thalamus master point, the Phase II Ankle is located near the Lung point, and the Phase II Foot is found near the Chinese Spleen point. The Phase II Shoulder is located near the Chinese Prostate point, the Phase II Elbow is located near the Bladder point, the Phase II Wrist is located near the Chinese Kidney point, and the Phase II Hand is located near the European Spleen point.

In Nogier's Phase III, the ear points for the upper and lower limbs shift to the ear lobe, the antitragus, and the antihelix of Territory 3. The Phase III Hip is located on the lowest regions of the antihelix tail and the scaphoid fossa, the Phase II Knee is located on the middle section of the antitragus near the original Temples point, the Phase III Ankle is located near the antitragus Forehead point, and the Phase III Foot is found on the intertragic notch. The Phase III Shoulder is located at approximately the same scaphoid fossa area as the Shoulder Joint point or Master Shoulder; the Phase III Elbow is located lower on the peripheral ear lobe, near the Face point; the Phase III Wrist is located on the central ear lobe near the Master Sensorial point; and the Phase III Hand is located on the central ear lobe near the Master Cerebral point.

Head and Skin Dermatomes: The auricular points that represent areas of the Head include the Skull, Jaw, and Tongue. The original ear points for the Forehead, Temples, and Occiput are arranged on three different sections of the antitragus, but in Nogier's Phase I, these Head points are found on the internal helix region of Territory 1 and the Tongue is represented on the helix arch. In Phase II, these Head points are found in the superior concha of Territory 2, with other musculoskeletal points. In Phase III, they are represented on the ear lobe of Territory 3. The different dermatomes of the skin are represented by a single scaphoid fossa point in the Chinese auricular system, by a range of points over the helix tail in Nogier's Phase I, in the superior concha in Phase II, and on the peripheral ear lobe in Phase III.

Mesodermal Internal Organs: Although most tissue that is derived from the mesoderm of the developing embryo becomes part of the musculoskeletal body, some internal visceral organs are also derived from mesodermal tissue. These mesodermal internal organs include the Heart, the Spleen, the Kidney, the Adrenal Gland, and Genital organs such as the Vagina, the Uterus, the Prostate, the Ovaries, and the Testes. In the Nogier phases, this set of internal organs is found in the same territories in each of the phases that the musculoskeletal tissue is found for that phase. In Phase I, these ear points are found in Territory 1, they are found in Phase II in Territory 2, and in Phase III they are found in Territory 3.

As previously noted, the Chinese Heart point is located at the very center of the inferior concha, whereas Nogier placed the mesodermal tissue of the Heart on the antihelix body. Although Nogier originally suggested that the Chinese Heart point in the inferior concha might correspond to a different phase in the Nogier system, the Phase II Heart was located on the superior concha near the Chinese Kidney point and the Phase III Heart was located on the ear lobe near the Lower Jaw point. The Phase IV control of cardiac muscle is represented on the posterior groove immediately behind the Phase I Heart point on the antihelix body.

There are five primary zang organs in Oriental medicine—the Heart, the Lungs, the Liver, the Spleen, and the Kidney. The phase location of the mesodermal Heart point has just been described, and the Lung and Liver organs are discussed with other endodermal tissue. The auricular locations of the mesodermal Spleen and Kidney organs are of considerable controversy. The Chinese ear charts localize the Spleen in the inferior concha, below the Liver point at LM_20, and the Chinese ear maps show the Kidney as located in the superior concha, below LM_16. In the Nogier system, the Spleen is represented on the concha wall in Phase I, in the peripheral superior concha in Phase II, and on the ear lobe in Phase III. These points would only be reactive when there was physiological spleen pathology, not when there was some spleen qi dysfunction as described in Oriental medicine. The Phase I Kidney is represented on the internal helix above LM_18, the Phase II Kidney is located on the inferior concha near the Chinese Spleen point, and the Phase III Kidney is found on the inferior regions of the antihelix. As with the Spleen, the Nogier representations of the Kidney would be reactive only when there was a urinary disorder, not when there was an imbalance of kidney qi.

In the Chinese auricular system, both the pituitary hormone ACTH and the adrenal hormone cortisol are represented by the same ear point labeled Adrenal Gland, which is located at LM_10 on the tragus. This Chinese Adrenal Gland point has been found to be very clinically effective for a variety of stress-related disorders. In the Nogier system, there are three locations for ACTH and three locations for cortisol. The locations of ear points representing the Pituitary hormone ACTH are found on the helix arch in Phase I, on the inferior concha in Phase II, and on the ear lobe in Phase III. The locations of ear points representing the Adrenal Gland hormone cortisol are found on the antihelix in Phase I, on the superior concha in Phase II, and on the tragus in Phase III.

The final set of mesodermal, internal organs includes the reproductive organs of the Ovaries, Testes, Prostate, and Uterus. The female gonads, the Ovaries, are found in the same auricular area of women that corresponds to the location of the male gonads, the Testes, that are found in men. Both gonads are associated with problems related to sexual desire, sexual dysfunctions, genital infections, and fertility, but only the Ovaries in women are a major factor in perimenstrual disorders, fertility, or menopause. The Chinese ear point for the Ovaries and the Testes on the concha wall behind the antitragus does not make any logical sense from an inverted fetus because all nearby ear points are related to organs located in the head.

However, if one reinterprets the findings of many Chinese practitioners of auricular acupuncture, the Chinese ear points for the Ovaries and Testes could actually represent the gonadal pituitary hormones, FSH and LH. Because the pituitary is located in the head, the release of pituitary FSH and LH which then activate the Ovaries or the Testes could thus account for the Chinese utilization of this ear point. The Chinese Uterus point located in the triangular fossa and the Chinese Prostate point located in the most upper tip of the superior concha are found far removed from the Chinese location for the Ovaries and the Testes. In physical anatomy, these organs would occur very close together. The Nogier ear charts do show the Ovaries, Testes, Prostate, and Uterus points as occurring relatively close together in the upper auricle, whereas Nogier represents the pituitary hormones FSH and LH gonadotrophin organs as occurring lower in the auricle. The ear points for the Phase I reproductive organs are all found on the internal helix, the Phase II ear points for these organs are found on the inferior concha of Territory 2, and the Phase III ear points are found on the ear lobe or the tragus of Territory 3 (Table 7.2).

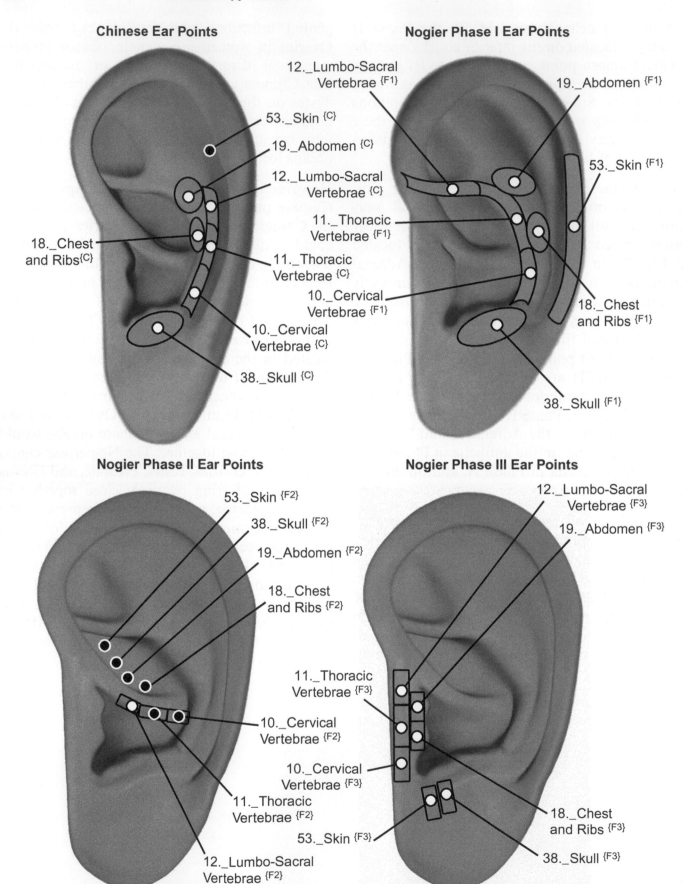

FIGURE 7.35 Spinal vertebrae represented in the auricular mesodermal phase.

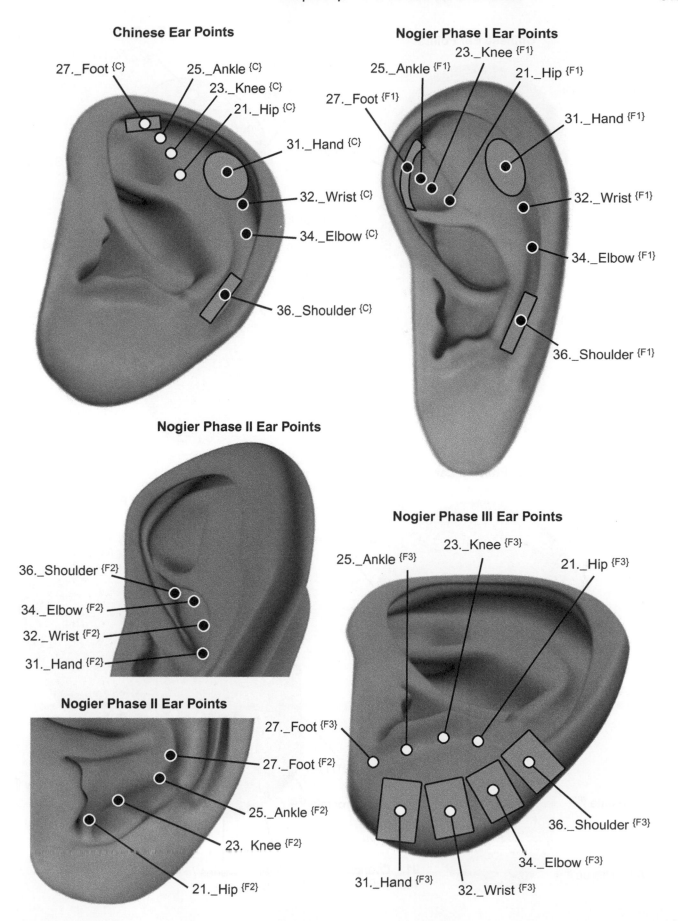

Chinese Ear Points

27._Foot {C}
25._Ankle {C}
23._Knee {C}
21._Hip {C}
31._Hand {C}
32._Wrist {C}
34._Elbow {C}
36._Shoulder {C}

Nogier Phase I Ear Points

23._Knee {F1}
25._Ankle {F1}
21._Hip {F1}
27._Foot {F1}
31._Hand {F1}
32._Wrist {F1}
34._Elbow {F1}
36._Shoulder {F1}

Nogier Phase II Ear Points

36._Shoulder {F2}
34._Elbow {F2}
32._Wrist {F2}
31._Hand {F2}

Nogier Phase II Ear Points

27._Foot {F2}
25._Ankle {F2}
23. Knee {F2}
21._Hip {F2}

Nogier Phase III Ear Points

25._Ankle {F3}
23._Knee {F3}
21._Hip {F3}
27._Foot {F3}
36._Shoulder {F3}
34._Elbow {F3}
31._Hand {F3}
32._Wrist {F3}

FIGURE 7.36 Lower and upper extremities represented in the auricular mesodermal phase.

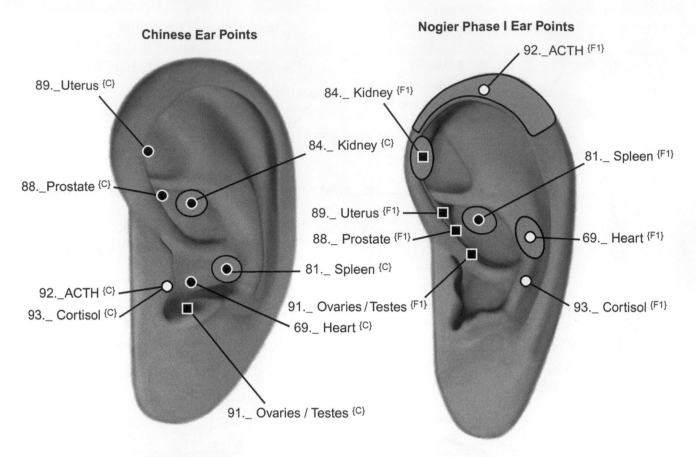

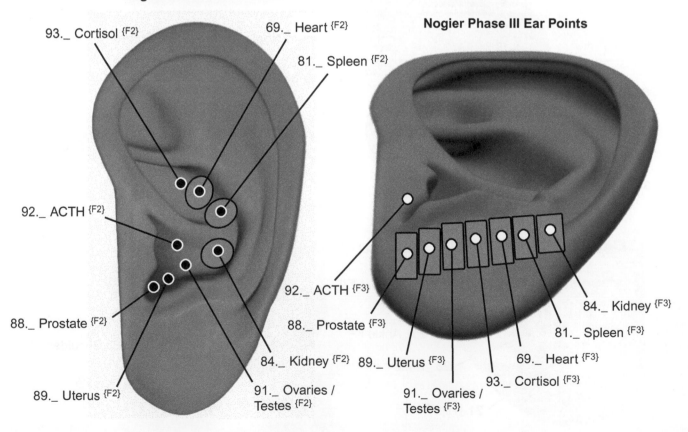

FIGURE 7.37 Internal organs represented in the auricular mesodermal phase.

TABLE 7.2	**Auricular Zones Related to Musculoskeletal System in Nogier Phases.**				
No.	**Musculoskeletal Points**	**Chinese**	**Phase I**	**Phase II**	**Phase III**
		Territory 1	*Territory 1*	*Territory 2*	*Territory 3*
10	Cervical Vertebrae	AH 1	AH 1	CR 2	TG 1–TG 2
11	Thoracic Vertebrae	AH 2–AH 3	AH 3–AH 4	CR 1	TG 2–TG 3
12	Lumbosacral Vertebrae	AH 4	AH 5–AH 6	HX 1	TG 4–TG 5
18	Chest and Ribs	AH 10	AH 10	SC 1	TG 3
19	Abdomen	AH 11	AH 11	IH 1	TG 4
21	Hip and Buttocks	AH 13	TF 1	IC 1–IC 2	AH 1, AT 3
23	Knee and Thigh	AH 15	TF 4	IC 2–IC 4	AT 2
25	Ankle and Calf	AH 17	TF 5	IC 5	AT 1
26	Foot, Heel, and Toes	AH 17	TF 5–TF 6	IC 8	IT 1
30	Hand and Fingers	SF 6	SF 6	SC 8	LO 1
32	Wrist and Forearm	SF 5	SF 5	SC 7	LO 1
34	Elbow and Arm	SF 4	SF 4	SC 5–SC 6	LO 5
36	Shoulder	SF 2	SF 2	SC 4	LO 7, SF 1
38	Head and Skull	AT 1–AT 3	IH 7–IH 9	SC 3	LO 4
49	Tongue	LO 4	HX 8–HX 11	IC 7	LO 2
53	Skin	SF 6	HX 12–HX 15	SC 4	LO 4
69	Heart	IC 4	AH 3–AH 11	SC 7	LO 8
76	Diaphragm	HX 2	AH 11	SC 2	TG 4
81	Spleen	IC 8	CW 9	SC 8	LO 8
84	Kidney and Ureter	SC 6	IH 5, IH 6	IC 7–IC 8	AH 3, AH 8
88	Prostate	SC 4	IH 3, IH 4	IC 1	LO 2
89	Uterus	TF 5, TF 6	IH 3, IH 4	IC 2	LO 2
91	Ovaries/Testes	CW 1	IH 1, IH 2	IC 4–IC 5	LO 4
92	ACTH	TG 2–TG 3	HX 2–HX 7	IC 3–IC 6	LO 6
93	Cortisol	TG 2–TG 3	AH 9	SC 6	TG 2

Auricular Zones for Different Phases of Endodermal Tissue

Almost all ear reflex points for the endodermal internal organs are found in the Concha of Territory 2 for both the Chinese system and Phase I of Nogier's system. The Phase I internal organ points include ear reflex points for the digestive system, such as the Stomach and Intestines; respiratory points such as the Lungs and Bronchi; abdominal organs such as the Bladder, Gall Bladder, Pancreas, and Liver; and the endocrine glands, such as the Thymus, Thyroid, and Parathyroid. All of these endodermal points shift to the Lobe and the Tragus of Territory 3 in Phase II and to the helix and antihelix areas of Territory 1 in Phase III.

The Chinese auricular system and the Nogier Phase I system both show the digestive system beginning in the inferior concha below the helix root, rising up to the Stomach on the concha ridge peripheral to LM_0, and then rising further into the superior concha, where the Duodenum, Small Intestines, and Large Intestines are found. The Chinese ear points and the Phase I auricular points for the Lung and Bronchi are found on the inferior concha; the Liver on the peripheral concha ridge; and the Pancreas, Gall Bladder, and Bladder on the superior concha. The Phase II internal organs are mostly located on the ear lobe, and the Phase III endodermal organs are mostly found on the scaphoid fossa, triangular fossa, and antihelix.

TABLE 7.3	Auricular Zones Related to Internal Organs in Nogier Phases.			
No.	Internal Organ Points	Chinese	Phase I	Phase II	Phase III
		Territory 2	*Territory 2*	*Territory 3*	*Territory 1*
61	Esophagus	IC 6–IC 7	IC 6–IC 7	LO 1	HX 1
63	Stomach	CR 1	CR 1	LO 3	HX 2–HX 5
64	Duodenum	SC 1	SC 1	LO 5	TF 4
65	Small Intestines	SC 2	SC 2	LO 4	IH 3–IH 9
66	Large Intestines	SC 3	SC 3, SC 4	AT 1–AT 3	HX 10–HX 14
67	Rectum	HX 3	IH 3	IT 1	HX 15
68	Circulatory System	AT 2	CW 4–CW 8	CW 1–CW 3	CW 9–CW 10
70	Lungs	IC 4	IC 4, IC 5	LO 8	SF 2–SF 3
71	Bronchi	IC 6	IC 3	LO 7, LO 8	SF 1
74	Larynx	ST 4	ST 1	LO 8	AH 4
79	Liver	CR 2	CR 2, SC 8	LO 7	SF 4, SF 5
82	Gall Bladder	SC 8	SC 8	LO 2	AH 13, AH 14
83	Pancreas	SC 7	SC 7	LO 1	TF 3–TF 5
86	Urinary Bladder	SC 5	SC 5, SC 6	LO 6	SF 6, AH 18
87	Urethra	HX 4	SC 4	LO 1	TF 6
94	Thymus Gland	—	IC 8	LO 5	HX 6–HX 8
96	Thyroid Gland	AH 8	IC 2	AH 1, AH 8	AH 2
97	Parathyroid Gland	—	IC 1	HX 15	AH 1

The Chinese ear charts do not show representation of the Thymus Gland or the Parathyroid Gland, but they do place the Thyroid Gland in its appropriate anatomical location near the region of the Neck ear points on the antihelix tail. The Nogier Phase I location for these three endocrine glands is shown on the inferior concha, and the Phase II location is shown on the region where the antihelix tail, the helix tail, and the peripheral ear lobe all come together. The Phase II and Phase III locations for the Thyroid and Parathyroid glands better conform to where these endocrine glands had been previously described than does the Phase I location for these three glands. In contrast, the Phase I location for the Thymus Gland is similar to previous descriptions of where this gland is represented on the auricle. The whole circulatory system is found along different sections of the concha wall (Table 7.3).

Auricular Zones for Different Phases of Ectodermal Tissue

Chinese Neuroendocrine Points: The nervous system and the endocrine system are mostly represented on the concha wall of Territory 3 in the Chinese ear charts. Chinese ear acupuncturists have not focused on the location of nervous system points on the ear as much as have the European schools of auriculotherapy. A most notable example of this lack of neurological emphasis is that the Chinese ear charts refer to one ear point as the "Brain" point, not at all specifying which part of the brain this point represents. At the same time, this "Brain" point turns out to be a very important point for the treatment of many disorders, particularly addictions. The master point that Nogier and colleagues first identified as the "Thalamus" point was independently discovered by the Chinese, which they labeled the "Subcortex" point. Although the Chinese ear charts do in fact describe the location of the Pituitary Gland, the master gland for the control of all endocrine hormones, they do not go into as much detail regarding the specific pituitary hormones that regulate hormone release by the peripheral endocrine glands.

Phase I Neuroendocrine Points: The central nervous system is represented on the ear lobe of Territory 3 in Nogier's Phase I. Whereas the Chinese ear charts seem overly minimal about the location of different brain areas, the European descriptions of the auricular location for specific areas of the nervous system are amazingly detailed. By advanced utilization of the VAS pulse, specific pulse reactions were obtained in response to biochemical filters that contained specific extracts of brain tissue. The lobes of the Cerebral Cortex in Phase I essentially correspond to how they have been previously described in this text, but the subcortical nuclei sometimes have rather different locations. The Thalamus and Hypothalamus in Phase I are found on the surface of the antitragus and the adjacent regions of the lobe rather than where they were previously described on the concha wall and inferior concha.

Phase II Neuroendocrine Points: The Neuroendocrine system shifts to the helix, the antihelix, and the triangular fossa regions of Territory 1 in Phase II. The Pituitary point for Gonadotrophins in Phase II is located in the triangular fossa region, near the Chinese Uterus point. The Thalamus in Phase II corresponds to the auricular location for the Chinese master point Shen Men. The Cerebral Cortex in Phase II is found along the antihelix superior crus, scaphoid fossa, and triangular fossa.

Phase III Neuroendocrine Points: The Neuroendocrine system shifts to the Territory 2 concha in Phase III. The Cortical areas are located in the superior concha and the subcortical Limbic and Striatal areas in the inferior concha. The location of the Phase III Thalamus occurs with its original designation on the concha wall, whereas the Phase III Hypothalamus is found in the inferior concha, which coincides with the location of the Chinese Lung points used in the treatment of narcotic detoxification and drug abuse. Although the stimulation of the Lung meridian for substance abuse makes sense from a TCM perspective, the utilization of the Hypothalamus in the treatment of addiction makes better sense from a Western medicine view point (Table 7.4).

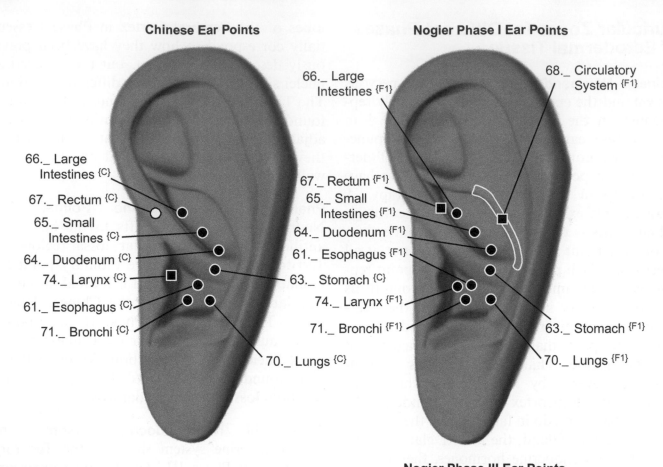

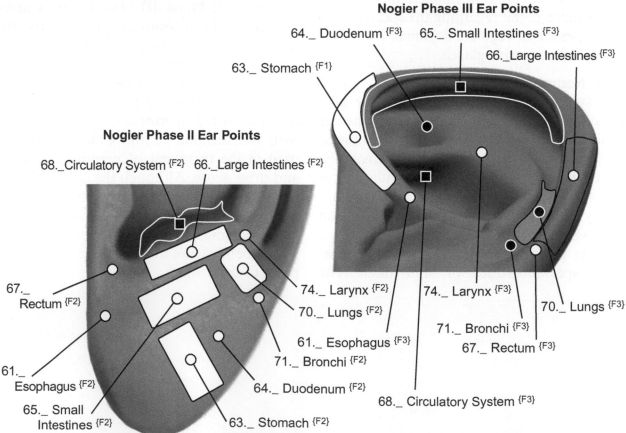

FIGURE 7.38 Thoracic organs represented in the auricular endodermal phase.

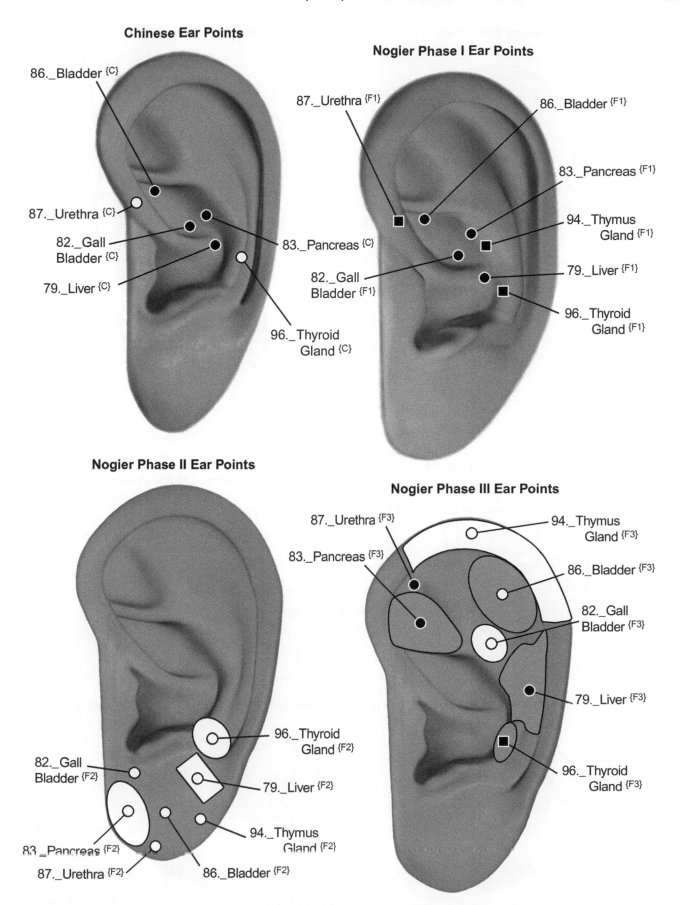

Chinese Ear Points

86._Bladder {C}

87._Urethra {C}

82._Gall Bladder {C}

79._Liver {C}

83._Pancreas {C}

96._Thyroid Gland {C}

Nogier Phase I Ear Points

87._Urethra {F1}

86._Bladder {F1}

83._Pancreas {F1}

94._Thymus Gland {F1}

82._Gall Bladder {F1}

79._Liver {F1}

96._Thyroid Gland {F1}

Nogier Phase II Ear Points

82._Gall Bladder {F2}

83._Pancreas {F2}

87._Urethra {F2}

86._Bladder {F2}

94._Thymus Gland {F2}

79._Liver {F2}

96._Thyroid Gland {F2}

Nogier Phase III Ear Points

87._Urethra {F3}

83._Pancreas {F3}

94._Thymus Gland {F3}

86._Bladder {F3}

82._Gall Bladder {F3}

79._Liver {F3}

96._Thyroid Gland {F3}

FIGURE 7.39 Abdominal organs represented in the auricular endodermal phase.

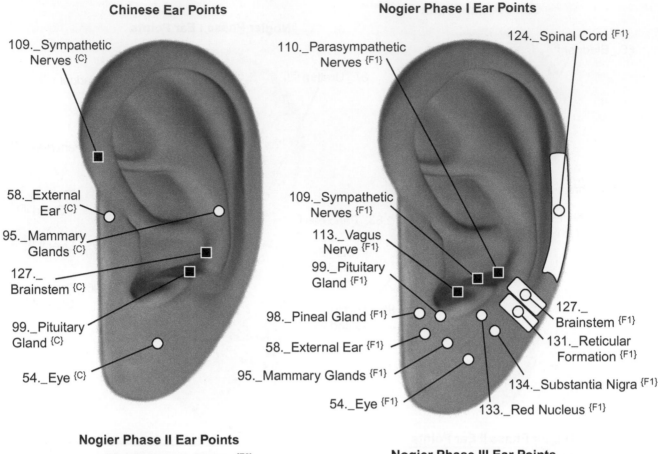

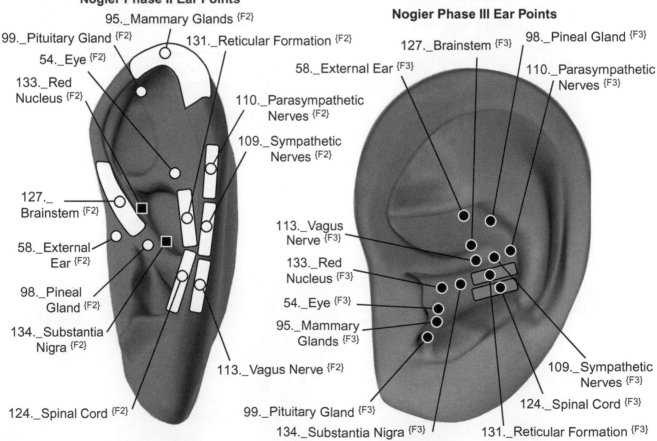

Chinese Ear Points

109._Sympathetic Nerves {C}

58._External Ear {C}

95._Mammary Glands {C}

127._Brainstem {C}

99._Pituitary Gland {C}

54._Eye {C}

Nogier Phase I Ear Points

110._Parasympathetic Nerves {F1}

124._Spinal Cord {F1}

109._Sympathetic Nerves {F1}

113._Vagus Nerve {F1}

99._Pituitary Gland {F1}

98._Pineal Gland {F1}

58._External Ear {F1}

95._Mammary Glands {F1}

54._Eye {F1}

127._Brainstem {F1}

131._Reticular Formation {F1}

134._Substantia Nigra {F1}

133._Red Nucleus {F1}

Nogier Phase II Ear Points

95._Mammary Glands {F2}

99._Pituitary Gland {F2}

131._Reticular Formation {F2}

54._Eye {F2}

133._Red Nucleus {F2}

110._Parasympathetic Nerves {F2}

109._Sympathetic Nerves {F2}

127._Brainstem {F2}

58._External Ear {F2}

98._Pineal Gland {F2}

134._Substantia Nigra {F2}

113._Vagus Nerve {F2}

124._Spinal Cord {F2}

Nogier Phase III Ear Points

127._Brainstem {F3}

98._Pineal Gland {F3}

58._External Ear {F3}

110._Parasympathetic Nerves {F3}

113._Vagus Nerve {F3}

133._Red Nucleus {F3}

54._Eye {F3}

95._Mammary Glands {F3}

109._Sympathetic Nerves {F3}

124._Spinal Cord {F3}

99._Pituitary Gland {F3}

134._Substantia Nigra {F3}

131._Reticular Formation {F3}

FIGURE 7.40 Brainstem, spinal cord, and nerves represented in the auricular ectodermal phase.

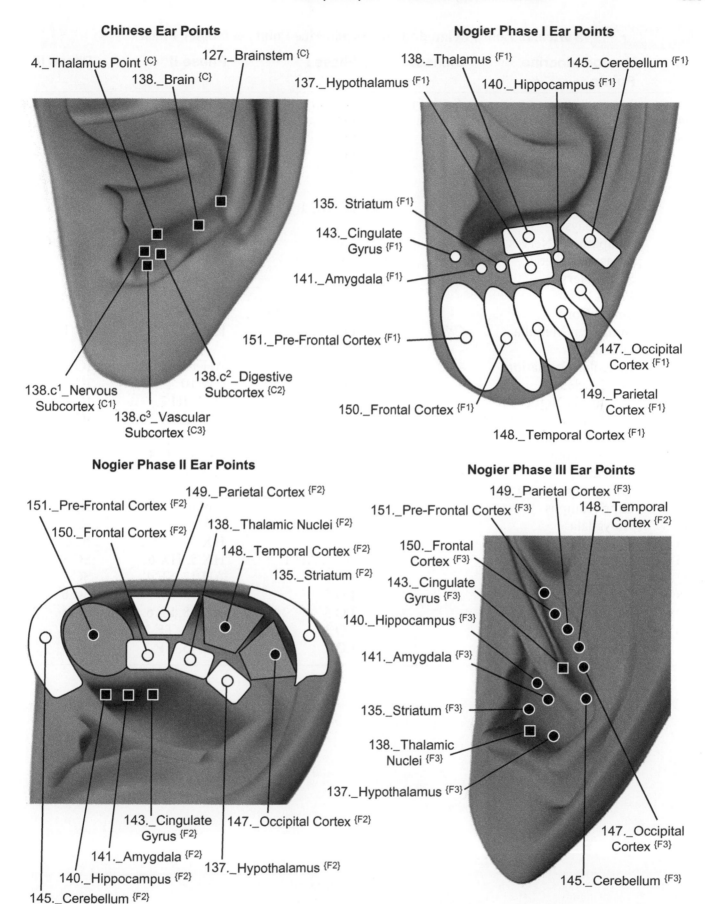

Chinese Ear Points

4._Thalamus Point {C}

127._Brainstem {C}

138._Brain {C}

138.c¹_Nervous Subcortex {C1}

138.c³_Vascular Subcortex {C3}

138.c²_Digestive Subcortex {C2}

Nogier Phase I Ear Points

138._Thalamus {F1}

145._Cerebellum {F1}

137._Hypothalamus {F1}

140._Hippocampus {F1}

135. Striatum {F1}

143._Cingulate Gyrus {F1}

141._Amygdala {F1}

151._Pre-Frontal Cortex {F1}

147._Occipital Cortex {F1}

149._Parietal Cortex {F1}

150._Frontal Cortex {F1}

148._Temporal Cortex {F1}

Nogier Phase II Ear Points

151._Pre-Frontal Cortex {F2}

149._Parietal Cortex {F2}

150._Frontal Cortex {F2}

138._Thalamic Nuclei {F2}

148._Temporal Cortex {F2}

135._Striatum {F2}

143._Cingulate Gyrus {F2}

147._Occipital Cortex {F2}

141._Amygdala {F2}

137._Hypothalamus {F2}

140._Hippocampus {F2}

145._Cerebellum {F2}

Nogier Phase III Ear Points

149._Parietal Cortex {F3}

148._Temporal Cortex {F2}

151._Pre-Frontal Cortex {F3}

150._Frontal Cortex {F3}

143._Cingulate Gyrus {F3}

140._Hippocampus {F3}

141._Amygdala {F3}

135._Striatum {F3}

138._Thalamic Nuclei {F3}

137._Hypothalamus {F3}

147._Occipital Cortex {F3}

145._Cerebellum {F3}

FIGURE 7.41 Cerebral cortex and forebrain nuclei represented in the auricular ectodermal phase.

TABLE 7.4 Auricular Zones Related to Neuroendocrine Points in Nogier Phases.

No.	Neuroendocrine Points	Chinese	Phase I	Phase II	Phase III
		Territory 3	*Territory 3*	*Territory 1*	*Territory 2*
54	Eye	LO 4	LO 4	AH 11	IC 3
58	External Ear	TG 5	LO 1	TG 5	SC 6
95	Mammary Gland	AH 10	LO 1	HX 7–HX 9	IC 1
98	Pineal Gland (Epiphysis)	—	TG 1	HX 1	SC 5
99	Pituitary Gland (Hypophysis)	IC 1	IT 2/IC 1	AH 17, AH 18	CW 1
109	Sympathetic Nerves	IH 4	CW 2	HX 12, HX 13	CR 1, CR 2
110	Parasympathetic Sacral Nerves	—	CW 3	HX 15	CR 2
113	Vagus Nerve	—	CW 1	HX 12	CR 1
124	Spinal Cord	—	HX 14, HX 15	AH 9, SF 2	IC 5
127	Brainstem Medulla Oblongata	CW 4	LO 7, LO 8	HX 2, HX 3	SC 1
131	Reticular Formation	—	LO 8	AH 12, SF 3	IC 8
133	Red Nucleus	—	LO 6	CW 10	IC 6
134	Substantia Nigra	—	LO 6	IH 1, IH 2	IC 7
135	Striatum (Basal Ganglia)		LO 4/AT 1	HX 9, HX 10	IC 3, IC 4
137	Hypothalamus	—	LO 6	AH 3, AH 4	IC 4
138	Thalamus (Subcortex, Brain)	CW 2	AT 2, AT 3	AH 11	CW 2, CW 3
140	Hippocampus	—	LO 2	CW 9	IC 6
141	Amygdala	—	LO 2, IT 1	CW 8	IC 7
143	Cingulate Gyrus		IT 1	HX 7	IC 6
145	Cerebellum		AT 3, AH 1	HX 5, HX 6	SC 8
147	Occipital Cortex		LO 7	AH 12, SF 4	SC 7
148	Temporal Cortex		LO 5	AH 14, SF 5	SC 6
149	Parietal Cortex		LO 5	AH 18, SF 6	SC 6
150	Frontal Cortex		LO 3	AH 13, TF 2	SC 5
151	Prefrontal Cortex		LO 1	AH 15, TF 3	SC 4

■ KEY TERMS FOR CHAPTER 7

Abdominal organs: The auricular points associated with other internal organs located in the abdomen reflect other visceral dysfunctions. These organs include the liver, which converts blood glucose into glycogen, incorporates amino acids into proteins, releases enzymes to metabolize toxic substances in the blood, and produces bile. Another such organ is the gall bladder, which releases bile into the small intestines to facilitate the digestion of fats. The spleen is a lymphatic organ next to the stomach that filters the blood and removes defective blood cells and bacteria. The pancreas produces digestive enzymes such as the hormone insulin to facilitate energy inside cells and the hormone glucagon to raise blood sugar levels. Finally, the appendix near the large intestine contains lymphatic tissue.

Autonomic Nervous System: This division of the peripheral nervous system consists of those nerves that connect the spinal cord to the visceral organs of the body.

Central Nervous System: The core of the nervous system consists of the brain and spinal cord, which respond to and regulate all other parts of the body. All auricular acupuncture points ultimately work through the central nervous system through reflex arcs in the spinal cord or the brainstem. The brain is represented on the ear lobe and the antitragus.

Circulatory System: The auricular points associated with pathology in this hydraulic fluid system include the cardiac heart muscle located in the thoracic chest cavity. The purpose of the heart is to send oxygen-rich blood through the arteries to deliver oxygen to all parts of the body and then receive oxygen-deficient blood from the veins. The lymphatic vessels collect excess fluid, metabolic wastes, and immune system breakdown products so that they can be eliminated from the body. Reactive ear points reflect pathology in cardiovascular organs.

Digestive System: The auricular points associated with problems in the gastrointestinal system refer to pathological conditions associated with the conversion of food that has been chewed by the mouth into smaller fragments, designed to become the basic nutrients absorbed by the body to provide metabolic energy and to form the basic building blocks for muscles, bones, and cellular tissue. The opening to the digestive system in the mouth passes food to the esophagus, which then allows the food to be stored in the stomach and broken down. The digestive food is then passed to the small intestines, where food is absorbed, and then to the large intestines and then released at the rectum. Ear points show reactive responses when this system of food processing is disrupted or when there is pain or pathology in any of the associated organs.

Functional Auricular Points: These auricular points are associated with a specific health problem rather than a specific part of the body and are used to treat that health disorder.

Master Auricular Points: These auricular points have mastery over the physiological and energetic function of many parts of the body and are used to treat a variety of health disorders.

Musculoskeletal System: The musculoskeletal system affected by somatotopic ear acupoints refers to the bones, muscles, tendons, ligaments, and fascia that comprise the physical body. However, the somatotopic auricular points that are associated with the musculoskeletal system represent specific pathological disorders associated with specific movements, muscles, tendons, ligaments, and the skeletal bone structures of the corresponding body area. Impaired blood vessel circulation to that somatotopic area is also represented on the auricle. These ear reflex points for the musculoskeletal body affect somatic nervous system reflexes that affect pathological maintenance of spinal reflex arcs. Somatic ear points also affect autonomic sympathetic reflexes associated with impaired vascular supply to the corresponding body region.

Parasympathetic Nervous System: This subdivision of the autonomic nervous system consists of those autonomic nerves that leave the central nervous system from either the cranium or the sacral vertebrae. Auricular points tend to improve underactivity in the parasympathetic nervous system.

Peripheral Nervous System: The peripheral nerves consist of (1) sensory neurons that send messages to the spinal cord from the skin, muscles, and visceral organs and (2) motor neurons that travel from the spinal cord out to the muscles and organs of the body. Like other peripheral organs, the auricle is functionally connected with the brain and with other areas of the body through peripheral nerves. Sensory neurons from a pathological organ send messages to the spinal cord and the brain, and from the brain messages are sent to the skin covering the auricle, forming an organocutaneous reflex. Sensory neurons from the reactive skin covering the auricle send messages to the brain, and from the brain messages are sent to heal the pathological organ, forming a cutaneo-organic reflex.

Respiratory System: The auricular points associated with pathology in this system reflect internal organ problems related to the exchange of air and carbon dioxide. The lungs absorb oxygen with each inhalation and release other gases upon exhalation. The mouth leads to the pharynx, larynx, and trachea, which then allows passage of air into the lungs through bronchial tubes that lead to expandable alveoli sacs, where gases are exchanged.

Somatic Nervous System: This part of the nervous system includes sensory neurons that receive afferent messages from the skin and regulate motor neurons that control the activation of skeletal muscles, leading to normal function, muscle spasms, or muscle paralysis. Somatic nerves are represented in Territory 1 of the auricle, covering the antihelix, triangular fossa, and scaphoid fossa.

Somatotopic Auricular Points: These auricular points are reactive when there is pain or pathology in a specific area of the body and are stimulated to alleviate health disorders in the corresponding part of the body.

Sympathetic Nervous System: This subdivision of the autonomic nervous system consists of those autonomic nerves that leave the spinal cord in the region of the thoracic and lumbar vertebrae and travel to a chain of ganglia alongside the spinal vertebrae. Auricular points tend to reduce overactivity in the sympathetic nervous system.

Urogenital Organs: The auricular points associated with pelvic organs are associated with dysfunctions in the urinary system and the reproductive systems. The purpose of the kidney is to filter toxic substances from the blood and release them into the urine through the ureter, a tube that leads from each kidney to the bladder. The bladder receives urine from the ureter and holds it for later release. The urethra connects the bladder and gonads to the outside world. The accessory reproductive organ in males that contributes milky substances to the semen is the prostate. The uterus is the reproductive organ in females that potentially holds an egg that has become fertilized. If fertilization does not occur, the vascular lining of the uterus is discharged during the menstrual period. The vagina is the reproductive organ in females that serves as the external entrance to the uterus. The external genitals include the penis in the male and the clitoris in the female.

■ CHAPTER 7 REVIEW QUESTIONS

1. The Sympathetic Autonomic point on the auricle is located on the_____.

   a. superior crus of the antihelix
   b. concha wall behind the antitragus
   c. internal helix adjacent to the inferior crus of the antihelix
   d. helix tail near the ear lobe

2. The gate control of pain signals is best represented on the auricle at the_____.

   a. Sympathetic Autonomic point
   b. Master Oscillation point
   c. Endocrine Internal Secretion point
   d. Thalamus Subcortex point

3. The antihelix tail on the auricle represents the_____.

   a. Cervical Vertebrae
   b. Thoracic Vertebrae
   c. Lumbar Vertebrae
   d. Sacral Vertebrae

4. The European Knee point is represented on the_____.

   a. scaphoid fossa
   b. triangular fossa
   c. superior crus of the antihelix
   d. inferior crus of the antihelix

5. The Occiput point that is used to treat headaches is found on the_____.

   a. tragus
   b. antitragus
   c. helix root
   d. antihelix body

6. The Stomach ear point that is used to treat nausea is found on the_____.

   a. ear lobe near the scaphoid fossa
   b. triangular fossa near the internal helix
   c. concha wall near the antitragus
   d. concha ridge near the helix root

7. The Chinese Kidney point is found on the_____.

   a. superior crus below the internal helix
   b. inferior concha near the ear canal
   c. superior concha below the antihelix inferior crus
   d. intertragic notch

8. The European and the Chinese ear points for the Thyroid Gland are located on the_____.

   a. antihelix tail
   b. helix tail
   c. triangular fossa
   d. tragus

9. The Prefrontal Cortex and the Master Cerebral point are located at the same area of the auricle, which is the_____.

   a. ear lobe
   b. tragus
   c. helix root
   d. scaphoid fossa

10. The Muscle Relaxation point is located on the_____.

    a. superior concha near the inferior crus
    b. superior crus below the helix arch
    c. inferior concha near the concha ridge
    d. subtragus near the helix root

Answers

1 = c; 2 = d; 3 = a; 4 = b; 5 = b; 6 = d; 7 = c; 8 = a; 9 = a; 10 = c

Clinical Case Studies of Auriculotherapy

8

CONTENTS

[8.0 | Clinical Case Studies of Auriculotherapy

CHAPTER 8 LEARNING OBJECTIVES

1. To describe frequently used auriculotherapy treatment procedures.

2. To provide clinical examples of different medical disorders treated with auriculotherapy.

3. To demonstrate clinical application of ear acupuncture procedures.

8.1 Clinical Experiences with Auriculotherapy

My personal experience with auriculotherapy began at the UCLA Pain Management Clinic in 1975. As a licensed psychologist working in an interdisciplinary pain clinic, I was asked to work with the chronic pain patients who had not benefited from previous trials of opiate medications, antidepressants, localized nerve blocks, or trigger point injections. Patients were referred to me by other doctors in the UCLA Medical Center for biofeedback training or auriculotherapy. Biofeedback therapy allowed patients to gradually learn to reduce their pathological muscle spasms and to improve vascular circulation. Patients were referred for auriculotherapy as a more direct procedure for immediately alleviating chronic pain. Whereas licensed acupuncturists activate acupuncture points with the insertion of needles, my clinical practice with auriculotherapy has predominantly utilized transcutaneous, microcurrent stimulation of ear reflex points. Electronic equipment that was used at UCLA included the Stim Flex, the Electro-Acuscope, and the HMR stimulator. An electrical detecting probe was guided over specific regions of the auricle to identify electrically reactive ear points. When an active ear point was detected, a button was pressed on the same bipolar probe to briefly stimulate the reactive ear point. There is no invasion of the skin with needles; thus, this approach tends to be less painful than other forms of auricular stimulation. Adhesive ear seeds or magnetic pellets were often placed on the identified ear points for more prolonged stimulation of the points.

When I was first learning auriculotherapy, it was very helpful to have a wall chart of ear acupuncture points positioned on the wall immediately above the treatment table where patients were being examined. Electronic equipment, acupuncture needles, or ear pellets were available on a nearby stand. While the inverted fetus concept facilitates an easy comprehension of which portions of the auricle relate to a particular patient's problem, the ready access to seeing the ear points on a wall chart can assist in precise point location. One can quickly learn the identification of auricular acupoints that one uses in most treatment plans, but one may still need a reminder of the location of ear points that are used less frequently. It is not necessary that a patient lie on a treatment table because patients are treated very easily in an ordinary armchair or a reclining chair. However, it is best that the practitioner is either standing or sitting at eye level with the patient's ear. Comfort for the practitioner as well as the patient is important when one sees a large number of individuals.

The first several years of my practice of auriculotherapy required that I suspend my skeptical judgment of the lack of scientific explanations for this procedure. I would observe rather remarkable examples of the effective treatment of pain problems that defied ordinary medical conceptualizations, yet I continued to have doubts that there was any veracity to this strange technique. I would repeatedly see significant improvements in the health status of patients with previously intractable pain, but my internal disbelief remained. I was encouraged by the writings of Dr. Paul Nogier (1972) in his *Treatise of Auriculotherapy*, who stated that

any method should not be rejected out of hand merely because it remains unexplained and does not tie up with our present scientific knowledge. A discovery is rarely logical and often goes against the conceptions then in fashion. It is often the result of a basic observation which has been sufficiently clear and repeatable for it to be retained.

Nogier further commented that

the spinal column, like the limbs, is projected clearly and simply in the external ear. The therapeutic applications are free from ambiguity and ought to allow the beginner to achieve convincing results. Each doctor needs to be convinced of the efficacy of the method by personal results, and he is right.

I needed many observations of the clinical effectiveness of auriculotherapy before I was convinced. The words of Nogier reminded me of the biofeedback literature that has emphasized the pioneering research on stress by Dr. Hans Selye. In his classic text, *The Stress of Life*, Selye (1976) described the initial scientific opposition to his concept that "there is a 'nonspecific' factor which contributes to disease in addition to the 'specific' pathogens first discovered by Pasteur." Selye relayed the story that one senior professor whom he admired "reminded me for months that he had attempted to convince me that I must abandon this futile line of research" on generalized factors for stress.

Fortunately, Selye persevered in his research and discovered that chronic stress leads to an enlargement of the adrenal glands, atrophy of the thymus glands, and ulcers in the gastrointestinal tissue. These organic changes are now widely recognized as reliable indications of the biological response to a variety of nonspecific stressors. Pasteur himself had to overcome considerable opposition to the "germ theory," which postulated that invisible micro-organisms could be the sole source of an illness. Many of Pasteur's colleagues scoffed at the supposed dangers of these invisible agents, but today, sterilized techniques in surgery and in acupuncture are based on Pasteur's seemingly bizarre proposals. Pasteur's professional colleagues in the 1860s were very skeptical that invisible germs could be the originator of medical diseases, whereas Selye's professional colleagues in the 1960s were equally skeptical that nonspecific stressors could impair the body's immunity to diseases. Alternative theories and therapies often require patience and persistence before they become widely accepted by the medical profession as a whole.

In this chapter, I incorporate my own clinical findings with those of other health care practitioners who treat auricular acupuncture points with needles or who utilize the Nogier vascular autonomic signal in diagnosis and treatment. I have endeavored to select cases that provide insight into the underlying processes affecting auriculotherapy as well as provide examples of typical clinical results one might expect from such treatments. The order of presentation of specific clinical cases first focuses on myofascial pain disorders, health conditions related to internal organs, neuropathic dysfunctions, and the auricular treatments used for substance abuse disorders. The results of clinical surveys completed by certified practitioners in this field are presented to show auriculotherapy treatment plans that have been found to be the most effective with different health conditions. The treatment protocols presented in Chapter 9 are partly based on the findings of the Nanking Army Ear Acupuncture Research Team. In 1958, this team compiled the results of more than 2000 clinical cases using the ear acupuncture inverted fetus map that was introduced to them from the West. In more recent research in the United States, a similar analysis was conducted on more than 2000 clinical cases that were obtained from practitioners certified by the Auriculotherapy Certification Institute (ACI) from 1999 to 2011.

8.2 Survey of Clinical Cases Seen by ACI Practitioners

The ACI was formed in 1999 at the International Consensus Conference on Acupuncture, Auriculotherapy, and Auricular Medicine (ICCAAAM'99). ACI certification served to acknowledge the advanced training of health care practitioners who had developed special expertise in their knowledge of auricular acupuncture and auriculotherapy. Certification

| TABLE 8.1 | Demographic Characteristics of Clinical Cases Evaluated for ACI Survey. |

Total No. of Clinical Cases Evaluated	No.	%
Female patients	7,922	64.8
Male patients	4,297	35.2
Total	12,219	

Age of Patients Evaluated	Mean	Standard Deviation
Average age (years)	43.6	16.2
Age range of patients (years)	2–92	

requirements include a 70% pass rate on 75 multiple-choice questions on the ACI Written Exam and direct observation of ear point location by a trained instructor who administers the ACI Practicum Exam. Each applicant is required to submit 20 clinical cases that included ear acupuncture or auriculotherapy as part of the treatment. The data in this analysis were chosen from more than 6000 clinical cases obtained from 620 ACI-certified practitioners. The specific ear points that were used for different health disorders were tabulated for each case and are presented throughout this chapter.

As shown in Table 8.1, the 12,219 patients who were included in this sample were predominantly female, with a mean age of 43.6 years. Children as young as 2 years old and seniors as old as 92 years old were treated with auriculotherapy or auricular acupuncture.

Table 8.2 reveals that most of these patients were treated with the simple insertion of acupuncture needles into the external ear, the electrical stimulation (EAS) of ear acupoints through needles inserted into the auricle, or the activation of auricular points by transcutaneous electrical stimulation (TAS) by surface electrodes that do not penetrate the skin. A substantial portion of the patients were treated by the application of acubeads, ear vaccaria seeds, or small magnetic pellets fastened to the ear with adhesive tape. Only a small percentage of the patients in

TABLE 8.2	Frequency of Different Types of Auricular Treatments.		
Categories of Treatment Procedures Utilized		**No.**	**%**
Insertion of ear acupuncture needles alone		3,532	28.9
Electroacupuncture stimulation of ear points (EAS)		2,529	20.7
Transcutaneous auricular stimulation (TAS)		3,873	31.7
Laser auricular stimulation (LAS)		245	2.0
Acubeads, ear vaccaria seeds, adhesive magnetic pellets		1,857	15.2
Manual acupressure of auricle, ear reflexology		183	1.5
Total		12,219	100.0

TABLE 8.3	Number of Sessions Used for Auriculotherapy Treatment.	
Total No. of Sessions Provided	**No.**	**%**
1	6,342	51.9
2	2,000	16.4
3	1,035	8.5
4–6	1,397	11.4
7–10	852	7.0
>10	593	4.9
Total	12,219	100.0

TABLE 8.4	Clinical Results of All Patients Treated by ACI Practitioners.	
Treatment Results of Clinical Cases Evaluated	**No.**	**%**
Excellent results	1,992	16.3
Good results	4,194	34.3
Moderate results	2,773	22.7
Slight results	2,226	18.2
No improvement	1,034	8.5
Total	12,219	100.0

this sample were treated by laser stimulation of ear points or by manual acupressure applied to auricular acupoints. The high proportion of patients treated by TAS may be related to the relatively high presence of chiropractic doctors who applied for ACI certification, whereas licensed acupuncturists more often preferred needle insertion alone or EAS through inserted needles. In addition to the 1857 individuals who were treated with acubeads alone, an equal number of the patients in this sample were given acubeads after either EAS or TAS auriculotherapy treatment.

Table 8.3 shows that a majority of the clinical cases submitted for ACI certification required only one auriculotherapy treatment, with two-thirds of the sample requiring less than four treatment sessions. It is not necessarily the case that most auriculotherapy treatments require only one to three sessions, as these cases were not randomly chosen from the potential pool of patients treated by ACI applicants. At the same time, that such a large number of cases could

be resolved by one or two sessions supports the common clinical observation that auriculotherapy and ear acupuncture can achieve rapid clinical effectiveness.

The therapeutic improvement of clinical symptoms tabulated across all types of disorders that were treated with auriculotherapy is shown in Table 8.4. A majority of these ACI clinical cases showed good to excellent results. Although such statements of clinical effectiveness were subjective findings, these results nonetheless demonstrated very high levels of clinical improvement by the participating patients.

In order to tabulate the frequency of different types of clinical disorders that were treated with auricular acupuncture or auriculotherapy, all patients in the ACI sample were designated with a specific code number associated with specific clinical conditions. Most of these symptom categories are comparable to the diagnostic distinctions used in the *International Classification of*

TABLE 8.5	Frequency of Different Clinical Disorders Treated by ACI Practitioners.			
Code	**ACI Category of Clinical Disorders**	**ICD Codes**	**No.**	**%**
3.0	Substance Abuse Disorders	303–305	1,148	9.4
4.0	Chronic Pain Disorders	710–847	6,268	51.3
5.0	Mental Health Disorders	290–311	1,792	14.7
6.0	Neurological and Sensory Disorders	320–389	576	4.7
7.0	Internal Organ Disorders	390–629	1,347	11.0
8.0	Endocrine & Immune Disorders	010–279	1,087	8.9
	Total		12,219	100.0

Diseases, Ninth Revision (ICD-9), with several exceptions. Whereas the substance abuse disorders are categorized by *ICD* as a small subsection of mental health disorders, this classification is presented more prominently in these ACI cases because auricular acupuncture is frequently used for substance abuse disorders. Moreover, the same set of ear points are used to treat biochemically different addictive substances; thus, the grouping of the substance abuse disorders together made more sense in terms of showing the ear acupuncture points used to treat such disorders. Chronic pain problems are presented in multiple categories in *ICD*, but they are grouped into one set of disorders in the accompanying ACI table. The majority of chronic pain disorders are related to musculoskeletal dysfunctions, including myofascial spasms, ligament sprains, and bone fractures. The auriculotherapy treatments for such chronic pain disorders are primarily based on the corresponding area of the body where the problem occurs, not necessarily on the underlying tissue disorder that is involved.

The major categories of clinical disorders identified for the ACI survey are presented in Table 8.5, and subcategories of these primary conditions are presented in Tables 8.6 to 8.11. Patients treated with auriculotherapy for alcoholism, substance abuse, and drug dependence—*ICD* codes 303–305—were given the numerical categories "3.1" to "3.4." The identification code "3.5" was used for the treatment of obesity and overeating, comparable to the *ICD* code 278. Chronic pain disorders were given ACI identification codes beginning with the numeral "4," from "4.1" for

back pain and sciatica to "4.9" for post-surgical pain and wound care. These pain-related conditions are generally classified in *ICD* diagnoses as codes 710–739, disorders of the musculoskeletal and connective tissues, including spasms, sprains, and strains. Mental health disorders are identified in *ICD* with code numbers 290–302. They were given ACI code numbers beginning with the numeral "5," from "5.1" for anxiety disorders to "5.7" for irritability problems. Diseases affecting the nervous system and sensory organs are identified in *ICD* diagnoses with codes 390–450 and were categorized in this study with numbers beginning with the numeral "6." Dysfunctions in various internal organs, including digestive disorders, respiratory disorders, and circulatory disorders, were given numbers beginning with the numeral "7." Finally, the numeral "8" was used to categorize a variety of symptoms related to different endocrine glands or to problems with one's immune system, including neoplasms.

As revealed in Table 8.5, the great majority (51.3%) of clinical disorders treated in this sample were for the treatment of some type of pain disorder. The other categories of clinical problems that were treated by ACI practitioners in this study ranged from 9% to 15% for substance abuse disorders, mental health disorders, internal organ dysfunctions, and endocrine or immune disorders. Less than 5% of the disorders examined in this sample were for neurological or sensory disorders. In a retrospective evaluation of the National Health Insurance database of patients using acupuncture services in Taiwan, Lin *et al.* (2011) reported similar percentages for

TABLE 8.6	Frequency of Substance Abuse Disorders Included in ACI Survey.		
Code	**ACI Category of Clinical Disorders**	**No.**	**%**
3.1	Smoking Cessation, Nicotine Addiction, Tobacco Withdrawal	628	54.7
3.2	Alcohol Abuse, Sedative Abuse, Hangovers	61	5.3
3.3	Opioid Abuse, Heroin, Vicodin, Oxycontin Abuse	36	3.2
3.4	Stimulant Abuse, Poly Drug Abuse	80	7.0
3.5	Appetite Control, Obesity, Weight Loss, Anorexia, Bulimia	343	29.9
	Total	1148	100.0

TABLE 8.7	Frequency of Chronic Pain Disorders Included in ACI Survey.		
Code	**ACI Category of Clinical Disorders**	**No.**	**%**
4.1	Back Pain, Sciatica, Hip Pain, Buttocks Spasms	1814	28.9
4.2	Tension Headaches, Migraine Headaches	815	13.0
4.3	Neck and Shoulder Pain	1474	23.5
4.4	Pain in Leg, Knee, Ankle, Foot, and Toes	832	13.3
4.5	Pain in Arm, Elbow, Wrist, Hand, and Fingers	654	10.4
4.6	Dental Pain, TMJ, Toothache, Gum Gingivitis, Facial Tics	331	5.3
4.7	Osteoarthritis, Rheumatoid Arthritis	144	2.3
4.8	Fibromyalgia, General Body Aches, Muscle Tension	180	2.9
4.9	Anesthesia, Post-Surgical Pain, Wound Care	24	0.4
	Total	6268	100.0

prostate cancer patients. The prevalence of acupuncture use from 2002 to 2008 by 2413 cancer patients revealed that 51.2% reported chronic pain disorders (*ICD* codes 710–739), 29.1% reported injury disorders (*ICD* codes 800–999), 9.2% reported circulatory system disorders (*ICD* codes 390–459), 4.3% reported neoplasm disorders (*ICD* codes 140–239), and 3.0% reported nervous system disorders (*ICD* codes 320–389).

A further breakdown of the specific disorders within each major category of this ACI sample is first shown for substance abuse disorders in Table 8.6. Within the category of substance abuse disorders, the most common clinical problem treated with auricular acupuncture was for smoking cessation (54.7%). The next most frequent clinical problem treated by auriculotherapy was for appetite control and weight loss (29.9%). Less than 10% of this ACI sample was treated for alcohol abuse, opioid abuse, or poly substance abuse. Two of the most common health conditions seen with auriculotherapy and

auricular acupuncture were for the treatment of nicotine addiction and for the alleviation of obesity problems. One reason why this ACI coding system was developed was to tabulate the variety of terms presented in clinical treatment notes for each of these conditions, such as the terms "smoking cessation," "nicotine addiction," or "tobacco dependence," all indicating the same condition, or the terms "weight loss," "eating disorder," or "obesity problems" referring to the same health problem. Because there were just a few examples of other eating disorders, such as "anorexia" or "bulimia," they were grouped into the same category as individuals seeking to limit their food intake in order to reduce their weight. Similar ear points were used for all of the conditions placed in a particular category.

Presented in Table 8.7 are the frequency distributions of different chronic pain disorders treated with auriculotherapy. Within this subcategory, the most frequent types of medical problems that were treated were back pain (28.9%), neck

TABLE 8.8	Frequency of Mental Health Disorders Included in ACI Survey.		
Code	**ACI Category of Clinical Disorders**	**No.**	**%**
5.1	Anxiety, Worry, Panic, Stress-Related Disorders	552	30.8
5.2	Sleep Disorders, Insomnia, Sleep Apnea	506	28.2
5.3	Fatigue, Chronic Fatigue Syndrome, Exhaustion	263	14.7
5.4	Depressed Mood, Bipolar Mood Disorders	292	16.3
5.5	Psychosis, Schizophrenia, Delusions	11	0.6
5.6	Attention Deficit Disorder, Dyslexia, Memory	90	5.0
5.7	Irritable, Agitated, Frustrated	78	4.4
	Total	1792	100.0

TABLE 8.9	Frequency of Neurological and Sensory Disorders Included in ACI Survey.		
Code	**ACI Category of Clinical Disorders**	**No.**	**%**
6.1	Stroke, Concussion, Head Trauma	109	19.0
6.2	Epileptic Seizures, Convulsions	63	11.0
6.3	Tremors, Palsy, Parkinson's Disease, Post-Polio Syndrome	46	8.0
6.4	Neuropathy, Peripheral Neuralgia, Shingles	39	6.8
6.5	Dermatitis, Skin Disorders, Acne, Hives, Hair Loss	63	11.0
6.6	Hearing Impaired, Sensorineural Deafness, Tinnitus	109	19.0
6.7	Dizziness, Vertigo, Balance Problems	63	11.0
6.8	Visual Impairment, Blurry Vision, Eye Disorder, Dry Eyes	46	8.0
6.9	Olfactory Disorders, Taste, Dry Mouth, Xerostomia	36	6.3
	Total	576	100.0

and shoulder pain (23.5%), tension headaches and migraine headaches (13.0%), pain in the lower extremities (13.3%), and pain in the upper extremities (10.4%). The frequencies of other pain disorders treated in this sample, such as dental pain, arthritic pain, fibromyalgia, or surgical anesthesia, were all less than 10%.

As revealed in Table 8.8, the most frequent mental health disorders that were treated by auriculotherapy were anxiety or stress-related symptoms (30.8%), insomnia or sleep disturbance (28.2%), depressed mood (16.3%), and chronic fatigue (14.7%). The other mental health disorders that were treated in this sample were attention deficit disorder, impaired memory, and irritability or agitation, but they comprised less than 5% each of this mental health subcategory. There were even fewer examples of the use of auricular acupuncture for the treatment of psychosis or schizophrenia.

Table 8.9 shows the distribution of different neurological disorders and sensory disorders that were treated with auriculotherapy. Within this subcategory, the most frequent types of neurological problems examined were the 19% incidence of strokes, concussion, deafness, or tinnitus. The next most frequent neurological disorders observed were for seizures or convulsions at 11%, but similar frequencies were found for dermatological conditions, dizziness, or vertigo. Motor dysfunctions, such as tremors, cerebral palsy, and Parkinson's disease, and disorders related to visual impairment were the next most frequently treated conditions at 8%. The other neurological disorders that were treated in this sample included peripheral neuropathies and olfactory dysfunctions, taste problems, and dry mouth problems such as xerostomia.

The frequency of internal organ disorders treated with auriculotherapy in this sample is

TABLE 8.10	Frequency of Internal Organ Disorders Included in ACI Survey.		
Code	ACI Category of Clinical Disorders	No.	%
7.1	Nausea, Vomiting, Heartburn, Acid Reflux	241	17.9
7.2	Intestinal Disorders, Constipation, Diarrhea	350	26.0
7.3	Asthma, Bronchitis, Coughs, Hiccups	309	22.9
7.4	Coronary Disorders, Angina, Cardiac Arrhythmias	53	4.0
7.5	Circulatory Disorder, Hypertension, Low Blood Pressure	163	12.1
7.6	Abdominal Pain, Liver Disease, Gall Stones, Appendicitis	88	6.5
7.7	Urinary Disorders, Kidney Stones, Bladder Infections	143	10.6
	Total	1347	100.0

TABLE 8.11	Frequency of Endocrine and Immune Disorders included in ACI Survey.		
Code	ACI Category of Clinical Disorders	No.	%
8.1	Thyroid Disorders, Adrenal Disorders, Grave's Disease	39	3.6
8.2	Pancreatic Disorders, Diabetes, Hypoglycemia	66	6.0
8.3	Sexual Dysfunctions, Impotency, Prostate Problems	32	2.9
8.4	Gynecology, Menstrual Pain, Menopausal Disorders, PMS	297	27.3
8.5	Obstetrics, Infertility, Labor, Post-Partum Pain	51	4.7
8.6	Common Cold, Flu, Sneezing, Sore Throats, Tonsillitis	343	31.5
8.7	Allergies, Infections, Inflammations	178	16.3
8.8	Cancer, Cancer Pain, AIDS/HIV Disease, Med. Side Effects	83	7.6
	Total	1087	100.0

presented in Table 8.10. Within this subcategory, the most frequent types of medical problems that were treated included gastrointestinal disorders affecting the stomach and the intestines (43.9%); cardiovascular disorders related to the heart and circulatory system (16.1%); respiratory disorders such as asthma, coughs, and hiccups (22.9%); and dysfunctions related to other abdominal organs (17.1%).

The final categories consist of disorders for endocrine dysfunctions and immune system problems, which are presented in Table 8.11. The greatest number of such disorders in this sample was utilized for symptoms of the common cold or influenza, such as sneezing and sore throats (31.3%); allergic symptoms, infections, or inflammations (16.3%); and gynecological problems, such as perimenstrual distress or menopause (27.3%). The specific protocols of auricular points that were used for the auriculotherapy treatment of each of these clinical conditions are presented in Chapter 9.

8.3 Auriculotherapy for Reducing Myofascial Trigger Points

During my tenure in the Pain Management Clinic at the UCLA Medical Center in the 1970s and 1980s, residents in the UCLA Department of Anesthesiology were offered training in pain management as one of their elective rotations. These residents were routinely shown demonstrations of trigger point injections as an alternative procedure to the nerve blocks that anesthesiologists conventionally utilized to treat chronic pain. Myofascial pain could be alleviated by intravenous injection of a local anesthetic into a specific trigger point, thus blocking the neurological reflex arcs that sustain chronic muscle spasms. On one occasion, a group of UCLA residents first observed the primary clinic physician palpate the trapezius muscle of patient CN, who was suffering from chronic shoulder pain. Hypersensitive trigger points were identified on the patient's right trapezius muscle, and

CN had significant limitation in the range of motion of his right arm. The attending physician suggested that the residents observe a demonstration of auriculotherapy prior to their practice with trigger point injections. I examined the patient's right ear, and localized reactive points were found on the shoulder region of the auricle. Electrical stimulation of these reactive ear points led to an immediate reduction in the patient's subjective sense of discomfort. The range of motion in his arm was no longer limited. When the original physician again palpated CN's trapezius muscle, he could no longer objectively identify the previously detected trigger points. The success of the auriculotherapy eliminated the need for any other treatment. Because the presence of the trigger points had been evaluated by another doctor who was not present when the auriculotherapy was conducted, this anecdotal observation was comparable to a double-blind assessment of patient improvement.

One of the most common conditions recently seen in many pain clinics is the diagnosis of fibromyalgia, literally defined as the presence of pain in many groups of muscle fibers. JM was a 43-year-old female who reported pain in multiple parts of her body. She exhibited hypersensitive trigger points in her jaw, neck, shoulders, upper back, hips, and legs. Reactive auricular points were evidenced throughout the ear. The auricular points corresponding to the Jaw, Cervical Vertebrae, Thoracic Vertebrae, Shoulders, and Hips were electrically stimulated at 10 Hz, on both the anterior and the posterior regions of the external ear. Bilateral, transcutaneous stimulation was also applied to Point Zero, Shen Men, Thalamus point, Endocrine point, and Muscle Relaxation. After each auriculotherapy treatment, JM reported feeling very relaxed and experienced a profound decrease in her various pain symptoms. Unfortunately, the aches in her spine and in her limbs gradually returned several days following the treatment. Biofeedback relaxation training and individual psychotherapy were also integral to the progressive improvement over 14 weeks of treatment. Complex pain disorders, such as fibromyalgia, require more than the alleviation of nociceptive sensations. Successful treatment of fibromyalgia also required attention to the management of daily stressors and helping the individual to resolve deeper, psychodynamic, emotional conflicts.

Someone who did not respond so favorably to interdisciplinary treatment was patient EJ, a 45-year-old married mother of two teenage children. She complained of chronic pain in many parts of her body and only reluctantly discussed that she had problems in her marriage. She had been referred to me by a fibromyalgia support group that met in a Los Angeles hospital. EJ reported severe tenderness and discomfort at trigger points found all over her body. For each of the multiple sites of pain perception in the body, there were tender points on her external ear that corresponded to these areas of body discomfort. Stimulation of the electrically reactive auricular points successfully led to profound reductions in perceived pain and also led to enhanced feelings of comfort and relaxation. EJ seemed very grateful for this immediate treatment effect, but unfortunately, the therapeutic effects only lasted several days. She also indicated that there were ongoing conflicts regarding her marriage. She was afraid of being alone, yet she was also quite frustrated by the continued lack of personal attention from her husband. The stress of this indecision seemed to reinitiate her fibromyalgia pain each week. Besides the musculoskeletal ear points and master points that are typically used for the treatment of pain, EJ also received stimulation of the ear acupoints related to psychosomatic disorders, nervousness, and depression. However, when it was suggested that she might consider the option of more directly asserting her personal needs to her husband, she became first defensive and then very quiet. She did not return for any other auriculotherapy sessions, complaining that she only wanted to focus on her pain problem, not on these psychological issues in her life. There are certain patients who are not ready to fully engage in health care procedures that might reduce their physical pain when it would also require that they address some of the psychosocial sources of their emotional discomfort.

8.4 Auriculotherapy Treatment of Back Pain

One of the most frequent applications of auriculotherapy is for the treatment of back pain. DF was a 43-year-old married mother of two adult children who had been injured on the playground at the elementary school where she taught. Various medical procedures by four other doctors at UCLA led to partial but inconsistent relief of her back pain. Auriculotherapy treatment produced a marked release of the tightness in her back, but her pain gradually returned after each session. Despite the persistent aching in her back, DF continued to go to work regularly as a high school teacher and to do the household chores and cooking for her husband, son, and daughter when she got home. It was not until DF also learned biofeedback relaxation and assertiveness skills that the pain subsided for longer durations. She needed to be strongly encouraged to verbally express to her family that she needed assistance around the house and that she needed to take time for herself to rest and relax. Sometimes a pain problem is present for secondary gain issues that must be corrected before the effects of auriculotherapy can be sustained. Auriculotherapy can dramatically alleviate back pain, but the patient's lifestyle that puts additional stress on that individual must also be addressed.

Patient CJ was a 38-year-old male airline pilot who attributed his chronic back pain to the 2-hour commute from his home in Santa Barbara, California, to the airline headquarters based at Los Angeles International Airport. The patient's drawings of the exact location of his discomfort indicated that intense pain was localized to his left buttocks. Although there were several reactive acupoints on CJ's right and left external ears, it was the Buttocks and Lumbago points on the left ear that were indeed the highest in perceived tenderness and were the highest in electrical conductivity. Even though his job stress remained unchanged, five auriculotherapy treatments led to pronounced relief of the pain in his buttocks.

While talking with him during the course of an auriculotherapy session, CJ divulged that he was in constant arguments with his wife, who was divorcing him after she found out that he was having an extramarital affair. He felt quite guilty about having the affair, but he also expressed that his now ex-wife was being "a real pain in the ass" during the divorce proceedings. He did not make the immediate connection between the pain he was experiencing in his gluteus maximus muscles and his description of his wife, but he ultimately did arrive at that understanding.

Several weeks after the pain in his lower back was gone, CJ reported that he had a new pain problem, which was focused on the left side of his neck. Sometimes, when the primary problem is successfully treated, a secondary issue may become more prominent than the pain problem that was originally observed. Not just a coincidence, CJ also commented on the stressful weekend he had with his new girlfriend, the woman for whom he had left his wife. He was complaining that she had been a "real pain in the neck" over the weekend. Although the Buttocks and Lumbago points on the ear were no longer tender to palpation, the Neck region of the left auricle was now very sensitive. It required only two auriculotherapy sessions to ease the pain and tightness in CJ's neck. Treatment primarily consisted of electrical stimulation of the Neck point (10 Hz, 60 μA, 20 sec). The master points Shen Men, Point Zero, Thalamus point, and Muscle Relaxation were also stimulated. It was further suggested that he needed to discuss his angry feelings with his new girlfriend rather than unconsciously somatize his emotions.

Although his original motivation to seek treatment was for generalized anxiety, AC had called to cancel an appointment because of acute back pain. He was encouraged to come in for treatment just the same. As a 33-year-old male public relations executive, AC could not get out of his bed the day after he had been in an automobile accident. He had already missed 2 days of work on the day he contacted me about his condition. I was able to bring a portable electronic device in order to see him in his home. Auricular stimulation was applied to extremely tender and electrically reactive points on the anterior antihelix points and on the posterior groove points that correspond to the Lumbar Vertebrae. Stimulation (10 Hz, 20 µA, 30 sec) of the corresponding body points on the right and left external ears was accompanied by treatment of the master points Shen Men, Point Zero, Thalamus, and Master Cerebral point. The response to this treatment was immediate and profound. At the conclusion of the auricular stimulation procedures, AC was able to arise from his bed without any discomfort in his back. He could bend and turn in ways that were impossible just 15 minutes earlier. Because the cause of his problem was so recent, the auriculotherapy treatment led to dramatic improvement with just a single session. Auricular pellets were placed on the front and the back of the Lumbar Vertebrae points. By the next day, he was able to fully return to work. The ear pellets were removed after 1 day and his back problems were completely gone.

Sciatica is the medical condition that first brought the possibilities of auriculotherapy to the attention of Dr. Nogier in the 1950s. As noted by Nogier more than 50 years ago, and as observed by many ear acupuncturists since, sciatica pain can be greatly alleviated by auricular acupuncture. BH was a 23-year-old male with complaints of sciatica and shooting pains down the left hip and left leg. When pressure was applied to the L5–S1 joint on the inferior crus of the left antihelix, BH exclaimed that that area of the ear was excruciatingly tender. It was also the most electrically responsive region of his left ear. Reactive points were also found in the triangular fossa of BH, the auricular region that Nogier indicated corresponds to the location for the leg. Electrical stimulation of reactive points on the front and back of the auricle led to an 85% reduction in pain level that he recorded on a visual analogue scale (VAS). Ear seeds were placed on the Sciatica point and on the Thigh point to sustain the treatment effects.

Although he was usually very athletic, MJ, a 26-year-old male patient, had become incapacitated by severe back pain. On the first auriculotherapy session for his back pain problems, I also noticed that MJ had an open scar on the region of the helix root that adjoins the face. Two months of antibiotic medications prescribed by his primary physician had failed to heal this scar. The scar was located on a part of the external ear that Chinese auricular charts depict as the External Genitals. For MJ's back pain, bipolar electrical stimulation was applied to the Lumbar Vertebrae points on the antihelix inferior crus of his left auricle. To facilitate wound healing, monopolar electrical probes were placed across the edges of the scar on the ear. The patient was told that electrical stimulation could potentially heal skin lesions as well as relieve back pain. At his appointment the next week, MJ came into the treatment room very upbeat. He was amazed that not only was there a decrease in his back pain but also his previously undisclosed scrotal pain had also diminished. I had not been informed that pain in his genital region was even a problem. The rapid improvement in his genital pain was a surprise to both of us. These results are explained by microsystem theory as organocutaneous reflexes producing the mysterious scar on MJ's ear. The auriculotherapy treatment of that scar activated a cutaneo-organic reflex that alleviated the discomfort in the genital region.

Although it is impressive to observe the many patients successfully treated with auriculotherapy, it is also important to distinguish the possible origins of treatment failures. Two different cases of back pain illustrate the limitations of this procedure. RT was a 33-year-old male art dealer and EE was a 41-year-old male executive at a Hollywood movie studio. They both suffered from recurrent back pain that was at times manageable but at other times prevented them from going to work. Both men had received nerve blocks and physical therapy. Only periodic treatment with opioid medications produced temporary alleviation of their discomfort. Both men were contemplating surgery for the removal of bone spurs that were discovered by MRI scans along the spine. RT and EE both expressed that they were interested in trying auriculotherapy before the possibly risky surgical procedures were initiated. They were each given several auriculotherapy sessions in which reactive points that represent the back were electrically stimulated. RT reported that the auricular stimulation produced a brief reduction of his back pain, but engaging in any body movement reactivated intense discomfort. Although EE did not initially report very severe pain, he also did not exhibit much relief from that pain after receiving auricular stimulation. Both men ultimately underwent surgical procedures to remove the bone spurs, and their back conditions were almost completely eliminated.

From these two examples, one can reasonably conclude that auriculotherapy is not particularly effective when there is a physical structure that is the source of the pain—in these instances a bone spur. Auriculotherapy can be more helpful when the problem is due to muscle tension and the pathological functioning of neuromuscular control of muscle spasms. Failure to provide satisfactory pain relief to another male patient was also best explained by the presence of a structural problem. MB was a 34-year-old computer graphics artist who had been to four different physicians for chronic neck pain before being referred to me. After five sessions in which auriculotherapy did not alleviate his pain problem, MB discontinued treatment. A year later, he contacted me to inform me that a subsequent physician had diagnosed a constriction in his cervical spine that was corrected by surgery, which also alleviated his persistent neck pain. Although osteopathic surgery can sometimes lead to further complications of a chronic pain condition, it is at other times the only effective solution.

8.5 Auriculotherapy Alleviation of Peripheral Neuropathies and Neuralgias

One of the most distinctive demonstrations that I had ever witnessed of the specificity of auriculotherapy was with the treatment of HR, a 46-year-old female diabetic patient with peripheral neuropathy. HR had accumulated three volumes of UCLA medical records that described in detail her multiple treatments for multiple conditions resulting from a life history of diabetes mellitus. In addition to the severe pain in her feet, HR experienced severe glaucoma, chronic back pain, and felt a great deal of bitterness and despair that modern medicine had not been able to help her. She had developed a rather resentful, pessimistic, hostile attitude toward the medical profession for failing to adequately relieve her varied sources of discomfort. Her negative reactions toward conventional medical treatments made it seem unlikely that she would respond any more favorably to alternative therapies, but auriculotherapy was recommended nonetheless.

When HR entered the pain clinic, she walked with a limp, requiring the assistance of her husband, and there was a pronounced scowl on her face. After the initial interview, she lay down on the examination table and her external ears were scanned for areas of decreased electrical resistance. There were reactive points on her right ear in auricular regions that corresponded to the feet. These auricular points for the Foot were electrically stimulated first (10 Hz, 40 μA, 30 sec), followed by stimulation of the master points on the right ear identified as Shen Men (10 Hz, 40 μA, 10 sec), Point Zero (10 Hz, 40 μA, 10 sec), and Thalamus point (80 Hz, 40 μA, 20 sec). Within 2 minutes of the completion of this stimulation of acupoints on the right auricle, a marked change appeared on the patient's face. Her negative frown turned into an almost peaceful smile. HR quietly exclaimed that the pain in her right foot was completely gone. She noted that it was the first time in more than 7 years that she did not feel any discomfort at all in her right foot. Interestingly, the pain in her left foot and the pain on the left side of her back remained approximately the same. It was not until I then stimulated the reactive Foot points on her left external ear that there was a reduction of pain in her left foot and left spine.

The theoretical as well as clinical significance of this differential effect observed in HR are profound. If the auriculotherapy were due to a general systemic effect, such as occurs after an injection of morphine or some other opioid medication, the pain relief should have been experienced equally in both feet. Moreover, if HR had been given an intravenous injection of morphine, it would have taken 10–20 minutes for her to notice any significant analgesia. Numerous scientific studies in humans and animals indicate that there is a systemic release of endorphins following auricular acupuncture, but this effect also requires 10–20 minutes to appear. Localized pain relief in only one of HR's feet following the treatment of the first ear suggests that specific neurological reflex circuits more appropriately account for this selective action of auriculotherapy, rather than general endorphin release. Patient HR continued to improve during the next several months of weekly treatments. The pain in both her feet gradually returned to some degree, but with each successive auriculotherapy treatment the pain was diminished for longer periods of time. Her back pain and her ability to walk without assistance also improved, and there was a pronounced enhancement of her mood. By the 15th session, there was only minimal, recurrent pain in her feet, and HR became more pleasant for everyone to interact with. She reported feeling very optimistic about her health, even though she still suffered from diabetes and glaucoma.

Treatment by auriculotherapy is not limited to pain relief but also affects motor neuron controlled behavioral reflexes. JJ, a 57-year-old white male, reported muscular atrophy and persistent pain in his left arm, which he attributed to the stress and strain related to his work activities. Reactive ear points were electrically detected on the auricle at the Cervical Vertebra region along the antihelix tail and at the Elbow point and the Wrist point on the scaphoid fossa of the left ear. JJ observed an immediate warm, tingly sensation throughout his left arm and hand after microcurrent stimulation of these three ear points. In the Nogier school of auriculotherapy, musculoskeletal disorders are stimulated with a frequency of 10 Hz, usually at 40 µA for 20 seconds. Moreover, because muscle tension or muscle weakness is related to a pathological disturbance within motor neurons, the Cervical Vertebrae region on the posterior groove was also stimulated on the back of the ear. These posterior ear points lie immediately behind the acupoints found on the front surface of the auricle. After only 3 weeks of once-a-week sessions, JJ reported a 70% reduction in pain, as measured by the VAS. By three treatments, he was able to return to his

position as an accountant for a restaurant chain. Whereas the alleviation of pain had been fairly rapid, the improvement in muscular atrophy was initially just slight. Satisfactory improvement in motor function required 8 more weeks of auriculotherapy.

Patient TM was a 28-year-old male graduate student who had been severely injured by faulty wiring in a piece of electronic equipment. A lethal jolt of electricity flowed from the wall cord of the equipment up his left hand, spreading to his head and down the left side of his body. His shoe was completely melted around his left foot. When I first saw him, he walked with a limp, dragging his partially paralyzed left leg, and he could not fully use the fingers of his left hand. Auriculotherapy treatment of his left external ear included points corresponding to the Hand, the Arm, the Leg, and the Thalamus point. These sessions were continued for more than 3 months. The reduction in pain sensations in his hand and the enhancement of his motor abilities and his memory were gradual but steady. By the last session, auriculotherapy had assisted TM in being able to write more legibly and without feeling pain in his fingers. His leg movements were more fluid, and he could remember more details of the academic topics he had studied before the accident. He was by no means completely healed because the neurological damage he had suffered seemed to result in permanent motor dystrophy. Nonetheless, auriculotherapy had led to far greater improvements than any of his medical doctors had expected.

Auriculotherapy has been effectively used for neuropathic pain related to either diabetes or HIV disease. JT was a 37-year-old man who has been diagnosed with AIDS and had suffered from neuropathic pain in his feet and lower legs for more than 8 months, whereas RB was a 58-year-old man who suffered from diabetic neuropathy that affected his feet. Although the source of their neuropathy was very different, the auricular treatment of the neuropathic pain was almost identical. For both JT and RB, reactive ear points were identified on the uppermost regions of the auricle, which represent the Chinese and European localizations of the Feet.

Ear acupoints were also stimulated on the uppermost region of the helix tail, which corresponds to the Lumbar Spinal Cord. The somatic region of the auricle, which represents control of the musculoskeletal tissues of the feet, is stimulated at 10 Hz. The helix tail region, which represents neurological spinal cord tissue, is stimulated at 40 Hz. Higher frequencies of stimulation are used for neurological tissue than are used for muscular tissue according to the auriculotherapy model first proposed by Nogier (1983). Similar to the findings with MRI scans, resonant waveforms occur at different frequencies for different types of tissue. More recently evolved tissue, such as that of the nervous system, is said to best respond to higher resonance frequencies than more primitive tissue, such as muscles and internal organs. Stimulation of the Foot points and the Lumbar Spinal Cord points on the auricle contributed to the complete elimination of the peripheral neuralgia pain in the feet. Both JT and RB reported maintained relief of their peripheral neuralgia after six sessions of auriculotherapy.

Herpes zoster, or shingles, is a different type of neuropathic pain that is found in many AIDS patients as well as patients with diabetes. TP was a 32-year-old man who had been diagnosed with AIDS 5 years prior to my first examination of him. He was initially seen for the possible relief of the stress and anxiety associated with his HIV infection. At a group therapy session, TP became extremely distressed after he openly revealed his positive HIV status to other group members. Although the psychotherapy group was very supportive, TP felt enormous shame and a deep sense of rejection and that no one would want to associate with him. The next day, TP came down with shingles. The acute inflammation of the T4 dermatome abruptly appeared on the right side of his chest, upper abdomen, and upper back. The reactive ear points for this individual were appropriately found on the antihelix body which represents the Chest and on the Thoracic Spinal Cord region of the helix tail. After the first session of auriculotherapy, the pain sensations in his body were eliminated, and there was a rapid reduction in the bumpy, swelling, red regions of skin that had been irritated by the herpes virus. After several more auriculotherapy sessions, over the course of 2 weeks, the herpes reaction had completely subsided.

An almost identical response was exhibited by EO, a 76-year-old woman who became affected by shingles as a reaction to her anti-hypertensive medications. The herpes zoster affected the L1 dermatome on her right side, manifested by red, blotchy, hypersensitive skin. She was given bipolar auricular stimulation (10 Hz, 40 μA, 60 sec) to the antihelix crus and antihelix body regions which represent the musculoskeletal tissue of the Lumbar Vertebrae. Faster frequency auricular stimulation (40 Hz, 40 μA, 60 sec) was applied to the Lumbar Spinal Cord region found on the upper helix tail. In addition, monopolar electrodes were held on each side of the dermatomal zone on her actual body that was inflamed. Low-frequency transcutaneous electrical nerve stimulation was applied across the skin of the body for another 10 minutes. Electroacupuncture through needles inserted into the skin surrounding a wound, sometimes referred to as "surrounding the dragon," is a similar technique. The shingles reaction by EO showed gradual reduction of skin sensitivity; by 2 days, the reddish, blotchy skin had almost completely returned to normal. Combining transcutaneous electrical stimulation of the actual body with electrical stimulation of the auricle is a very effective procedure for treating both neuropathies and neuralgia.

Several case studies on the effect of auriculotherapy for healing leg wounds were reported by Fred Swing at the ICCAAAM'99. JC was a 68-year-old male admitted to a Texas hospital for sepsis, pneumonia, and multiple large ulcerations on both lower legs. Because of the sensitivity of the wounds on the patient's legs, only ear acupuncture was allowed. The day after auriculotherapy, an increased presence of fluids and redness in the wound areas was observed by the attending nurse, the feet were warmer, and the patient reported greater sensations in his lower legs. Auriculotherapy and traditional wound care treatment were continued for the next 4 months. After 50 ear treatments, the right leg was completely healed and the left leg was sufficiently improved to permit successful skin grafting. The ear acupoints for the Leg, Shen Men, Sympathetic, Lungs, and Dermatitis points were electrically stimulated. Because wound healing requires that sufficient oxygen and body nutrients be delivered to the wound site, auriculotherapy can improve vasodilation of the small arterioles that leads to a greater delivery of oxygenated blood to the lower legs.

The total number of points treated in each clinical case can vary from 5 to 10 ear points, depending on how many anatomic and master points were stimulated. The whole auricle is first examined with a point locator, often revealing more than 20 reactive ear points. Only the most electrically conductive and most tender of the points that specifically correspond to the patient's complaints are finally used. With transcutaneous electrical nerve stimulation on the auricle, each point is stimulated with 20–40 microamps for only 10–30 seconds. The practitioner then moves onto the next point. Needles are inserted into the selected ear points and left in place for approximately 20 minutes, similar to body acupuncture. Treatments are offered twice a week for several weeks and then reduced to once a week for several more weeks until there is satisfactory improvement in symptoms. Both practitioners and patients continue to be amazed that these different sites on the ear can have such a profound pain-relieving effect on complaints from other parts of the body.

8.6 Auriculotherapy for Relief of Nausea and Abdominal Discomfort

As originally suggested by Dr. Paul Nogier in his early writings, what may be most persuasive to a beginning practitioner is the relief of a symptom that the doctor himself or herself has experienced. I learned auriculotherapy from Dr. Richard Kroening and Dr. David Bresler at the UCLA Medical Center. They asked me to be the Research Director at the UCLA Pain Control Center, and our first research project was on auricular diagnosis. I myself, however, had never received any auricular acupuncture treatment. At one of the first lecture presentations of our auricular diagnosis research, I had the firsthand opportunity to assess the clinical effectiveness of ear acupuncture. I had eaten something for breakfast that began to greatly disagree with me. By the time the lecture was set to begin, the discomforting stomach sensations were getting worse. I told this to Dr. Kroening, who noticed the unpleasant grimaces on my face. He promptly pulled a sterilized needle out of the pocket of his lab coat and inserted it into the Stomach point on my left ear. To my surprise, the nausea in my stomach disappeared within 1 minute. Because the skeptical, scientific side of my personality wondered whether this sudden relief of pain was simply a placebo effect, I removed the needle. The uncomfortable nausea feelings immediately returned and I almost started to vomit. Somewhat embarrassed by my lack of faith in his medical skills, I had to then ask Dr. Kroening to put the acupuncture needle back into my ear. He compassionately smiled and complied with my request. Almost immediately after he re-inserted the acupuncture needle into the Stomach point on my external ear, the feelings of discomfort in my abdomen quickly subsided. Only after leaving the needle in place for another 20 minutes was I able to remove the acupuncture needle from my ear and not feel any nauseating discomfort.

What this experience clearly taught me was that auriculotherapy could be very fast-acting, but without sufficient stimulation of the appropriate ear acupuncture point, the benefits could rapidly fade. The changes in nausea sensations were directly related to the original needle insertion, then needle removal, and then the re-insertion of the acupuncture needle. Since this initial observation, I have used the Stomach point for myself and for many clients with whom I have worked. Both needle insertion and transcutaneous electrical stimulation can quickly relieve stomachaches, not only in response to disagreeable foods but also from the side effects of various medications. It is also possible to produce a more gradual reduction in nauseous feelings by just the tactile pressure of rubbing one's own finger over the Stomach point. Acupressure at an ear point is not as rapid as electrical stimulation, usually requiring several minutes of maintained pressure against the ear points, but it is easily available for patients to do on themselves.

Pain complaints related to internal organs are represented in a different region of the ear than are musculoskeletal complaints. The central concha of the auricle is associated with diffuse representation of the vagus nerve control of internal organs. The surrounding ridges of the antihelix and the antitragus are more associated with precise control of musculoskeletal movements. For this reason, one can find a broad area of the concha that could affect the stomach but only a small set of specific antihelix points that could affect a particular Thoracic Vertebra. Auriculotherapy is also very effective for the relief of gastrointestinal distress that has not been successfully alleviated by conventional medications. I have treated nausea in many patients with HIV/AIDS who had been administered antiviral medications or cancer patients who were undergoing chemotherapy. In most of these cases, stimulation of the auricular Stomach point dramatically alleviated their gastrointestinal reactions. There are more than 20 controlled clinical trials demonstrating that needling of the body acupuncture point PC6 on the wrist has a significant anti-emetic effect. The relief of nausea by stimulating the auricular Stomach point can be just as profound, and recent research on auricular acupressure at the Stomach point has confirmed these clinical case observations.

Patient PL was a 28-year-old male who had been diagnosed with HIV disease 6 years previous to my seeing him. The advent of triple-combination therapy had yielded a great improvement in his T-helper cell count and a dramatic drop in viral load, but PL continued to suffer from agonizing stomach discomfort related to his HIV medications. Weekly treatment of the Stomach point (5 Hz, 40 μA, 30 sec) and master points (10 Hz, 40 μA, 10 sec) on both ears allowed PL to feel substantially more comfortable for the next several months. The Thymus Gland point on his auricle was very reactive, and although auriculotherapy stimulation of this point led to a temporary improvement in stamina, it did not reverse the progressive deterioration of his immune system from AIDS. He only stopped coming for treatments in the several weeks before his death, when he was too weak to get out of bed.

A different AIDS patient reported a similar positive experience with auriculotherapy. LR was a 30-year-old male who continued to lose weight from his lack of desire to eat. His HIV medications gave him such severe stomachaches that he needed to periodically stop so that the side effects of these drugs did not further compromise his health. When he did take his HIV medications, LR reported that the auriculotherapy treatment was the only medical procedure that provided him any sense of comfort. He continued to positively respond to stimulation of the Stomach point, to the auricular master points Shen Men and Point Zero, and to stimulation of the Vitality point on the upper tragus of the ear.

A comparable experience was reported by patient AS, a 47-year-old female diagnosed with liver cancer. Her health had not improved after three different trials of chemotherapy. She also was greatly distressed by nausea from the chemotherapy medications she was taking. Stimulation of the Stomach point on the concha ridge of the ear produced pronounced alleviation of her chronic stomachaches. Electrical detection indicated a broad spread of reactive points related to the Stomach region of the ear, not just a single point. The determination of auricular points for internal organs does not need to be as precise as is necessary for the identification of musculoskeletal ear points. Internal, visceral organs have diffuse receptive fields that are not as specific as somatic areas of the body. When using microcurrent transcutaneous stimulation, the concha region of the ear is stimulated at 5 Hz for 30 seconds; needles are left in place for approximately 30 minutes. For both forms of stimulation, the treatment effect is augmented by the placement of ear seeds over the Stomach point, which are left in place for the next week.

Ongoing clinical studies of auriculotherapy continuously reveal amazing new discoveries. At the 2011 Conference of the American Academy for

Medical Acupuncture, I had the opportunity to interact with a long-time practitioner of auricular acupuncture, Dr. Fred Swing. While working with a woman suffering from kidney stones, Dr. Swing noticed a distinct red spot on the external ear of this patient, in the region of the Chinese location for the Kidney point in the superior concha of the auricle. Needling this point produced some reduction in abdominal pain, but the kidney problem, as well as the patient's pain, persisted. Over the course of the next several days, however, Dr. Swing had the opportunity to continue his observations of this female patient with kidney stones. The distinct red surface of the skin that he had originally observed over the more peripherally located Kidney point on the superior concha gradually moved, appearing closer and closer each day to the more centrally located region of the superior concha that represents the Urinary Bladder. Dr. Swing observed that the skin surface reaction on the auricle that corresponded to the region of the Ureter moved along, day by day, directly corresponding to the position of the actual kidney stone in her body as it moved down the ureter tube. Although X-rays were not taken to confirm this correspondence between the location of the moving kidney stone and the daily changes in location of the red skin spot on the auricle, there was a correspondence in clinical reports by this patient. It would be very interesting to learn of more such examples by practitioners in the field.

8.7 Auricular Acupuncture for Weight Control

An intriguing potential of auricular acupuncture has been its clinical application for weight control. Sun and Xu (1993) treated obesity patients with "otoacupoint" stimulation, which is another term for ear acupressure. All patients were also given body acupuncture for the 3-month study period. The acupuncture group consisted of 110 patients diagnosed as at least 20% over ideal weight. They were compared to 51 obesity patients in a control group given an oral medication for weight control. An electrical point finder was used to determine the following

auricular points: Mouth, Esophagus, Stomach, Abdomen, Appetite Control (Hunger point), Shen Men, Lung, and the Endocrine point. Pressure pellets made from vacarria seeds were applied to the appropriate points of both ears. The body acupuncture points that were needled included ST 25, ST 36, ST 40, SP 6, and PC 6. The acupuncture group exhibited an average reduction of body weight of 5 kg, which was significantly greater than the average 2 kg reduction of body weight shown for the control group. The percentage of body fat was reduced by 3% in the acupuncture group and by 1.54% in the control group, whereas the triglyceride blood lipid levels were diminished 67 units in the acupuncture group and 38 units in the control group.

A randomized controlled trial by Richards and Marley (1998) also found that weight loss was significantly greater for women in an auricular acupuncture group than in a control group. Women in the auricular group were given surface electrical stimulation to the ear acupoints for the Stomach and for Shen Men; women in the control group were given transcutaneous electrical stimulation to the first joint of the thumb. Auricular acupuncture was theorized to suppress appetite by stimulating the auricular branch of the vagal nerve, which can increase smooth muscle tone in the gastric wall. Rather than examine changes in weight measurements, Choy and Eidenschenk (1998) examined the effect of tragus clips on gastric peristalsis in 13 volunteers. The duration of single peristaltic waves was measured before and after the application of ear clips to the tragus. The frequency of peristalsis was reduced by one-third with clips on the ear and returned to normal levels with clips off. The ear clips were said to produce inhibition of vagal nerve activity, leading to a delay of gastric emptying; the latter could then lead to a sense of fullness and satiety. These obesity studies on human subjects have received potential validation from neurophysiological research in animals.

Niemtzow (1998) evaluated blood assays in 42 obesity patients given a high-protein diet and weekly treatments with auricular acupuncture. Needles were inserted into the following ear points: Appetite Control, Shen Men, Point Zero, and Tranquilizer Point, all left in both ears for 15 minutes. During a 12-week period, mean weight decreased significantly from 206 pounds to 187 pounds, triglycerides significantly changed as well, and there was a marked but statistically significant reduction in total cholesterol. Patients commented after the study that the auriculotherapy treatments helped them to feel more comfortable while they coped with their cravings for eating foods not on their diet plan.

8.8 The NADA Protocol for Addiction and Drug Detoxification

One of the fastest-growing applications of auriculotherapy in the health care field is the use of ear acupuncture points for the treatment of various additions. The National Detoxification and Addiction Association (NADA) was founded on the pioneering work of Dr. H. L. Wen of Hong Kong and the early application of this procedure by Dr. Michael Smith of New York City. Dr. Wen (Wen and Cheung, 1973; Wen, 1997) found that placing one needle in just the Lung point was sufficient to withdraw a heroin addict from his addiction, but he also added the Shen Men point to produce general calming. Dr. Smith (1979, 1980) developed a five point protocol for substance abuse recovery that included the Lung, Shen Men, Sympathetic Autonomic point, Kidney, and Liver points on the ear (Figure 8.1). NADA was formed in 1985 (Brewington et al., 1994) so that there would be an organization and increased opportunity for training beyond what was offered by Dr. Smith at Lincoln Hospital. The first open meeting of NADA was held in Washington, DC, and the NADA board was formed. The first NADA conference occurred in Miami in 1990 because many people were interested in seeing the Drug Court that had been established in Miami in 1989. Similar drug courts that incorporate referral to NADA practitioners have now occurred in many other states. NADA's official website is http://www. acudetox.com. Controlled clinical trials have shown that the five ear points used in the NADA protocol are effective in the treatment of alcoholism (Bullock et al., 1989), cocaine addiction (Margolin et al., 1993a, 1993b), and morphine withdrawal (Yang and Kwok, 1986).

To obtain training and certification in NADA, one must complete a 70-hour course. This training includes 30 didactic hours of instruction and 40 clinical hours working with clients. The trainings also includes attendance at 12-step meetings. High emphasis is placed on the clinical experience so that NADA practitioners can become comfortable working with an addict population. At New York City Lincoln Recovery Center, most trainees are chemical dependency counselors. They spend much of their time getting comfortable with doing acupuncture as a physical procedure. Students learn about the "yin nature" of the NADA environment, which is intended to be supportive and nonconfrontive. For acupuncturists, the training utilizes more time covering definitions of addiction and mental health treatments. Acupuncturists are instructed to speak the same language as the chemical dependency counselors, the criminal justice system, and medical professionals in those environments.

One of the most important lessons that both groups have to learn is to be quiet and let the acupuncture needles do the work. Both groups are used to spending time talking to evaluate patient progress. One of the most important pieces of the NADA protocol is that it offers a nonverbal alternative among the treatment modalities. Substance abusers often feel shame, guilt, anger, or other issues that they do not know how to cope with verbally. Without acupuncture, the only other therapy that is often made available is talk therapy, either individually or in a group setting. NADA training also includes learning about various recreational drugs, their pharmacological effects, and various types of settings into which acupuncture has been integrated. NADA continues to be a grassroots movement. Most NADA programs were started because administrators were convinced of the value rather than as a result of a request from the treatment providers. More than 4000 practitioners throughout the world have been

Five Point NADA Protocol

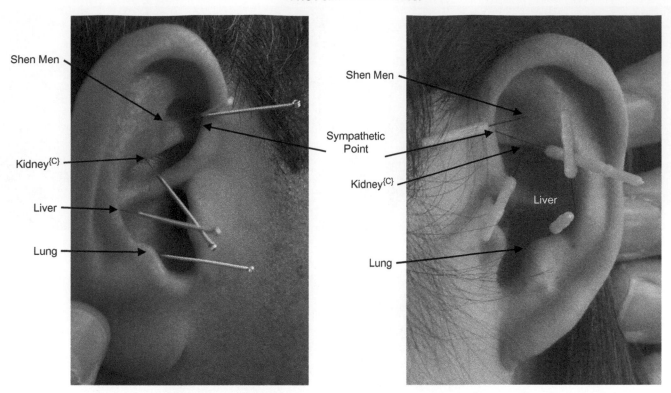

[**FIGURE 8.1** Photographs of the five ear points that are part of the NADA protocol.

taught the five point NADA protocol for the treatment of various types of substance abuse.

Although the five point NADA protocol has become the most commonly employed treatment program in the United States, it is not the only auriculotherapy procedure that has been developed for substance abuse treatment. The ear points developed for NADA are principally based on Chinese ear acupuncture systems, but additional auricular points for addiction have been derived from European treatment plans. Oriental medicine focuses on the use of the auricular Lung point for detoxification, the Kidney point for yin deficiency, and the Liver point for nourishment. The Shen Men and Sympathetic points are intended to alleviate psychological distress and an imbalance of one's spirit. European practitioners of auricular medicine have focused on selecting ear points to treat based on their reactivity. These European practitioners utilize the Nogier vascular autonomic signal to determine which ear points to treat. Repeated experience with many substance abuse

patients has led to the discovery of additional ear points besides those that were developed at Lincoln Hospital. Dr. Jay Holder (Holder *et al.*, 2001) and Dr. Kenneth Blum (Blum *et al.*, 2000) were instrumental in developing the American College of Addictionology and Compulsive Disorders (ACACD) based in Miami Beach, Florida. The ACACD protocol includes a total of six auricular points: Point Zero, Shen Men, Sympathetic Autonomic point, Kidney, Brain, and Limbic point. Two addiction axis lines were emphasized that connect these different treatment points. A primary axis could be vertically drawn between the Shen Men, Kidney, Point Zero, and Brain points, whereas a secondary axis line could be indicated that connected the Sympathetic Autonomic point and Limbic point. This system still emphasizes that only reactive ear points are stimulated. There has been no controlled scientific research to verify whether the NADA protocol or the ACACD treatment is more effective in working with addicts. Clinical experience from multiple practitioners supports the utilization of both approaches.

(A)

(B)

(C)

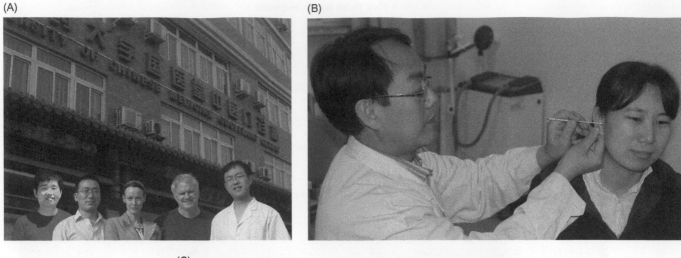

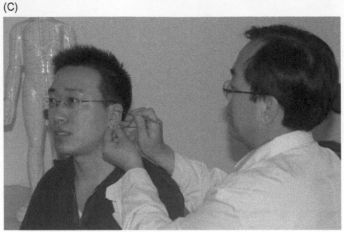

[**FIGURE 8.2** (A) Photograph of Dr. Baixiao Zhao with three of his graduate students at the Beijing University of Chinese Medicine meeting with Dr. Terry Oleson. (B and C) Photographs showing Dr. Zhao conducting auricular acupuncture treatment of several patients.

8.9 Auricular Acupuncture Treatments in Contemporary China

Although there are multiple treatment approaches for both substance abuse disorders and chronic pain problems, there are some conditions for which neither conventional Western medicine nor complementary and alternative medicine seem to have any adequate solutions. On my most recent visit to acupuncture clinics in China, I had the opportunity to observe the effectiveness of auricular acupuncture treatments for neurological problems that would seem beyond any health care treatment facility. In May 2010, I was able to attend an international meeting in Beijing, China,

that was sponsored by the World Federation of Acupuncture–Moxibustion Societies (WFAS). In addition to the exchange of scientific information at this meeting, I was able to observe acupuncture practices in hospitals and clinics throughout Beijing (Figures 8.2–8.4).

Dr. Zhao Baixiao is the director of the Ear Acupuncture Program at the Beijing University of Chinese Medicine. I first met Dr. Zhao at an acupuncture conference in Hong Kong in 2005 and then again when he spoke at the ICCAAAM conference in the United States in 2006. While I was in China in 2010, I had the opportunity to follow Dr. Zhao at an evening clinic that he offered at the Beijing University of Chinese Medicine. When we

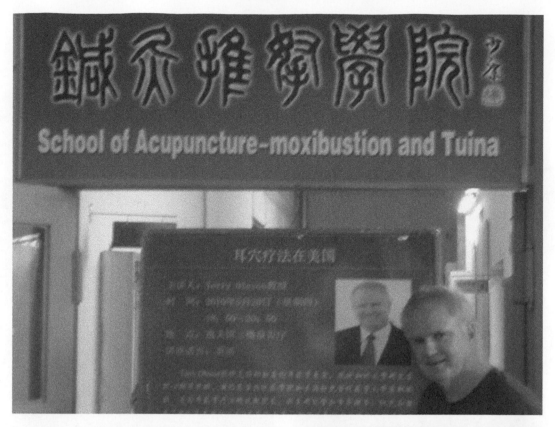

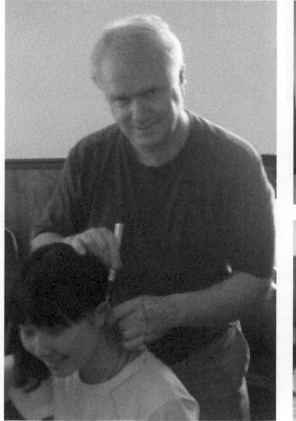

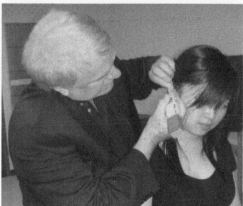

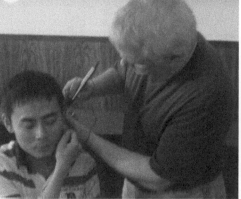

[FIGURE 8.3 (Top) Photograph of Dr. Terry Oleson presenting an auriculotherapy lecture at the Beijing University of Chinese Medicine in 2010. Other photographs show Dr. Oleson treating several students who attended the 2010 lecture in Beijing.

(A)

(B)

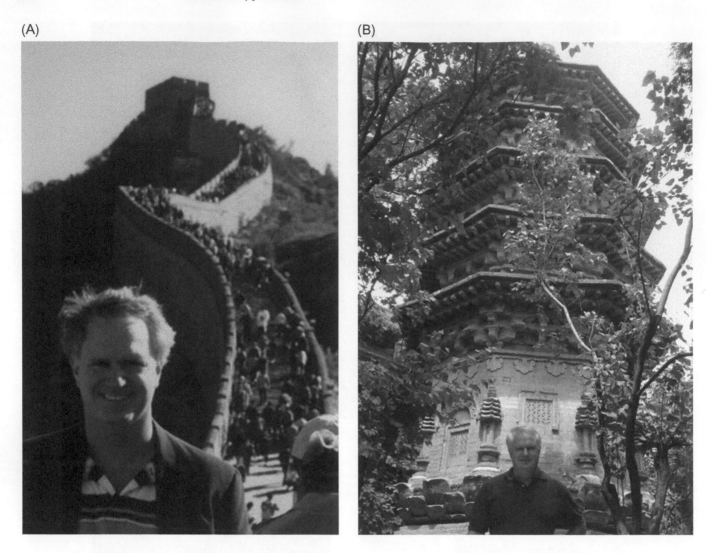

[**FIGURE 8.4** Photographs of Dr. Terry Oleson (A) at the Great Wall of China while attending an international auricular acupuncture symposium in 1995 and (B) in front of a Buddhist pagoda while attending the 2010 WFAS conference on auricular nomenclature.

arrived, more than 20 patients were seated in plain chairs along both sides of a narrow hallway leading to his office. Some had been waiting there for several hours because clinical appointments with him were so highly valued. Rather than expressing frustration or impatience at the long wait ahead of them, all of these patients broke into broad smiles upon seeing Dr. Zhao arrive. He, in turn, warmly smiled upon seeing them. Although eight of his more senior graduate students were there to assist him, he individually saw almost 30 patients in one evening.

The clinic itself was very minimal—a small room cramped with four beds separated from each other by curtains hung from a high bar. Anyone

who has been exposed to American hospitals in the 1950s, or to acupuncture clinics in the United States in the 1970s, would readily recognize these surroundings. Each patient's physical symptoms, pulse, and tongue were evaluated by the traditional diagnostic procedures of classical Oriental medicine. Dr. Zhao then determined the type of treatment each patient would receive, whether it be long acupuncture needles inserted into the back, moxa sticks heated over areas of discomfort, or massage of painful muscles or joints. Dr. Zhao's particular specialty is ear acupuncture. He is considered one of the most prestigious ear acupuncture practitioners throughout China. Most patients who came for treatment suffered from chronic pain, and the insertion of acupuncture needles into their skin was itself visibly uncomfortable. However, following their initial flinching and grimacing upon needle insertion, their suffering was gradually replaced by the development of profound relaxation and by the relief of their pain. It was very apparent that a special, spiritual energy accompanied his healings in addition to his acupuncture expertise. Dr. Zhao's warm sense of humor seemed to disarm the negativity of their pain, and his encouraging reassurance decidedly calmed the worries of their mind.

Of all the different patients who came to his clinic that night, one patient was the most memorable. A mother had brought her 4-year-old daughter to Dr. Zhao and stayed with her child throughout the whole procedure. Her daughter looked up at Dr. Zhao with an awkward, blank gaze that indicated some type of mental impairment. I was informed that the child had accidentally fallen out the window of a three-story building more than 1 year ago. The initial diagnosis was severe brain damage, and her condition was not alleviated by any of the Western medical hospitals that exist in China. The mother stopped all other activities in her life and dedicated herself to finding someone who might be able to treat her little girl. One should remember that in the "one child policy" of overpopulated China, children are held especially dear. One could readily see the caring concern in the mother's face as she calmed the screams of her child when acupuncture needles were inserted into the girl's scalp and her external ear. Acupuncture needles are sometimes quite painful upon insertion, especially for a child. After several minutes, however, the tears ceased, and the child became less fidgety and restless. By 20 minutes, the child was able to hold her head steady and could show more appropriate eye gaze in reacting to others. I do not know that I have ever seen such joy demonstrated by a mother upon seeing such behavioral improvement in the health of her child. I did not need to understand any Chinese words to perceive her expressions of gratitude to Dr. Zhao. Although I have personally observed the clinical benefits of auricular acupuncture for the past 35 years, I continue to be amazed at some of the most surprising results from this approach.

8.10 Auricular Medicine Treatments in Modern Europe

For the most part, the clinical training of European practitioners of auriculotherapy has followed one of three principle influences, with some practitioners integrating all three forms:

1. The classical teachings of Dr. Paul Nogier as practiced by the Group Lyonaise Études Medicales (GLEM), which he founded. This approach utilizes the vascular autonomic signal for determining reactive ear points and then treats just those reactive points with either a press needle or laser stimulation.

2. The primary teachings of Dr. Paul Nogier and the supplemental teachings of Dr. Frank Bahr as practiced by the German Academy of Auricular Medicine. This approach also utilizes the vascular autonomic signal for determining reactive ear points but includes many treatment approaches that are not utilized by the GLEM organization.

3. The primary teachings of Paul Nogier and the supplemental teachings of Chinese practitioners of auricular acupuncture. This approach typically does not utilize the vascular autonomic signal for determining reactive ear points, but these practitioners do typically include TCM pulse diagnosis. Auriculotherapy treatments include the full range of procedures discussed in Chapter 6, including acupuncture needles, electroacupuncture, transcutaneous electrical stimulation, and acubeads.

There are no scientific studies that systematically compare these three approaches, nor are there any controlled scientific studies that systematically compare the European auriculotherapy system with the Chinese auriculotherapy system. Practitioners in both Europe and the United States who have learned both systems seem to report positive clinical experiences with either approach. From the accounts of many acupuncture physicians who I have met, auricular medicine in European countries is in some respects similar but in other respects quite different to how ear acupuncture is practiced in either China or the United States. There is a growing interest in incorporating both body acupuncture and auricular acupuncture as an important modality for improving health care throughout the world.

The 7th International Symposium of Auriculotherapy was held in Lyon, France, in June 2012. Speakers from different countries in Europe, South America, and Asia and from the United States presented their most recent scientific and clinical findings that have advanced the field of auricular acupuncture. Claudie Terral from Montpellier, France, utilized very sophisticated electronic equipment to identify specific patterns of electrical resistance that characterize the cardiac auricular reflex. From the Acupuncture Center of the U.S. Department of the Air Force, Richard Niemtzow (2012) introduced his expanding work on functional magnetic resonance imaging (fMRI) neurological measurements obtained in patients receiving Battlefield Acupuncture. Semipermanent, gold ASP needles were placed in the auricular points Cingulate Gyrus, Thalamus point, Omega 2, Shen Men, and Point Zero. The measured increase in fMRI activity of the anterior cingulate gyrus, thalamus, hypothalamus, and periaqueductal gray was prominently reduced after stimulation of the Battlefield Acupuncture points on the auricle. Infrared, 50-channel mapping of the central nervous system by the placement of multiple sensors over the scalp revealed distinctive changes in brain oxygen distribution following Battlefield Acupuncture. Through the use of infrared camera technology, Michel Marignan demonstrated neurophysiological changes in blood flow to the vertebral spine that specifically corresponded to changes in blood flow within areas of the auricle that represent the spinal vertebrae.

One of the most intriguing clinical studies presented at the 2012 auriculotherapy symposium was by Daniel Asis and colleagues from Sao Paulo, Brazil. They examined patients suffering from severe post-traumatic stress disorder (PTSD). The treatment that these practitioners examined was referred to as auricular chromotherapy, which consists of the application of a specific color to reactive microsystem points on the external ear. After the external ears of 50 PTSD patients were evaluated for their most reactive ear acupoints, typically the Hippocampus point and the Amygdala on the ear lobe region below the antitragus, a yellow felt pen was used to color these points on the ear a yellow color. Compared to their pretreatment emotional reactions when they were asked to recall their traumatic memory, there was a dramatic reduction in emotional reactivity following the auricular chromotherapy. A different auriculotherapy protocol for the treatment of PTSD was shown by Jim Chalmers of Carsphairn, Scotland. The specific European auricular points that were stimulated included Point Zero at LM_0 on the helix root, Point Zero Prime at LM_23 on the tragus, Point R below LM_1 on the helix, and Point E at LM_9 at the intertragic notch. Similar to Niemtzow's work with military personnel on the battlefield, the authors stimulated the ear points for the Cingulate Gyrus and Omega points and sometimes stimulated the Sympathetic Autonomic point, Tranquilizer point, Shen Men, and Insomnia points. Auriculotherapy treatments were typically integrated with sessions of cognitive behavioral therapy (CBT) and eye movement desensitization and reprocessing (EMDR). The combination of stimulating the most reactive auriculotherapy points to facilitate a relaxing neurophysiological state with psychotherapy sessions that ask the patient to recall traumatic events was found to be very effective for a large number of patients suffering from PTSD.

Raphael Nogier, the son of auriculotherapy pioneer Paul Nogier, evaluated auricular acupuncture points that were perceived as tender or painful to applied pressure. Other ear acupoints were identified by the measurement of electrical resistance but were not labeled painful by the patient being examined. In his assessment of the 24 patients, Nogier (2012) found that only 46% of the 207 ear acupoints detected with an electrical point finder were reported to be painful, whereas 54% of the electrically reactive ear points were non-painful. The clinical conclusion from Nogier's work was that although some reactive ear acupoints show both lowered electrical skin resistance and heightened tenderness to touch, there are a large number of ear acupuncture points that are electrically conductive but not painful.

A related study by Marco Romoli and colleagues in Florence, Italy, compared the somatotopic representation of the Knee point on the antihelix of the Chinese auricular system versus representation in the triangular fossa of the European auricular system. The electric skin resistance test (ESRT), the pain pressure test (PPT), and the needle contact test (NCT) were all utilized in patients with chronic knee disorders. Measurement of perceived knee pain by the VAS was employed to assess reductions in pain by the different knee points. The broader purpose of a series of studies by this Italian group was to determine if auricular diagnosis of patients with chronic knee disorders was more commonly found in the Chinese auricular acupuncture system or the European auriculotherapy system. The primary conclusion was that after the examination of several hundred individuals with knee disorders, active auricular points were found in both the triangular fossa and the nearby superior crus of the antihelix, thus supporting both Chinese and European auricular maps. Significant reduction in perceived knee pain was obtained with needle insertion into either the Chinese Knee points or the European Knee points.

A double blind, crossover study by Guiseppe Gagliadi and colleagues from Padua, Italy, examined 16 individuals who were given the State-Trait Anxiety Inventory (STAI) and the VAS measure of anxiety before and after real or sham auricular acupuncture. These investigators found a significantly greater reduction in the measures of anxiety following the insertion of real acupuncture needles in specific auricular acupoints as contrasted with the application of sham acupuncture needles.

Of all the different applications of auriculotherapy, one of the most popular is for the treatment of weight reduction in patients diagnosed as obese. Etsutaro Ikezono from Tokyo, Japan, reported on his study of 37 obese subjects given ear acupuncture needling of the Stomach point and the Shen Men point. On randomly determined, alternative days, all subjects were given either true needle acupuncture or false (placebo) needle acupuncture. Patients were asked to rate their personal sense of feeling satiated on a VAS. In this within-subject design, in which each participant served as his or her own control, the satiety score was significantly higher after true needle stimulation than after placebo needle stimulation. The clinical value of this finding is for obese patients who commit to a low-caloric diet but who have difficulty dealing with their hunger cravings while on such a diet. With auriculotherapy, they can feel more satiated when they are simultaneously stimulated by true needling of the Stomach and Shen Men points on the auricle.

At the 2012 Lyon symposium, Raphael Nogier led a panel discussion of different systems for identifying anatomical subdivisions of the auricle. I presented the auricular zone system that was previously described in Chapter 4 of this book; Romoli Marco from Florence, Italy, presented the diagnostic usefulness of his auricular sectogram system; and David Alimi from Paris, France, revealed a different sectogram system that utilized the midtragus auricular landmark as the center of radiating lines that spread across the auricle, with circular rings dividing each subsection of the auricle. The more rectilinear auricular zone system developed by Winfried Wojak from Meinberg, Germany, and the International Standard of Auricular Acupuncture Points created by Baixiao Zhao and Liqun Zhou of Beijing were also evaluated. The primary conclusion of this panel was that further discussion of the relative value of each of these auricular systems would need to be debated at future international conferences.

Auriculotherapy Treatment Protocols

9

Key to Abbreviations Used with Ear Points

Corresponding Area: This term refers to the name of a reactive ear acupoint that shows somatotopic correspondence to a part of the body where there is pain or pathology.

{C} or {E}: Superscript that indicates whether an auricular point is somatotopically represented in the Chinese {C} ear acupuncture system or in the European {E} system.

{C, F1, F2, F3, F4}: Superscript that indicates whether an auricular point is somatotopically represented in the Chinese {C} system or in Phase I, Phase II, Phase III, or Phase IV of the Nogier French {F} system of auriculotherapy.

Alternative Terms for the Names of Some Ear Points Used in These Treatment Plans

Sympathetic Autonomic Point is replaced with the term *Sympathetic Point*

Master Endocrine Point is replaced with the term *Endocrine Point*

Cheek {C} is replaced with the term *Face* {C}

Lesser Occipital Nerve {C} is replaced with the term *Windstream* {C}

Triple Warmer {C} is replaced with the term *San Jiao*

Aggressivity Point {E} is replaced with the term *Irritability Point* {E}

External Genitals {C or E} is replaced with the term *Genitals* {C or E}

Ovaries {C} is replaced with the term *Gonadotrophins* {E}

[9.0 | Auriculotherapy Treatment Protocols

CHAPTER 9 LEARNING OBJECTIVES

1. To demonstrate knowledge of auriculotherapy treatment protocols for the alleviation of substance abuse.

2. To demonstrate knowledge of auriculotherapy treatment protocols for the alleviation of musculoskeletal pain disorders.

3. To demonstrate knowledge of auriculotherapy treatment protocols for the alleviation of internal organ disorders.

4. To demonstrate knowledge of auriculotherapy treatment protocols for the alleviation of psychological disorders.

5. To demonstrate knowledge of auriculotherapy treatment protocols for the alleviation of neurological and immunological disorders.

9.1 Standard Treatment Plan Guidelines

The following list of treatment plans indicates those ear reflex points that have previously been used for effective treatment of that health condition. This selection of ear points was originally derived from treatment plans developed in China, but it was modified by auriculotherapy discoveries in Europe and the United States. Practitioners of auricular acupuncture should *not treat all the ear points listed* for a given disorder. Only stimulate those ear points that are both reactive and associated with a patient's symptoms and underlying conditions. Consider the ear points listed for each treatment plan as guidelines, not definite requirements that must be rigidly followed. Moreover, some patients may have other ear points needing treatment that are not listed on these pages.

Primary Auricular Points (PAP) are the most effective set of auricular points for the treatment of a health disorder in a particular body organ or for a physiological dysfunction.

Master Auricular Points (MAP) are those specific master points on the auricle that are most effectively used for that particular health condition.

SupplementalAuricular Points (SAP) are those points on the ear that are used as alternative or additional auricular treatment points for facilitation of the action of the primary ear points and master auricular points.

Reactive Ear Reflex Points: For all of the treatment plans listed, the practitioner should limit the treatment to only those auricular points that are most reactive, as indicated by increased skin conductance or heightened tenderness to applied pressure. If a point that is listed in these treatment protocols is not electrically reactive nor tender to touch, then it should *not* be included in the treatment plan.

Functional Ear Points in Oriental Medicine: For many auricular acupuncture treatments, there are six internal organ points that serve the purpose of master points from the perspective of Oriental medicine. The Chinese location for ear points corresponding to the Heart [C], Liver, Lung [C], Spleen [C], Kidney [C], and San Jiao [C] (Triple Warmer) are often added to many clinical protocols. In addition, the Chinese ear points Adrenal Gland [C], Brain [C], Occiput, and Windstream [C] are utilized as supportive points in many auriculotherapy treatments.

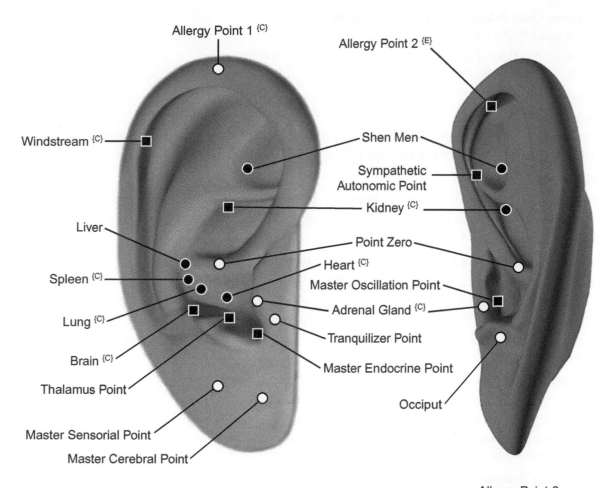

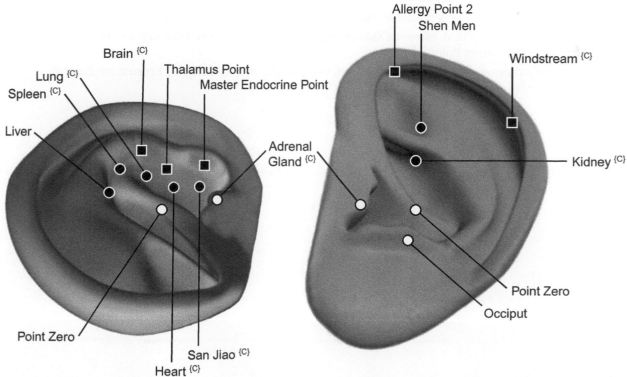

FIGURE 9.1 Master points and supplemental points represented on the auricle.

9.2 Addictive Behaviors and Drug Detoxification

9.2.1 Substance Abuse, Drug Addiction, or Drug Detoxification
PAP: Lung 2, Liver, Kidney {C}, Brain {C}, Nucleus Accumbens
MAP: Shen Men, Sympathetic Point, Nervous Subcortex, Master Cerebral Point
SAP: Adrenal Glands {C}, Anxiety Point, Occiput, Internal Nose

9.2.2 Alcohol Abuse
PAP: Alcoholic Point {C}, Thirst Point {C}, Liver, Lung 2, Kidney {C}, Brain {C}
MAP: Shen Men, Sympathetic Point, Nervous Subcortex, Point Zero, Tranquilizer Point, Master Cerebral Point
SAP: Occiput, Irritability Point {E}, Anti-Depressant Point {E}, Anxiety Point

9.2.3 Nervous Drinking
PAP: Alcoholic Point {C}, Thirst Point {C}, Kidney {C}, Brain {C}, Anxiety Point
MAP: Point Zero, Shen Men, Sympathetic Point, Nervous Subcortex, Tranquilizer Point, Master Cerebral Point
SAP: Limbic Brain

9.2.4 Nicotine Dependence, Smoking Cessation, or Tobacco Withdrawal
PAP: Nicotine Point {E}, Lung 1, Lung 2, Mouth, Palate {C}, Brain {C}
MAP: Point Zero, Shen Men, Sympathetic Point, Nervous Subcortex, Master Sensorial
SAP: Anxiety Point, Irritability Point {E}, Prostaglandin Point {E}, Psychosomatic Point {E}
             (*When using electrical stimulation to activate Lung points, stimulate at 80 Hz for at least 2 minutes each, stimulating both right and left auricles*)

9.2.5 Appetite Control, Weight Reduction, or Obesity Treatment
PAP: Appetite Control Point {C}, Stomach, Mouth, Small Intestines, Omega 1
MAP: Point Zero, Shen Men, Endocrine Point, Master Sensorial, Master Cerebral Point
SAP: Anti-Depressant Point {E}, Occiput, Adrenal Glands {C}, Psychosomatic Point {E}, Master Point for Metabolism {E}

9.2.6 Anorexia Nervosa or Bulimia
PAP: Appetite Control Point {C}, Stomach, Mouth, Small Intestines, Omega 1
MAP: Master Cerebral Point, Nervous Subcortex, Point Zero, Shen Men, Endocrine Point, Master Oscillation Point {E}
SAP: Anti-Depressant Point {E}, Anxiety Point, Occiput, Adrenal Glands {C}, Frustration Point {E}, Master Point for Metabolism {E}

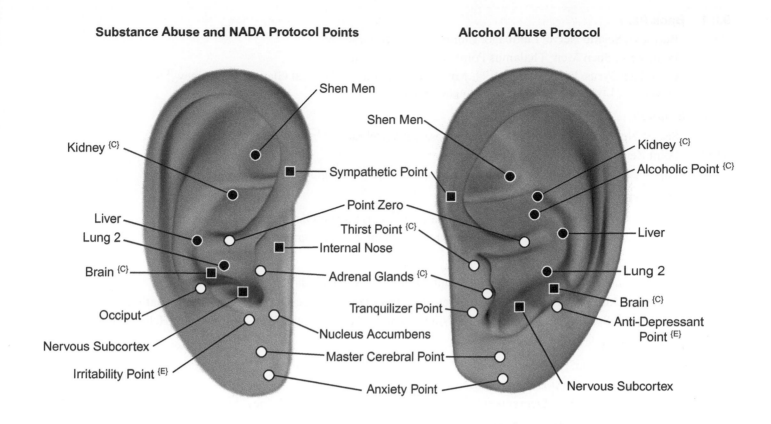

Substance Abuse and NADA Protocol Points

Shen Men

Kidney {C}

Sympathetic Point

Point Zero

Thirst Point {C}

Internal Nose

Liver

Lung 2

Brain {C}

Adrenal Glands {C}

Occiput

Tranquilizer Point

Nervous Subcortex

Nucleus Accumbens

Irritability Point {E}

Master Cerebral Point

Anxiety Point

Alcohol Abuse Protocol

Shen Men

Kidney {C}

Alcoholic Point {C}

Point Zero

Liver

Lung 2

Brain {C}

Anti-Depressant Point {E}

Nervous Subcortex

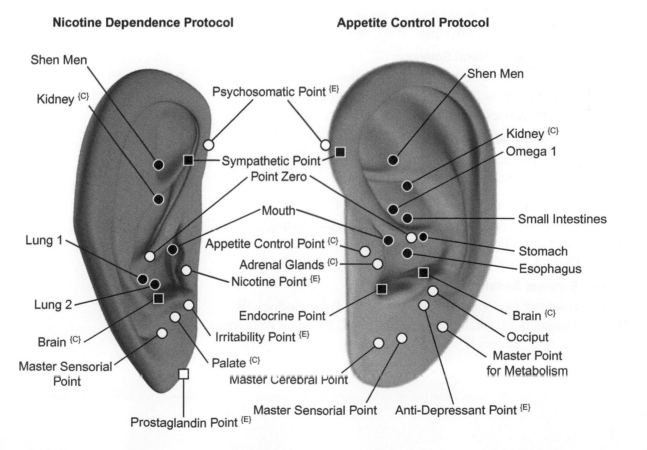

Nicotine Dependence Protocol

Shen Men

Kidney {C}

Psychosomatic Point {E}

Sympathetic Point

Point Zero

Mouth

Lung 1

Appetite Control Point {C}

Adrenal Glands {C}

Nicotine Point {E}

Lung 2

Endocrine Point

Brain {C}

Irritability Point {E}

Master Sensorial Point

Palate {C}

Master Cerebral Point

Prostaglandin Point {E}

Appetite Control Protocol

Shen Men

Kidney {C}

Omega 1

Small Intestines

Stomach

Esophagus

Brain {C}

Occiput

Master Point for Metabolism

Master Sensorial Point

Anti-Depressant Point {E}

FIGURE 9.2 Addiction and substance abuse auricular treatment protocols.

9.3 Back Pain and Body Aches

9.3.1 Back Pain
PAP: Buttocks, Sciatic Nerve, Lumbago, Lumbosacral Vertebrae [C, F1, F2, F3, F4]

MAP: Point Zero, Shen Men, Thalamus Point, Tranquilizer Point

SAP: Cingulate Gyrus, Darwin's Point [E], Muscle Relaxation [C], Adrenal Glands [C], Kidney [C], Spleen [C], Liver, Sympathetic Postganglionic Nerves

9.3.2 Sciatica
PAP: Sciatic Nerve, Buttocks, Lumbago, Lumbosacral Vertebrae [C, F1, F2, F3, F4]

MAP: Point Zero, Shen Men, Thalamus Point

SAP: Hip [C], Hip [E], Kidney [C], Bladder, Adrenal Glands [C], Cingulate Gyrus

9.3.3 Osteoarthritis or Osteoporosis
PAP: *Corresponding Area*, Omega 2, Adrenal Glands [C], Parathyroid Glands [E], Kidney [C]

MAP: Allergy 1, Allergy 2, Endocrine Point, Shen Men, Point Zero, Thalamus Point

9.3.4 Rheumatoid Arthritis or Gout
PAP: *Corresponding Area*, Omega 2, Prostaglandin Point [E], Adrenal Glands [C]

MAP: Allergy 1, Allergy 2, Point Zero, Shen Men, Thalamus Point, Endocrine Point, Master Oscillation Point

SAP: Kidney [C], Spleen [C], Liver, San Jiao, Windstream [C], Helix 1, Helix 2, Helix 3, Helix 4, Helix 5, Helix 6

9.3.5 Fibromyalgia
PAP: Thoracic, Lumbar, Sacral Vertebrae [C, F1, F2, F3, F4], Psychosomatic Point [E]

MAP: Thalamus Point, Point Zero, Shen Men, Master Oscillation Point

SAP: Cingulate Gyrus, Anti-Depressant Point [E], Vitality Point [E], Liver, Kidney [C], Windstream [C]

9.3.6 Abdominal Pain or Pelvic Pain
PAP: Abdomen, Pelvis, Vagus Nerve, Omega 1

MAP: Thalamus Point, Sympathetic Point, Shen Men, Point Zero

9.3.7 Amyotrophic Lateral Sclerosis
PAP: *Corresponding Area*, Spinal Motor Neurons, Brain [C], Brainstem [C], Brainstem [E]

MAP: Shen Men, Point Zero, Sympathetic Point, Endocrine Point

SAP: Occiput, Kidney [C], San Jiao

9.3.8 Intercostal Neuralgia
PAP: Chest, Thoracic Vertebrae [C, F1, F2, F3, F4], Thoracic Spinal Cord, Cingulate Gyrus

MAP: Point Zero, Shen Men, Thalamus Point

9.3.9 Surgical Anesthesia
PAP: Chest, Abdomen, Analgesia Point [E], Lung 2, Occiput

MAP: Point Zero, Shen Men, Thalamus Point

SAP: Occiput, Liver, Spleen [C], Gall Bladder, Stomach, San Jiao

9.3.10 Surgical Sedation
PAP: Forehead, Occiput, Barbiturate Point [E], Hypnotic Point [E]

MAP: Tranquilizer Point, Master Cerebral Point, Thalamus Point, Point Zero, Shen Men

SAP: Heart [C], Kidney [C], Cingulate Gyrus

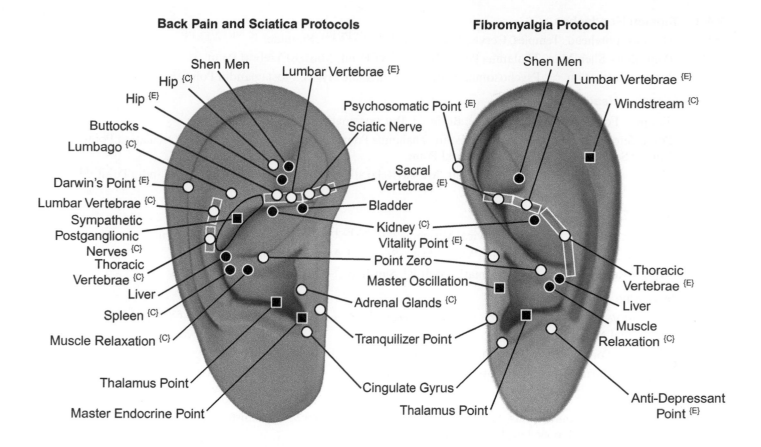

Back Pain and Sciatica Protocols

Shen Men
Hip {C}
Hip {E}
Buttocks
Lumbago {C}
Darwin's Point {E}
Lumbar Vertebrae {C}
Sympathetic
Postganglionic
Nerves {C}
Thoracic
Vertebrae {C}
Liver
Spleen {C}
Muscle Relaxation {C}

Lumbar Vertebrae {E}
Psychosomatic Point {E}
Sciatic Nerve
Sacral
Vertebrae {E}
Bladder
Kidney {C}
Vitality Point {E}
Point Zero
Master Oscillation
Adrenal Glands {C}
Tranquilizer Point

Thalamus Point
Master Endocrine Point

Cingulate Gyrus
Thalamus Point

Fibromyalgia Protocol

Shen Men
Lumbar Vertebrae {E}
Windstream {C}

Thoracic
Vertebrae {E}
Liver
Muscle
Relaxation {C}

Anti-Depressant
Point {E}

Osteoarthritis and Rheumatoid Arthritis Protocols

Allergy Point 1
Allergy Point 2
Omega 2
Shen Men
Windstream {C}
Helix 1
Kidney {C}
Helix 2
Liver
Helix 3
Spleen {C}
Helix 4
Helix 5
Helix 6

Point Zero
Master
Oscillation Point
Adrenal Gland {C}
Endocrine Point
Prostaglandin Point {E}

Parathyroid Gland
Helix 6
Thalamus Point
Endocrine Point
Helix 5
San Jiao {C}
Helix 4
Adrenal Gland {C}
Master
Oscillation Point
Helix 3
Helix 2
Omega 2
Helix 1
Windstream {C}
Shen Men
Allergy Point 1

FIGURE 9.3 Back pain auricular treatment protocols.

9.4 Headaches and Neck Pain

9.4.1 Tension Headaches
PAP: Occiput, Forehead, Temples, Cervical Vertebrae $^{\{C, F1, F2, F3, F4\}}$, Shoulder $^{\{C, F1, F2, F3, F4\}}$

MAP: Point Zero, Shen Men, Thalamus Point, Tranquilizer Point, Master Cerebral Point

SAP: Muscle Relaxation $^{\{C\}}$, Psychosomatic Point $^{\{E\}}$, Cingulate Gyrus, Prostaglandin Point $^{\{E\}}$

9.4.2 Migraine Headaches
PAP: Temples, Forehead, Windstream $^{\{C\}}$, Brain $^{\{C\}}$, Psychosomatic Point $^{\{E\}}$

MAP: Point Zero, Shen Men, Sympathetic Point, Thalamus Point, Tranquilizer Point, Master Oscillation Point, Master Sensorial Point, Master Cerebral Point

SAP: Shoulder $^{\{C, F1, F2, F3, F4\}}$, Shoulder Joint, Muscle Relaxation $^{\{C\}}$, Cingulate Gyrus, Prostaglandin Point $^{\{E\}}$, Kidney $^{\{C\}}$, Irritability Point $^{\{E\}}$

9.4.3 TMJ or Bruxism
PAP: TMJ, Upper Jaw, Lower Jaw, Cervical Vertebrae $^{\{C, E, F2, F3, F4\}}$, Occiput, Trigeminal Nucleus

MAP: Thalamus Point, Point Zero, Shen Men, Master Sensorial, Master Cerebral Point

SAP: Muscle Relaxation $^{\{C\}}$, Psychosomatic Point $^{\{E\}}$, San Jiao

9.4.4 Torticollis or Whiplash
PAP: Cervical Vertebrae $^{\{C, F1, F2, F3, F4\}}$, Occiput, Clavicle $^{\{C\}}$, Clavicle $^{\{E\}}$, Shoulder $^{\{C, F1, F2, F3, F4\}}$, Trigeminal Nucleus

MAP: Thalamus Point, Point Zero, Shen Men, Endocrine Point, Master Cerebral Point

SAP: Cingulate Gyrus, Muscle Relaxation $^{\{C\}}$, Adrenal Glands $^{\{C\}}$, Liver

9.4.5 Sinusitis
PAP: Internal Nose, Frontal Sinus, Forehead, Lung 1, Lung 2, Asthma $^{\{C\}}$, Antihistamine $^{\{C\}}$, External Ear $^{\{C\}}$, External Ear $^{\{E\}}$, Upper Jaw, Lower Jaw

MAP: Allergy 1, Allergy 2, Point Zero, Shen Men, Thalamus Point

SAP: ACTH, Adrenal Glands $^{\{C\}}$, Adrenal Glands $^{\{E\}}$, San Jiao, Thymus Gland

9.4.6 Facial Spasms
PAP: Trigeminal Nucleus, Facial Nerve, Face, Occiput, Temples, Forehead, Brainstem $^{\{C\}}$, Brainstem $^{\{E\}}$

MAP: Thalamus Point, Master Sensorial, Point Zero, Shen Men, Master Cerebral Point

SAP: Cervical Vertebrae $^{\{C, F1, F2, F3, F4\}}$, Windstream $^{\{C\}}$, Liver, Spleen $^{\{C\}}$, Helix 4

9.4.7 Facial Tics
PAP: Trigeminal Nucleus, Face, Forehead, Eye, Brainstem $^{\{C\}}$, Lower Jaw, Upper Jaw, Cervical Vertebrae $^{\{C, F1, F2, F3, F4\}}$

MAP: Thalamus Point, Master Cerebral Point, Point Zero, Shen Men

SAP: Stomach, Liver, Muscle Relaxation $^{\{C\}}$

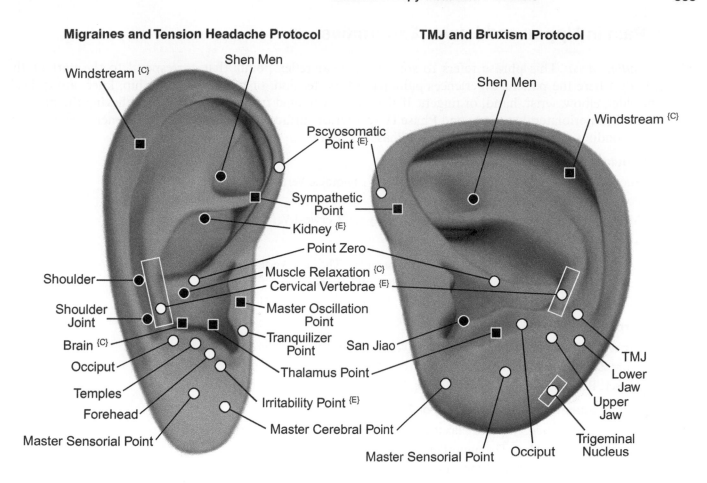

Migraines and Tension Headache Protocol

Windstream {C}
Shen Men
Pscyosomatic Point {E}
Sympathetic Point
Kidney {E}
Point Zero
Muscle Relaxation {C}
Cervical Vertebrae {E}
Shoulder
Shoulder Joint
Master Oscillation Point
Brain {C}
Tranquilizer Point
Occiput
Thalamus Point
Temples
Irritability Point {E}
Forehead
Master Cerebral Point
Master Sensorial Point

TMJ and Bruxism Protocol

Shen Men
Windstream {C}
Point Zero
San Jiao
TMJ
Lower Jaw
Upper Jaw
Trigeminal Nucleus
Master Sensorial Point
Occiput

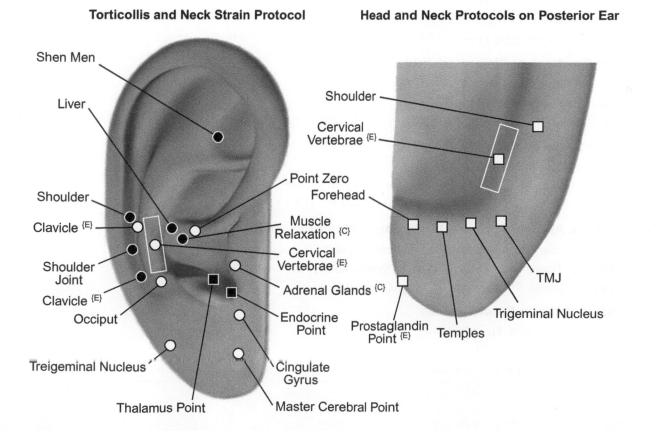

Torticollis and Neck Strain Protocol

Shen Men
Liver
Shoulder
Clavicle {E}
Shoulder Joint
Clavicle {E}
Occiput
Point Zero
Muscle Relaxation {C}
Cervical Vertebrae {E}
Adrenal Glands {C}
Endocrine Point
Treigeminal Nucleus
Thalamus Point
Cingulate Gyrus
Master Cerebral Point

Head and Neck Protocols on Posterior Ear

Shoulder
Cervical Vertebrae {E}
Forehead
TMJ
Trigeminal Nucleus
Prostaglandin Point {E}
Temples

FIGURE 9.4 Head and neck pain auricular treatment protocols.

9.5 Pain in Upper and Lower Extremities

Corresponding Area: This phrase refers to somatotopic ear reflex points that correspond to the part of the actual body where the patient experiences pain, pathology, tension, or weakness in the hip, knee, ankle, heel, toes, shoulder, elbow, wrist, hand, or fingers. If there is only limited treatment success for relieving the problem with Phase I (anteriolateral surface) and Phase IV (posterior surface) ear points, the practitioner should stimulate corresponding ear points on Phase II and Phase III charts.

9.5.1 Shoulder Pain, Frozen Shoulder, or Bursitis
PAP: Shoulder [C, F1, F2, F3, F4], Clavicle [C], Clavicle [E], Thoracic Vertebrae [C, F1, F2, F3, F4]

MAP: Point Zero, Shen Men, Thalamus Point

SAP: Muscle Relaxation [C], Cingulate Gyrus, Kidney [C], Cervical Vertebrae [E], Adrenal Glands [E]

9.5.2 Tennis Elbow
PAP: Elbow [F1, F2, F3, F4], Forearm, Arm, Windstream [C], Thoracic Vertebrae [F1, F4]

MAP: Point Zero, Point Zero Prime, Shen Men, Thalamus Point

SAP: Muscle Relaxation [C], Adrenal Glands [C], Kidney [C], San Jiao, Helix 3, Helix 4

9.5.3 Carpal Tunnel Syndrome or Wrist Pain
PAP: Wrist [C, F1, F2, F3, F4], Forearm, Thoracic Vertebrae [C, F1, E, F2, F3, F4]

MAP: Point Zero, Shen Men, Thalamus Point

SAP: Muscle Relaxation [C], Cingulate Gyrus, Helix 1, Helix 2

9.5.4 Muscle Spasms, Muscle Tension, or Muscle Cramp
PAP: *Corresponding Area*, Muscle Relaxation [C], Cerebellum, Spleen [C], Striatum

MAP: Point Zero, Shen Men, Thalamus Point

SAP: Frontal Cortex, Striatum, Cingulate Gyrus, Sciatic Nerve, Heat Point [C]

9.5.5 Battlefield Acupuncture
PAP: *Corresponding Area*, Cingulate Gyrus, Omega 2

MAP: Point Zero, Point Zero Prime [E1, E2], Thalamus Point [C, F1, E, F2, F3, F4], Shen Men

9.5.6 Bone Fractures or Dislocated Joints
PAP: *Corresponding Area*, Kidney [C], Kidney [E], Parathyroid Glands

MAP: Point Zero, Shen Men, Thalamus Point

SAP: Liver, Spleen [C], Adrenal Glands [C]

9.5.7 Joint Inflammation or Joint Swelling
PAP: *Corresponding Area*, Omega 2, Kidney [C]

MAP: Allergy 1, Allergy 2, Point Zero, Shen Men, Endocrine Point

SAP: Occiput, Prostaglandin Point [E], Adrenal Glands [C], Helix 1, Helix 2, Helix 3, Helix 4, Helix 5, Helix 6

9.5.8 Muscular Atrophy, Muscular Dystrophy, or Motor Paralysis
PAP: *Corresponding Area*, Spinal Motor Neurons, Frontal Cortex, Cerebellum

MAP: Thalamus Point, Point Zero, Shen Men, Sympathetic Point

SAP: Striatum, Spleen [C], Parathyroid Glands, Sciatic Nerve

9.5.9 Muscle Sprain or Sports Injuries
PAP: *Corresponding Area*, Heat Point [C]

MAP: Point Zero, Shen Men, Thalamus Point

SAP: Striatum, Liver, Spleen [C], Kidney [C], Adrenal Glands [C], Helix 4

Frozen Shoulder or Bursitis Protocols

Tennis Elbow or Carpal Tunnel Syndrome Protocols

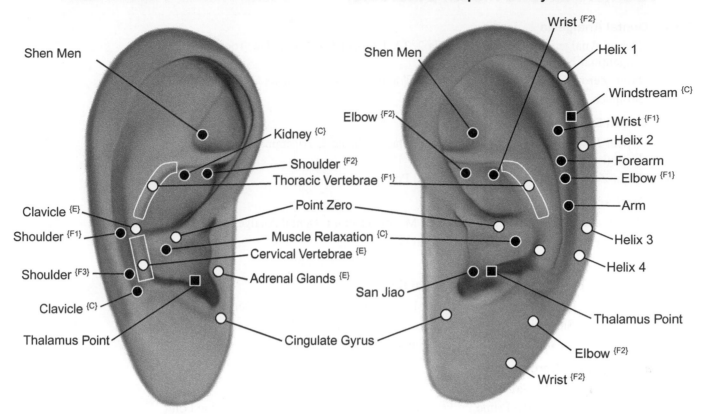

Shen Men

Kidney {C}

Shoulder {F2}

Thoracic Vertebrae {F1}

Point Zero

Clavicle {E}

Shoulder {F1}

Muscle Relaxation {C}

Cervical Vertebrae {E}

Shoulder {F3}

Adrenal Glands {E}

Clavicle {C}

Thalamus Point

Cingulate Gyrus

Wrist {F2}

Shen Men

Helix 1

Windstream {C}

Elbow {F2}

Wrist {F1}

Helix 2

Forearm

Elbow {F1}

Arm

Helix 3

Helix 4

San Jiao

Thalamus Point

Elbow {F2}

Wrist {F2}

Lower Limbs Muscle Spasms Protocols

External Limb Protocols on Posterior Ear

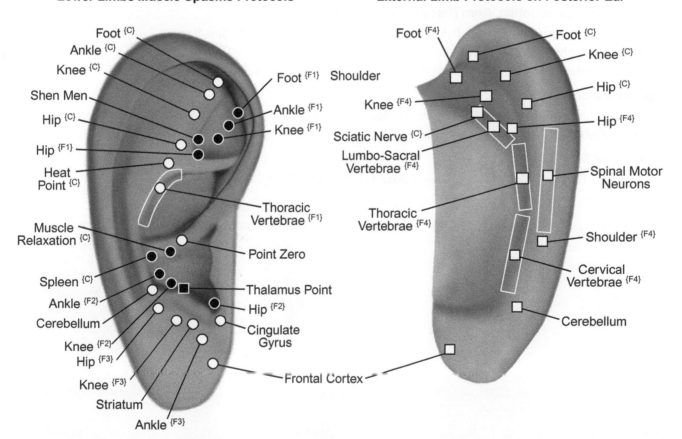

Foot {C}

Ankle {C}

Knee {C}

Shen Men

Hip {C}

Hip {F1}

Heat Point {C}

Muscle Relaxation {C}

Spleen {C}

Ankle {F2}

Cerebellum

Knee {F2}

Hip {F3}

Knee {F3}

Striatum

Ankle {F3}

Foot {F1}

Ankle {F1}

Knee {F1}

Thoracic Vertebrae {F1}

Point Zero

Thalamus Point

Hip {F2}

Cingulate Gyrus

Frontal Cortex

Foot {F4}

Shoulder

Knee {F4}

Sciatic Nerve {C}

Lumbo-Sacral Vertebrae {F4}

Thoracic Vertebrae {F4}

Foot {C}

Knee {C}

Hip {C}

Hip {F4}

Spinal Motor Neurons

Shoulder {F4}

Cervical Vertebrae {F4}

Cerebellum

FIGURE 9.5 Leg and arm pain auricular treatment protocols.

9.6 Dental Pain and Mouth Disorders

9.6.1 Dental Analgesia

PAP: Dental Analgesia 1, Dental Analgesia 2, TMJ, Upper Jaw, Lower Jaw, Toothache[1, 2, 3], Trigeminal Nerve, Occiput

MAP: Point Zero, Shen Men, Thalamus Point, Tranquilizer Point, Master Sensorial Point

SAP: Stomach, Kidney [C]

9.6.2 Dental Surgery

PAP: Upper Jaw, Lower Jaw, Toothache[1, 2, 3], Palate 1, Palate 2, Trigeminal Nerve, Dental Analgesia 1, Dental Analgesia 2

MAP: Point Zero, Shen Men, Master Sensorial Point

9.6.3 Toothache

PAP: Toothache[1, 2, 3], Upper Jaw, Lower Jaw, Mouth, Occiput, Dental Analgesia 1, Dental Analgesia 2

MAP: Point Zero, Shen Men, Master Sensorial Point

SAP: Cervical Vertebrae [E], Trigeminal Nerve, Kidney [C], San Jiao

9.6.4 Trigeminal Neuralgia or Facial Neuralgia

PAP: Trigeminal Nerve, Trigeminal Nucleus, Face, Upper Jaw, Lower Jaw, Occiput

MAP: Point Zero, Shen Men, Master Oscillation, Master Sensorial, Master Cerebral Point

SAP: Brainstem [C], Windstream [C], Liver, San Jiao, Large Intestines

9.6.5 Dry Mouth or Xerostomia

PAP: Salivary Gland [C], Salivary Gland [E], Thirst Point [C], Mouth

MAP: Point Zero, Point Zero Prime [E1, E2], Shen Men, Sympathetic Point, Endocrine Point

SAP: Posterior Pituitary [E], Vagus Nerve

9.6.6 Gingivitis, Periodontitis, Gum Disease, or Bleeding of Gums

PAP: Upper Jaw, Lower Jaw, Mouth, Palate 1, Palate 2, Kidney [C], Spleen [C], San Jiao

MAP: Point Zero, Shen Men, Thalamus Point

SAP: Adrenal Glands [C], Adrenal Glands [E], Large Intestines, Helix 3, Helix 4

9.6.7 Mouth Ulcer

PAP: Mouth, Lips, Palate 1, Palate 2, Tongue [C], Tongue [E], Adrenal Glands [C], Adrenal Glands [E]

MAP: Point Zero, Shen Men, Thalamus Point

9.6.8 Mercury Toxicity

PAP: Mercury Toxicity Point [E], Upper Jaw, Lower Jaw, Thymus Gland

MAP: Point Zero, Shen Men, Thalamus Point

Dental Analgesia Protocol

Toothache Protocol

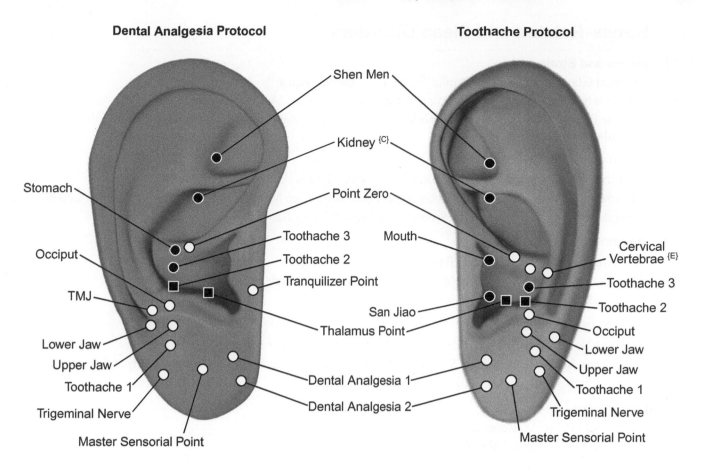

Trigeminal Neuralgia Protocol

Dry Mouth or Xerostomia Protocol

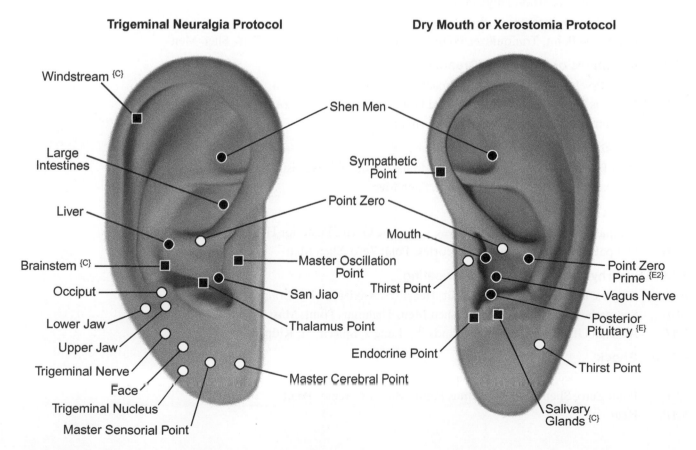

FIGURE 9.6 Dental pain and mouth disorders auricular treatment protocols.

9.7 Stress-Related and Sleep Disorders

9.7.1 Stress and Strain
PAP: Adrenal Glands {C}, Adrenal Glands {E}, ACTH, Occiput, Heart {C}

MAP: Nervous Subcortex, Tranquilizer Point, Point Zero, Shen Men, Master Cerebral Point

SAP: Muscle Relaxation {C}, Posterior Hypothalamus, Psychosomatic Point {E}, Prostaglandin Point {E}, Cingulate Gyrus

9.7.2 Chronic Fatigue Syndrome
PAP: Vitality Point {E}, Anti-Depressant Point {E}, Adrenal Glands {C}, Adrenal Glands {E}

MAP: Nervous Subcortex, Master Oscillation Point, Point Zero, Shen Men, Sympathetic Point, Master Cerebral Point

SAP: Cingulate Gyrus, Brain {C}, Liver, Spleen {C}, Kidney {C}, San Jiao

9.7.3 Insomnia
PAP: Insomnia 1, Insomnia 2, Pineal Gland

MAP: Nervous Subcortex, Master Cerebral Point, Point Zero, Shen Men, Tranquilizer Point

SAP: Forehead, Occiput, Brain {C}, Heart {C}, Kidney {C}

9.7.3 Snoring or Sleep Apnea
PAP: Internal Nose, Trachea, Throat {E}, Tongue {C}, Tongue {E}, Lower Jaw

MAP: Point Zero, Shen Men, Nervous Subcortex, Sympathetic Point, Tranquilizer Point, Endocrine Point

SAP: Chest, Adrenal Glands {C}, Lung 1, Lung 2, San Jiao

9.7.4 Drowsiness
PAP: Excitement Point {C}, Reticular Formation, Insomnia 1, Insomnia 2

MAP: Master Cerebral Point, Point Zero, Shen Men

9.7.5 Jet Lag or Circadian Rhythm Dysfunction
PAP: Pineal Gland, Insomnia 1, Insomnia 2

MAP: Endocrine Point, Tranquilizer Point, Master Cerebral Point, Point Zero, Shen Men

9.7.6 Nightmares or Disturbing Dreams
PAP: Pons, Psychosomatic Point {E}, Anxiety Point, Heart {C}, Occiput

MAP: Nervous Subcortex, Master Cerebral Point, Shen Men, Point Zero

SAP: Insomnia 1, Insomnia 2, Reticular Formation

9.7.7 Heat Stroke
PAP: Heat Point {C}, Occiput, Heart {C}, Adrenal Glands {C}, Windstream {C}

MAP: Sympathetic Point, Thalamus Point, Shen Men

9.7.8 Reflex Sympathetic Dystrophy
PAP: Sympathetic Postganglionic Nerves, Cingulate Gyrus, Posterior Hypothalamus

MAP: Sympathetic Point, Nervous Subcortex, Point Zero, Shen Men

9.7.9 Hyperhydrosis or Excessive Sweating
PAP: Fingers, Hand, Forehead, Occiput, Heart {C}, Anxiety Point, Brain {C}

MAP: Sympathetic Point, Point Zero, Shen Men, Thalamus Point, Master Cerebral Point

SAP: Adrenal Glands {C}, Adrenal Glands {E}, Lung 2, Spleen {C}, Kidney {C}

9.7.10 Shock
PAP: Brain {C}, Occiput, Adrenal Glands {C}, Adrenal Glands {E}

MAP: Point Zero, Shen Men, Thalamus Point, Master Cerebral Point

SAP: Heart {C}

Stress and Strain Protocol

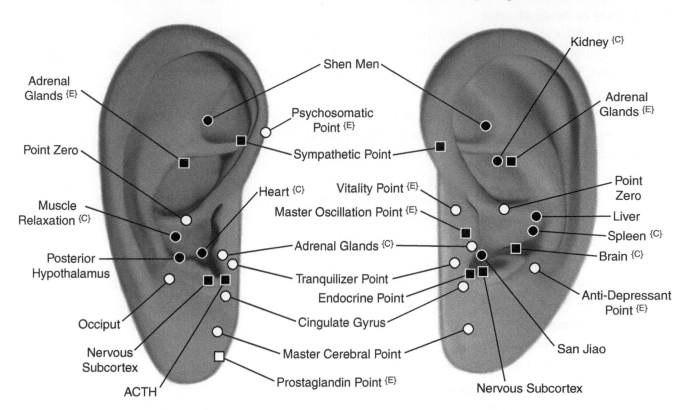

Shen Men

Adrenal Glands {E}

Psychosomatic Point {E}

Sympathetic Point

Point Zero

Heart {C}

Muscle Relaxation {C}

Adrenal Glands {C}

Posterior Hypothalamus

Tranquilizer Point

Endocrine Point

Occiput

Cingulate Gyrus

Nervous Subcortex

Master Cerebral Point

ACTH

Prostaglandin Point {E}

Chronic Fatigue Syndrome Protocol

Kidney {C}

Adrenal Glands {E}

Point Zero

Vitality Point {E}

Master Oscillation Point {E}

Liver

Spleen {C}

Brain {C}

Anti-Depressant Point {E}

San Jiao

Nervous Subcortex

Insomnia Protocol

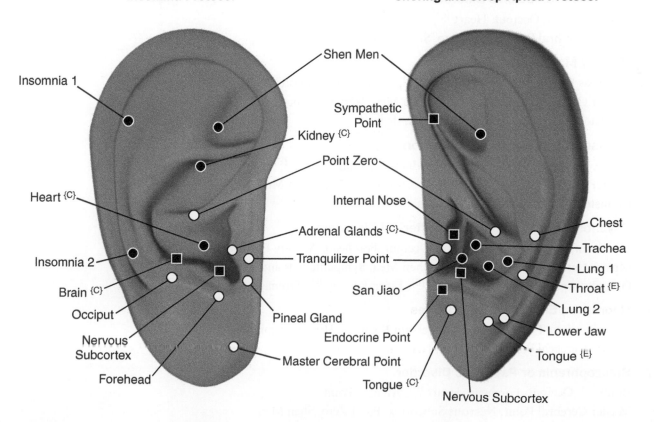

Shen Men

Insomnia 1

Sympathetic Point

Kidney {C}

Point Zero

Heart {C}

Internal Nose

Adrenal Glands {C}

Insomnia 2

Tranquilizer Point

Brain {C}

San Jiao

Occiput

Pineal Gland

Nervous Subcortex

Master Cerebral Point

Forehead

Snoring and Sleep Apnea Protocol

Chest

Trachea

Lung 1

Throat {E}

Lung 2

Lower Jaw

Tongue {E}

Endocrine Point

Tongue {C}

Nervous Subcortex

FIGURE 9.7 Stress-related and sleep disorders auricular treatment protocols.

9.8 Mental Health Disorders

9.8.1 Anxiety or Panic Attacks

PAP: Anxiety Point, Adrenal Glands {C}, Adrenal Glands {E}, Brain {C}, Heart {C}, Heart {E}

MAP: Tranquilizer Point, Master Cerebral Point, Sympathetic Point, Shen Men, Point Zero, Nervous Subcortex

SAP: Occiput, Kidney {C}, Stomach, Vagus Nerve, Psychosomatic Point {E}

9.8.2 Depression or Dysthymia

PAP: Anti-Depressant {E}, Brain {C}, Cingulate Gyrus, Excitement Point {C}, Heart {C}, Occiput

MAP: Master Cerebral Point, Nervous Subcortex, Point Zero, Shen Men, Tranquilizer Point

SAP: Reticular Formation, Pineal Gland, Gonadotrophins {E}, Ovaries/Testes {E}

9.8.3 Mania or Bipolar Disorder

PAP: Mania Point, Irritability Point {E}, Anti-Depressant Point {E}, Brain {C}, Occiput

MAP: Master Cerebral Point, Nervous Subcortex, Tranquilizer Point, Shen Men, Point Zero

9.8.4 Attention Deficit Hyperactivity Disorder (ADHD)

PAP: Brain {C}, Excitement Point {C}, Prefrontal Cortex, Hippocampus, Occiput

MAP: Shen Men, Master Cerebral, Master Oscillation Point, Point Zero, Nervous Subcortex

SAP: Forehead, Anxiety Point, Thyroid Glands {C}, Thyroid Glands {E}, Kidney {C}, Liver

9.8.5 Memory Problems

PAP: Memory 1, Memory 2, Memory 3, Hippocampus, Brain {C}, Heart {C}

MAP: Master Cerebral Point, Point Zero, Shen Men, Nervous Subcortex

9.8.6 Irritability or Overly Aggressive Behaviors

PAP: Irritability Point {E}, Mania Point {E}, Frustration Point {E}, Cingulate Gyrus, Heart {C}

MAP: Master Cerebral Point, Point Zero, Shen Men, Thalamus Point

9.8.7 Obsessive–Compulsive Disorder

PAP: Frontal Cortex, Occiput, Heart {C}

MAP: Master Cerebral Point, Point Zero, Shen Men, Nervous Subcortex

9.8.8 Difficulty Maintaining Alertness

PAP: Alertness Point {E}, Excitement Point {C}, Frontal Cortex, Forehead, Heart {C}

MAP: Master Cerebral Point, Point Zero, Shen Men, Nervous Subcortex, Endocrine Point

SAP: Brainstem {C}, Kidney {C}, Adrenal Glands {C}

9.8.9 Neurasthenia or Nervous Exhaustion

PAP: Anxiety Point, Occiput, Heart {C}, Kidney {C}, Vitality Point {E}

MAP: Master Cerebral Point, Nervous Subcortex, Point Zero, Shen Men, Tranquilizer Point

SAP: Brainstem {C}, Stomach, Liver, Spleen {C}

9.8.10 Psychosomatic Disorders or Hysterical Disorders

PAP: Psychosomatic Point {E}, Brain {C}, Occiput, Forehead, Anxiety Point, Heart {C}

MAP: Master Cerebral Point, Point Zero, Shen Men, Sympathetic Point, Nervous Subcortex

SAP: Gonadotrophins {E}, Ovaries/Testes {E}, Liver, Kidney {C}, Stomach, Windstream {C}

9.8.11 Repressed Emotional Experiences

PAP: Psychosomatic Point {E}, Anti-Depressant Point {E}, Hippocampus, Heart {C}

MAP: Master Cerebral Point, Shen Men, Nervous Subcortex

9.8.12 Schizophrenia or Psychotic Disorder

PAP: Brain {C}, Occiput, Forehead, Heart {C}, Anxiety Point

MAP: Master Cerebral Point, Nervous Subcortex, Point Zero, Shen Men

SAP: Brainstem {C}, Kidney {C}, Windstream {C}, Stomach, Liver

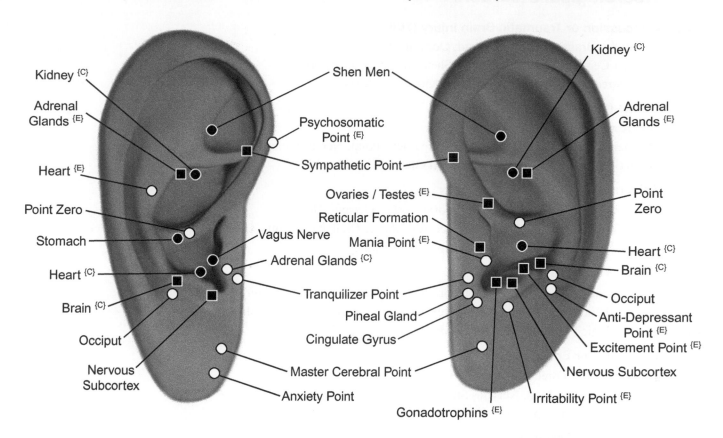

Anxiety or Panic Attack Protocols

Kidney {C}
Adrenal Glands {E}
Shen Men
Psychosomatic Point {E}
Sympathetic Point
Heart {E}
Point Zero
Stomach
Vagus Nerve
Heart {C}
Adrenal Glands {C}
Brain {C}
Tranquilizer Point
Occiput
Nervous Subcortex
Master Cerebral Point
Anxiety Point

Depression or Bipolar Disorder Protocols

Kidney {C}
Adrenal Glands {E}
Shen Men
Point Zero
Ovaries / Testes {E}
Reticular Formation
Mania Point {E}
Heart {C}
Brain {C}
Occiput
Anti-Depressant Point {E}
Tranquilizer Point
Pineal Gland
Cingulate Gyrus
Excitement Point {E}
Nervous Subcortex
Master Cerebral Point
Irritability Point {E}
Gonadotrophins {E}

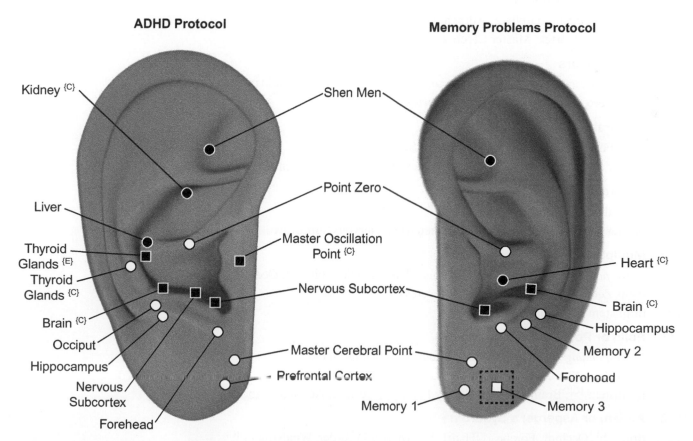

ADHD Protocol

Kidney {C}
Shen Men
Liver
Point Zero
Thyroid Glands {E}
Master Oscillation Point {C}
Thyroid Glands {C}
Nervous Subcortex
Brain {C}
Occiput
Hippocampus
Nervous Subcortex
Master Cerebral Point
Prefrontal Cortex
Forehead

Memory Problems Protocol

Shen Men
Point Zero
Heart {C}
Brain {C}
Hippocampus
Memory 2
Forehead
Memory 1
Memory 3

FIGURE 9.8 Mental health disorders auricular treatment protocols.

9.9 Neurological Disorders

9.9.1 Concussion or Traumatic Brain Injury (TBI)
PAP: Brain [C], Brainstem [C], Forehead, Occiput, Heart [C]
MAP: Master Cerebral Point, Point Zero, Shen Men, Nervous Subcortex
SAP: Windstream [C], Adrenal Glands [C], Kidney [C], Liver

9.9.2 Stroke (Cerebral Vascular Accident)
PAP: Corresponding Brain Area, Brain [C]
MAP: Master Cerebral Point, Shen Men, Sympathetic Point, Nervous Subcortex
SAP: Heart [C], Adrenal Glands [C], Adrenal Glands [E], Kidney [C]

9.9.3 Seizures, Convulsions, or Epilepsy
PAP: Epilepsy Point [C], Amygdala, Temporal Cortex, Occiput, Heart [C]
MAP: Point Zero, Shen Men, Nervous Subcortex, Master Oscillation Point
SAP: Brain [C], Brainstem [C], Stomach, Spleen [C], Kidney [C]

9.9.4 Peripheral Neuralgia
PAP: *Corresponding Body Area*, Spinal Cord Sensory Neurons, Cingulate Gyrus
MAP: Sympathetic Point, Nervous Subcortex, Master, Sensorial Point Zero, Shen Men
SAP: Sympathetic Postganglionic Nerves, Brain [C], Adrenal Glands [C]

9.9.5 Meningitis or Encephalitis
PAP: Brainstem [C], Forehead, Occiput, Windstream [C], Heart [C]
MAP: Point Zero, Shen Men, Nervous Subcortex, Master Cerebral Point
SAP: Kidney [C], Stomach, Heart [C], Vitality Point [E]

9.9.6 Parkinsonian Tremors
PAP: Striatum, Substantia Nigra, Adrenal Glands [C], Adrenal Glands [E]
MAP: Nervous Subcortex, Master Cerebral Point, Point Zero, Shen Men

9.9.7 Motor Tremors
PAP: Spinal Motor Neurons, Frontal Cortex, Striatum, Cerebellum, Brainstem [C]
MAP: Point Zero, Shen Men, Nervous Subcortex

9.9.8 Bell's Palsy
PAP: Face, Forehead, Facial Nerve, Brain [C], Striatum, Occiput
MAP: Point Zero, Shen Men, Nervous Subcortex, Master Cerebral Point

9.9.9 Cerebral Palsy
PAP: Frontal Cortex, Brain [C], Brainstem [C], Striatum, Occiput
MAP: Master Cerebral Point, Point Zero, Shen Men, Nervous Subcortex

9.9.10 Multiple Sclerosis
PAP: *Corresponding Area*, Brain [C], Thymus Gland, Vitality Point [E], Occiput
MAP: Point Zero, Shen Men, Nervous Subcortex
SAP: Brainstem [C], Kidney [C]

9.9.11 Polio or Post-Polio Syndrome
PAP: *Corresponding Area*, Spinal Motor Neurons, Thymus Gland
MAP: Point Zero, Shen Men, Nervous Subcortex, Master Cerebral Point
SAP: Brainstem [C], Brainstem [E], Vitality Point [E], Occiput, Adrenal Glands [C]

9.9.12 Autism or Asperger's Syndrome
PAP: Brain [C], Occiput, Forehead, Heart [C], Anxiety Disorder, Windstream [C]
MAP: Master Cerebral Point, Nervous Subcortex, Point Zero, Shen Men, Endocrine Point
SAP: Brainstem [C], Kidney [C]

Concussion Protocol

Stroke Protocol

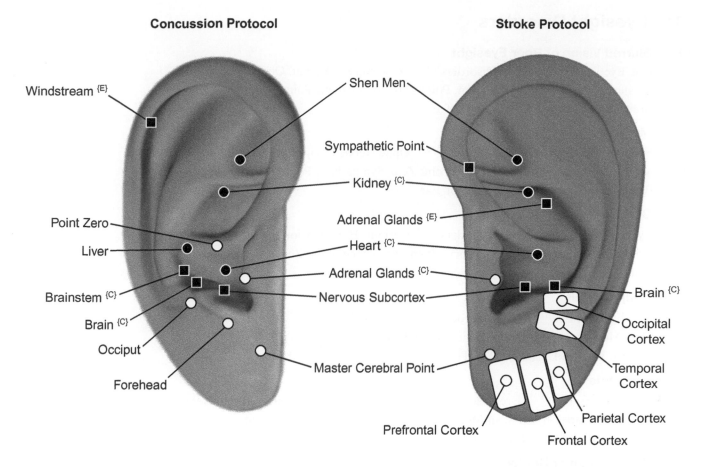

Windstream {E}

Shen Men

Sympathetic Point

Kidney {C}

Adrenal Glands {E}

Point Zero

Liver

Heart {C}

Adrenal Glands {C}

Brainstem {C}

Nervous Subcortex

Brain {C}

Brain {C}

Occiput

Occipital Cortex

Forehead

Master Cerebral Point

Temporal Cortex

Prefrontal Cortex

Parietal Cortex

Frontal Cortex

Seizures or Convulsions Protocols

Neuralgias or Neuropathies Protocols

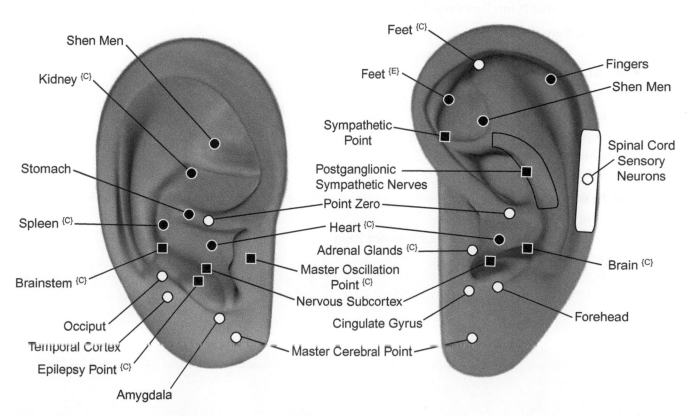

Feet {C}

Shen Men

Feet {E}

Fingers

Kidney {C}

Shen Men

Sympathetic Point

Stomach

Postganglionic Sympathetic Nerves

Spinal Cord Sensory Neurons

Spleen {C}

Point Zero

Heart {C}

Adrenal Glands {C}

Brainstem {C}

Master Oscillation Point {C}

Brain {C}

Nervous Subcortex

Occiput

Cingulate Gyrus

Temporal Cortex

Forehead

Epilepsy Point {C}

Master Cerebral Point

Amygdala

FIGURE 9.9 Neurological disorders auricular treatment protocols.

9.10 Eyesight Disorders

9.10.1 Blurred Vision or Poor Eyesight
PAP: Eye, Eye [F2], Eye [F3], Eye Disorders[1, 2, 3], Optic Nerve, Occiput, Occipital Cortex
MAP: Master Sensorial Point, Shen Men, Point Zero, Sympathetic Point
SAP: Brain [C], Kidney [C], Liver, Apex of Ear

9.10.2 Myopia
PAP: Eye, Eye [F2], Eye [F3], Eye Disorders[1, 2, 3], Optic Nerve, Occiput
MAP: Master Sensorial Point, Shen Men, Point Zero, Sympathetic Point
SAP: Brain [C], Kidney [C], Liver, Apex of Ear

9.10.3 Glaucoma
PAP: Eye, Eye [F2], Eye [F3], Eye Disorders[1, 2, 3], Occiput, Hypertension[1, 2, 3]
MAP: Nervous Subcortex, Master Sensorial Point, Shen Men, Point Zero
SAP: Kidney [C], Liver

9.10.4 Conjunctivitis
PAP: Eye, Eye [F2], Eye [F3], Eye Disorders[1, 2, 3], Adrenal Glands [C]
MAP: Shen Men, Nervous Subcortex, Endocrine Point
SAP: Lung 1, Lung 2, Dermatitis [C], Thymus Gland, Occiput, Liver, Kidney [C]

9.10.5 Cataracts
PAP: Eye, Eye [F2], Eye [F3], Eye Disorders[1, 2, 3], Adrenal Glands [C], Adrenal Glands [E]
MAP: Master Sensorial Point, Shen Men, Nervous Subcortex, Endocrine Point
SAP: Dermatitis [C], Occiput, Liver, Kidney [C]

9.10.6 Eye Irritation or Dry Eyes
PAP: Eye, Eye [F2], Eye [F3], Eye Disorders[1, 2, 3]
MAP: Master Sensorial Point, Endocrine Point, Shen Men, Point Zero

9.10.7 Astigmatism
PAP: Eye, Eye [F2], Eye [F3], Eye Disorders[1, 2, 3], Optic Nerve
MAP: Master Sensorial Point, Shen Men
SAP: Kidney [C], Liver, Occiput

9.10.8 Stye
PAP: Eye, Eye [F2], Eye [F3], Eye Disorders[1, 2, 3]
MAP: Shen Men, Master Sensorial Point
SAP: Liver, Spleen [C]

9.10.9 Night Blindness
PAP: Eye, Eye [F2], Eye [F3], Vitamin A
MAP: Master Sensorial Point, Shen Men, Endocrine Point
SAP: Liver, Spleen [C]

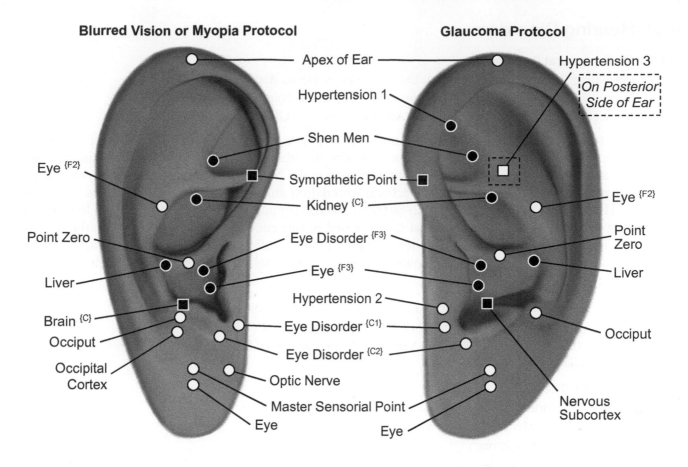

Blurred Vision or Myopia Protocol

- Apex of Ear
- Hypertension 1
- Shen Men
- Eye {F2}
- Sympathetic Point
- Kidney {C}
- Point Zero
- Eye Disorder {F3}
- Liver
- Eye {F3}
- Brain {C}
- Hypertension 2
- Occiput
- Eye Disorder {C1}
- Occipital Cortex
- Eye Disorder {C2}
- Optic Nerve
- Master Sensorial Point
- Eye

Glaucoma Protocol

- Hypertension 3
- *On Posterior Side of Ear*
- Eye {F2}
- Point Zero
- Liver
- Occiput
- Nervous Subcortex
- Eye

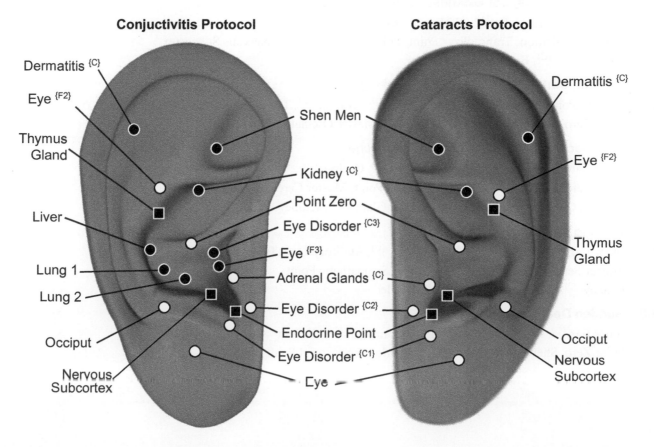

Conjuctivitis Protocol

- Dermatitis {C}
- Eye {F2}
- Thymus Gland
- Shen Men
- Kidney {C}
- Point Zero
- Liver
- Eye Disorder {C3}
- Eye {F3}
- Lung 1
- Adrenal Glands {C}
- Lung 2
- Eye Disorder {C2}
- Occiput
- Endocrine Point
- Eye Disorder {C1}
- Nervous Subcortex
- Eye

Cataracts Protocol

- Dermatitis {C}
- Eye {F2}
- Thymus Gland
- Occiput
- Nervous Subcortex

FIGURE 9.10 Visual disorders auricular treatment protocols.

9.11 Hearing Disorders

9.11.1 Sensorineural Deafness

PAP: Inner Ear {C}, Inner Ear {E}, External Ear {C}, Auditory Nerve, Auditory Line {E}

MAP: Master Sensorial Point, Shen Men, Point Zero, Sympathetic Point, Nervous Subcortex

SAP: Kidney {C}, Occiput, Temples, San Jiao, Adrenal Glands {C}, Gall Bladder

(In addition to stimulating the previously mentioned ear points, treat the four walls of the ear canal directly with a probe or needle. When using TAS (transauricular stimulation) with pulsing electrical stimulation, first fill the ear canal with saline. Use a monopolar auricular probe placed into the saline solution within the ear canal, not touching the skin. Turn on the electrical stimulation and treat a range of frequencies, from 1 Hz to 2.5 Hz to 5 Hz to 10 Hz to 20 Hz to 40 Hz to 80 Hz to 160 Hz, stimulating each point at 150 μA for 30 seconds, then moving on to the next frequency. Treat the ear canal of one ear, have the patient compare the differences between the two ears, and then treat the other ear canal. Patients suffering from deafness need to make a minimum commitment of 20 sessions of 30-minute treatments in order to show distinct improvement.)

9.11.2 Tinnitus

PAP: Inner Ear {C}, Inner Ear {E}, External Ear {C}, Auditory Nerve, Auditory Line, Kidney {C}

MAP: Master Sensorial Point, Point Zero, Shen Men, Sympathetic Point

SAP: Temples, Occiput, Forehead, Cervical Vertebrae {E}, Shoulder, Gall Bladder, Windstream {C}, Adrenal Glands {C}, Vagus Nerve

9.11.3 Dizziness or Vertigo

PAP: Dizziness {E}, Inner Ear {C}, Inner Ear {E}, Kidney {C}, Occiput, Cerebellum

MAP: Point Zero, Shen Men, Nervous Subcortex, Sympathetic Point

SAP: Forehead, Liver, Windstream {C}, Gall Bladder, San Jiao

9.11.4 Motion Sickness, Car Sickness, or Seasickness

PAP: Inner Ear {C}, Inner Ear {E}, Stomach, Occiput

MAP: Master Oscillation, Tranquilizer Point, Point Zero, Shen Men, Nervous Subcortex

SAP: Windstream {C}, Esophageal Sphincter

9.11.5 Mutism, Stuttering, or Difficulty Speaking

PAP: Mutism Point {C}, Inner Ear {C}, Inner Ear {E}, Tongue {C}, Tongue {E}, Kidney {C}, Heart {C}

MAP: Point Zero, Shen Men, Nervous Subcortex, Master Oscillation Point

9.11.6 Ear Infection, Ear Inflammation, or Earache

PAP: Inner Ear {C}, Inner Ear {E}, External Ear {C}, Occiput

MAP: Point Zero, Shen Men, Master Oscillation Point, Master Cerebral Point

SAP: Thymus Gland, Windstream {C}, Adrenal Glands {C}, Kidney {C}, San Jiao, Helix 5

9.11.7 Hearing Impairment

PAP: Inner Ear {C}, Inner Ear {E}, External Ear {C}, Auditory Line, Temples

MAP: Master Sensorial, Point Zero, Shen Men, Sympathetic Point

SAP: Kidney {C}, Occiput, San Jiao, Gall Bladder

9.11.8 Sudden Deafness

PAP: Inner Ear {C}, Inner Ear {E}, Brain {C}, Brainstem {C}, Occiput

MAP: Point Zero, Shen Men, Thalamus Point, Master Sensorial Point

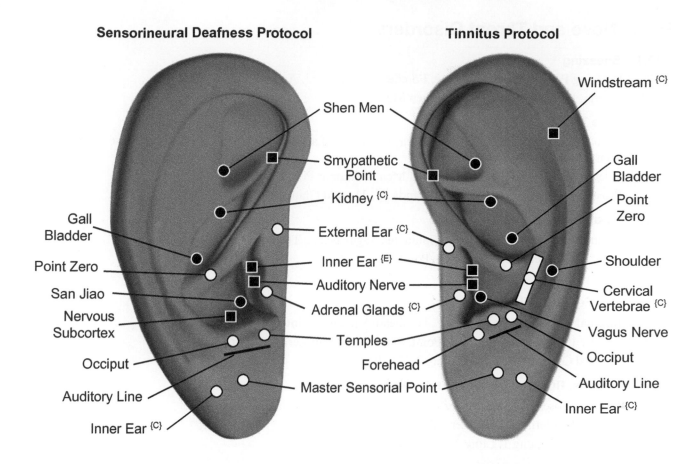

Sensorineural Deafness Protocol

- Shen Men
- Smypathetic Point
- Kidney {C}
- External Ear {C}
- Inner Ear {E}
- Auditory Nerve
- Adrenal Glands {C}
- Temples
- Forehead
- Master Sensorial Point
- Gall Bladder
- Point Zero
- San Jiao
- Nervous Subcortex
- Occiput
- Auditory Line
- Inner Ear {C}

Tinnitus Protocol

- Windstream {C}
- Gall Bladder
- Point Zero
- Shoulder
- Cervical Vertebrae {C}
- Vagus Nerve
- Occiput
- Auditory Line
- Inner Ear {C}

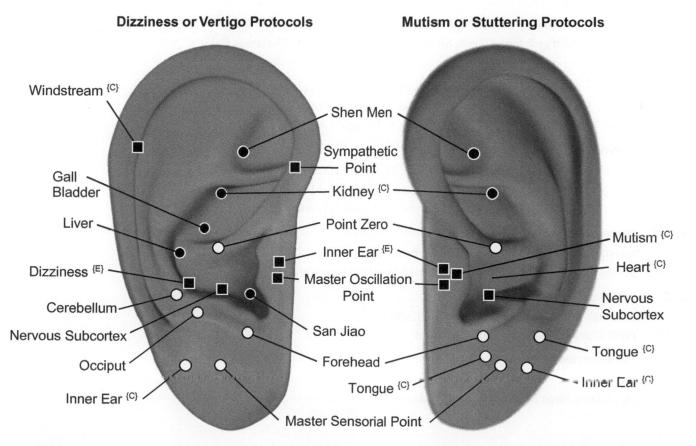

Dizziness or Vertigo Protocols

- Windstream {C}
- Gall Bladder
- Liver
- Dizziness {E}
- Cerebellum
- Nervous Subcortex
- Occiput
- Inner Ear {C}
- Shen Men
- Sympathetic Point
- Kidney {C}
- Point Zero
- Inner Ear {E}
- Master Oscillation Point
- San Jiao
- Forehead
- Master Sensorial Point

Mutism or Stuttering Protocols

- Shen Men
- Sympathetic Point
- Kidney {C}
- Point Zero
- Mutism {C}
- Heart {C}
- Nervous Subcortex
- Tongue {C}
- Inner Ear {C}
- Tongue {C}

FIGURE 9.11 Auditory disorders auricular treatment protocols.

9.12 Nose and Throat Disorders

9.12.1 Sneezing
PAP: Sneezing Point {E}, Internal Nose, Forehead, Asthma {C}, Antihistamine {C}
MAP: Allergy 1, Allergy 2, Point Zero, Shen Men

9.12.2 Sore Throat or Hoarse Throat
PAP: Throat {C}, Throat {E}, Mouth, Trachea, Larynx {C}, Larynx {E}, Lung 1, Lung 2, Adrenal Glands {C}, Tonsil 1, Tonsil 2, Tonsil 3, Tonsil 4
MAP: Allergy 1, Allergy 2, Point Zero, Shen Men, Thalamus Point, Endocrine Point
SAP: Prostaglandin Point {E}, Thyroid Glands {C}, Thyroid Glands {E}

9.12.3 Swallowing Difficulties
PAP: Mouth, Esophagus, Esophageal Sphincter, Vagus Nerve, Throat {C}, Throat {E}
MAP: Point Zero, Shen Men, Thalamus Point
SAP: Diaphragm {C}

9.12.4 Hay Fever or Allergic Rhinitis
PAP: Internal Nose, External Nose {C}, Forehead, Sneezing Point {E}, Windstream {C}
MAP: Allergy 1, Allergy 2, Endocrine Point, Shen Men, Point Zero, Sympathetic Point
SAP: Adrenal Glands {C}, Lung 1, Lung 2, Vitality Point {E}

9.12.5 Rhinitis, Running Nose, or Stuffy Nose
PAP: Internal Nose, Forehead, Sneezing Point {E}, Kidney {C}, Adrenal Glands {C}
MAP: Allergy 1, Allergy 2, Point Zero, Shen Men, Endocrine Point
SAP: External Ear, Lung 1, Lung 2, Windstream {C}

9.12.6 Pharyngitis
PAP: Throat {C}, Throat {E}, Trachea, Mouth, Lung 1, Lung 2, Adrenal Glands {C}
MAP: Allergy 1, Allergy 2, Point Zero, Shen Men, Endocrine Point, Thalamus Point

9.12.7 Tonsillitis
PAP: Throat {C}, Throat {E}, Larynx {C}, Larynx {E}, Mouth, Trachea
MAP: Allergy 1, Allergy 2, Point Zero, Shen Men, Thalamus Point, Endocrine Point
SAP: Tonsil 1, Tonsil 2, Tonsil 3, Tonsil 4, Helix 6, Thyroid Glands {C}, Thyroid Glands {E}

9.12.8 Laryngitis
PAP: Larynx {C}, Larynx {E}, Palate 1, Palate 2, Thymus Gland
MAP: Allergy 1, Allergy 2, Endocrine Point, Point Zero, Shen Men
SAP: Heart {C}, Lung 1, Lung 2, Tonsil 1, Tonsil 2, Tonsil 3, Tonsil 4

9.12.9 Nose Bleed
PAP: Internal Nose, External Nose {C}, Forehead, Lung 1, Lung 2, Adrenal Glands {C}
MAP: Sympathetic Point, Shen Men, Endocrine Point, Master Cerebral Point, Vascular Subcortex

9.12.10 Broken Nose
PAP: External Nose {C}, External Nose {E}, Kidney {C}
MAP: Point Zero, Shen Men, Thalamus Point

9.12.11 Sunburned Nose
PAP: External Nose {C}, External Nose {E}, Face, Dermatitis {C}, Lung 1, Lung 2
MAP: Point Zero, Shen Men, Thalamus Point

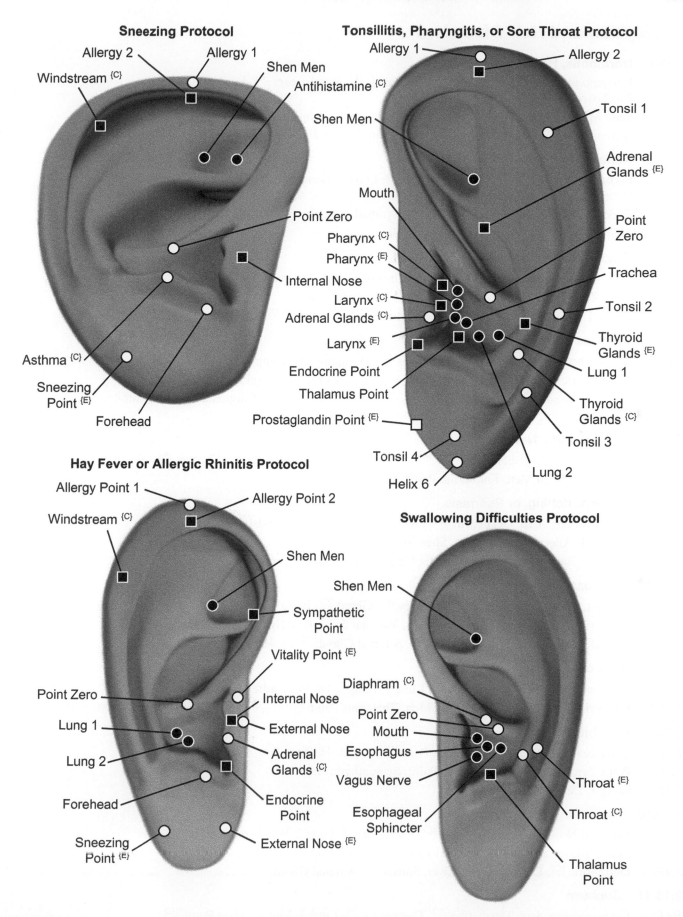

Sneezing Protocol

Allergy 2 — Allergy 1
Windstream {C}
Shen Men
Antihistamine {C}
Point Zero
Internal Nose
Asthma {C}
Sneezing Point {E}
Forehead

Tonsillitis, Pharyngitis, or Sore Throat Protocol

Allergy 1 — Allergy 2
Shen Men
Tonsil 1
Adrenal Glands {E}
Mouth
Point Zero
Pharynx {C}
Pharynx {E}
Trachea
Larynx {C}
Tonsil 2
Adrenal Glands {C}
Thyroid Glands {E}
Larynx {E}
Lung 1
Endocrine Point
Thalamus Point
Thyroid Glands {C}
Prostaglandin Point {E}
Tonsil 3
Tonsil 4
Lung 2
Helix 6

Hay Fever or Allergic Rhinitis Protocol

Allergy Point 1 — Allergy Point 2
Windstream {C}
Shen Men
Sympathetic Point
Vitality Point {E}
Point Zero
Internal Nose
Lung 1
External Nose
Lung 2
Adrenal Glands {C}
Forehead
Endocrine Point
Sneezing Point {E}
External Nose {E}

Swallowing Difficulties Protocol

Shen Men
Diaphram {C}
Point Zero
Mouth
Esophagus
Vagus Nerve
Esophageal Sphincter
Throat {E}
Throat {C}
Thalamus Point

[FIGURE 9.12 Nose and throat disorders auricular treatment protocols.

9.13 Skin and Hair Disorders

9.13.1 Dermatitis, Hives, or Urticaria
PAP: *Corresponding Area*, Dermatitis {C}, Dermatitis {E}, Windstream {C}, Lung 1, Lung 2, Psychosomatic Point {E}, Vitamin E

MAP: Shen Men, Point Zero, Endocrine Point, Sympathetic Point

SAP: Adrenal Glands {C}, Spleen {C}, Occiput, Brain {C}, San Jiao, Thyroid Glands {C}, Thyroid Glands {E}

9.13.2 Acne
PAP: Face, Dermatitis {C}, Dermatitis {E}, Lung 1, Lung 2, Genitals {C}, Genitals {E}, Gonadotrophins {E}, Ovaries {E}/Testes {E}

MAP: Endocrine Point, Point Zero, Shen Men, Sympathetic Point

SAP: Adrenal Glands {C}, Large Intestines, Liver

9.13.3 Cold Sores or Herpes Simplex
PAP: Lips, Mouth, Lung 1, Lung 2, Occiput, Thymus Gland, Adrenal Glands {C}

MAP: Point Zero, Shen Men, Thalamus Point, Sympathetic Point

SAP: Palate 1, Palate 2, Dermatitis {C}, Dermatitis {E}, Windstream {C}, San Jiao

9.13.4 Shingles or Herpes Zoster
PAP: Chest, Thoracic Vertebrae {E}, Dermatitis {C}, Dermatitis {E}, Lung 1, Lung 2

MAP: Sympathetic Point, Endocrine Point, Point Zero, Shen Men, Thalamus Point

SAP: Adrenal Glands {C}, Pituitary Gland {C}, Occiput, Thymus Gland, Cingulate Gyrus, Brain {C}, Windstream {C}, Gall Bladder, Psychosomatic Point {E}

9.13.5 Post-Herpetic Neuralgia
PAP: Chest, Thoracic Vertebrae {C, F1, F2, F3, F4}, Dermatitis {C}, Dermatitis {E}, Thymus Gland

MAP: Point Zero, Shen Men, Endocrine Point, Thalamus Point

9.13.6 Eczema, Itching, or Psoriasis
PAP: *Corresponding Area*, Dermatitis {C}, Dermatitis {E}, Occiput, Windstream {C}

MAP: Allergy 1, Allergy 2, Point Zero, Shen Men, Endocrine Point

SAP: Adrenal Glands {C}, Lung 2, Gall Bladder, Psychosomatic Point {E}

9.13.7 Hair Loss, Baldness, or Alopecia
PAP: Occiput, Vertex, Lung 1, Lung 2, Kidney {C}, Gland {C}, Brain {C}, Vitamin E

MAP: Endocrine Point, Point Zero, Shen Men, Vascular Subcortex, Sympathetic Point

SAP: Gonadotrophins {E}, Ovaries/Testes {E}, Adrenal Glands {C}, Spleen {C}, Gall Bladder

9.13.8 Boils or Carbuncles
PAP: *Corresponding Area*, Dermatitis {C}, Lung 1, Lung 2, Occiput, Adrenal Glands {C}

MAP: Endocrine Point, Point Zero, Shen Men, Thalamus Point

9.13.9 Frostbite
PAP: *Corresponding Area*, Occiput, Heat Point {C}, Adrenal Glands {C}

MAP: Point Zero, Shen Men, Thalamus Point, Sympathetic Point

SAP: Lung 1, Lung 2, Spleen {C}

9.13.10 Rosacea
PAP: External Nose {C}, External Nose {E}, Face, Lung 1, Lung 2, Windstream {C}

MAP: Endocrine Point, Shen Men, Point Zero, Thalamus Point

SAP: Dermatitis {C}, Dermatitis {E}, Liver, Spleen {C}, Adrenal Glands {C}

9.13.11 Sunburn
PAP: *Corresponding Area*, Dermatitis {C}, Dermatitis {E}, Lung 1, Lung 2, Heat Point {C}

MAP: Point Zero, Shen Men, Endocrine Point, Thalamus Point

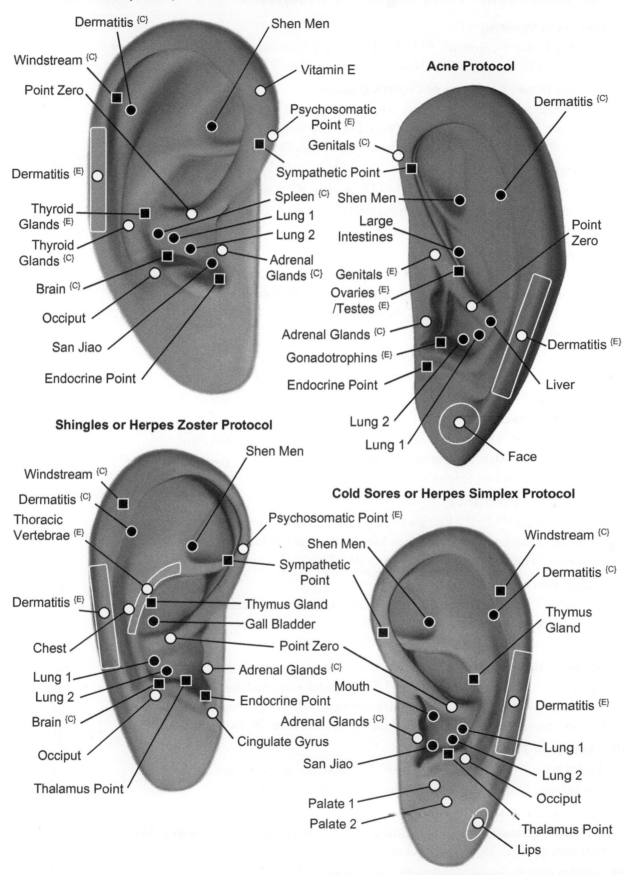

Dermatitis, Hives, or Urticaria Protocol

Dermatitis {C}
Shen Men
Windstream {C}
Point Zero
Vitamin E
Psychosomatic Point {E}
Genitals {C}
Sympathetic Point
Dermatitis {E}
Spleen {C}
Lung 1
Lung 2
Thyroid Glands {E}
Thyroid Glands {C}
Adrenal Glands {C}
Brain {C}
Occiput
San Jiao
Endocrine Point

Acne Protocol

Dermatitis {C}
Point Zero
Shen Men
Large Intestines
Genitals {E}
Ovaries /Testes {E}
Adrenal Glands {C}
Gonadotrophins {E}
Endocrine Point
Dermatitis {E}
Liver
Lung 2
Lung 1
Face

Shingles or Herpes Zoster Protocol

Windstream {C}
Shen Men
Dermatitis {C}
Psychosomatic Point {E}
Thoracic Vertebrae {E}
Sympathetic Point
Thymus Gland
Gall Bladder
Dermatitis {E}
Point Zero
Chest
Adrenal Glands {C}
Lung 1
Endocrine Point
Lung 2
Brain {C}
Cingulate Gyrus
Occiput
Thalamus Point

Cold Sores or Herpes Simplex Protocol

Shen Men
Windstream {C}
Dermatitis {C}
Thymus Gland
Mouth
Dermatitis {E}
Adrenal Glands {C}
Lung 1
San Jiao
Lung 2
Occiput
Palate 1
Thalamus Point
Palate 2
Lips

FIGURE 9.13 Skin and hair disorders auricular treatment protocols.

9.14 Gastrointestinal and Digestive Disorders

9.14.1   Nausea or Vomiting
PAP: Vomiting Reflex [E], Stomach [F1, F2, F3], Esophageal Sphincter, Omega 1, Occiput, Liver
MAP: Sympathetic Point, Digestive Subcortex, Shen Men, Point Zero

9.14.2   Irritable Bowel Syndrome or Crohn's Disease
PAP: Large Intestines [F1, F2, F3], Stomach, Abdomen, Omega 1, Constipation [C]
MAP: Point Zero, Shen Men, Sympathetic Point, Digestive Subcortex, Endocrine Point
SAP: Rectum [C], Rectum [E], Pancreas, Spleen [C], San Jiao, Psychosomatic Point [E]

9.14.3   Constipation
PAP: Constipation [C], Large Intestines [F1, F2, F3], Rectum [C], Rectum [E], Omega 1
MAP: Digestive Subcortex, Shen Men, Sympathetic Point
SAP: Abdomen, San Jiao, Stomach, Spleen [C]

9.14.4   Diarrhea
PAP: Large Intestines [F1, F2, F3], Rectum [C], Rectum [E], Omega 1, Abdomen, San Jiao
MAP: Point Zero, Shen Men, Digestive Subcortex, Sympathetic Point
SAP: Rectum [C], Rectum [E], Spleen [C], Adrenal Glands [C]

9.14.5   Hemorrhoids
PAP: Hemorrhoids 1, Hemorrhoids 2, Rectum [C], Rectum [E], Large Intestines
MAP: Digestive Subcortex, Point Zero, Shen Men, Master Cerebral Point
SAP: Adrenal Glands [C]

9.14.6   Gastritis or Gastric Spasm
PAP: Stomach [F1, F2, F3], Esophageal Sphincter, Duodenum, Abdomen, San Jiao
MAP: Point Zero, Shen Men, Sympathetic Point, Digestive Subcortex
SAP: Large Intestines, Liver, Spleen [C], Gall Bladder, Windstream [C]

9.14.7   Colitis or Gastroenteritis
PAP: Large Intestines [F1, F2, F3], Rectum [C], Rectum [E], Hypogastric Plexus
MAP: Digestive Subcortex, Point Zero, Shen Men, Sympathetic Point, Endocrine Point
SAP: Abdomen, Small Intestines [F1, F2, F3], San Jiao, Spleen [C], Liver, Occiput

9.14.8   Indigestion or Bloated Stomach
PAP: Stomach [F1, F2, F3], Esophageal Sphincter, Duodenum, Small Intestines, Abdomen
MAP: Sympathetic Point, Digestive Subcortex, Shen Men, Point Zero
SAP: Omega 1, Pancreas, Spleen [C], San Jiao, Liver, Occiput

9.14.9   Stomach Ulcer or Duodenal Ulcer
PAP: Stomach [F1, F2, F3], Small Intestines [F1, F2, F3], Duodenum, Abdomen
MAP: Shen Men, Sympathetic Point, Digestive Subcortex, Master Cerebral Point
SAP: Psychosomatic Point [E], Irritability Point [E], Vitality Point [E], Occiput, Spleen [C]

9.14.10   Ascites or Flatulence
PAP: Ascites Point [C], Large Intestines [F1, F2, F3], Small Intestines, Abdomen, San Jiao
MAP: Sympathetic Point, Digestive Subcortex, Endocrine Point, Shen Men

9.14.11   Fecal Incontinence
PAP: Rectum [C], Rectum [E], Large Intestines [F1, F2, F3], Stomach, Omega 1, Spleen [C]
MAP: Sympathetic Point, Digestive Subcortex, Shen Men

9.14.12   GERD (Gastroesophageal Reflux Disease)
PAP: Esophageal Sphincter, Esophagus, Stomach, Hypogastric Plexus
MAP: Digestive Subcortex, Shen Men, Sympathetic Point, Tranquilizer Point

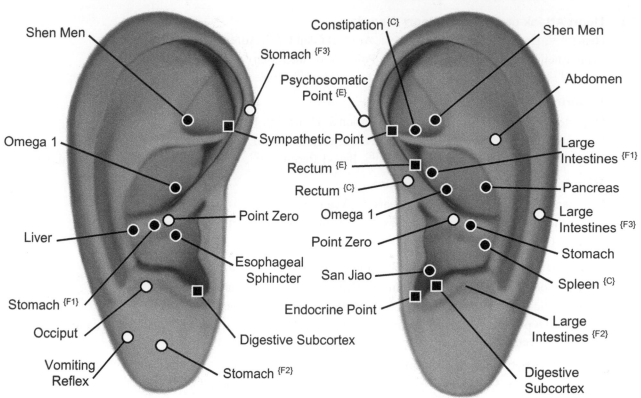

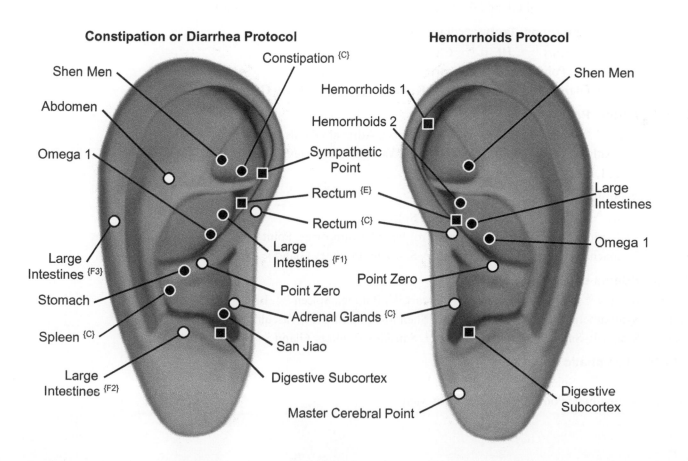

FIGURE 9.14 Gastrointestinal disorders auricular treatment protocols.

9.15 Heart and Circulatory Disorders

9.15.1 Heart Attack or Coronary Heart Disorder

PAP: Heart {C1}, Heart {C2}, Heart {F1}, Chest, Adrenal Glands {C}, Adrenal Glands {E}

MAP: Sympathetic Point, Vascular Subcortex, Point Zero, Shen Men

SAP: Heart {F2}, Heart {F3}, Small Intestines, Liver, Kidney {C}, Spleen {C}

9.15.2 Hypertension or High Blood Pressure

PAP: Hypertension 1, Hypertension 2, Hypertension 3, Heart {C1}, Heart {C2}, Heart {F1}

MAP: Sympathetic Point, Vascular Subcortex, Point Zero, Shen Men

SAP: Heart {F2}, Heart {F3}, Wonderful Point {E}, Beta-1 Receptor {E}, Vagus Nerve, Occiput, Forehead, Kidney {C}

9.15.3 Hypotension or Low Blood Pressure

PAP: Hypotension Point {C}, Heart {C1}, Heart {E}, Vagus Nerve

MAP: Sympathetic Point, Vascular Subcortex, Shen Men, Endocrine Point

SAP: Adrenal Glands {C}, Occiput, Brain {C}, Liver, Spleen {C}

9.15.4 Raynaud's Disease or Impaired Circulation to Hands or Feet

PAP: Fingers, Foot {C}, Foot {E}, Heat Point {C}, Heart {E}, Sensory Spinal Cord

MAP: Sympathetic Point, Point Zero, Shen Men, Vascular Subcortex, Endocrine Point

SAP: Posterior Hypothalamus, Sympathetic Postganglionic Nerves, Windstream {C}, Adrenal Glands {C}, Occiput, Spleen {C}, Liver

9.15.5 Cardiac Arrhythmias or Premature Ventricular Contractions

PAP: Heart {C1}, Heart {C2}, Heart {E}, Chest, Vagus Nerve, Adrenal Glands {C}

MAP: Sympathetic Point, Vascular Subcortex, Point Zero, Shen Men

SAP: Kidney {C}, Adrenal Glands {E}, Occiput, Liver, Stomach, Pituitary Gland {C}

9.15.6 Heart Palpitations, Tachycardia, or Bradycardia

PAP: Heart {C1}, Heart {C2}, Heart {E}, Chest, Occiput

MAP: Sympathetic Point, Vascular Subcortex, Point Zero, Shen Men

SAP: Adrenal Glands {C}, Small Intestines, Kidney {C}, Liver, Pituitary Gland {C}

9.15.7 Angina Pain

PAP: Heart {C1}, Heart {C2}, Heart {E}, Vagus Nerve, Adrenal Glands {C}

MAP: Sympathetic Point, Point Zero, Shen Men, Vascular Subcortex

SAP: Lung 1, Lung 2, Stomach

9.15.8 Anemia

PAP: Heart {C1}, Heart {C2}, Heart {E}, Liver, Spleen {C}

MAP: Endocrine Point, Shen Men, Point Zero, Vascular Subcortex, Point Zero

SAP: Stomach, Small Intestines, Kidney {C}, San Jiao, Pituitary Gland {C}

9.15.9 Edema or Swelling

PAP: Kidney {C}, Kidney {E}, Heart {C1}, Heart {E}, Bladder, Spleen {C}, Liver

MAP: Sympathetic Point, Endocrine Point, Shen Men, Point Zero, Vascular Subcortex

SAP: Stomach, Small Intestines, Kidney {C}, San Jiao, Pituitary Gland {C}, Prostaglandin Point {E}

9.15.10 Lymphatic Disorders

PAP: Spleen {C}, Spleen {E}, Thymus Gland, Vitality Point {E}

MAP: Sympathetic Point, Point Zero, Shen Men

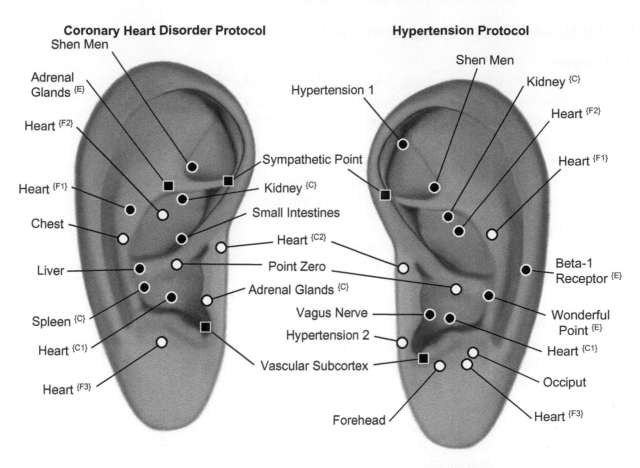

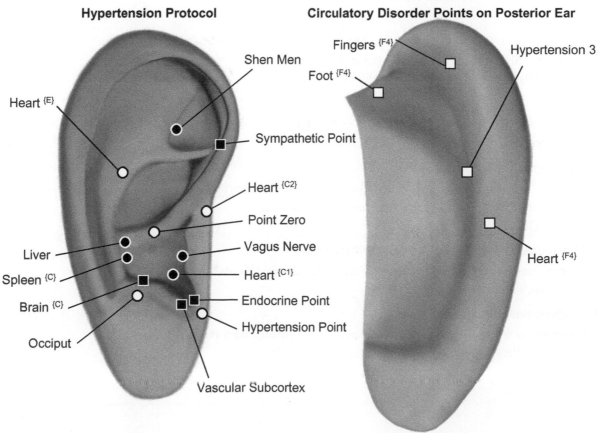

FIGURE 9.15 Cardiovascular disorders auricular treatment protocols.

9.16 Lung and Respiratory Disorders

9.16.1 Coughing
PAP: Cough Reflex [E], Asthma [C], Antihistamine [C], Pharynx [C], Pharynx [E], Bronchi

MAP: Sympathetic Point, Shen Men, Point Zero, Allergy 1, Allergy 2

SAP: Lung 1, Lung 2, Adrenal Glands [C], Brain [C], Occiput, Spleen [C]

9.16.2 Hiccups
PAP: Diaphragm [C], Esophageal Sphincter, Vagus Nerve

MAP: Point Zero, Shen Men, Thalamus Point, Sympathetic Point

SAP: Solar Plexus, Vagus Nerve, Stomach, Liver, Occiput, San Jiao

9.16.3 Asthma
PAP: Asthma [C], Antihistamine [C], Lung 1, Lung 2, Bronchi, Chest, Windstream [C]

MAP: Allergy 1, Allergy 2, Sympathetic Point, Point Zero, Shen Men, Tranquilizer Point, Thalamus Point, Master Cerebral Point

SAP: Psychosomatic Point [E], Occiput, Kidney [C], Spleen [C], Adrenal Glands [C]

9.16.4 Emphysema
PAP: Lung 1, Lung 2, Bronchi, Chest, Asthma [C], Antihistamine [C], Windstream [C]

MAP: Point Zero, Shen Men, Sympathetic Point, Thalamus Point

SAP: Adrenal Glands [C], Occiput, Kidney [C]

9.16.5 Bronchitis
PAP: Bronchi, Asthma [C], Antihistamine [C], Trachea, Lung 1, Lung 2, Windstream [C]

MAP: Allergy 1, Allergy 2, Shen Men, Point Zero, Sympathetic Point, Endocrine Point

SAP: Adrenal Glands [C], Adrenal Glands [E], Occiput, Spleen [C], Vitality Point [E]

9.16.6 Pneumonia
PAP: Lung 1, Lung 2, Bronchi, Asthma [C], Antihistamine [C]

MAP: Point Zero, Shen Men, Sympathetic Point, Endocrine Point

SAP: Adrenal Glands [C], Adrenal Glands [E], Occiput

9.16.7 Pleurisy
PAP: Lung 1, Lung 2, Chest, Adrenal Glands [C], San Jiao

MAP: Point Zero, Shen Men, Endocrine Point

9.16.8 Chest Pain or Chest Heaviness
PAP: Asthma [C], Lung 1, Lung 2, Chest, Heart [C1], Heart [C2], Heart [E]

MAP: Sympathetic Point, Point Zero, Shen Men, Thalamus Point

SAP: Adrenal Glands [C], Adrenal Glands [E]

9.16.9 Shortness of Breath or Breathing Difficulties
PAP: Internal Nose, Lung 1, Lung 2, Chest, Forehead, Adrenal Glands [C]

MAP: Shen Men, Point Zero, Thalamus Point

9.16.10 Tuberculosis
PAP: Tuberculosis [C], Lung 1, Lung 2, Windstream [C], Prostaglandin Point [E]

MAP: Allergy 1, Allergy 2, Point Zero, Shen Men, Thalamus Point

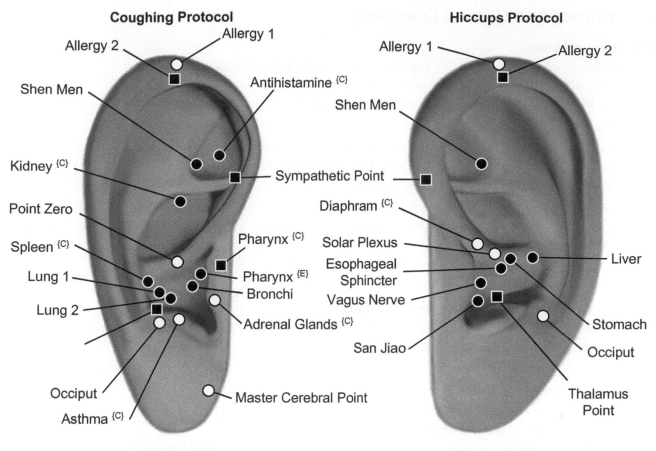

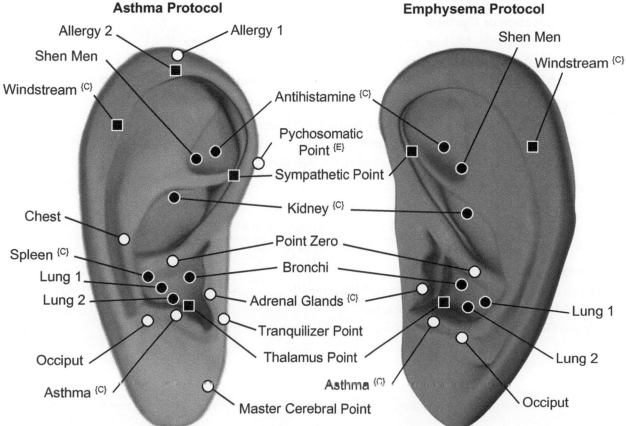

FIGURE 9.16 Respiratory disorders auricular treatment protocols

9.17 Kidney and Urinary Disorders

9.17.1 Kidney Stones

PAP: Kidney {C, F1, F2, F3}, Urethra {C}, Urethra {E}, Bladder, Posterior Pituitary {E}, Abdomen

MAP: Sympathetic Point, Vascular Subcortex, Point Zero, Shen Men

SAP: Nephritis Point {C}, Excitement Point, Occiput, Omega 1

9.17.2 Diabetes Insipidus

PAP: Kidney {C}, Kidney {E}, Bladder, Mouth, Thirst Point {C}, Posterior Pituitary {E}

MAP: Point Zero, Shen Men, Sympathetic Point, Endocrine Point, Vascular Subcortex

SAP: Brain {C}, Adrenal Glands {C}, Spleen {C}, Liver

9.17.3 Frequent Urination or Enuresis Problems

PAP: Bladder {C, F1, F2, F3}, Kidney {C, F1, F2, F3}, Urethra {C}, Urethra {E}, Posterior Pituitary {E}, Nephritis Point {C}, Excitement Point {C}

MAP: Sympathetic Point, Endocrine Point, Vascular Subcortex, Point Zero

SAP: Hypogastric Plexus, Occiput, Adrenal Glands {C}

9.17.4 Urinary Incontinence or Urinary Retention

PAP: Urethra {C}, Urethra {E}, Bladder, Kidney {C}, Kidney {E}, San Jiao, Brain {C}

MAP: Sympathetic Point, Shen Men, Vascular Subcortex, Endocrine Point, Point Zero

SAP: Hypogastric Plexus, Gonadotrophins {E}, Genitals {C}, Genitals {E}, Lumbago

9.17.5 Antidiuresis or Water Imbalance

PAP: Bladder, Kidney {C}, Kidney {E}, San Jiao, Posterior Pituitary {E}, Occiput

MAP: Point Zero, Shen Men, Sympathetic Point, Endocrine Point

SAP: Anterior Hypothalamus, Heart {C}, Spleen {C}, Adrenal Glands {C}, Adrenal Glands {E}

9.17.6 Urinary Infection or Cystitis

PAP: Kidney {C}, Kidney {E}, Bladder, Urethra {C}, Urethra {E}, Ureter {C}, Ureter {E}

MAP: Sympathetic Point, Shen Men, Endocrine Point, Point Zero

SAP: Hypogastric Plexus, Thymus Gland, Gonadotrophins {E}, Genitals {C}, Genitals {E}, Adrenal Glands {C}

9.17.7 Bladder Control Problems

PAP: Bladder, Kidney {C}, Kidney {E}, Posterior Pituitary {E}, Urethra {C}, Urethra {E}

MAP: Vascular Subcortex, Shen Men, Point Zero

SAP: Gonadotrophins {E}, Ovaries/Testes {E}, Spleen {C}, San Jiao, Liver

9.17.8 Nephritis

PAP: Nephritis Point {C}, Kidney {C}, Kidney {E}, Bladder, Occiput

MAP: Endocrine Point, Sympathetic Point, Vascular Subcortex, Shen Men, Point Zero

SAP: Adrenal Glands {C}, Adrenal Glands {E}, Spleen {C}, Liver, San Jiao, Brain {C}

9.17.9 Kidney Pyelitis

PAP: Kidney {C}, Kidney {E}, Bladder, Urethra {C}, Urethra {E}

MAP: Point Zero, Shen Men, Vascular Subcortex

SAP: Adrenal Glands {C}, Adrenal Glands {E}, Spleen {C}, Liver

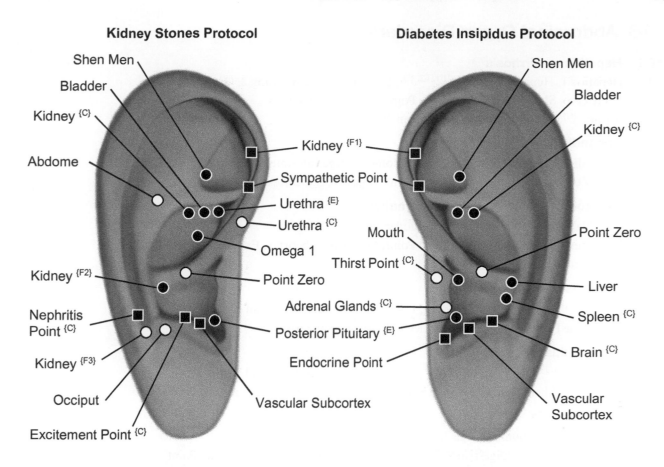

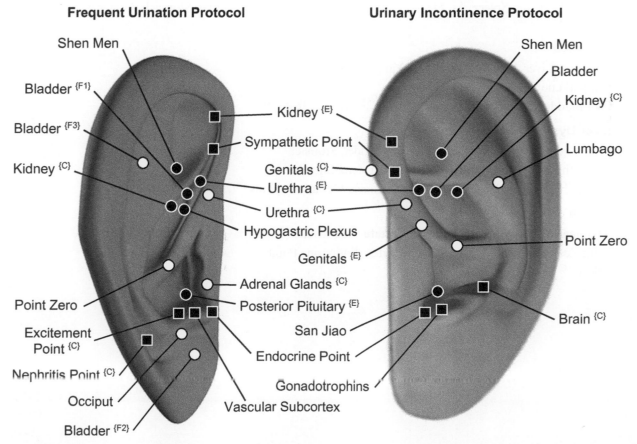

FIGURE 9.17 Urinary disorders auricular treatment protocols.

9.18 Abdominal Organ Disorders

9.18.1 Hepatitis or Cirrhosis
PAP: Hepatitis 1, Hepatitis 2, Liver [F1, F2, F3], Liver Yang 1, Liver Yang 2, Omega 1
MAP: Point Zero, Shen Men, Sympathetic Point, Digestive Subcortex
SAP: Kidney [C], Gall Bladder, Stomach, San Jiao

9.18.2 Appendicitis
PAP: Appendix, Appendix Disorder[1, 2, 3], Abdomen, Large Intestines, San Jiao
MAP: Point Zero, Shen Men, Sympathetic Point, Digestive Subcortex, Endocrine Point

9.18.3 Gallstones or Gall Bladder Inflammation
PAP: Gall Bladder [F1, F2, F3], Stomach, Duodenum
MAP: Point Zero, Shen Men, Sympathetic Point, Digestive Subcortex, Endocrine Point
SAP: Liver, Lung 1, Lung 2, San Jiao

9.18.4 Diabetes Mellitus
PAP: Pancreas [F1, F2, F3], Pancreatitis [C], Liver, Pituitary Gland [C], San Jiao
MAP: Endocrine Point, Point Zero, Shen Men, Digestive Subcortex

9.18.5 Pancreatitis
PAP: Pancreas [F1, F2, F3], Pancreatitis [C], Liver, Omega 1, San Jiao, Gall Bladder
MAP: Point Zero, Shen Men, Endocrine Point, Digestive Subcortex, Sympathetic Point

9.18.6 Hypoglycemia
PAP: Pancreas, Duodenum, Omega 1, Stomach
MAP: Sympathetic Point, Digestive Subcortex, Point Zero, Shen Men, Endocrine Point
SAP: Kidney [C], Liver, Spleen [C], Heart [C], Pituitary Gland [C], Gall Bladder, Stomach, Gonadotrophins [E], Ovaries/Testes [E]

9.18.7 Jaundice
PAP: Hepatitis, Liver, Liver Yang 1, Liver Yang 2, Spleen [C]
MAP: Sympathetic Point, Shen Men
SAP: Gall Bladder, Stomach, Gonadotrophins [E], Ovaries/Testes [E]

9.18.8 Liver Dysfunction
PAP: Liver, Liver Yang 1, Liver Yang 2, Gall Bladder, Stomach
MAP: Sympathetic Point, Endocrine Point, Point Zero, Shen Men
SAP: Spleen [C], Kidney [C], Gall Bladder, Stomach, Gonadotrophins [E], Ovaries/Testes [E]

9.18.9 Hernia
PAP: Abdomen, Large Intestines, Pelvis, Prostate [C], Prostate [E]
MAP: Point Zero, Shen Men, Digestive Subcortex, Endocrine Point
SAP: Spleen [C], Pituitary Gland [C]

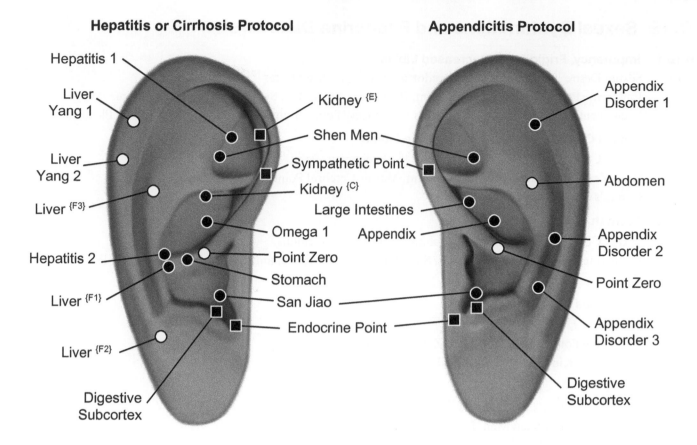

Hepatitis or Cirrhosis Protocol

- Hepatitis 1
- Liver Yang 1
- Liver Yang 2
- Liver {F3}
- Hepatitis 2
- Liver {F1}
- Liver {F2}
- Digestive Subcortex
- Kidney {E}
- Shen Men
- Sympathetic Point
- Kidney {C}
- Omega 1
- Point Zero
- Stomach
- San Jiao
- Endocrine Point

Appendicitis Protocol

- Appendix Disorder 1
- Abdomen
- Large Intestines
- Appendix
- Appendix Disorder 2
- Point Zero
- Appendix Disorder 3
- Digestive Subcortex

Gallstones Protocol

- Gall Bladder {F3}
- Stomach
- Liver
- Lung 1
- Lung 2
- Digestive Subcortex
- Shen Men
- Sympathetic Point
- Gall Bladder {F1}
- Duodenum
- Point Zero
- San Jiao
- Endocrine Point
- Gall Bladder {F2}

Diabetes Mellitus Protocol

- Shen Men
- Pancreas {F3}
- Sympathetic Point
- Omega 1
- Pancreas {F1}
- Pancreatitis
- Liver
- Point Zero
- Pituitary Gland {C}
- Digestive Subcortex
- Pancreas {F2}

FIGURE 9.18 Abdominal organ disorders auricular treatment protocols.

9.19 Sexual Dysfunctions and Endocrine Disorders

9.19.1 Impotency, Frigidity, or Decreased Libido
PAP: Sexual Desire [E], Genitals [C], Gonadotrophins [E], Ovaries/Testes [E]
MAP: Endocrine Point, Master Cerebral Point, Point Zero, Shen Men, Sympathetic Point, Thalamus Point
SAP: Excitement Point [E], Uterus [C], Uterus [E], Anxiety Point, Brain [C], Forehead, Hypogastric Plexus, Kidney [C]

9.19.2 Sexual Compulsiveness or Excessive Libido
PAP: Sexual Compulsion [E], Irritability Point [E], Excitement Point [C], Ovaries/Testes [E]
MAP: Point Zero, Shen Men, Tranquilizer Point, Master Cerebral Point, Thalamus Point
SAP: Genitals [C], Gonadotrophins [E]

9.19.3 Premature Ejaculation
PAP: Sexual Compulsion [E], Gonadotrophins [E], Testes [E], Genitals [C], Genitals [E]
MAP: Endocrine Point, Tranquilizer Point, Shen Men, Point Zero, Thalamus Point, Master Cerebral Point
SAP: Kidney [C]

9.19.4 Prostatitis
PAP: Prostate [C, F1, F2, F3], Urethra [C, F1, F2, F3], Bladder, Pelvis
MAP: Endocrine Point, Shen Men, Point Zero, Thalamus Point
SAP: Kidney [C], Kidney [E], Pituitary Gland [C], Adrenal Glands [C]

9.19.5 Testitis
PAP: Testes [E], Genitals [C], Genitals [E], Gonadotrophins [E], Adrenal Glands [C]
MAP: Endocrine Point, Shen Men, Point Zero
SAP: Prostate [C], Prostate [E], Hip [C], Hip [E], Occiput

9.19.6 Scrotal Rash
PAP: Genitals [C], Genitals [E], Urethra [C], Urethra [E], Dermatitis [C], Dermatitis [E]
MAP: Sympathetic Point, Master Sensorial, Shen Men, Thalamus Point, Point Zero

9.19.7 Hypergonadism or Hypogonadism
PAP: Genitals [C], Genitals [E], Gonadotrophins [E], Ovaries/Testes [E], Brain [C], San Jiao, Pituitary Gland [C]
MAP: Point Zero, Shen Men, Endocrine Point, Thalamus Point
SAP: San Jiao, Liver, Kidney [C]

9.19.8 Hyperthyroidism or Hypothyroidism
PAP: Thyroid Glands [C, F1, F2, F3], Brain [C], Liver, Pituitary Gland [C]
MAP: Endocrine Point, Point Zero, Shen Men, Thalamus Point, Sympathetic Point
SAP: Excitement Point [C], San Jiao

9.19.9 Goiter
PAP: Thyroid Glands [C], Thyroid Glands [E], Brain [C], San Jiao, Liver, Kidney [C]
MAP: Endocrine Point, Point Zero, Shen Men, Thalamus Point

9.19.10 Calcium Metabolism
PAP: Parathyroid Glands, Parathormone, Kidney [C]
MAP: Endocrine Point, Shen Men, Point Zero

9.19.11 Dwarfism
PAP: Anterior Pituitary, Kidney [C], Kidney [E]
MAP: Endocrine Point, Point Zero, Shen Men

Impotency or Frigidity Protocols

Sexually Compulsive Protocol

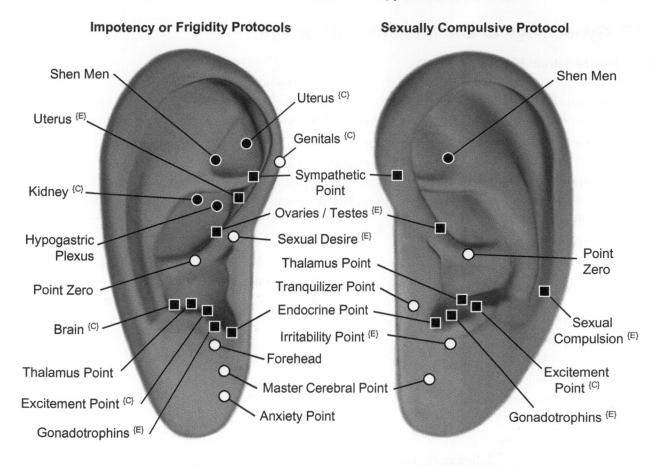

Prostatitis Protocol

Hyperthyroidism Protocol

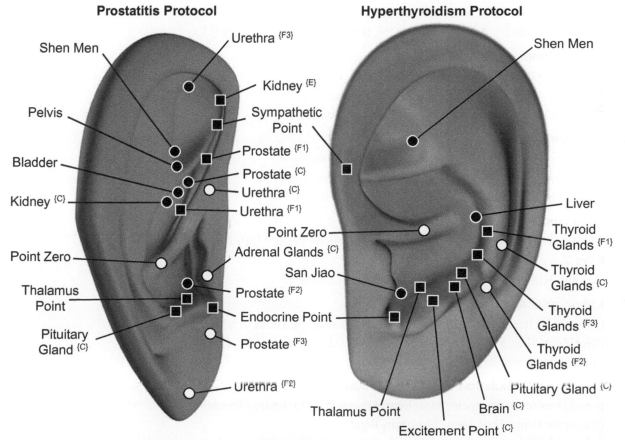

FIGURE 9.19 Sexual and endocrine disorders auricular treatment protocols.

9.20 Gynecological and Menstrual Disorders

9.20.1 Perimenstrual Syndrome (PMS)
PAP: Uterus $^{\{C\}}$, Uterus $^{\{E\}}$, Gonadotrophins $^{\{E\}}$, Ovaries $^{\{E\}}$, Abdomen

MAP: Endocrine Point, Shen Men, Point Zero, Sympathetic Point, Thalamus Point, Master Cerebral Point

SAP: Pituitary Gland $^{\{C\}}$, Brain $^{\{C\}}$, Kidney $^{\{C\}}$, Liver, Adrenal Glands $^{\{C\},}$ Irritability Point $^{\{E\}}$, Frustration Point $^{\{E\}}$

9.20.2 Dysmenorrhea or Irregular Menstruation
PAP: Uterus $^{\{C\}}$, Uterus $^{\{E\}}$, Gonadotrophins $^{\{E\}}$, Ovaries $^{\{E\}}$, Genitals $^{\{C\}}$, Genitals $^{\{E\}}$

MAP: Endocrine Point, Point Zero, Shen Men, Sympathetic Point, Thalamus Point

SAP: Brain $^{\{C\}}$, Kidney $^{\{C\}}$, Abdomen, Pelvis, Vagus Nerve, Prostaglandin Point $^{\{E\}}$, Irritability Point $^{\{E\}}$, Frustration Point $^{\{E\}}$, Pituitary Gland $^{\{C\}}$

9.20.3 Menopause
PAP: Gonadotrophins $^{\{E\}}$, Ovaries $^{\{E\}}$, Uterus $^{\{C\}}$, Uterus $^{\{E\}}$

MAP: Endocrine Point, Shen Men, Point Zero, Sympathetic Point, Master Cerebral Point

SAP: Pituitary Gland $^{\{C\}}$, Kidney $^{\{C\}}$, Liver, Vagus Nerve, Muscle Relaxation $^{\{C\}}$, Irritability Point $^{\{E\}}$, Frustration Point $^{\{E\}}$

9.20.4 Infertility
PAP: Uterus $^{\{C\}}$, Uterus $^{\{E\}}$, Gonadotrophins $^{\{E\}}$, Ovaries $^{\{E\}}$, Genitals $^{\{C\}}$, Genitals $^{\{E\}}$

MAP: Endocrine Point, Point Zero, Shen Men, Thalamus Point, Master Cerebral Point

SAP: Kidney $^{\{C\}}$, Adrenal Glands $^{\{C\}}$, Abdomen, Brain $^{\{C\}}$, Pituitary Gland $^{\{C\}}$, San Jiao, Irritability Point $^{\{E\}}$, Frustration Point $^{\{E\}}$

9.20.5 Breast Tenderness
PAP: Mammary Glands $^{\{C\}}$, Mammary Glands $^{\{E\}}$, Breast

MAP: Endocrine Point, Shen Men, Thalamus Point, Point Zero

SAP: Adrenal Glands $^{\{C\}}$, Adrenal Glands $^{\{E\}}$, Brain $^{\{C\}}$, Occiput, Kidney $^{\{C\}}$

9.20.6 Breast Tumor or Ovarian Cancer
PAP: Mammary Glands $^{\{C\}}$, Mammary Glands $^{\{E\}}$, Breast, Ovaries $^{\{C\}}$, Ovaries $^{\{E\}}$

MAP: Shen Men, Point Zero, Endocrine Point, Thalamus Point

SAP: Thymus Gland, Vitality Point $^{\{C\}}$, Kidney $^{\{C\}}$, Liver, San Jiao

9.20.7 Endometriosis
PAP: Uterus $^{\{C\}}$, Uterus $^{\{E\}}$, Gonadotrophins $^{\{E\}}$, Ovaries $^{\{E\}}$

MAP: Shen Men, Endocrine Point, Point Zero, Thalamus Point

SAP: Pelvis, Abdomen, Adrenal Glands $^{\{C\}}$, Adrenal Glands $^{\{E\}}$

9.20.8 Vaginismus
PAP: Vagina, Gonadotrophins $^{\{E\}}$, Ovaries $^{\{E\}}$, Abdomen, Brain $^{\{C\}}$, Prostaglandin Point $^{\{E\}}$

MAP: Point Zero, Shen Men, Endocrine Point

SAP: Occiput, Kidney $^{\{C\}}$, Lung 1, Lung 2, Adrenal Glands $^{\{C\}}$

9.20.9 Labor Induction or Postpartum Pain
PAP: Uterus $^{\{C\}}$, Uterus $^{\{E\}}$, Gonadotrophins $^{\{E\}}$, Ovaries $^{\{E\}}$, Pelvis, Abdomen

MAP: Point Zero, Shen Men, Sympathetic Point, Thalamus Point, Point Zero

SAP: Lumbar Vertebrae $^{\{C, F1, F2, F3\}}$, Spleen $^{\{C\}}$

9.20.10 Lactation Stimulation or Milk Secretion
PAP: Breast, Prolactin, Oxytocin, Mammary Glands $^{\{C\}}$, Mammary Glands $^{\{E\}}$

MAP: Endocrine Point, Shen Men, Thalamus Point

SAP: Spleen $^{\{C\}}$, Kidney $^{\{C\}}$, Liver, Stomach, San Jiao, Pituitary Gland $^{\{C\}}$

Peri-Menstrual or Dysmenorrhea Protocols

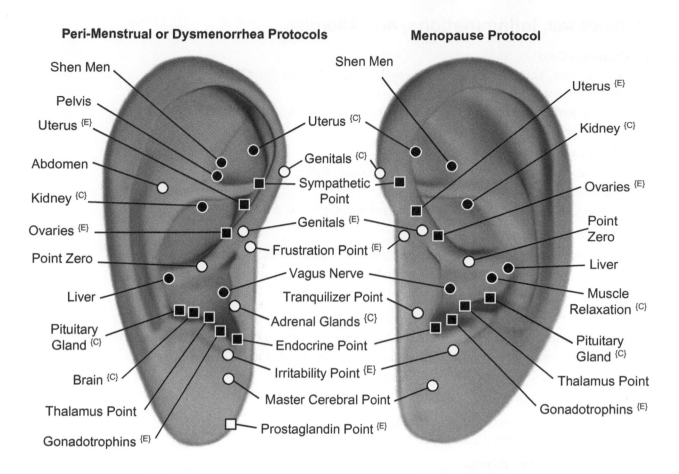

Shen Men
Pelvis
Uterus {E}
Abdomen
Kidney {C}
Ovaries {E}
Point Zero
Liver
Pituitary Gland {C}
Brain {C}
Thalamus Point
Gonadotrophins {E}

Uterus {C}
Genitals {C}
Sympathetic Point
Genitals {E}
Frustration Point {E}
Vagus Nerve
Tranquilizer Point
Adrenal Glands {C}
Endocrine Point
Irritability Point {E}
Master Cerebral Point
Prostaglandin Point {E}

Menopause Protocol

Shen Men

Uterus {E}
Kidney {C}
Ovaries {E}
Point Zero
Liver
Muscle Relaxation {C}
Pituitary Gland {C}
Thalamus Point
Gonadotrophins {E}

Infertility Protocol

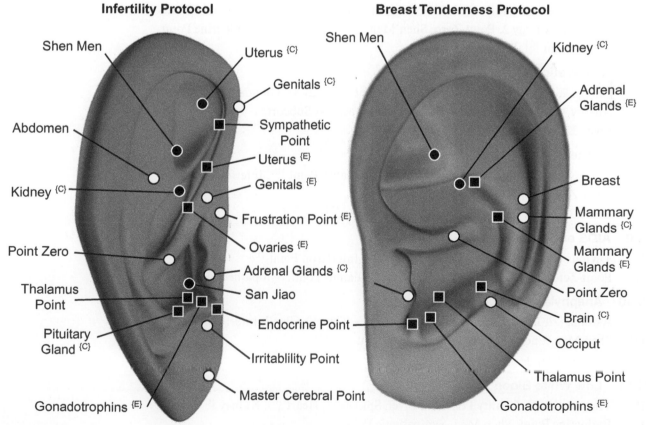

Shen Men
Abdomen
Kidney {C}
Point Zero
Thalamus Point
Pituitary Gland {C}
Gonadotrophins {E}

Uterus {C}
Genitals {C}
Sympathetic Point
Uterus {E}
Genitals {E}
Frustration Point {E}
Ovaries {E}
Adrenal Glands {C}
San Jiao
Endocrine Point
Irritablility Point
Master Cerebral Point

Breast Tenderness Protocol

Shen Men

Kidney {C}
Adrenal Glands {E}
Breast
Mammary Glands {C}
Mammary Glands {E}
Point Zero
Brain {C}
Occiput
Thalamus Point
Gonadotrophins {E}

FIGURE 9.20 Menstrual and gynecological disorders auricular treatment protocols.

9.21 Illnesses, Inflammations, and Allergies

9.21.1 Common Cold
PAP: Internal Nose, Throat {E}, Forehead, Lung 1, Lung 2, Asthma {C}, Antihistamine {C}
MAP: Allergy 1, Allergy 2, Point Zero, Shen Men, Endocrine Point
SAP: Sneezing Reflex {C}, Cough Reflex {C}, Adrenal Glands {C}, Adrenal Glands {E}, Windstream {C}, Occiput, Spleen {C}, Vitamin C

9.21.2 Influenza (Flu)
PAP: Forehead, Lung 1, Lung 2, Thymus Gland, Sneezing Reflex {C}, Cough Reflex {C}
MAP: Point Zero, Shen Men, Thalamus Point
SAP: Vitamin C, Asthma {C}, Omega 2, Prostaglandin Point {E}, Adrenal Glands {C}

9.21.3 Fever or Malaise
PAP: Heat Point {C}, Vitality Point {E}, Occiput, Thymus Gland, Vitamin C
MAP: Point Zero, Shen Men, Thalamus Point, Endocrine Point, Sympathetic Point
SAP: Omega 2, Prostaglandin Point {E}, Adrenal Glands {C}, Adrenal Glands {E}

9.21.4 Allergies
PAP: Omega 2, Internal Nose, Asthma {C}, Antihistamine {C}, Adrenal Glands {C}, Windstream {C}
MAP: Allergy 1, Allergy 2, Point Zero, Shen Men, Sympathetic Point, Endocrine Point
SAP: Thymus Gland, Thyroid Glands {C}, Thyroid Glands {E}, Spleen {C}, San Jiao

9.21.5 Weather Changes
PAP: Weather Point {E}, Lung 1, Lung 2, Frontal Sinus
MAP: Allergy 1, Allergy 2, Point Zero, Shen Men

9.21.6 Anti-Inflammatory Effects
PAP: Omega 2, Prostaglandin Point {E}, Occiput, Adrenal Glands {C}, Adrenal Glands {E}
MAP: Allergy 1, Allergy 2, Point Zero, Shen Men, Sympathetic Point, Endocrine Point
SAP: Windstream {C}, Spleen {C}

9.21.7 Antipyretic Effects
PAP: Omega 2, Heat Point {C}, Prostaglandin Point {E}, Adrenal Glands {C}
MAP: Allergy 1, Allergy 2, Shen Men, Point Zero, Vascular Subcortex
SAP: Liver, Large Intestines, Interferon Point {E}

9.21.8 Cancer
PAP: *Corresponding Organ Area*, Thymus Gland, Vitality Point {E}, Interferon Point {E}
MAP: Point Zero, Shen Men, Thalamus Point
SAP: Breast, Ovaries/Testes {E}, Prostate {C}, Prostate {E}

9.21.9 AIDS or HIV Disease
PAP: Thymus Gland, Vitality Point {E}, Heart {C}, Interferon Point {E}
MAP: Point Zero, Shen Men, Endocrine Point, Thalamus Point, Sympathetic Point

9.21.10   Anaphylaxis Hypersensitivity
PAP: Asthma {C}, Lung 1, Lung 2, Large Intestines, Thymus Gland, Interferon Point {E}
MAP: Shen Men, Endocrine Point, Thalamus Point
SAP: Adrenal Glands {C}, Adrenal Glands {E}

9.21.11   Low White Blood Cells
PAP: Thymus Gland, Vitality Point {E}, Liver, Spleen {C}, Heart {C}, Kidney {C}
MAP: Endocrine Point, Shen Men, Sympathetic Point
SAP: Adrenal Glands {C}, Diaphragm {C}, Occiput

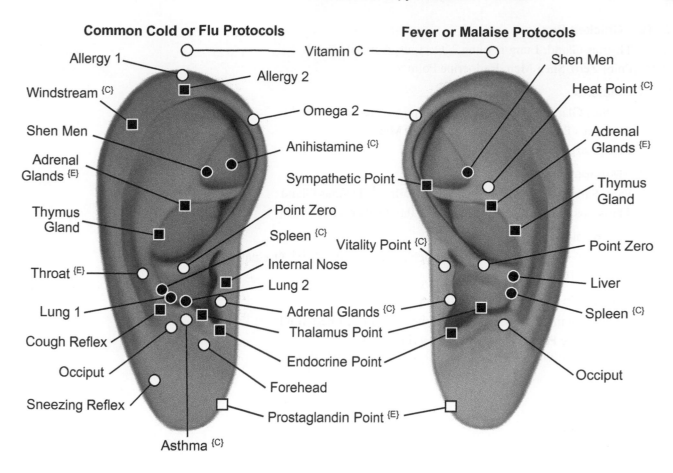

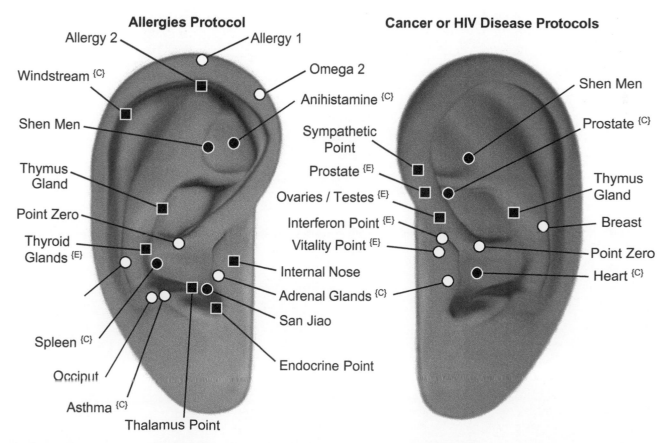

FIGURE 9.21 Allergies and immune system disorders auricular treatment protocols.

9.21.12   Chicken Pox

PAP: Thymus Gland, Lung 1, Lung 2, Occiput, Adrenal Glands {C}

MAP: Point Zero, Shen Men, Endocrine Point

9.21.13   Malaria

PAP: Thymus Gland, Lung 1, Lung 2, Occiput, Adrenal Glands {C}

MAP: Thalamus Point, Endocrine Point, Shen Men

SAP: Liver, Large Intestines, Spleen {C}

9.21.14   Mumps

PAP: Face, Salivary Glands {C}, Salivary Glands {E}, Thymus Gland

MAP: Thalamus Point, Endocrine Point, Thalamus Point, Shen Men

9.21.15   Whooping Cough

PAP: Asthma {C}, Antihistamine {C}, Bronchi, Adrenal Glands {C}, Occiput

MAP: Sympathetic Point, Shen Men

9.21.16   Systemic Lupus Erythematosus

PAP: Thymus Gland, Dermatitis {C}, Forehead, Lung 2, Interferon Point {E}

MAP: Sympathetic Point, Shen Men, Endocrine Point

SAP: Windstream {C}, Adrenal Glands {C}, Liver, Spleen {C}, Kidney {C}

Index of Ear Reflex Points

No.	Name of Ear Point	Chinese Ear Zones	European Ear Zones	Posterior Zones	Page No.
0.0	Point Zero	HX 1/CR 1	HX 1/CR 1		227
1.0	Shen Men (Spirit Gate)	TF 2	TF 2		227
2.0	Sympathetic Autonomic Point	IH 4/AH 7	IH 4/AH 7		228
3.0	Allergy Point	AH 7/AH 8	IH 7/IH 8		228
4.0	Thalamus Point (Subcortex)	CW 2/IC 4	CW 2/IC 4		228
5.0	Master Endocrine Point	IT 2	IT 2		229
6.0	Master Oscillation Point	ST 3	ST 3		229
7.0	Tranquilizer Point (Valium Analog Point)	TG 2	TG 2		229
8.0	Master Sensorial Point	LO 4	LO 4		229
9.0	Master Cerebral Point	LO 1	LO 1		229
10.0	Cervical Vertebrae	AH 8	AH 1–AH 2	PG 2	238
11.0	Thoracic Vertebrae	AH 9–AH 10	AH 3–AH 4	PG 3, PG 4	238
12.0	Lumbar Vertebrae	AH 11	AH 5–AH 6	PG 5, PG 6	238
13.0	Sacral Vertebrae	AH 11	AH 7	PG 7	238
14.0	Buttocks	AH 5	AH 5	PG 5	238
15.0	Throat (Neck muscles)		AH 8 & AH 9	PP 1	240
16.0	Clavicle (Collarbone)	SF 1	AH 9	PP 3	240
17.0	Breast	AH 10	AH 10	PP 3	240
18.0	Chest and Ribs	AH 10	AH 10	PP 3	240
19.0	Abdomen	AH 11	AH 11 & AH 12	PP 5	240
20.0	Pelvis (Pelvic Girdle)	TF 1	TF 1	PG 8	240
21.0	Hip	AH 13	TF 1	PT 1	242
22.0	Thigh (Upper Leg)	TF 3	TF 3	PT 1	242
23.0	Knee (Patella)	AH 15	TF 3, TF 4	PT 2	242
24.0	Calf (Lower Leg)		TF 5	PT 3	242
25.0	Ankle	AH 17	TF 5/TF 6	PT 3	242
26.0	Heel	AH 17	TF 5	PT 3	242
27.0	Foot	AH 17 & AH 18	TF 5 & TF 6	PT 3	242
28.0	Toes	AH 18	TF 6	PT 3	243
29.0	Thumb		AH 14 & AH 16	PP 9	244
30.0	Fingers	SF 6	SF 6	PP 10	244
31.0	Hand	SF 5	SF 5	PP 9	244
32.0	Wrist	SF 5	SF 5	PP 7	244
33.0	Forearm	SF 4	SF 4	PP 7	244

No.	Name of Ear Point	Chinese Ear Zones	European Ear Zones	Posterior Zones	Page No.
34.0	Elbow	SF 3	SF 3	PP 5	244
35.0	Upper Arm	SF 3	SF 3	PP 5	244
36.0	Shoulder	SF 2	SF 2	PP 3	244
37.0	Shoulder Joint	SF 1	SF 1	PP 1	244
38.0	Occiput	AT 3	AT 3	PL 4	246
39.0	Temple	AT 2	AT 2	PG 1	246
40.0	Forehead	AT 1	AT 1	PL 2	246
41.0	Frontal Sinus	LO 1	LO 1		246
42.0	Vertex	LO 6	LO 6	PL 4	246
43.0	TMJ	LO 8	LO 8	PL 6	246
44.0	Lower Jaw (Mandible)	LO 8	LO 8	PL 6	246
45.0	Upper Jaw (Maxilla)	LO 8	LO 8	PL 6	248
46.c	Toothache 1, 2, 3	LO 8, CW 3, IC 5	LO 8		248
47.c	Dental Analgesia 1 & 2	LO 1, LO 2			248
48.0	Palate 1 & 2	LO 4			248
49.0	Tongue	LO 4	LO 5	PL 5	248
50.0	Lips		LO 5	PL 5	248
51.0	Chin		LO 7	PL 5	248
52.0	Face (Cheeks)	LO 5	LO 5	PL 5	248
53.0	Dermatitis (Urticaria)	SF 5/IH 11	HX 12–HX 15		250
54.0	Eye (Retina)	LO 4	LO 4	PL 4	250
55.c	Eye Disorders 1, 2, 3	IT 1 & AT 1			250
56.0	Internal Nose	ST 2	ST 2		250
57.0	External Nose	TG 3	LO 1		250
58.0	Inner Ear (Cochlea)	LO 5	ST 3		250
59.0	External Ear (Auricle)	TG 5	LO 5		250
60.0	Mouth (Soft Palate)	IC 6	IC 6		261
61.0	Esophagus	IC 7	IC 7	PC 2	261
62.0	Esophageal Sphincter	IC 7	IC 7	PC 2	261
63.0	Stomach	CR 1	CR 1	PC 2	261
64.0	Duodenum	SC 1	SC 1	PC 3	261
65.0	Small Intestines	SC 2	SC 2	PC 3	261
66.0	Large Intestines (Colon)	SC 3, SC 4	SC 3, SC 4	PC 2	262
67.0	Rectum (Anus)	HX 3	IH 2/SC 4	PC 4	262
68.0	Circulatory System		CW 2–CW 9	PG 3	264
69.0	Heart.c^1, .c^2, .e	IC 4 & TG 5	AH 3	PG 4	264
70.c	Lung 1 & 2	IC 4 & IC 5	IC 2–IC 5	PC 2	264
71.c	Bronchi	IC 7		PC 2	265
72.0	Trachea (Windpipe)	IC 3	IC 3		265
73.0	Pharynx (Throat Lining)	ST 4	IC 3		265
74.0	Larynx (Voice Box)	ST 4	IC 3	PC 2	265
75.c	Tonsil Point 1, 2, 3, 4	HX 9–HX 15	SF 1	LO 3	266
76.0	Diaphragm	HX 2	IC 8/CR 2		266
77.0	Appendix	SC 1/SC 2	SC 1/SC 2		268
78.c	Appendix Disorder 1, 2, & 3	SF 6, 3, 1			268
79.0	Liver	CR 2	CR 2	PC 3	268
80.c	Liver Yang 1 & 2	HX 10 & HX 11			268
81.0	Spleen	IC 8	SC 8 & SC 6	PC 3	268
82.0	Gall Bladder	SC 8	SC 8	PC 3	268
83.0	Pancreas	SC 7 & CW 7	SC 7 & CW 7	PC 3	268
84.0	Kidney	SC 6/CW 8	IH 5	PP 10	270
85.0	Ureter	SC 6	IH 4		270
86.0	Bladder (Urinary Bladder)	SC 5	SC 5	PC 3	270

No.	Name of Ear Point	Chinese Ear Zones	European Ear Zones	Posterior Zones	Page No.
87.0	Urethra	HX 3	SC 4	PC 3	270
88.0	Prostate/Vagina	SC 4	IH 2		270
89.0	Uterus	TF 5/6	IH 3		272
90.0	Genitals (Penis or Clitoris)	HX 4	HX 1		272
91.0	Ovaries/Testes (Gonads)	CW 1	IH 1		277
92.0	Adrenal Glands	TG 2/TG 3	CW 7	PG 5	277
93.0	Cortisol		SC 6	PG 5	277
94.0	Thymus Gland		CW 6	PG 4	277
95.0	Mammary Glands	AH 10	CW 5	PG 3	278
96.0	Thyroid Glands	AH 8	CW 5	PG 3	278
97.0	Parathyroid Glands		CW 4	PG 4	279
98.0	Pineal Gland (Epiphysis)		TG 1		279
99.0	Anterior Pituitary (Adenohypophysis)	CW 3	IC 1	PC 1	279
100.0	Posterior Pituitary (Neurohypophysis)		IC 3		279
101.0	Gonadotrophins (FSH, LH)		CW 1		279
102.0	Thyrotrophins (TSH)		IT 2		279
103.0	Parathyrotrophins		IT 2		279
104.0	ACTH		ST 1		279
105.0	Prolactin (LTH)		IC 1		280
106.0	Salivary Gland	CW 2/LO 8			279
107.0	Sciatic Nerve	AH 6/AH 7	AH 6/AH 7		286
108.0	Sympathetic Preganglionic Nerves		HX 12–HX 14		286
109.0	Sympathetic Postganglionic Nerves		CW 5–CW 9	PG 4	286
110.0	Parasympathetic Cranial & Sacral Nerves		IC 1 & IC 6	PG 7	286
111.0	Hypogastric Plexus		SC 4/SC 5		286
112.0	Solar Plexus (Celiac Plexus)		HX 1		286
113.0	Vagus Nerve		IC 3	PG 1	286
114.0	Auditory Nerve (Cochleovestibular Nerve)		ST 3		286
115.0	Facial Nerve			PL 6	286
116.0	Trigeminal Nerve		LO 5	PL 5	287
117.0	Oculomotor Nerve			PL 3	287
118.0	Optic Nerve	LO 1	LO 1		287
119.0	Olfactory Nerve	LO 2	LO 2		287
120.0	Inferior Cervical Ganglia (Stellate Ganglion)		CW 5		287
121.0	Middle Cervical Ganglia (Marvelous Point)		CR 2/CW 4		287
122.0	Superior Cervical Ganglia		CW 4		287
123.c	Lesser Occipital Nerve	IH 11/SF 5			287
124.0	Lumbosacral Spinal Cord		HX 12	PP 8	288
125.0	Thoracic Spinal Cord		HX 13	PP 6	288
126.0	Cervical Spinal Cord		HX 14	PP 4	288
127.0	Brainstem (Medulla Oblongata)	CW 4	LO 8	PP 2	288
128.0	Pons		LO 7	PL 6	288
129.0	Midbrain Tectum (Superior & Inferior Colliculus)		LO 6		288

No.	Name of Ear Point	Chinese Ear Zones	European Ear Zones	Posterior Zones	Page No.
130.0	Midbrain Tegmentum (Periaqueductal Gray)		LO 5	PL 5	290
131.0	Reticular Formation		ST 2 & ST 3	PL 5	290
132.0	Trigeminal Nucleus		LO 7	PL 6	290
133.0	Red Nucleus		LO 6	PL 4	290
134.0	Substantia Nigra		LO 6	PL 6	290
135.0	Striatum (Basal Ganglia)		LO 4	PL 4	291
136.0	Anterior Hypothalamus		IC 2	PG 2	291
137.0	Posterior Hypothalamus		IC 4, IC 5	PP 1	291
138.0	Brain	CW 3	CW 3	PG 2	291
139.0	Limbic Brain		LO 2	PL 2	292
140.0	Hippocampus		LO 6/LO 8	PL 6	292
141.0	Amygdala		LO 2/AT 1	PL 2	292
142.0	Nucleus Accumbens		LO 2/IT 1		292
143.0	Cingulate Gyrus		IT 1		292
144.0	Olfactory Bulb		LO 2		292
145.0	Cerebellum		AH 1/AT 3	PL 4	292
146.0	Corpus Callosum		TG 2–TG 4		293
147.0	Occipital Cortex (Visual Cortex)		AT 3/LO 8		293
148.0	Temporal Cortex (Auditory Cortex)		LO 6/LO 8		293
149.0	Parietal Cortex (Post-Central Gyrus)		LO 3/LO 5		293
150.0	Frontal Cortex (Pre-Central Gyrus)		LO 3	PL 3	293
151.0	Prefrontal Cortex (Executive Brain)		LO 1	PL 1	293
152.c	Asthma Point (Ping Chuan)	AT 2			295
153.c	Antihistamine Point	TF 3/TF 4			295
154.c	Constipation	TF 3			295
155.c	Hepatitis 1 & 2	TF 4 & CR 2			295
156.c	Hypertension 1, 2, & 3	TF 6 & TG 2		PG 4	295
157.c	Hypotension Point	IT 1			295
158.c	Lumbago	AH 11 & AH 12			295
159.c	Muscle Relaxation	IC 7/IC 8			295
160.c	San Jiao (Triple Warmer)	IC 1			297
161.c	Appetite Control Point (Hunger Point)	TG 3			297
162.c	Thirst Point	TG 4			297
163.c	Alcoholic Point (Drunk Point)	SC 2/SC 6			297
164.0	Anxiety Point	LO 1	LO 1		297
165.c	Excitement Point	CW 2			297
166.c	Tuberculosis	IC 5			298
167.c	Bronchitis	IC 6/IC 7			298
168.c	Heat Point	AH 11			298
169.c	Cirrhosis	CR 2			298
170.c	Pancreatitis	SC 7			298
171.c	Nephritis	SF 1/HX 15			298
172.c	Ascites Point	SC 6			298

No.	Name of Ear Point	Chinese Ear Zones	European Ear Zones	Posterior Zones	Page No.
173.c	Mutism Point (Dumb Point)	ST 3			298
174.c	Hemorrhoids 1 & 2	IH 6 & SC 4			298
175.c	Windstream	IH 11			299
176.c	Central Rim (Pituitary Gland)	CW 3			299
177.c	Apex of Tragus	TG 5			299
178.c	Apex of Antitragus	AT 2			299
179.c	Apex of Auricle	HX 7			299
180.c	Helix Points 1, 2, 3, 4, 5, 6	HX 11–HX 15			299
181.e	Auditory Line		LO 6		302
182.e	Irritability Point		LO 2/IT 1		302
183.e	Psychosomatic Point (Bourdiol Point)		HX 4		302
184.e	Sexual Desire (Bosch Point)		HX 1/TG 5		302
185.e	Sexual Suppression (Jerome Point)		HX 15		302
186.e	Master Omega		LO 1		302
187.e	Omega 1		SC 2		302
188.e	Omega 2		HX 6		302
189.e	Marvelous Point (Wonderful Point)		CW 4/CR 2		302
190.e	Anti-Depressant Point		LO 8		303
191.e	Mania Point		TG 2		303
192.e	Nicotine Point		TG 2		303
193.e	Vitality Point		TG 4		303
194.e	Alertness Point		HX 12/HX 13		303
195.e	Insomnia 1 & 2		SF 1 & SF 5		303
196.e	Dizziness Point (Vertigo Point)		CW 4		303
197.e	Sneezing Point		LO 5		303
198.e	Weather Point		HX 3		303
199.e	Laterality Point		Jaw		303
200.e	Darwin's Point		HX 11		305
201.e	Prostaglandin Point		LO 1/PL 1		305
202.e	Progesterone		IH 6		305
203.e	Oxytocin		CW 3		305
204.e	Angiotensin Point		IH 6		305
205.e	Analgesia Point		SC 7		305
206.e	Hypnotic Point		HX 13		305
207.e	Barbiturate Point		SF 3		305
208.e	Beta-1 Receptor		SF 4/IH 12		305
209.e	Frustration Point		TG 5/HX 2		305
210.e	Interferon Point		TG 5/HX 1		305
211.e	Mercury Toxicity Point		SC 6		305
212.e	Vomiting Reflex		LO 7		307
213.e	Cough Reflex		CW 4		307
214.e	Memory Points 1, 2, 3		LO 1 & LO 6	PL 2	307
215.e	Vitamin C		Head		307
216.e	Vitamin E		HX 9		307
217.e	Vitamin A		Neck		307

No.	Name of Ear Point	Chinese Ear Zones	European Ear Zones	Posterior Zones	Page No.
218.e	Master Point for Metabolism		LO 7		307
219.e	Master Point for Lower Limbs		HX 2		307
220.e	Master Point for Upper Limbs		HX 15		307
221.e	Master Point for Endodermal Tissue		PG 7/HX 4		307
222.e	Master Point for Mesodermal Tissue		LO 7		307
223.e	Master Point for Ectodermal Tissue		IH 1		308
224.e	Point Zero Prime 1 & 2		TG 3 & CR 2		308
225.c	Epilepsy Point	CW 2			308

Ear Point Names Listed Alphabetically	No.	Chinese Ear Zones	European Ear Zones	Posterior Zones	Page No.
Abdomen	19	AH 11	AH 11 & AH 12	PP 5	240
Achilles Tendon	25.e	AH 17	TF 5/TF 6	PT 3	242
ACTH	104.e		ST 1		279
Adrenal Glands	92.c/92.e	TG 2/TG 3	CW 7	PG 5	277
Alcoholic Point	163.c	SC 2			297
Alertness Point	194.e		HX 12/HX 13		303
Allergy Point	3.c/3.e	AH 7/AH 8	IH 7/IH 8		228
Amygdala	141		LO 2/AT 1	PL 2	292
Analgesia Point	205.e		SC 7		305
Angiotensin Point	204.e		IH 6		305
Ankle	25.c	AH 17	TF 5/TF 6	PT 3	242
Anti-Aggressivity Point	182.e		LO 2/IT 1		302
Anti-Depressant Point	190.e		LO 8		303
Antihistamine Point	153.c	TF 3/TF 4			295
Anus	67	HX 3	IH 2/SC 4	PC 4	262
Anxiety Point	164.c	LO 1	LO 1		297
Apex of Antitragus	178.c	AT 2			299
Apex of Auricle	179.c	HX 7			299
Apex of Head	42	LO 6	LO 6	PL 4	246
Apex of Tragus	177.c	TG 5			299
Appendix	77	SC 1/SC 2	SC 1/SC 2		268
Appendix Disorder	78.c^1/c^2/c^3	SF 6, SF 3, SF 1			268
Appetite Control Point	161.c	TG 3			297
Arm, Upper	35	SF 3	SF 3	PP 5	244
Ascites Point	172.c	SC 6			298
Asthma Point	152.c	AT 2			295
Atlas of Head	38	AT 3	AT 3	PL 4	246
Auditory Cortex	148.e		LO 6/LO 8		293
Auditory Line	181.e		LO 6		302
Auditory Nerve	114.e		ST 3		286
Auricle	59.c	TG 5	LO 5		250
Autonomic Point	2.0	IH 4/AH 7	IH 4/AH 7		228
Barbiturate Point	207.e		SF 3		305
Basal Ganglia	135		LO 4	PL 4	291
Beta-1 Receptor	208.e		SF 4/IH 12		305
Biceps muscle	35	SF 3	SF 3	PP 5	244
Bladder	86	SC 5	SC 5	PC 3	270
Blood Vessels	68.e		CW 2–CW 9	PG 3	264
Bosch Point	184.e		HX 1/TG 5		302
Bourdiol Point	183.e		HX 4		302
Brachioradialis Muscle	33	SF 4	SF 4	PP 7	244
Brain	138.c	CW 3	CW 3	PG 2	291
Brainstem	127.c	CW 4	LO 8	PP 2	288
Breast	17	AH 10	AH 10	PP 3	240
Bronchi	71.c	IC 7		PC 2	265
Bronchitis	167.c	IC 6/IC 7			298
Buttocks	14	AH 5	AH 5	PG 5	238
Calf	24.e		TF 5	PT 3	242
Cardia	62	IC 7	IC 7	PC 2	261
Cardiac Orifice	62	IC 7	IC 7	PC 2	261
Caudate Nucleus	135.e1		LO 4	PL 4	291
Celiac Plexus	112.e		HX 1		286
Central Rim	176.c	CW 3			299

Ear Point Names Listed Alphabetically	No.	Chinese Ear Zones	European Ear Zones	Posterior Zones	Page No.
Cerebellum	145.e		AH 1/AT 3	PL 4	292
Cervical Ganglia, Inferior	120.e		CW 5		287
Cervical Ganglia, Middle	121.e		CR 2/CW 4		287
Cervical Ganglia, Superior	122.e		CW 4		287
Cervical Vertebrae	10.c	AH 8	AH 1–AH 2	PG 2	238
Cheeks	52	LO 5	LO 5	PL 5	248
Chest and Ribs	18	AH 10	AH 10	PP 3	240
Chin	51.e		LO 7	PL 5	248
Cingulate Gyrus	143.e		IT 1		292
Circulatory System	68.e		CW 2–CW 9	PG 3	264
Cirrhosis	169.c	CR 2			298
Clavicle	16.c/16.e	SF 1	AH 9	PP 3	240
Clitoris	90.c	HX 4	HX 1		272
Coccyx	13.e	AH 11	AH 7	PG 7	238
Cochlea	58.e	LO 5	ST 3		250
Cochleovestibular Nerve	114.e		ST 3		286
Collarbone	16.c	SF 1	AH 9	PP 3	240
Colon	66	SC 3, SC 4	SC 3, SC 4	PC 2	262
Constipation	154.c	TF 3			295
Corpus Callosum	146.e		TG 2–TG 4		293
Cortisol	93.e		SC 6	PG 5	277
Cough Reflex	213.e		CW 4		307
Cranial Nerve, 10th	113.e		IC 3	PG 1	286
Cranial Nerve, 1st	119.e	LO 2	LO 2		287
Cranial Nerve, 2nd	118.e	LO 1	LO 1		287
Cranial Nerve, 3rd	117.e			PL 3	287
Cranial Nerve, 5th	116.e		LO 5	PL 5	287
Cranial Nerve, 7th	115.e			PL 6	286
Crown of Head	42	LO 6	LO 6	PL 4	246
Darwin's Point	200.e		HX 11		305
Deltoid Muscles	36	SF 2	SF 2	PP 3	244
Dental Analgesia	47.c/c^2	LO 1, LO 2			248
Dermatitis	53.c/53.e	SF 5/IH 11	HX 12–HX 15		250
Diaphragm	76.c/76.e	HX 2	IC 8/CR 2		266
Dizziness Point	196.e		CW 4		303
Dorsal Vertebrae	11	AH 9–AH 10	AH 3–AH 4	PG 3, PG 4	238
Drunk Point	163.c	SC 2/SC 6			297
Dumb Point	173.c	ST 3			298
Duodenum	64	SC 1	SC 1	PC 3	261
Ear, External	59.c/59.e	TG 5	LO 5		250
Ear, Inner	58.c/58.e	LO 5	ST 3		250
Elbow	34	SF 3	SF 3	PP 5	244
Epilepsy Point	225.c	CW 2			308
Epiphysis	98		TG 1		324
Esophageal Sphincter	62	IC 7	IC 7	PC 2	261
Esophagus	61	IC 7	IC 7	PC 2	261
Excitement Point	165.c	CW 2			297
Extrapyramidal Motor System	135		LO 4	PL 4	291
Eye (Retina)	54	LO 4	LO 4	PL 4	250
Eye Disorders	55.c^1/55.c^2	IT 1			250
Face	52	LO 5	LO 5	PL 5	248
Facial muscles	52	LO 5	LO 5	PL 5	248

Ear Point Names Listed Alphabetically	No.	Chinese Ear Zones	European Ear Zones	Posterior Zones	Page No.
Facial Nerve	115.e			PL 6	286
Fallopian Tubes	89.e	TF 5/TF 6	IH 3		272
Femur Bone	22	TF 3	TF 3	PT 1	242
Fibula Bone	24.e		TF 5	PT 3	242
Fingers	30	SF 6	SF 6	PP 10	244
Foot	27.e	AH 17 & AH 18	TF 5 & TF 6	PT 3	242
Forearm	33	SF 4	SF 4	PP 7	244
Forehead	40	AT 1	AT 1	PL 2	246
Frontal Cortex	150.e		LO 3	PL 3	293
Frontal Sinus	41	LO 1	LO 1		246
Frontal Skull	40	AT 1	AT 1	PL 2	246
Frustration Point	209.e		TG 5/HX 2		305
Gall Bladder	82	SC 8	SC 8	PC 3	268
Gastrocnemius Muscle	24.e		TF 5	PT 3	242
Genitals, External	90.e	HX 4	HX 1		272
Genitals, Internal	91.c	CW 1	IH 1		277
Globus Pallidus	135.e^3		LO 4	PL 4	291
Gluteus Maximus Muscle	14	AH 5	AH 5	PG 5	238
Gonadal Glands	91	CW 1	IH 1		277
Gonadotrophins (FSH, LH)	101.e		CW 1		279
Groin	20	TF 1	TF 1	PG 8	240
Hand	31	SF 5 & AH 14	SF 5	PP 9	244
Heart	69.c^1/c^2/c^3	IC 4 & TG 5	AH 3	PG 4	264
Heat Point	168.c	AH 11			298
Heel	26.c/26.e	AH 17	TF 5	PT 3	242
Helix Points	180.c	HX 11–HX 15	LO 3, LO 7		299
Hemorrhoids	174.c/c^2	IH 6 & SC 4			298
Hepatitis	155.c/c^2	TF 4 & CR 2			295
Hip	21.c/21.e	AH 13	TF 1	PT 1	242
Hippocampus	140.e		LO 6/LO 8	PL 6	292
Hives	53.c	SF 5/IH 11			250
Humerus Bone	35	SF 3	SF 3	PP 5	244
Hunger Point	161.c	TG 3			297
Hypertension	156.c/c^2/c^3	TF 6 & TG 2		PG 4	295
Hypnotic Point	206.e		HX 13		305
Hypogastric Plexus	111.e		SC 4/SC 5		286
Hypophysis, Adenohypophysis	99	CW 3	IC 1	PC 1	279
Hypophysis, Neurohypophysis	100		IC 3		279
Hypotension Point	157.c	IT 1			295
Hypothalamus, Anterior	136.e		IC 2	PG 2	291
Hypothalamus, Posterior	137.e		IC 4, IC 5	PP 1	291
Insomnia Point	195.e^1/.e^2		SF 1 & SF 5		303
Interferon Point	210.e		TG 5/HX 1		305
Internal Secretion Point	5	IT 2	IT 2		279
Irritability Point	182.e		LO 2/IT 1		302
Ischium	107	AH 6/AH 7	AH 6/AH 7		286
Jaw, Lower	44	LO 8	LO 8	PL 6	246
Jaw, Upper	45	LO 8	LO 8	PL 6	246
Jerome Point	185.e		HX 15		302
Kidney	84.c/84.e	SC 6/CW 8	IH 5	PP 10	270
Knee	23.c/23.e	AH 15	TF 3, TF 4	PT 2	242

Ear Point Names Listed Alphabetically	No.	Chinese Ear Zones	European Ear Zones	Posterior Zones	Page No.
Large Intestines	66	SC 3, SC 4	SC 3, SC 4	PC 4	262
Larynx	74.c/74.e	ST 4	IC 3	PC 2	265
Laterality Point	199.e		Jaw		303
Leg, Lower	24		TF 5	PT 3	242
Leg, Upper	22	TF 3	TF 3	PT 1	242
Lesser Occipital Nerve	123.c	IH 11/SF 5			287
Libido Point	184.e		HX 1/TG 5		302
Limbic Brain	139.e		LO 2	PL 2	292
Lips	50.e		LO 5	PL 5	248
Liver	79	CR 2	CR 2	PC 6	268
Liver Yang	80.c^1/c^2	HX 10 & HX 11			268
Lumbago	158.c	AH 11 & AH 12			295
Lumbar Vertebrae	12.c	AH 11	AH 5–AH 6	PG 5, PG 6	238
Lung	70.c	IC 4 & IC 5	IC 2–IC 5	PC 2	264
Lymph Vessels	68		CW 2–CW 9	PG 3	264
Mammary Glands	95.c/95.e	AH 10	CW 5	PG 3	278
Mandible	44	LO 8	LO 8	PL 6	246
Mania Point	191.e		TG 2		303
Marvelous Point	189.e		CW 4/CR 2		302
Masseter Muscle	44	LO 8	LO 8	PL 6	246
Master Cerebral Point	9	LO 1	LO 1		229
Master Endocrine Point	5	IT 2	IT 2		229
Master Omega Point	186.e		LO 1		302
Master Oscillation Point	6.e	ST 3	ST 3		229
Master Point for Ectodermal Tissue	223.e		IH 1		309
Master Point for Endodermal Tissue	221.e		PG 7/HX 4		307
Master Point for Lower Limbs	219.e		HX 2		307
Master Point for Mesodermal Tissue	222.e		LO 7		307
Master Point for Metabolism	218.e		LO 7		307
Master Point for Upper Limbs	220.e		HX 15		307
Master Sensorial Point	8	LO 4	LO 4		229
Maxilla	45	LO 8	LO 8	PL 6	246
Medulla Oblongata	127.e	CW 4	LO 8	PP 2	288
Memory Point	214.e^1/e^2/e^3		LO 1 & LO 6	PL 2	307
Mercury Toxicity	211.e		SC 6		305
Midbrain Periaqueductal Gray (PAG)	130.e		LO 5	PL 5	290
Midbrain Tectum	129.e		LO 6		288
Midbrain Tegmentum	130.e		LO 5	PL 5	290
Midbrain Ventral Tegmental Area	130		LO 5	PL 5	290
Minor Occipital Nerve	123.c	IH 11/SF 5			287
Motor Cortex	150.e		LO 3	PL 3	293
Mouth (Soft Palate)	60	IC 6	IC 6		261
Muscle Relaxation	159.c	IC 7/IC 8			295
Mutism Point	173.c	ST 3			298
Nasal Cavity	56.c	ST 2	ST 2		250
Neck Muscles	15		AH 8 & AH 9	PP 1	240

Ear Point Names Listed Alphabetically	No.	Chinese Ear Zones	European Ear Zones	Posterior Zones	Page No.
Nephritis	171.c	SF 1/HX 15			298
Nicotine Point	192.e		TG 2		303
Nose, External	57.c	TG 3	LO 1		250
Nose, Internal	56.c	ST 2	ST 2		250
Nucleus Accumbens	142.e		LO 2/IT 1		292
Occipital Cortex	147.e		AT 3/LO 8		293
Occiput (Occipital Skull)	38	AT 3	AT 3	PL 4	246
Oculomotor Nerve	117.e			PL 3	287
Olfactory Bulb	144.e		LO 2		292
Olfactory Nerve	119.e	LO 2	LO 2		287
Omega 1 Point	187.e		SC 2		302
Omega 2 Point	188.e		HX 6		302
Optic Nerve	118.e	LO 1	LO 1		287
Ovaries	91.c/.e	CW 1	IH 1		277
Oxytocin	203.e		CW 3		305
Palate	48.c^1/c^2	LO 4			248
Paleocortex	143.e		IT 1		292
Palm	31	SF 5	SF 5	PP 9	244
Pancreas	83	SC 7 & CW 7	SC 7 & CW 7	PC 4	268
Pancreatitis	170.c	SC 7			298
Parasympathetic Cranial Nerves	110.e		IC 1 & IC 6	PG 7	286
Parathyroid Glands	97.e		CW 4	PG 4	278
Parathyrotrophins	103.e		IT 2		279
Parietal Cortex	149.e		LO 3/LO 5/LO 6		293
Patella	23.e	AH 15	TF 3, TF 4	PT 2	242
Pectoral Girdle	36	SF 2	SF 2	PP 3	244
Pelvic Girdle	20	TF 1	TF 1	PG 8	240
Pelvis	20	TF 1	TF 1	PG 8	240
Penis	90	HX 4	HX 1		272
Phalanges	30	SF 6	SF 6	PP 10	244
Pharynx	73.c/e	ST 4	IC 3		265
Pineal Gland	98.e		TG 1		279
Ping Chuan	152.c	AT 2			295
Pituitary, Anterior	99.e	CW 3	IC 1	PC 1	279
Pituitary, Posterior	100.e		IC 3		279
Point E	98.e		TG 1		279
Point R	183.e		HX 4		302
Point Zero (Point of Support)	0	HX 1/CR 1	HX 1/CR 1		227
Point Zero Prime 1	224.e^1		TG 3		308
Point Zero Prime 2	224.e^2		CR 2		308
Pons	128.e		LO 7	PL 6	288
Post-Central Gyrus	149.e		LO 3/LO 5		293
Pre-Central Gyrus	150.e		LO 3	PL 3	293
Prefrontal Cortex	151.e		LO 1	PL 1	293
Progesterone	202		IH 6		305
Prolactin (LTH)	105.e		IC 1		280
Prostaglandin Point	201.e		LO 1/PL 1		305
Prostate	88.c/.e	SC 4	IH 2		270
Psychosomatic Point	183.e		HX 4/HX 5		302
Putamen	135.e^2		LO 4	PL 4	291
Pyramidal Motor System	150.e		LO 3	PL 3	293

Ear Point Names Listed Alphabetically	No.	Chinese Ear Zones	European Ear Zones	Posterior Zones	Page No.
Quadricep Muscles	22	TF 3	TF 3	PT 1	242
Radius Bone	33	SF 4	SF 4	PP 7	244
Rectum	67.c/e	HX 3	IH 2/SC 4	PC 4	262
Red Nucleus	133.e		LO 6	PL 6	290
Reticular Formation	131.e		ST 2 & ST 3	PL 5	290
Sacral Vertebrae	13.e	AH 11	AH 7	PG 7	238
Sacroiliac	12.c/e	AH 11	AH 5–AH 6	PG 5, PG 6	238
Salivary Gland	106.0	CW 2/LO 8			297
San Jiao	160.c	IC 1			297
Scalene Muscles	15		AH 8 & AH 9	PP 1	240
Scapula	37	SF 1	SF 1	PP 1	244
Sciatic Nerve	107	AH 6	AH 6		286
Sciatica	107	AH 6/AH 7	AH 6/AH 7		286
Septal Nucleus	142.e		LO 2/IT 1		292
Sexual Desire Point	184.e		HX 1/TG 5		302
Sexual Suppression Point	185.e		HX 15		302
Shen Men (Spirit Gate)	1	TF 2	TF 2		227
Shoulder	36	SF 2	SF 2	PP 3	244
Shoulder Joint	37	SF 1	SF 1	PP 1	244
Skin Disorders	53.c/e	SF 5/IH 11	HX 12–HX 15		250
Sleep Disorder Point	195.e		SF 1 & SF 5		303
Small Intestines	65	SC 2	SC 2	PC 3	261
Sneezing Point	197.e		LO 5		303
Solar Plexus	112.e		HX 1		286
Somatic Cortex	149.e		LO 3/LO 5		293
Spinal Cord, Cervical	126.e	HX 14	HX 14	PP 4	288
Spinal Cord, Lumbosacral	124.e	HX 12	HX 12	PP 8	288
Spinal Cord, Thoracic	125.e	HX 13	HX 13	PP 6	288
Spleen	81.c/e/e^2	IC 8	SC 8 & SC 6	PC 3	268
Stellate Ganglion	120.e		CW 5		287
Sternum	18	AH 10	AH 10	PP 3	240
Stomach	63	CR 1	CR 1	PC 2	261
Striatum	135.e		LO 4	PL 4	291
Subcortex Point	4	CW 2/IC 4	CW 2/IC 4		228
Subcortex, Digestive	138.c^2	CW 2			291
Subcortex, Nervous	138.c^1	CW 2			291
Subcortex, Vascular	138.c^3	CW 2			291
Substantia Nigra	134.e		LO 6	PL 6	290
Sympathetic Autonomic Point	2	IH 4/AH 7	IH 4/AH 7		228
Sympathetic Postganglionic Chain	109.e		CW 5–CW 9	PG 4	286
Sympathetic Preganglionic Nerves	108.e		HX 12–HX 14		286
Teeth, Lower	44	LO 8	LO 8	PL 6	246
Teeth, Upper	45	LO 8	LO 8	PL 6	246
Temple	39	AT 2	AT 2	PG 1	246
Temporal Cortex	148.e		LO 6/LO 8		293
Testes	91.c/e	CW 1	IH 1		277
Thalamic Relay Nuclei	138.e	CW 3	CW 3	PG 2	291
Thalamus Point	4	CW 2/IC 4	CW 2/IC 4		228
Thigh	22	TF 3	TF 3	PT 1	242
Thirst Point	162.c	TG 4			297
Thoracic Cavity	18	AH 10	AH 10	PP 3	240

Ear Point Names Listed Alphabetically	No.	Chinese Ear Zones	European Ear Zones	Posterior Zones	Page No.
Thoracic Vertebrae	11.c	AH 9–AH 10	AH 3–AH 4	PG 3, PG 4	238
Throat	15		AH 8 & AH 9	PP 1	240
Throat Lining	73.c/e	ST 4	IC 3		265
Thumb	29		AH 14 & AH 16	PP 9	244
Thymus Gland	94.e		CW 6	PG 4	277
Thyroid Glands	96.c/.e	AH 8	CW 5	PG 3	278
Thyrotrophins (TSH)	102.e		IT 2		279
Tibia Bone	24.e		TF 5	PT 3	242
TMJ	43	LO 8	LO 8	PL 6	246
Toes	28.c/e	AH 18	TF 6	PT 3	243
Tongue	49.c/e	LO 4	LO 5	PL 5	248
Tonsils	75.c/c^2/c^3/c^4/e	HX 9–HX 15	SF 1	LO 3	266
Toothache	46.c/c^2/c^3	LO 8	CW 3/IC 5		248
Trachea	72	IC 3	IC 3		265
Tranquilizer Point	7	TG 2	TG 2		229
Trapezius Muscles	37	SF 1	SF 1	PP 1	244
Triceps Muscle	35	SF 3	SF 3	PP 5	244
Trigeminal Nerve	116		LO 5	PL 5	287
Trigeminal Nucleus	132.e		LO 7	PL 5	290
Triple Warmer	160.c	IC 1			297
Tuberculosis	166.c	IC 5			298
Ulna Bone	33	SF 4	SF 4	PP 7	244
Ureter	85.e/.c	SC 6	IH 4		270
Urethra	87.e/.c	HX 3	SC 4	PC 3	270
Urinary Bladder	86	SC 5	SC 5	PC 3	270
Urticaria	53.c	SF 5/IH 11			250
Uterus	89.c/.e	TF 5/6	IH 3		272
Vagina	88.e	SC 4	IH 2		270
Vagus Nerve	113.e		IC 3	PG 1	286
Valium Analog Point	7	TG 2	TG 2		229
Vertex	42	LO 6	LO 6	PL 4	246
Vertigo Point	196.e		CW 4		303
Visual Cortex	147		AT 3/LO 8		293
Vitality Point	193.e		TG 4		303
Vitamin A	217.e		Neck		307
Vitamin C	215.e		Head		307
Vitamin E	216.e		HX 9		307
Voice Box	74	ST 4	IC 3	PC 2	265
Vomiting Reflex	212.e		LO 7		307
Weather Point	198.e		HX 3		303
Windpipe	72	IC 3	IC 3		265
Windstream	175.c	IH 11			299
Wonderful Point	189.e		CW 4/CR 2		287
Wrist	32	SF 5	SF 5	PP 7	244

Index of Treatment Protocols

Auriculotherapy Protocols Listed in Numerical Order

Auriculotherapy Protocols Listed in Numerical Order

Auriculotherapy Protocols Listed in Numerical Order

Auriculotherapy Protocols Listed Alphabetically

Auriculotherapy Protocols Listed Alphabetically

Protocol	Code No.	Page No.
Chronic Fatigue Syndrome	9.7.2	368
Circadian Rhythm Dysfunction	9.7.5	368
Circulatory Disorders	9.15	384
Cirrhosis	9.18.1	390
Cold Sores	9.13.3	380
Colitis or Gastroenteritis	9.14.7	382
Common Cold	9.21.1	396
Concussion	9.9.1	372
Conjunctivitis	9.10.4	374
Constipation	9.14.3	382
Convulsions	9.9.3	372
Coronary Heart Disorder	9.15.1	384
Coughing	9.16.1	386
Crohn's Disease	9.14.2	382
Cystitis	9.17.6	388
Dental Analgesia	9.6.1	366
Dental Surgery	9.6.2	366
Depression or Dysthymia	9.8.2	370
Dermatitis	9.13.1	380
Diabetes Insipidus	9.17.2	388
Diabetes Mellitus	9.18.4	390
Diarrhea	9.14.4	382
Difficulty Maintaining Alertness	9.8.8	370
Difficulty Speaking	9.11.5	376
Digestive Disorders	9.14	382
Dislocated Joints	9.5.6	364
Dizziness	9.11.3	376
Drowsiness	9.7.5	368
Drug Addiction	9.2.1	358
Drug Detoxification	9.2.1	358
Dry Eyes	9.10.6	374
Dry Mouth	9.6.5	366
Duodenal Ulcer	9.14.9	382
Dwarfism	9.19.11	392
Dysmenorrhea	9.20.2	394
Ear Infection or Earache	9.11.6	376
Eczema	9.13.6	380
Edema or Swelling	9.15.9	384
Emphysema	9.16.4	386
Endocrine Disorders	9.19	392
Endometriosis	9.20.7	394
Enuresis	9.17.3	388
Epilepsy	9.9.3	372
Eye Irritation	9.10.6	374
Eyesight Disorders	9.10	374
Facial Neuralgia	9.6.4	366
Facial Spasms	9.4.6	362
Facial Tics	9.4.7	362
Fecal Incontinence	9.14.11	382
Fever or Malaise	9.21.3	396

Auriculotherapy Protocols Listed Alphabetically

Auriculotherapy Protocols Listed Alphabetically

Auriculotherapy Protocols Listed Alphabetically

Auriculotherapy Protocols Listed Alphabetically

Auriculotherapy Protocols Listed Alphabetically

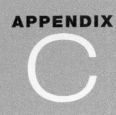
Resources

The following organizations and companies provide additional books and supplies that can be used with auriculotherapy, auricular acupuncture, and auricular medicine treatments.

Company or Organization   Service or Product

American Academy of Medical Acupuncture (AAMA)   Professional organization
1970 E. Grand Ave., #330, El Segundo, CA 90245
Tel.: (310) 364-0193
Fax: (323) 937-0959
Website: http://www.medicalacupuncture.org

American Association of Acupuncture & Oriental Medicine (AAAOM)   Professional organization
9650 Rockville Pike, Bethesda, MD 20814
Tel.: (866) 455-7999
Fax: (301) 634-7099
Website: http://www.aaaomonline.org

Auriculotherapy Certification Institute (ACI)   Certification and training in auriculotherapy
8033 Sunset Blvd., PMB #270, Los Angeles, CA 90046-2427
Tel.: (323) 656-2084
Fax: (323) 656-2085
Website: http://www.auriculotherapy.org

Electrotherapy Association   Stim Flex equipment
P.O. Box 33189, Tulsa, OK 74153
Tel.: (877) 382-7246
Fax: (918) 663-0298
Website: http://www.electrotherapy.com

Health Care Alternatives, Inc. (HCA)   Books, tapes, and seminars on auriculotherapy
8033 Sunset Blvd., PMB #265, Los Angeles, CA 90046-2427
Tel.: (323) 656-2084
Fax: (323) 656-2085
Website: http://www.auriculotherapy.com

Helio Medical Supplies   Acupuncture supplies
2076 Zanker Rd., San Jose, CA 95131
Tel.: (800) 672-2726
Fax: (408) 433-5566
Website: http://www.heliomed.com

IQUIM Quantum University   Online training
735 Bishop St., # 337, Honolulu, HI 96813
Tel.: (877) 888-8970
Fax: (818) 864-3388
Website: http://iquim.org

Lhasa OMS   Acupuncture books, products
230 Libbey Parkway, Weymouth, MA 02189
Tel.: (800) 722-8775
Fax: (718) 335-5779
Website: http://www.lhasaoms.com

National Acupuncture Detoxification Association (NADA)   Substance abuse certification
P.O. Box 1066, Laramie, WY 82073
Tel.: (888) 765-6232
Fax: (573) 777-9956
Website: http://www.acudetox.com

National Certification Commission for Acupuncture and Oriental Medicine (NCCAOM)
76 South Laura Street, Suite 1290 Jacksonville, FL, 32202, USA
Tel.: (904) 598-1005
Fax: (904) 598-5001
Website: http://www.nccaom.org

PBS International   Acuscope equipment, Myopulse equipment
2981 S. Pebble Beach Ave., Pahrump, NV 89048
Tel.: (714) 843-1183
Fax: (714) 843-1192

Redwing Book Company   Books on Oriental medicine
202 Bendix Drive, Taos, NM 87571
Tel.: (575) 758-7758
Fax: (617) 738-4620
Website: http://www.redwingbooks.com

Clinical Forms

The clinical forms included with this manual are copyrighted by the author, but free permission to reproduce these forms for your own use may be granted by writing to Health Care Alternatives (HCA) at 8033 Sunset Blvd., PMB #265, Los Angeles, CA 90046. You may also email HCA at terry.oleson@gmail.com or you may contact our website at http://www.auriculotherapy.com. Original copies of each form can be sent to you upon request.

For collecting clinical research data, it is recommended that therapists complete the **Auricular Diagnosis Form** and the **Auriculotherapy Treatment Form** each time they see a patient for auriculotherapy. In order to collect systematic information for treatment outcome studies, you may have the patient fill out the **Health Distress Index** (HDI-40) on the first day of treatment and then complete the **Health Distress Index Diary** (HDID-45) each day during the week following treatment. The HDI-40-C is used for clinical purposes, and the HDI-40-R is used for research. The HDI-40-R items have been randomly sorted rather than presented together in each clinical category. The **Health Distress Index Visual Analogue Scale** (HDI-VAS) is to be filled out at the beginning and at the end of the treatment provided on a given day. The **Participant Demographic Form** (PDI) and the **Health History Inventory** (HHI) should be completed by patients only on the first day they are seen.

Scoring of items for the HDI-40 and HDID-45 is evaluated as follows:

None = 0, Mild = 1, Moderate = 2, High = 3, and Highest = 4

Add the sums of the scores for the items designated as subscales S, P, V, I, A, D, W, and T.

Health Distress Index and Diary Symptom Scales

1	Sleep Disturbance (S):	Add items # 1, 2, 3, 4.
2	Somatic Pain (P):	Add items # 11, 12, 13, 14, 15, 16.
3	Visceral Distress (V):	Add items # 17, 18, 19, 20.
4	Illness Condition (I):	Add items # 21, 22, 23, 24.
5	Anxiety (A):	Add items # 25, 26, 27, 28, 29, 30, 31, 32, 33.
6	Depression (D):	Add items # 34, 35, 36, 37, 38, 39, 40.
7	Positive Well-Being (W):	Add items # 5, 6, 7, 8, 9, 10.
8	Total Distress Score (T):	Add the total scores for scales 1, 2, 3, 4, 5, and 6, then subtract the total score for scale 7.

Health Distress Visual Analogue Scale Scoring

The Health Distress Visual Analogue Scale (HDI-VAS) is scored by placing a 10-cm ruler along the line that runs from "No Discomfort" to "Extreme Discomfort" or "Very Relaxed" to "Very Tense." An X mark crossing the line is used to obtain a numerical score for each person's subjective rating of discomfort or tension. In the example shown on the HDI-VAS page, the top line would be given a score of 9.0, and the lower line of the example would be given a score of 1.5. Divide the total score by the number of items in that scale.

Auricular Diagnosis Form						
No.	**AZ**	**Ear Acupoint Name**	**Left Ear**		**Right Ear**	
			T	**E**	**T**	**E**
0.0	HX 1	Point Zero				
1.0	SF 2	Shen Men				
2.0	IH 4	Sympathetic Autonomic point				
3.0	IH 7	Allergy point				
4.0	CW 3	Thalamus point				
5.0	IT 2	Endocrine point				
6.E	ST 3	Oscillation, Inner Ear				
7.E	TG 2	Tranquilizer point				
8.E	LO 4	Master Sensorial				
9.E	LO 1	Master Cerebral				
10.E	AH 1	Upper Cervical Spine				
10.E	AH 2	Lower Cervical Spine				
11.E	AH 3	Upper Thoracic, Heart.F				
11.E	AH 4	Lower Thoracic Spine				
12.E	AH 5	Upper Lumbar Spine				
12.E	AH 6	Lower Lumbar Spine				
13.E	AH 7	Sacral Spine				
10.C	AH 8	Lower Neck, Thyroid.C				
10.C	AH 9	Upper Neck, Clavicle.E				
11.C	AH 10	Chest, Breast				
11.C	AH 11	Abdomen				
12.C	AH 12	Abdomen, Lumbago				
21.C	AH 13	Hip.C				
23.C	AH 15	Knee.C				
27.C	AH 17	Ankle.C, Foot.C				
21.E	TF 1	Hip.E				
22.E	TF 3	Thigh, Constipation				
23.E	TF 4	Knee.E				
25.E	TF 5	Ankle.F, Uterus.C				
27.E	TF 6	Toes.E				
37.C	SF 1	Master Shoulder				
36.0	SF 2	Shoulder				
35.0	SF 3	Arm				
34.0	SF 4	Elbow, Forearm				
32.0	SF 5	Wrist				
30.0	SF 6	Hand, Fingers				
40.0	AT 1	Forehead				
39.0	AT 2	Temples, Asthma.C				
38.0	AT 3	Occiput				
43.0	LO 8	TMJ, Antidepressant				
44.0	LO 7	Jaw, Trigeminal n.				

No.	AZ	Ear Acupoint Name	Left Ear		Right Ear	
			T	E	T	E
60.0	IC 6	Mouth				
61.0	IC 7	Esophagus				
63.0	CR 1	Stomach				
64.0	SC 1	Duodenum				
65.0	SC 2	Small Intestines				
66.0	SC 3	Large Intestines				
87.E	SC 4	Urethra.E				
86.0	SC 5	Bladder				
84.C	SC 6	Kidney.C				
83.0	SC 7	Pancreas				
81.E	SC 8	Spleen.E				
79.0	CR2	Liver				
81.C	IC 8	Spleen.C, Relaxation				
70.0	IC 5	Lung 1				
69.C	IC 4	Heart.C, Lung 1				
70.0	IC 2	Lung 2				
113.E	IC 3	Vagus n., Trachea				
160.C	IC 1	San Jiao				
101.E	CW 1	Gonadotropins				
138.0	CW 2–3	Thalamus, Brain.C				
127.C	CW 4	Brainstem.C				
96.C	CW 5	Thyroid Gland.E				
95.C	CW 6	Mammary Gland.E				
94.C	CW 7	Thymus Gland.E				
92.C	CW 8	Adrenal Gland.E				
109.E	CW 9	Sympathetic n.				
91.E	IH 1–2	Ovaries/Testes				
89.E	IH 3–4	Uterus.E				
84.E	IH 5–6	Kidney.E				
76.C	HX 2	Diaphragm.C				
67.C	HX 3	Rectum.C				
90.0	HX 4	Genitals.C				
179.C	HX 7	Apex of Ear, Allergy.C				
124.E	HX 12	Lumbar Sp. Cord				
125.E	HX 13	Thoracic Sp. Cord				
126.E	HX 14	Cervical Sp. Cord				
127.E	HX 15	Brainstem.E				
98.E	TG 1	Pineal Gland				
161.C	TG 3	Appetite, Adrenal Gland				
193.E	TG 4	Vitality point				
182.E	LO 4	Aggressivity				

T, tenderness; E, electrical diagnosis

Auriculotherapy Treatment Form

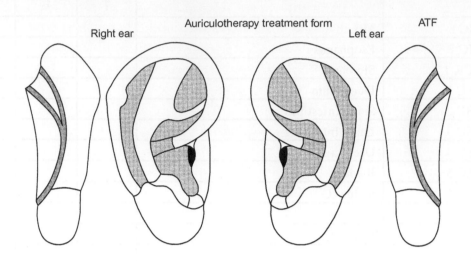

Indicate on pictures above the ear areas where reactive ear reflex points were found.

1. Patient ID _____   2. Therapist name _____   3. Date _____

4. Age_____   5. Sex: ☐ Male ☐ Female   6. Handedness: ☐ Right ☐ Left   7. Session No. _____

8. Patient complaints prior to treatment: _____

_____

9. Objective body assessments prior to treatment: (*e.g., Limitations in range of motion*)

_____

_____

10. Auricular diagnosis observations: (*e.g., Regions of tenderness and electrodermal conductance*)

_____

_____

11. Auriculotherapy treatments used: ☐ Acupuncture needles ☐ Transcutaneous stimulation

☐ Electroacupuncture ☐ Acupoint pellets ☐ Acupressure ☐ Other: _____

12. Auricular points treated: _____

_____

13. Duration of treatment and electrical frequencies used: _____

14. Patient experience following treatment: _____

_____

15. Objective body assessments following treatment: _____

_____

_____

Health Distress Index Instructions

Overview: The purpose of these two health surveys is to have you personally evaluate your typical symptoms of stress, pain, tension, and mood changes during the week. The Health Distress Index (HDI-40) survey asks you to evaluate 40 symptoms averaged over a whole week, whereas the Health Distress Index Diary (HDID-45) asks you to evaluate your experience on 45 items rated each day of the week for 7 consecutive days.

Ratings: For items #1 to #40, please rate your most typical daily experience for each of the items indicated, using a subjective rating scale that combines the degree, intensity, frequency, and duration of that symptom. The numeric values of the rating are as follows:

4 = Highest level of the presence of that
    symptom or experience
3 = High level of the presence of that symptom
    or experience
2 = Moderate level of the presence of that
    symptom or experience
1 = Mild level of the presence of that symptom
    or experience
__ (leave blank)=None of that experience.

Example ratings: These items are very subjective. You should compare your rating to the range of such experiences that you have had in your life. A rating of 4, for example, would be reserved for the worst time that you have ever had in either falling asleep or remaining asleep, the most severely painful headache or back pain that you have ever had, the most bothersome experience of feeling nervous or depressed that you can remember, or the best times of feeling good or working productively that you can remember. A rating of 3, 2, or 1 would indicate progressively less severity or pressure of that symptom.

Number of HDID experiences: For items #41 to #45 on the Health Distress Index Diary (HDID-45), please show the number of minutes you engaged in that activity or the number of times you took that item.

Physical exercise or sports activity: Item #41 refers to any physical exercise, such as walking, jogging, going to the gym, or playing a sport. Indicate whether you spent 2 hours engaged in strenuous physical exercise or athletics or you spent even 15 minutes of doing light exercise.

Closed-eyes, deep relaxation: Item #42 refers to any deep relaxation technique or meditation process that you do with your eyes closed. It includes practices such as abdominal breathing, progressive relaxation, guided imagery, autogenic training, self-hypnosis, prayer, or transcendental meditation (TM). Indicate if during the day you spent 60 minutes engaged in a deep relaxation process, or if you spent just 10 minutes taking the time to relax deeply. Relaxation does not include open-eyed activities such as watching television or reading a book.

Number of cigarettes or alcoholic drinks: Items #43 and #44 refer to the total number of cigarettes smoked that day or the total number of drinks consumed that day. One drink could be a can of beer, a glass of wine, a shot of liquor, or an alcoholic cocktail.

Number of hours of a symptom: Item #45 refers to the number of hours each day that you experienced a specific symptom that bothers you. Identify the symptom at the bottom of the page. This symptom could include the number of hours inebriated by alcohol, "high" on a drug, "craving" a chemical substance, skin irritation, menstrual or menopausal symptoms, or generalized body aches. The symptoms identified in item #45 should focus on experiences not already covered in items #1 to #40.

Menstrual period: Item "M" is to be filled out only by women. Please show the days that you experienced your menstrual period over the past week, if at all, by writing an M in that column.

	Health Distress Index Clinical Form					HDI-40-C

Name or ID_____   Age _____   Sex: ☐ Male   ☐ Female   Date _____

	Symptoms or experiences during the past week	Degree or frequency of experience				
	Place a check mark in the column that applies to you.	Never	Low	Middle	High	Highest
1	Difficulty falling asleep at night					
2	Difficulty remaining asleep at night					
3	Felt sleep duration was inadequate or insufficient					
4	Felt tired, drowsy, or fatigued during the day					
5	Felt full of energy and vitality during the day					
6	Felt joyful, happy, euphoric					
7	Engaged in fun or enjoyable activities					
8	Socialized with people you like to be with					
9	Felt confident or optimistic about things					
10	Able to work productively and accomplish tasks					
11	Back pain					
12	Headaches					
13	Shoulder tension or stiff neck					
14	Aches or stiffness in hands, feet, arms, or legs					
15	Movements or activities limited by pain					
16	Chest pain, chest tightness, breast tenderness					
17	Nausea, stomachache, abdominal discomfort					
18	Constipation or diarrhea					
19	Excessive overeating or binge eating					
20	Undereating or low appetite					
21	Runny nose, sneezing, nasal congestion					
22	Difficulty breathing, coughing, lung congestion					
23	Sore throat, mouth sores, swollen lymph glands					
24	Felt ill, sick, chills, feverish, or malaise					
25	Sweaty palms or general sweating					
26	Heart pounding, rapid heartbeats, palpitations					
27	Felt dizzy, weak, or faint					
28	Trembling, shaking, or easily startled					
29	Felt tense, restless, agitated, or on edge					
30	Nervous or anxious					
31	Felt scared or panicked for no apparent reason					
32	Afraid something bad will happen beyond my control					
33	Difficulty concentrating or unable to make decisions					
34	Felt depressed, hopeless, or discouraged					
35	Felt worthless or miserable					
36	Felt lonely, isolated, or withdrawn					
37	Sad, tearful, or cried easily					
38	Felt little interest or satisfaction in doing things					
39	Felt irritated, annoyed, or resentful					
40	Recurrent, self-critical, negative thoughts					

Health Distress Index Research Form		HDI-40-R

Name or ID _____   Age _____   Sex: ☐ Male   ☐ Female   Date _____

	Symptoms or experiences during the past week	Degree or frequency of experience				
	Place a check mark in the column that applies to you.	Never	Low	Middle	High	Highest
1	Felt depressed, hopeless, or discouraged					
2	Shoulder tension or stiff neck					
3	Have self-critical, negative thoughts unable to stop					
4	Felt full of energy and vitality during the day					
5	Difficulty falling asleep at night					
6	Felt ill, feverish, sick, or malaise					
7	Felt irritated, annoyed, or resentful					
8	Nausea or vomiting					
9	Socialized with people you like to be with					
10	Sore throat, runny nose, or swollen lymph glands					
11	Felt lonely, isolated, or withdrawn					
12	Abdominal pain or discomfort					
13	Coughing, lung congestion, or difficulty breathing					
14	Felt tired, drowsy, or fatigued during the day					
15	Sad, tearful, or cried easily					
16	Aches or stiffness in hands, feet, arms, or legs					
17	Felt worthless or miserable					
18	Felt confident or optimistic about things					
19	Nervous or anxious					
20	Sweaty palms or moist forehead					
21	Difficulty remaining asleep at night					
22	Felt dizzy, weak, or faint					
23	Able to work productively and accomplish tasks					
24	Chest pain, chest tightness, or tenderness in breasts					
25	Heart pounding or rapid heartbeats					
26	Took time to engage in fun activities					
27	Felt scared or panicked					
28	Felt little interest or satisfaction in doing things					
29	Back pain					
30	Felt happy, joyful, elated					
31	Undereating or low appetite					
32	Constipation or diarrhea					
33	Felt sleep duration was inadequate or insufficient					
34	Shaking, trembling, or jittery					
35	Excessive overeating or binge eating					
36	Cold hands or cold feet					
37	Worried about finances or work pressures					
38	Afraid of losing control or being overwhelmed					
39	Headaches					
40	Felt tense, agitated, or restless					

Health Distress Visual Analogue Scale   HDI-VAS

Mark an X on the line that indicates a range of feelings. For instance, if you were feeling "Very happy," you would indicate it on the line below as follows:

Unhappy |_____ X ____| Happy

However, if you were feeling somewhat "Unhappy," you would indicate it on the line below as follows:

Unhappy |_____ X _____| Happy

Visual Analogue Scale

On the lines below, which represent the degree to which you experience a particular symptom, please rate the intensity of your experience on that item by marking an X on that part of the line which most corresponds to your experience. Identify two distinct areas of the body where you feel your most severe pain or discomfort, or feel some other distinct symptom, and rate those two areas for items #1 and #2.

Pre-treatment

Area or problem #1:_____   Area or symptom #2:_____

1.   No pain in #1 |_____| High pain in area #1
2.   No symptom #2 |_____| High symptom #2
3.   Very relaxed |_____| Very tense

Post-treatment

Area or problem #1:_____   Area or symptom #2:_____

1.   No pain in #1 |_____| High pain in area #1
2.   No symptom #2 |_____| High symptom #2
3.   Very relaxed |_____| Very tense

Participant Demographic Inventory   **PDI-25**

1. Name or ID_____   2. Date_____   3. Age_____   4. Sex: ☐ Male   ☐ Female

5. Current health complaints: _____

_____

_____

6. Date of onset of primary condition_____   7. Handedness: ☐ right ☐ left

8. Ethnicity: ☐ Caucasian, not Hispanic ☐ Hispanic ☐ Black ☐ Asian ☐ Other_____

9. Place of birth_____   10. Date of birth_____

11. Marital status: ☐ single ☐ married ☐ intimate relationship ☐ separated or divorced ☐ widowed

12. Are you currently pregnant? ☐ yes ☐ no   13. Date of last menstrual period_____

14. Highest level of education: ☐ high school ☐ some college ☐ bachelor's degree ☐ graduate degree

15. Occupation_____

16. Occupational status: ☐ working full-time ☐ part-time work ☐ student ☐ disability ☐ not working

17. Physical body: height_____ weight_____

18. Health care providers seen in last year: ☐ medical doctor ☐ chiropractic doctor ☐ acupuncturist
☐ dentist ☐ naturopath ☐ nurse ☐ physical therapist ☐ psychotherapist ☐ other_____

19. Are you involved with any litigation? ☐ no ☐ insurance co. ☐ disability ☐ workman's comp. ☐ personal
injury

☐ other_____ comments_____

20. Please list the drug or herb name and daily (dosage) of all medications or herbs that you are taking.

Drug #1_____ (_____ mg/day)   Drug #5_____ (_____ mg/day)
Drug #2_____ (_____ mg/day)   Drug #6_____ (_____ mg/day)
Drug #3_____ (_____ mg/day)   Drug #7_____ (_____ mg/day)
Drug #4_____ (_____ mg / day)   Drug #8_____ (_____ mg/day)

21. Average number of minutes engaged in physical exercise each day   _____ minutes

22. Average number of minutes did closed-eyes relaxation process each day   _____ minutes

23. Average number of cigarettes smoked each day   _____ cigarettes

24. Average number of alcoholic drinks consumed each day   _____ drinks

25. Average number of hours per day that you experienced primary symptoms   _____ hours

Health History Inventory   HHI-4

Name or ID_____ Date _____

Please mark an X in the boxes (☐) below for those items that apply to you.

1. Health history: Have you ever been diagnosed by a licensed health care practitioner for any of the following?

☐ Tension headaches
☐ Coronary disorder or heart attack
☐ Stroke
☐ Migraine headaches
☐ Liver disease or hepatitis
☐ Cancer
☐ Cluster headaches
☐ Urinary or bladder disorder
☐ Concussion or head trauma
☐ TMJ disorder or jaw pain
☐ Kidney disorder or stones
☐ Brain seizures or epilepsy
☐ Chronic back pain or sciatica
☐ Gall bladder disorder or stones
☐ Multiple sclerosis or palsy
☐ Rheumatoid arthritis
☐ Asthma or bronchitis

☐ Polio
☐ Osteoarthritis
☐ Tuberculosis or pneumonia
☐ Mononucleosis
☐ Fibromyalgia
☐ Irritable bowel syndrome
☐ AIDS or HIV disease
☐ Muscle tremors or tics
☐ Hypertension
☐ Deafness
☐ Tendonitis or bursitis
☐ Hemorrhoids or hernia
☐ Tinnitus
☐ Carpal tunnel syndrome
☐ Diabetes mellitus
☐ Anorexia or bulimia
☐ Bone fracture or joint sprain

☐ Thyroid disorder
☐ Chronic fatigue syndrome
☐ Radiculopathy
☐ Dysmenorrhea
☐ Attention deficit disorder
☐ Neuralgia
☐ Premenstrual syndrome
☐ Panic attacks or phobias
☐ Peripheral neuropathy
☐ Menopause problems
☐ Depressed Mood
☐ Shingles (herpes zoster)
☐ Prostate or genital disorder
☐ Alcohol abuse problems
☐ Dermatitis, eczema, or hives
☐ Allergies or hay fever
☐ Substance abuse problems

2. Accidents: Have you ever been left injured or impaired by any of the following types of accident?

☐ Automobile accident
☐ Work-related accident

☐ Surgical complication
☐ Athletic injury

☐ Accident in daily living
☐ Medication side effects

3. Current conditions: In the past 3 months, have you experienced any of the following symptoms?

☐ Pain in elbows, or hands
☐ Pain in hips, knees, or feet
☐ Abdominal distension
☐ Sinus congestion
☐ More than 10 pounds underweight
☐ More than 20 pounds overweight
☐ Chills or aversion to cold
☐ Stiff, aching, or swollen joints
☐ Night sweats
☐ Dry skin
☐ Diarrhea or loose stools
☐ Frequent colds or flu

☐ Dry mouth or dry throat
☐ Constipation or dry stools
☐ Heart palpations
☐ Bleeding gums
☐ Heartburn or indigestion
☐ Excessive sexual activity
☐ Grinding teeth at night
☐ Craving for sweets
☐ Low sex drive
☐ Shortness of breath
☐ Difficulty making decisions
☐ Insomnia or poor sleep

☐ Hearing impairment
☐ Difficulty concentrating
☐ Lethargy, tiredness
☐ Ringing in ears
☐ Poor memory
☐ Disturbing dreams
☐ Blurry vision
☐ Bored or uninterested
☐ Unable to relax
☐ Overstrain or overstressed
☐ Thoughts of killing yourself
☐ Crave a recreational drug

4. Substances or medications: In the past 3 months, have you regularly used any of the following items

☐ Several cigarettes per day
☐ Several aspirin pills
☐ Sleeping pills

☐ Several cups of coffee per day
☐ Prescribed pain reliever
☐ Anti-anxiety medication

☐ More than 3 alcoholic drinks per day
☐ Blood pressure medication
☐ Antidepressant medication

References

Abbate, D., et al. 1980. Beta-endorphin and electroacupuncture. Lancet 16, 13–31.

Ackerman, J., 1999. Navach's biochemical and neurophysical aspects of the VAS. International Consensus Conference on Acupuncture, Auriculotherapy, and Auricular Medicine, Las Vegas, NV, 51–57.

Akerele, O., 1991. WHO and the development of acupuncture nomenclature: overcoming a tower of Babel. Am. J. Chin. Med. 1, 89–94.

Alimi, D., 2000. Effects of auricular stimulation on functional magnetic resonance imaging of the cerebral cortex. Third International Symposium of Auriculotherapy and Auricular Medicine, Lyon, France.

Alimi, D., Geissmann, A., Gardeur, D., 2002. Auricular acupuncture stimulation measured on functional magnetic resonance imaging. Med. Acupunct. 13, 18–21.

Alimi, D., et al., 2003. Analgesic effect of auricular acupuncture for cancer pain: a randomized blinded controlled trial. J. Clin. Oncol. 21, 4120–4126.

Andersson, E., Persson, A.L., Carlsson, C.P., 2007. Are auricular maps reliable for chronic musculoskeletal pain disorders? a double blind evaluation. Acupunct. Med. 25, 72–79.

Asamoto, S., Takeshige, C., 1992. Activation of the satiety center by auricular acupuncture point stimulation. Brain Res. Bull. 29, 157–164.

Asis, D., 2012. Auricular chromotherapy in the treatment of psychological trauma. Seventh International Symposium of Auriculotherapy, Lyon, France, 159–164.

Bahr, F., 1977. The Clinical Practice of Scientific Auricular Acupuncture. German Academy for Auricular Medicine, Kalamazoo, MI.

Basbaum, A.I., Fields, H.L., 1979. The origin of descending pathways in the dorsolateral funiculus of the spinal cord of the cat and rat: further studies on the anatomy of pain modulation. J. Comp. Neurol. 187, 513–531.

Basbaum, A.I., Fields, H.L., 1984. Endogenous pain control systems: brainstem spinal pathway and endorphin circuitry. Annu. Rev. Neurosci. 7, 309–338.

Becker, R.O., 1976. Electrophysiological correlates of acupuncture points and meridians. Psychoenergetic Syst. 1, 105–112.

Beinfield, H., Korngold, E., 1991. Between Heaven and Earth. Ballantine, New York.

Bergsmann, O., Hart, A., 1973. Differences in electrical skin conductivity between acupuncture points and adjacent skin areas. Am. J. Acupunct. 1, 27–32.

Birch, S.J., Felt, R.L., 1999. Understanding Acupuncture. Churchill Livingstone, London.

Blum, K., et al. 2000. Reward deficiency syndrome (RDS): a biogenic model for the diagnosis and treatment of impulsive, addictive, and compulsive behaviors. J. Psychoactive Drugs 32, 2.

Bohm, D., 1980. Wholeness and the Implicate Order. Routledge & Kegan Paul, London.

Bossy, J., 1979. Neural mechanisms in acupuncture analgesia. Minerva Med. 70, 1705–1715.

Bossy, J., 2000. Anatomical comparisons of the external ear. Third International Symposium of Auriculotherapy and Auricular Medicine. Lyon, France.

Bourdiol, R., 1982. Elements of Auriculotherapy. Maisonneuve, Moulins-les-Metz, France.

Brewington, V., Smith, M., Lipton, D., 1994. Acupuncture as a detoxification treatment: an analysis of controlled research. J. Subst. Abuse Treat. 11, 289–307.

Bullock, M., Culliton, P., Olander, R., 1989. Controlled trial of acupuncture for severe recidivist alcoholism. Lancet 1, 1435–1439.

Campbell, J., 1988. The Power of Myth. Doubleday, New York.

Ceccherelli, F., et al. 2006. The therapeutic efficacy of somatic acupuncture is not increased by auriculotherapy: a randomised blind control study in cervical myofascial pain. Complement Ther. Med. 14, 47–52.

Chan, W., et al. 1998. Comparison of substance P concentration in acupuncture points in different tissues in dogs. Am. J. Chin. Med. 26, 13–18.

Chapman, C., et al. 1983. Naloxone fails to reverse pain thresholds elevated by acupuncture: acupuncture analgesia reconsidered. Pain 16, 13–31.

Chen, G.S., 1995. On auricular acupuncture. Second International Symposium on Auricular Medicine. Beijing, China: 37–48.

Chen, G.S., Lu, P., 1999. History of auricular acupuncture in China. International Consensus Conference on Acupuncture, Auriculotherapy, and Auricular Medicine. Las Vegas, NV: 7–8.

Chen, H., 1993. Recent studies on auriculo acupuncture and its mechanism. J. Trad. Chin. Med. 13, 129–143.

Chen, Y.Y., et al. 2010. Effects of sympathetic histamine on vasomotor responses of blood vessels in rabbit ear to electrical stimulation. Neurosci. Bull. 26, 219–224.

Chien, C.H., et al. 1996. The composition and central projections of the internal auricular nerves of the dog. J. Anat. 189, 349–362.

Chiou, S., Chao, C., Yang, Y., 1998. Topography of low skin resistance points (LSRP) in rats. Am. J. Chin. Med. 26, 19–27.

Cho, Z.H., Wong, G., 1998. New findings of the correlation between acupoints and corresponding brain cortices using functional MRI. Proc. Natl. Acad. Sci. U. S. A. 95, 2670–2673.

Cho, Z.H., Wong, E.K., Falon, J.H., 2001. Neuro-acupuncture. Q-puncture, Los Angeles.

Choy, D., Eidenschenk, E., 1998. Effect of tragus clips on gastric peristalsis: a pilot study. J. Altern. Compl. Med. 4, 399–403.

Clement-Jones, V., et al. 1979. Acupuncture in heroin addicts: changes in met-enkephalin and beta-endorphin in blood and cerebrospinal fluid. Lancet 2, 380–382.

Clement-Jones, V., et al. 1980. Increased beta-endorphin but not met-enkephalin levels in human cerebrospinal fluid after acupuncture for recurrent pain. Lancet 3, 946–948.

Clemente, C., 1997. Anatomy: A Regional Atlas of the Human Body, fourth ed.. Williams & Wilkins, Baltimore, MD.

Dale, R., 1976. The micro-acupuncture systems, parts I & II. Am. J. Acupunct. 4 (7–24), 196–224.

Dale, R., 1985. The micro-acupuncture meridians. Intl. J. Chin. Med. 2, 31–49.

Dale, R., 1991. Acupuncture meridians and the homunculus principle. Am. J. Acupunct. 19, 73–75.

Dale, R., 1993. Addictions and acupuncture: the treatment methods, formulae, effectiveness and limitations. Am. J. Acupunct. 21, 247–266.

Dale, R., 1999. The systems, holograms and theory of micro-acupuncture. Am. J. Acupunct. 27, 207–242.

Debreceni, L., 1991. The effect of electrical stimulation of the ear points on the plasma ACTH and GH level in humans. Acupunct. Electrotherap. Res. 16, 45–51.

Dhond, R.P., Kettner, N., Napadow, V., 2007. Neuroimaging acupuncture effects in the human brain. J. Altern. Complement Med. 13, 603–616.

Dvorkin, E., 1999. Morphology of auricular reflex points. International Consensus Conference on Acupuncture, Auriculotherapy, and Auricular Medicine. Las Vegas, NV: 29–30.

Eckman, P., 1996. In the Footsteps of the Yellow Emperor. Cypress, San Francisco.

Ernst, M., Lee, M., 1987. Influence of naloxone on electro-acupuncture analgesia using an experimental pain test. Acupunct. Electrotherap. Res. 12, 5–22.

Fedoseeva, O., Kalyuzhnyi, L., Sudakov, K., 1990. New peptide mechanisms of auriculo-acupuncture electro-analgesia: role of angiotensin II. Acupunct. Electrotherap. Res. 15, 1–8.

Feely, R.A., 2010. Yamamoto New Scalp Acupuncture: Principles and Practice. Thieme, New York.

Fusumada, K., et al. 2007. C-Fos expression in the periaqueductal gray is induced by electroacupuncture in the rat, with possible reference to GABAergic neurons. Okajomas Folia Anat. Jpn. 84, 1–10.

Gao, X.Y., et al. 2008. Investigation of specificity of auricular acupuncture points in regulation of autonomic function in anesthetized rats. Auton. Neurosci. 138, 50–56.

Gao, X.Y., et al. 2011. Acupuncture-like stimulation at auricular point heart evokes cardiovascular inhibition via activating the cardiac-related neurons in the nucleus tractus solitaries. Brain Res. 1397, 19–27.

Gao, X.Y., et al. 2012. Brain-modulated effects of auricular acupressure on the regulation of autonomic function in healthy volunteers. Evid. Based Complement Alternat. Med. 2012, 1–8.

Greenwood, M.T., 2011. How do you treat menstrual cramps in your practice? Med. Acupunct. 23, 194–195.

Grobglas, A., Levy, J., 1986. Traité d'acupuncture Auriculaire. Maloine, Paris.

Group Lyonaise Études Medicales, 2012. International Symposium of Auriculotherapy, Seventh Symposium. Lyon, France.

Guimarases, A.P., Prado, W.A., 1999. Pharmacological evidence for a periaqueductal gray–nucleus raphe magnus connection mediating the antinociception induced by microinjecting carbachol into the dorsal periaqueductal gray of rats. Brain Res. 8, 152–159.

Han, J.S., 2001. Opioid and antiopioid peptides: a model of yin–yang balance in acupuncture mechanisms of pain modulation. In: Stux, G., Hammerschlag, R. (Eds.), Clinical Acupuncture: Scientific Basis. Springer, Heidelberg, pp. 29–50.

Hecker, H.U., Peuker, E., Steveling, A., 2006. Microsystems Acupuncture, the Complete Guide: Ear–Scalp–Mouth–Hand. Thieme, Stuttgart.

Helms, J., 1990. WHO adopts standard international acupuncture nomenclature. AAMA Review 2, 33.

Helms, J., 1995. Acupuncture Energetics: A Clinical Approach for Physicians. Medical Acupuncture, Berkeley, CA.

Hild, W., 1974. Atlas of Human Anatomy, ninth ed.. Macmillan, New York.

Ho, W., et al. 1978. The influence of electroacupuncture on naloxone induced morphine withdrawal in mice: elevation of brain opiate-like activity. Eur. J. Pharmacol. 49, 197–199.

Ho, W.K., Wen, H.L., 1989. Opioid-like activity in the cerebrospinal fluid of pain patients treated by electroacupuncture. Neuropharmacology 28, 961–966.

Holder, J., et al. 2001. Increasing retention rates among the chemically dependent in residential treatment: auriculotherapy and subluxation-based chiropractic care. Mol. Psychiatry 6, S8.

Hosobuchi, Y., et al. 1979. Stimulation of human periaqueductal gray for pain relief increases immunoreactive beta endorphin in ventricular fluid. Science 203, 279–281.

Hsieh, C., 1998. Modulation of cerebral cortex in acupuncture stimulation: a study using sympathetic skin response and somatosensory evoked potentials. Am. J. Chin. Med. 26, 1–11.

Hsieh, J., et al. 1995. Traumatic nociceptive pain activates the hypothalamus and the periaqueductal gray: a positron emission tomography study. Pain 64, 303–314.

Hsu, H., 1977. Peacher Chen's History of Chinese Medical Science. Modern Drug Publishing, Taipei, Taiwan.

Huan, Z., Rose, K., 1999. Who can Ride the Dragon?. Paradigm, Brookline, MA.

Huang, H., 1974. Ear Acupuncture. Rodale Press, Emmaus, PA.

Huang, L.C., 1996. Auriculotherapy Diagnosis and Treatment. Longevity Press, Bellaire, TX.

Huang, L.C., 1999. Auricular Diagnosis. Longevity Press, Bellaire, TX.

Huang, L.C., 2005. Auricular Diagnosis. Auricular International Research Center, Orlando, FL.

Hyvarinen, J., Karlsson, M., 1977. Low skin resistance skin points that may coincide with acupuncture loci. Med. Biol. 55, 88–94.

International Congress of Anatomists, 1977. Nomina Anatomica, fourth ed.. Excerpta Medica, Amsterdam.

Jaung-Geng, L., Salahin, H., Jung-Charng, L., 1995. Investigation on the effects of ear acupuncture on exercise-induced lactic acid levels and the implications for athletic training. Am. J. Acupunct. 23, 309–313.

Jung, C., 1964. Man and His Symbols. Dell, New York.

Kaptchuk, T., 1983. The Web that has No Weaver. Congdon & Weed, New York.

Kashiba, H., Ueda, Y., 1991. Acupuncture to the skin induces release of substance P and calcitonin gene-related peptide from peripheral terminals of primary sensory neurons in the rat. Am. J. Chin. Med. 19, 189–197.

Kawakaita, K., Kawamura, H., Keino, H., Hongo, T., Kitakohji, H., 1991. Development of the low impedance points in the auricular skin of experimental peritonitis rats. Am. J. Chin. Med. 19, 199–205.

Kenyon, J., 1983. Modern Techniques of Acupuncture: A Practical Scientific Guide to Electro-acupuncture. Thorsons, Wellingborough, UK.

Kho, H., Robertson, E., 1997. The mechanisms of acupuncture analgesia: review and update. Am. J. Acupunct. 25, 261–281.

Kitade, T., Hyodo, M., 1979. The effects of stimulation of ear acupuncture points on the body's pain threshold. Am. J. Chin. Med. 7, 241–252.

König, G., Wancura, I., 1993. Einführung in die chinesische ohrakupunktur. Haug, Heidelberg.

Krause, A., Clelland, J., Knowles, C., Jackson, J., 1987. Effects of unilateral and bilateral auricular transcutaneous electrical stimulation on cutaneous pain threshold. Physical Ther. 67, 507–511.

Kroening, R., Oleson, T., 1985. Rapid narcotic detoxification in chronic pain patients treated with auricular electroacupuncture and naloxone. Int. J. Addict. 20, 1347–1360.

Kropej, H., 1984. The fundamentals of Ear Acupuncture, second ed.. Haug, Heidelberg.

Kvirchishvili, V., 1974. Projections of different parts of the body on the surface of the concha auriculae in humans and animals. Am. J. Acupunct. 2, 208.

Landgren, K., 2008. Ear Acupuncture. Churchill Livingstone, Edinburgh, UK.

Lee, T., 1977. Thalamic neuron theory: a hypothesis concerning pain and acupuncture. Med. Hypoth. 3, 113–121.

Lee, T., 1994. Thalamic neuron theory: theoretical basis for the role played by the central nervous system (CNS) in the causes and cures of all disease. Med. Hypoth. 43, 285–302.

Leib, S., 1999. Nogier's three functional layers to evaluate conventional medications. International Consensus Conference on Acupuncture, Auriculotherapy, and Auricular Medicine. Las Vegas, NV: 59–60.

Li, L., et al. 2008. The human brain response to acupuncture on same-meridian acupoints: evidence from an fMRI study. J. Altern. Complement Med. 14, 673–678.

Lichstein, E., et al. 1974. Diagonal earlobe crease: prevalence and implications as a coronary risk factor. N. Engl. J. Med. 290, 615–616.

Liebeskind, J., Mayer, D., Akil, H., 1974. Central mechanisms of pain inhibition: studies of analgesia from focal brain stimulation. Advances in Neurology, 4. Raven Press, New York.

Lin, C., 1984. Use of auricular acupuncture for the relief of tooth pain. Am. J. Acupunct. 12, 239–244.

Lin, Y.H., Chen, K.K., Chiu, J.H., 2011. Use of Chinese medicine among prostate cancer patients in Taiwan: a retrospective longitudinal cohort study. Int. J. Urol. 18, 383–386.

Maciocia, G., 1989. The Foundations of Chinese Medicine. Churchill Livingstone, Edinburgh, UK.

Margolin, A., Avants, S., Chung, P., Kosten, T., 1993b. Acupuncture for the treatment of cocaine dependence in methadone-maintained patients. Am. J. Addict. 2, 194–201.

Margolin, A., Chung, P., Avants, S., Kosten, T., 1993a. Effects of sham and real auricular needling: Implications for trials of acupuncture for cocaine addiction. Am. J. Chin. Med. 221, 191–197.

Margolin, A., et al. 1996. Methodological investigations for a multisite trial of auricular acupuncture for cocaine addiction: a study of active and control auricular zones. J. Substance Abuse Treat. 13, 471–481.

Marignan, M., 1999. Dynamic and digital thermography of the ear. International Consensus Conference on Acupuncture, Auriculotherapy, and Auricular Medicine. Las Vegas, NV: 23.

Mayer, D.J., Liebeskind, J.C., 1974. Pain reduction by focal electrical stimulation of the brain: an anatomical and behavioral analysis. Brain Res. 68, 73–93.

Mayer, D.J., Price, D., Rafii, A., 1977. Antagonism of acupuncture analgesia in man by the narcotic antagonist naloxone. Brain Res. 121, 368–372.

Mayer, D.J., et al. 1971. Analgesia from electrical stimulation in the brainstem of the rat. Science 174, 1351–1354.

Mehta, J., Homby, R., 1974. Diagonal earlobe crease as a coronary risk factor. N. Engl. J. Med. 291, 260.

Melzack, R., Wall, P., 1965. Pain mechanisms: a new theory. Science 150, 197.

Mountcastle, V., Henneman, E., 1952. The representation of tactile sensibility in the thalamus of the monkey. J. Comp. Neurol. 97, 409–431.

Nahemkis, A., Smith, B., 1975. Ear Acupuncture Therapy. Alba Press, Long Beach, CA.

Ng, L., et al. 1975. Modification of morphine-withdrawal in rats following transauricular electrostimulation: an experimental paradigm for auricular electroacupuncture. Biol. Psychiatr. 10, 575–580.

Ng, L., et al. 1981. Alterations in rat central nervous system endorphins following transauricular acupuncture. Brain Res. 224, 83–93.

Niemtzow, R.C., 1998. A high-protein regimen and auriculomedicine for the treatment of obesity: a clinical observation. Med. Acupunct. 9, 15–21.

Niemtzow, R.C., 2012. Neurological measurements of the battlefield acupuncture technique: fMRI and Infrared 50 channel mapping of the central nervous system. Seventh International Symposium of Auriculotherapy. Lyon, France: 23–27.

Nogier, P., 1968. Handbook to Auriculotherapy. Maisonneuve, Moulins-les-Metz, France.

Nogier, P., 1972. Treatise of Auriculotherapy. Maisonneuve, Moulins-les-Metz, France.

Nogier, P., 1983. From Auriculotherapy to Auriculomedicine. Maisonneuve, Moulins-les-Metz, France.

Nogier, P., Nogier, R., 1985. The Man in the Ear. Maisonneuve, Moulins-les-Metz, France.

Nogier, P., Petitjean, F., Mallard, A., 1987. Points Réflexes Auriculaires. Maisonneuve, Moulins-les-Metz, France.

Nogier, P., Petitjean, F., Mallard, A., 1989. Compléments des Points Réflexes Auriculaires. Maisonneuve, Moulins-les-Metz, France.

Nogier, R., 1999. History of Dr. Paul Nogier's work in auricular medicine. International Consensus Conference on Acupuncture, Auriculotherapy, and Auricular Medicine. Las Vegas, NV: 19–22.

Nogier, R., 2009. Auriculotherapy. Thieme, Stuttgart.

Nogier, R. 2012. Are the electrically datable auricular points always painful? Seventh

International Symposium of Auriculotherapy. Lyon, France: 45–51.

Oleson, T., 1990. Auriculotherapy Manual: Chinese and Western Systems of Ear Acupuncture. Health Care Alternatives, Los Angeles.

Oleson, T., 1995. International Handbook of Ear Reflex Points. Health Care Alternatives, Los Angeles.

Oleson, T., 1996. Auriculotherapy Manual: Chinese and Western Systems of Ear Acupuncture, second ed.. Health Care Alternatives, Los Angeles.

Oleson, T., 1998. Differential application of auricular acupuncture for myofascial, autonomic, and neuropathic pain. Med. Acupunct. 9, 23–28.

Oleson, T., 2003. Auriculotherapy Manual: Chinese and Western Systems of Ear Acupuncture, third ed.. Churchill Livingstone, London.

Oleson, T., 2012a. Auricular landmarks identified on a three dimensional ear model. Seventh International Symposium of Auriculotherapy. Lyon, France: 53–59.

Oleson, T., 2012b. International standardization of auricular acupuncture nomenclature. Seventh International Symposium of Auriculotherapy. Lyon, France: 81–93.

Oleson, T., Flocco, W., 1993. Randomized controlled study of premenstrual symptoms treated with ear, hand, and foot reflexology. Obstet. Gynecol. 82, 906–911.

Oleson, T., Kirkpatrick, D., Goodman, S., 1980a. Elevation of pain threshold to tooth shock by brain stimulation in primates. Brain Res. 194, 79–95.

Oleson, T., Kroening, R., 1983a. A comparison of Chinese and Nogier auricular acupuncture points. Am. J. Acupunct. 11, 205–223.

Oleson, T., Kroening, R., 1983b. A new nomenclature for identifying Chinese and Nogier auricular acupuncture points. Am. J. Acupunct. 12, 325–344.

Oleson, T., Kroening, R., Bresler, D., 1980b. An experimental evaluation of auricular diagnosis: the somatotopic mapping of musculoskeletal pain at ear acupuncture points. Pain 8, 217–229.

Oleson, T., Liebeskind, J., 1978. Effect of pain-attenuating brain stimulation and morphine on electrical activity in the raphe nuclei of the awake rat. Pain 4, 211–230.

Oliveri, A., Clelland, J., Jackson, J., Knowles, C., 1986. Effects of auricular transcutaneous electrical stimulation on experimental pain threshold. Physical Ther. 66, 12–16.

Penfield, W., Rasmussen, T., 1950. The Cerebral Cortex of Man. Macmillan, New York.

Pert, A., et al. 1981. Alterations in rat central nervous system endorphins following transauricular electroacupuncture. Brain Res. 224, 83–93.

Peuker, E.T., Filler, T.J., 2002. The nerve supply of the human auricle. Clin. Anatomy 15, 35–37.

Peyron, R., Laurent, B., Carcia-Larrea, L., 2000. Functional imaging of brain responses to pain: a review and meta-analysis. Neurophysiol. Clin. 30, 263–268.

Pomeranz, B., 2001. Acupuncture analgesia—basic research. In: Stux, G., Hammerschlag, R. (Eds.), Clinical Acupuncture: Scientific Basis. Springer, Heidelberg, pp. 1–28.

Pomeranz, B., Chiu, D., 1976. Naloxone blockade of acupuncture analgesia: endorphin implicated. Life Sci. 19, 1757.

Pribram, K., 1993. Rethinking Neural Networks: Quantum Fields and Biological Data. Erlbaum, Hillsdale, NJ.

Rainville, P., et al. 1997. Pain affect encoded in anterior cingulate but not somatosensory cortex. Science 227, 968–971.

Reichmanis, M., Marino, A., Becker, R., 1975. Electrical correlates of acupuncture. IEEE Trans. Biomed. Eng. 22, 533–535.

Reichmanis, M., Marino, A., Becker, R., 1976. D.C. skin conductive variation at acupuncture loci. Am. J. Chin. Med. 4, 69–72.

Richards, D., Marley, J., 1998. Stimulation of auricular acupuncture points in weight loss. Aust. Fam. Physician 27 (Suppl. 2), S73–S77.

Rinaldi, S., et al. 2012. Psychometric evaluation of a radio electric auricular treatment for stress related disorders: a double-blinded, placebo-controlled pilot study. Health Qual. Life Outcomes 8, 31–37.

Romoli, M., 2009. Auricular Acupuncture Diagnosis. Churchill Livingstone, Edinburgh, UK.

Romoli, M., 2012. Verifying the somatotopic representation of the knee on the outer ear: is there a true difference between auricular maps? Seventh International Symposium of Auriculotherapy. Lyon, France: 133–138.

Romoli, M., Mazzoni, R., 2009. The validation of a new system of transcription of acupuncture points on the ear: the auricular sectogram. German J. Acupunct. 53, 3–7.

Romoli, M., Vettoni, F., 1982. Alterations in the skin of the auricle and correlation with chronic disease. Minerva Med. 73, 725–730.

Rubach, A., 2001. Principles of Ear Acupuncture: Microsystem of the Auricle. Thieme, Stuttgart.

Sabine, B., 2012. Finger phantom pain, auriculotherapy, and fMRI. Seventh International Symposium of Auriculotherapy. Lyon, France: 165–168.

Saku, K., Mukaino, Y., Ying, H., Arakwa, K., 1993. Characteristics of reactive electropermeable points on the auricles of coronary heart disease patients. Clin. Cardiol. 16, 415–419.

Schjelderup, V., 1982. The principle of holography: a key to holistic approach in medicine. Am. J. Acupunct. 10, 167–171.

Selye, H., 1976. The Stress of Life. McGraw-Hill, New York.

Shea, V.K., Perl, E.R., 1985. Sensory receptors with unmyelinated C fibers innervating the skin of the rabbit's ear. J. Neurophysiol. 54, 491–501.

Shiraishi, T., Onoe, M., Kojima, T., Sameshima, Y., Kageyama, T., 1995. Effects of auricular stimulation on feeding-related hypothalamic neuronal activity in normal and obese rats. Brain Res. Bull. 36, 141–148.

Simmons, M., Oleson, T., 1993. Auricular electrical stimulation and dental pain threshold. Anesth. Progr. 40, 14–19.

Sjolund, B., Eriksson, M., 1976. Electroacupuncture and endogenous morphines. Lancet 2, 1085.

Sjolund, B., Terenius, L., Eriksson, M., 1977. Increased cerebrospinal fluid levels of endorphins after electroacupuncture. Act. Physiol. Scand. 100, 382–384.

Smith, M., 1979. Acupuncture and healing in drug detoxification. Am. J. Acupunct. 7, 97–107.

Smith, M., 1988. Acupuncture treatment for crack: clinical survey of 1500 patients treated. Am. J. Acupunct. 16, 241–247.

Smith, M., 1990. Creating a substance abuse treatment program incorporating acupuncture. AAMA Rev. 2, 29–32.

Starwynn, D., 2002. Microcurrent Electroacupuncture. Desert Heart Press, Phoenix, AZ.

Strittmatter, B., 1998. Das Storfeld in Diagnostik und Therapie. Hippokrates, Stuttgart.

Strittmatter, B., 2001. Taschenatals Ohrakupunktur. Hippokrates, Stuttgart.

Strittmatter, B., 2003. Ear Acupuncture: A Precise Pocket Atlas. Thieme, Stuttgart.

Stux, G., Hammerschlag, R. (Eds.),, 2001. *Clinical Acupuncture: Scientific Basi*s. Springer, Heidelberg

Stux, G., Pomeranz, B., 1998. Basics of Acupuncture, fourth ed.. Springer, Heidelberg.

Sun, Q., Xu, Y., 1993. Simple obesity and obesity hyperlipema treated with otoacupoint pressure and body acupuncture. J. Trad. Chin. Med. 13, 22–26.

Takeshige, C., 2001. Mechanisms of acupuncture analgesia produced by low frequency electrical stimulation of acupuncture points. In: Stux, G., Hammerschlag, R. (Eds.), Clinical Acupuncture: Scientific Basis. Springer, Heidelberg, pp. 29–50.

Takeshige, C., Sato, T., Mera, T., Hisamit, T., Fang, J., 1992. Descending pain inhibitory system involved in acupuncture analgesia. Brain Res. Bull. 29, 617–634.

Talbot, M., 1991. The Holographic Universe. HarperCollins, New York.

Tang, J.S., Qu, C.L., Huo, F.Q., 2009. The thalamic nucleus submedius and ventrolateral orbital cortex are involved in nociceptive modulation: a novel pain modulation pathway. Prog. Neurobiol. 89, 383–389.

Tiller, W., 1997. Science and Human Transformation. Pavior, Walnut Creek, CA.

Tiller, W., 1999. Augmented electromagnetic waves and qi energy. International Consensus Conference on Acupuncture, Auriculotherapy, and Auricular Medicine. Las Vegas, NV: 34.

Travell, J.G., Simons, D.G., 1983. Myofascial Pain and Dysfunction: The Trigger Point Manual. Williams & Wilkins, Baltimore.

Unschuld, P., 1943. Medicine in China. University of California Press, Berkeley, CA.

Usichenko, T.I., et al. 2003. Auricular acupuncture for pain relief after total hip arthroplasty: a randomized controlled study. Pain 114, 320–327.

Usichenko, T.I., et al. 2005. Detection of ear acupuncture points by measuring the electrical skin resistance in patients before, during and after orthopedic surgery performed under general anesthesia. Acupunct. Electrother. Res. 28, 167–173.

Van Gelder, A., 1985. Strategieën in de ooracupunctuur. Deel 1: Chinese ooracupunctuur. Uitgeverij Lemma, Utrecht.

Van Gelder, A., 1992. Strategieën in de ooracupunctuur. Deel 2: Auriculotherapie. Uitgeverij Lemma, Utrecht.

Veith, I., 1972. The Yellow Emperor's Classic of Internal Medicine. University of California Press, Berkeley, CA.

Wang, D., 1984. Standard Acupuncture Nomenclature. WHO Regional Publications, Western Pacific Series, Manila.

Wang, M.C., et al. 2009. Effects of auricular acupressure on menstrual symptoms and nitric oxide for women with primary dysmenorrhea. J. Altern. Complement Med. 15, 235–242.

Wei, F., Dubner, R., Ren, K., 1999. Nucleus reticularis gigantocellularis and nucleus raphe magnus in the brain stem exert opposite effects on behavioral hyperalgia and spinal Fos protein expression after peripheral inflammation. Pain 80, 127–141.

Weintraub, M., 2001. Alternative and Complementary Treatment in Neurologic Illness. Churchill Livingstone, Philadelphia.

Wen, H.L., 1977. Fast detoxification of heroin addicts by acupuncture and electrical stimulation (AES) in combination with naloxone. Comp. Med. East West 5, 257–263.

Wen, H.L., Cheung, S., 1973. Treatment of drug addiction by acupuncture and electrical stimulation. Am. J. Acupunct. 1, 71–75.

Wen, H.L., Ho, K., Ling, N., Ma, L., Choa, G., 1979. The influence of electro-acupuncture on naloxone-induced morphine withdrawal: II. Elevation of immunoassayable beta-endorphin activity in the brain but not the blood. Am. J. Chin. Med. 7, 237–240.

Wexu, M., 1975. The Ear Gateway to Balancing the Body: A Modern Guide to Ear Acupuncture. ASI, New York.

Woerdeman, M., 1955. Standard Atlas of Human Anatomy. Butterworth, London. 106–189

Wojak, W., 2004. Introduction into systematics of diagnosis and therapy in auriculomedicine as used in the Germany. Medical Acupuncture Web Page. Available at <http://med-vetacupuncture.org/english/articles/wojak.html>.

Wojak, W., 2012. Proposal of a developed system for the description of the exact localization of ear acupuncture points as a necessary step for international cooperation of ear acupuncture research. Seventh International Symposium of Auriculotherapy. Lyon, France: 119–122.

Wong, E.K., Cho, Z.H., 1999. Acupuncture, brain function, and modern fMRI imaging techniques. International Consensus Conference on Acupuncture, Auriculotherapy, and Auricular Medicine. Las Vegas, NV: 31–33.

Woolsey, C.N., 1958. Organization of somatic sensory and motor areas of the cerebral cortex. In: Harlow, H.F., Woolsey, C.N. (Eds.), Biological and Biochemical Bases of Behavior. University of Wisconsin Press, Madison, WI

World Federation of Acupuncture–Moxibustion Societies (WFAS), 2010. Working group on nomenclature and location of auricular points standard. Beijing, China.

World Health Organization, 1985. Report on second WHO working group on the standardization of acupuncture nomenclature. Hong Kong.

World Health Organization, 1987. Report on third WHO working group on the standardization of acupuncture nomenclature. Seoul, Korea.

World Health Organization, 1990a. WHO report of the working group on auricular acupuncture nomenclature. Lyon, France.

World Health Organization, 1990b. A standard international acupuncture nomenclature: Memorandum from a WHO meeting. WHO Bulletin 68: 165–169.

Xianglong, H., Baohua, W., Xiaoqing, H., Jinsen, X., 1992. Computerized plotting of low skin impedance points. J. Trad. Chin. Med. 12, 277–282.

Xinnong, C., 1987. Chinese Acupuncture and Moxibustion. Foreign Language Press, Beijing.

Yang, M.M., Kwok, J.S., 1986. Evaluation on the treatment of morphine addiction by acupuncture Chinese herbs and opioid peptides. Am. J. Chin. Med. 14, 46–50.

Yoo, T., 1993. Koryo Hand Therapy. Eum Yang Maek, Seoul.

Young, M., McCarthy, P., 1998. Effect of acupuncture stimulation of the auricular sympathetic point on evoked sudomotor response. J. Altern. Compl. Med. 4, 29–38.

Zhang, Y.Q., 1980. A new micro-acupuncture system and another general law of distribution of acupoints besides that of the meridian-following distribution: the second metacarpal side therapy and the holographic law of distribution of acupoints [in Chinese]. Wulanchabu Sci. Tech 1, 38.

Zhang, Y.Q., 1992. A New View of the Organism: The ECIWO Theory and Its Solution of Some Challenging Problems in the Frontiers of Medicine and Biology. Peace Book, Hong Kong.

Zhang, Y.Q., et al. 1997. Inhibitory effects of electrically evoked activation of ventrolateral orbital cortex on the tail-flick reflex are mediated by periaqueductal gray in rats. Pain 72, 127–135.

Zhao, B., Zhou, L., Lei, W., 2012. Thoughts and Strategies of Developing an International Standard of Auricular Acupuncture Points (ISAAP). Seventh International Symposium of Auriculotherapy. Lyon, France: 95–105.

Zhao, Z.Q., 2008. Neural mechanism underlying acupuncture analgesia. Prog. Neurobiol. 85, 335–375.

Zhou, L., 1995. Supplementary comments on the standardization of auricular points. J. Trad. Chin. Med. 15, 132–134.

Zhou, L., 1999. The national standards of the People's Republic of China. International Consensus Conference on Acupuncture, Auriculotherapy, and Auricular Medicine. Las Vegas, NV: 11–18.

Index

Note: Page numbers followed by "*f*" and "*t*" refers to figures and tables respectively.